CANCER NURSING

CANCER NURSING

LISA BEGG MARINO, R.N., M.S., F.A.A.N.
Nurse Consultant,
Los Angeles, California

With **27** *contributors*

With **102** *illustrations*

The C. V. Mosby Company

ST. LOUIS • TORONTO • LONDON 1981

Printed in the United States of America

The C. V. Mosby Company
11830 Westline Industrial Drive, St. Louis, Missouri 63141

Library of Congress Cataloging in Publication Data

Main entry under title:

Cancer nursing.

Bibliography: p.
Includes index.
1. Cancer—Nursing. I. Marino, Lisa Begg.
RC266.C353 610.73′698 80-24705
ISBN 0-8016-3107-6

VT/CB/B 9 8 7 6 5 4 3 2 1 05/B/600

Contributors

Mary D. Bates, R.N., B.S.N., M.S.N.

Clinical Nurse Specialist—Leukemia,
The University of Texas System Cancer Center,
M. D. Anderson Hospital and Tumor Institute,
Houston, Texas

Carolyn St. John Elliott Battles, R.N., M.S.

Nurse Coordinator,
Consortium for Cancer Control Ohio;
Comprehensive Cancer Center,
Ohio State University,
Columbus, Ohio

Jeanne Quint Benoliel, R.N., D.N.Sc., F.A.A.N.

Professor,
School of Nursing,
Department of Community Health Care Systems,
University of Washington,
Seattle, Washington

Phyllis Palka Cullen, R.N., B.S.N.

Formerly Gastrointestinal Oncology
Nurse Clinician,
Department of Nursing,
University of Chicago Hospitals and Clinics,
Chicago, Illinois

Mary Jo Dropkin, R.N., M.S.N.

Research Associate,
Department of Nursing Research,
Memorial Sloan-Kettering Cancer Center,
New York, New York

Marilyn Frank-Stromborg, R.N., Ed.D., N.P.

Oncology Coordinator,
School of Nursing,
Northern Illinois University, DeKalb, Illinois

Mary H. Green, R.N., M.S.P.H.

Formerly Coordinator for Patient Education,
Ellis Fischel State Cancer Hospital,
Columbia, Missouri

Gary R. Houston, R.N., M.N., E.T.

Assistant Director of Nursing
for Developmental Therapeutics,
The University of Texas System Cancer Center,
M. D. Anderson Hospital and Tumor Institute,
Houston, Texas

Susan Molloy Hubbard, R.N., B.S.

Clinical Nurse Expert,
Medicine Branch and Department of Nursing,
Clinical Center,
National Institutes of Health,
Bethesda, Maryland

Ada K. Jacox, R.N., Ph.D.

Professor of Nursing, School of Nursing, University of Maryland, Baltimore, Maryland

Judith Bond Johnson, R.N., Ph.D.

Oncology Coordinator, North Memorial Medical Center, Minneapolis, Minnesota

Judith A. Kooser, R.N., M.S.

Formerly Clinical Nurse Specialist, Psychiatric Nursing, University of Chicago Hospitals and Clinics, Chicago, Illinois

Mary G. MacVicar, R.N., Ph.D.

Assistant Professor, School of Nursing, Ohio State University, Columbus, Ohio

Lisa Begg Marino, R.N., M.S., F.A.A.N.

Nurse Consultant, Los Angeles, California

Ida M. Martinson, R.N., Ph.D., F.A.A.N.

Professor of Nursing and Director of Research, School of Nursing, University of Minnesota, Minneapolis, Minnesota

Ruth McCorkle, R.N., Ph.D., F.A.A.N.

Associate Professor, School of Nursing, Department of Community Health Care Systems, University of Washington, Seattle, Washington

Pearl Moore, R.N., M.N.

Oncology Nurse Specialist, Montefiore Hospital, Pittsburgh, Pennsylvania

Mary Morrow, R.N., M.S.

Assistant Director of Nursing Education and Research, The Children's Hospital, Denver, Colorado

Mary Beth Orton, R.N.

Head Nurse for Cancer Clinical Research Center, The University of Texas System Cancer Center, M. D. Anderson Hospital and Tumor Institute, Houston, Texas

Pamela K. S. Patrick, R.N., Ph.D.

Clinical Psychologist, North Mississippi Medical Center, Tupelo, Mississippi

Dorothy Rodriguez, R.N., M.S., E.T.

Chief Enterostomal Therapist, Department of Nursing, The University of Texas System Cancer Center, M. D. Anderson Hospital and Tumor Institute, Houston, Texas

Ada G. Rogers, R.N.

Research Associate, Analgesic Studies Section, Sloan-Kettering Institute for Cancer Research, New York, New York

Saundra Elaine Saunders, R.N., M.S.N., M.Ed.

Clinical Nurse Specialist, Nursing Service, University of Wisconsin for the Health Services, Madison, Wisconsin

Corinne Ann Sovik, R.N., B.S.N.

Nurse Coordinator, Chest Oncology, University of Chicago Hospitals and Clinics, Chicago, Illinois

Deborah S. White, R.N.

Oncology Research Nurse, M. S. Hershey Medical Center, Hershey, Pennsylvania

Harry L. Wilson, M.D.

Fellow in Pediatric Pathology, The Children's Hospital, Denver, Colorado

James S. Woods, Ph.D., M.P.H.

Program Leader, Epidemiology and Environmental Health Research Program, Health and Population Study Center, Battelle Human Affairs Research Center, Seattle, Washington

Nancy Fugate Woods, R.N., Ph.D.

Associate Professor, Department of Physiological Nursing, School of Nursing, University of Washington, Seattle, Washington

To

my husband

Al

whose love, encouragement, and support

have enabled me to complete this book

Preface

Since you are reading this preface, I assume that you are interested in the specialty of cancer nursing. The purpose of this book is to present a comprehensive framework for cancer nursing practice and to aid in expanding the knowledge base about the nursing care of people with cancer. To meet this goal, I invited 27 contributors who are registered professional nurses in the forefront of oncology and others who are actively involved in cancer health care to author various chapters.

Although this may appear to be a large number of people, the specialty being defined as cancer nursing is sufficiently broad that meaningful content could only be achieved through a contributed book. Because of the knowledge and experience of these people, the reader has been presented with an *integrated approach* to the care of this population of clients. A common philosophy permeates this book. We believe nurses are very important providers of cancer health care. This care demands much of the nurse, but at the same time it offers numerous opportunities to achieve professional satisfaction by better meeting the needs of people afflicted with these catastrophic illnesses.

The previous statement is in no way intended to diminish the numerous contributions of other health care providers—quite the contrary. We repeatedly cite examples where truly multidisciplinary efforts are required. Further, we wish to encourage our nursing colleagues to become more involved so that they will assume greater responsibility for care in the various clinical settings and further explore intervention strategies for potential or existing areas of need.

Therefore the book is directed primarily at the practicing professional nurse and students interested in increasing knowledge and skills relative to cancer clients and their families. Interested nurse educators and researchers should also find value to the book in that content has been presented in both general and specific nursing care concepts along with numerous references to areas needing further research.

The book's specific goals are to provide a comprehensive discussion of the biologic, emotional, social, and economic issues operative in cancer health care; to increase the nurse's understanding of what constitutes professional cancer nursing practice; to offer suggestions for more effective nursing interventions on behalf of the client and family; and to offer encouragement and information to nurses relative to strategies for expanding their individual and collective contributions to cancer health care policymaking on local and national levels.

To accomplish these goals, the book has been divided into seven parts; each part contains several chapters that revolve around a common theme. Part I focuses on a conceptual framework for cancer nursing practice, the scope, economics, and organizational framework of cancer health care. Part II discusses issues that can hinder nursing's involvement in cancer health care or major areas that could benefit from more nursing involvement. Part III covers the increasingly important area of cancer prevention and early detection. Part IV discusses the scientific rationale and nursing interventions in the four major treatment modalities along with a chapter on cancer quackery. Part V focuses on important components of care relative to clients who have advanced cancer. All the previous sections lead up to Part VI, which presents information on areas of need or high-incidence problem areas for the client and family. Part VII concludes the book with a discussion of current achievements of this specialty as well as areas likely to undergo development in the future.

It is appropriate to emphasize that *Cancer Nursing* is a nursing book with medically oriented content kept to a minimum and included only when related to nursing interventions. The contributors and I have made special effort to be accurate with this content, but cancer therapy changes very quickly so the reader is cautioned to consult updated pharmacologic data rather than rely on the content of this book alone. Another qualification pertains to the use of the word "client" rather than "patient." This was done for consistency and in no way implies any value judgment regarding either term. I believe that labels of client and patient are less important than one's attitude and approach to care and that people are responsible individuals, capable of decision making and deserving of our respect. Moreover, no sexism connotation should be construed from the infrequent references to he or she. What needs to be reinforced is that all of us want to promote improved cancer health care, greater satisfaction, and involvement by you, our nursing colleagues. Through the content in this book, we intend to make you more aware of the important contributions that can be made to the nursing care of these individuals.

Lisa Begg Marino

Contents

I
OVERVIEW OF CANCER

1 **A conceptual framework for cancer nursing,** 3

Lisa Begg Marino

Historical perspective, 3
Changing attitudes, 4
New nursing roles in cancer, 5
A conceptual framework for cancer nursing, 5
Health-disease continuum, 6
General application of the health-disease continuum, 8
Continuum applied to the health care system, 8
Health care providers defined, 9
The nurse as provider defined, 10
Cancer nursing defined, 10
Integrating adaptation and rehabilitation with cancer nursing model, 11
Nursing opportunities in cancer prevention and carcinogenesis, 12
Nursing opportunities in cancer detection and diagnosis, 13
Nursing opportunities in cancer treatment, 16
Conclusion, 18

2 **The nature and scope of the cancer problem,** 20

Lisa Begg Marino

Defining cancer, 20
Definition of cancer, 20
Differentiating normal and malignant cells, 20
Cancer incidence, 25
Mortality or cause-of-death statistics, 25
Incidence statistics, 25
Types of cancers, 26
Characteristics of population affected, 26
Comparison with other diseases, 28
Survival following diagnosis of cancer, 28
Trends in survival data, 29
Costs of cancer, 31
Major categories of costs associated with cancer, 31
Calculation of direct costs associated with cancer, 31
Calculation of indirect costs associated with cancer, 34
Summary, 34

3 The organizational structure of cancer health care, 35

Lisa Begg Marino

United States government agencies and branches, 35
- National Cancer Institute, 36
- Food and Drug Administration, 40
- The legislative branch of the United States government, 41
- Environmental Protection Agency, 41
- Consumer Product Safety Commission, 42
- National Institute of Occupational Safety and Health, 42
- Occupational Safety and Health Administration, 42
- National Institute of Environmental Health Sciences, 42
- Office for Protection from Research Risks, 42

Cancer organizations, 43
- Voluntary agencies such as the American Cancer Society, 43
- Professional societies, 45
- Institutional and national organizations, 46

Local cancer efforts, 48
- Hospital Cancer Program of the American College of Surgeons, 48
- Institutional review boards, 48

Conclusion, 48

II

ISSUES IMPORTANT TO THE NURSE

4 The psychosocial care of cancer clients and their families: periods of high risk, 53

Lisa Begg Marino
Judith A. Kooser

Need for increased nursing involvement, 54
Concept of normality, 54
The family as the unit of care, 55
Risks to the nurse, 55
High-risk periods for the client and family, 56
- Prediagnostic period, 57
- Diagnostic period, 59
- Period of treatment, 61
- End of life, 65

Conclusion, 65

5 An ethical basis for cancer nursing practice, 67

Jeanne Quint Benoliel

Rationale for nursing practice as a moral art, 67
- Fundamental goals of nursing, 67
- Vulnerability of people with cancer, 68
- Conflicts between care and cure, 69
- Moral basis of nursing, 69

Conditions that inhibit ethical nursing practice, 70
- Value conflicts in the work context, 70
- Sexist stereotypes of nurses, 71
- Confusion between nonmedical questions and medical expertise, 71

A conceptual framework for cancer nursing practice, 72
- Protection of self-care agency, 72
- Problem analysis in clinical situations, 72
- A decision-making model to guide choice of action, 73

Organizations conducive to ethical decision making, 76
- Practitioners educated for accountable nursing practice, 76
- A context that promotes moral decisions, 76
- Public policy and moral accountability, 77

6 Client education: an integral part of cancer nursing, 79

Judith Bond Johnson
Mary H. Green

Overview and background of client education, 79
- Changing concepts, 79
- Aging of the population, 79
- The consumers' rights movement, 79
- Changes in the delivery of health care, 80

Increasing accountability of the health care provider, 80
Rationale for client education within cancer nursing practice, 80
Justification for client education: studies related to adapting to chronic illness, 81
Providing information, 81
Reducing anxiety, 82
Minimizing the sense of helplessness, 82
Fostering hope, 82
Step-by-step development of cancer client education, 83
Step I. Identify the educational needs of client and family, 83
Step II. Establish educational goals for client and family, 84
Step III. Select appropriate educational methods, 86
Step IV. Carry out the educational program, 88
Step V. Evaluate client and family education, 91
Principles of client education, 94
Conclusion, 95

7 Nursing research applied to cancer nursing practice, 98

Mary G. MacVicar

Rationale for research, 99
Research defined, 99
Research process, 100
Development of a research proposal: impact of cancer on the family, 100
Statement of the problem, 101
Review of the literature, 101
Formulation of the objectives and hypothesis, 101
Formulation of the theoretical framework, 103
Description of the research design, 103
Selection of variables, 104
Operationalizing the variables, 104
Identification of the target population, 105
Selection or development of methodological procedures, 105
Selection of data analysis techniques, 105
Research findings, 105
Implications for clinical practice, 107
General implications, 107
More specific assessment criteria, 107
Importance of client-family education, 108
Impediments to successful learning, 109
Minimum content of educational program, 109
Client-family counseling, 109
General findings, 109
Situations benefiting from counseling, 110
Client-family advocate, 110
Summary, 111
Conclusions, 111

8 Burnout: antecedents, manifestations, and self-care strategies for the nurse, 113

Pamela K. S. Patrick

Definition of burnout, 113
Antecedents of burnout: factors that increase burnout risk, 114
Nature of cancer nursing, 114
Environmental factors: the setting for care, 115
Psychologic and social factors: demands versus limits, 116
Manifestations of burnout, 119
Psychologic and behavioral signs and symptoms, 119
Physical signs and symptoms, 123
Strategies for burnout prevention and interruption, 125
The first step: looking inward, 125
Taking action: implementing individualized interventions, 127
Review cognitive basis for client care, 128
Revamp communication styles, 129
Recreate and relax for wellness, 131
Restore physical capacities, 132
Revitalize the work environment, 133
Miscellaneous essentials, 134
Summary, 134

III
CANCER CAUSES, PREVENTION, AND EARLY DETECTION

9 Epidemiology and the study of cancer, 139

Nancy Fugate Woods
James S. Woods

Concepts of epidemiology, 139
  Scope of epidemiology, 139
  Strategies used in epidemiologic investigations, 140
Epidemiology and the study of cancer, 140
  Descriptive approaches to the epidemiology of cancer, 141
  The cyclic nature of epidemiologic investigations, 146
Causation and association, 146
  Criteria for causal associations, 146
  Noncausal associations, 147
  Causal associations, 148
Analytic approaches to the etiology of cancer, 149
  Prospective studies, 149
  Historic or reconstructed cohort study, 153
  Retrospective studies, 154
  Cross-sectional studies, 159
  Analytic approaches to studying the effectiveness of interventions, 159
  Protocols, 162
Etiology of cancer, 162
Special problems in assessing causal relationships, 166
  Problems in animal-to-human extrapolation, 167
Screening, 169
Cancer surveillance programs, 171
Policy implications from epidemiologic studies, 172

10 Nursing's contribution to case finding and the early detection of cancer, 176

Marilyn Frank-Stromborg

Skin cancer, 177
  Risk factors, 177
  Nursing interventions, 178
Oral cancer, 183
  Risk factors, 183
  Nursing interventions, 184
Thyroid cancer, 186
  Risk factors, 186
  Nursing interventions, 187
Breast cancer, 187
  Risk factors, 187
  Nursing interventions, 189
Lung cancer, 193
  Risk factors, 193
  Nursing interventions, 194
Prostate cancer, 197
  Risk factors, 197
  Nursing interventions, 198
Colorectal cancer, 200
  Risk factors, 200
  Nursing interventions, 203
Bladder cancer, 204
  Risk factors, 204
  Nursing interventions, 205
Gastric cancer, 206
  Risk factors, 206
  Nursing interventions, 207
Testicular cancer, 208
  Risk factors, 208
  Nursing interventions, 208
Gynecologic cancer, 211
  Risk factors, 211
  Nursing interventions, 211
Leukemia, 221
  Risk factors, 221
  Nursing interventions, 221
Conclusion, 224

IV
MULTIMODALITY CANCER TREATMENT AND ITS IMPLICATIONS ON NURSING CARE

11 Multimodality cancer treatment—a challenge for nursing, 237

Lisa Begg Marino

Recent advances in cancer treatment, 237
  Breast cancer, 237
  Osteogenic sarcoma, 238

Nonseminomatous testicular cancer, 238
Small cell and epidermoid carcinoma of the lung, 238
Acute leukemia in adults, 239
Soft tissue sarcoma, 239
Non-Hodgkin's lymphoma, 239
Ovarian cancer, 239
Colorectal cancers, 239
Gastric cancer, 240
Bladder cancer, 240
Malignant melanoma, 240
Brain tumors, 240
Head and neck cancers, 240
Childhood cancers, 240
Reasons for improved client survival, 241
Improvements in the diagnosis and staging of cancer, 241
Benefits of combined or multimodality cancer treatment, 244
Models of multimodality cancer treatment, 247
Wilms' tumor, 247
Hodgkin's disease, 247
Conclusion, 250

12 Cancer surgery—its value, client-family needs, and nursing interventions, 251

Lisa Begg Marino

History, 251
Current surgical concepts, 252
Surgery as a diagnostic and staging procedure, 252
Definitive surgery, 254
Surgery as palliation, 256
Neurosurgical management of pain, 257
Conclusion, 259

13 Nursing management of the radiation therapy client, 260

Carolyn St. John Elliott Battles

Discovery, 260
Aims of radiation therapy, 261
Explanation of ionizing radiation and its effects, 261
Radioresponsiveness of various forms of cancers, 263
Factors determining responsiveness, 263
Methods of delivering radiation therapy, 265
External radiation therapy, 265
Internal radiation therapy, 270
Explanation of the components of radiation and its effect on the tissues, 270
Acute, intermediate, and late effects of radiation therapy, 272
Acute effects, 273
Intermediate effects, 273
Late effects, 273
Summary for nursing assessment, 273
Planning nursing interventions relative to diet in those clients receiving radiation therapy, 274
Gastrointestinal system, 274
Specific effects on head and neck cancer clients, 275
Specific effects on clients receiving radiation therapy to the chest area, 277
Specific effects on clients receiving radiation therapy to the abdominal area, 280
Planning nursing interventions relative to skin care in those clients receiving radiation therapy, 280
Planning nursing interventions relative to myelosuppression in those clients receiving radiation therapy, 283
Planning nursing interventions relative to psychosocial issues in those clients receiving radiation therapy, 283
Conclusion, 285

14 Chemotherapy and the cancer nurse, 287

Susan Molloy Hubbard

Biologic considerations, 289
Cellular replication, 289
Cell cycle, 289
Kinetic considerations in relation to cancer treatment, 291

Rationale for the use of drugs in cancer treatment, 294
Chemotherapeutic agents in clinical use, 295
Alkylating agents, 295
Antimetabolites, 308
Plant alkaloids, 311
Antitumor antibiotics, 312
Miscellaneous agents, 315
Endocrine therapy, 317
Ablative procedures, 317
Aminoglutethimide, 320
Estrogen, 320
Androgen, 320
Progestins, 320
Antiestrogens, 320
Corticosteroids, 321
Thyroid hormones, 321
Drug development and clinical trials, 321
General concepts and methodology, 321
The new drug-screening program, 322
Phase I clinical trials, 323
Calculation of dosage, 324
Phase II clinical trials, 325
Phase III clinical trials, 326
Combination chemotherapy: rationale for development, 328
Combination modality and "adjuvant" therapy, 332
Complications of therapy, 333
Immunosuppression, 336
Long-term effects of chemotherapy, 336
Research methodology, 337
Summary, 339

15 Nursing care of the client receiving tumor immunotherapy, 344

Deborah S. White

Scientific rationale, 344
Types of immunotherapy, 345
Active immunotherapy, 345
Passive immunotherapy, 346
Immunotherapy agents, 346
Bacillus Calmette-Guérin, 346
Corynebacterium parvum, 348
Levamisole, 349
Methanol-extracted residue, 349
Miscellaneous immunotherapeutic agents, 350
Nursing care, 350

16 Cancer quackery: information, issues, responsibility, action, 357

Pamela K. S. Patrick

Information: parameters of cancer quackery, 357
Definition of quackery, 357
Forms of cancer quackery, 358
Issues: why cancer quackery thrives, 361
Freedom to make choices, 361
Organizational supports, 362
Medical model limitations, 362
Promises and guarantees, 363
Need for future hopes, 364
Reduction of fears, 364
Reaction to multiple losses, 365
Mythical, magical beliefs, 365
Psychologic benefits, 366
Responsibility and action: the nurse's role, 366
Communication, 366
Information, 367
Emotional support, 367
Decision making, 368
Nonjudgmental attitude, 368
Education and community awareness, 369
Summary, 369

V

NURSING CARE OF THE CLIENT WITH ADVANCED CANCER

17 Control and comfort: caring for the client who has advanced cancer, 373

Lisa Begg Marino

Scope of the problem, 373
Scientific basis for treating advanced cancer, 374
Characteristics of client population, 374

Concept of comfort, 375
Psychologic comfort, 375
Physiologic comfort, 376
Conclusion, 380

18 The nursing management of pain, 381

Ada K. Jacox
Ada G. Rogers

Overview of pain and pain assessment, 381
Gate control theory of pain, 382
Selected factors influencing the pain experience, 383
Pain threshold and tolerance, 383
Chronic versus acute pain, 383
Individual perceptions of pain, 383
Pain and cancer, 384
Incidence of pain in cancer, 384
Causes of pain in cancer, 386
Pain assessment in cancer, 388
Interventions for controlling pain, 391
Biologically based techniques, 392
Psychosocially based interventions, 400
Conclusion, 402

19 Communication approaches to effective cancer nursing care, 405

Ruth McCorkle

The threat of cancer, 405
Delay and awareness, 406
Telling, 407
Uncertainty, 408
Nurse's specialized communication knowledge, 409
Preconditions for intercommunication, 410
Communication strategies, 410
Expectations, 411
Contracting—the art of negotiation, 411
Challenging situations, 412
Acting out, 412
Living with guilt, 413
The badgering family, 414
Nonpersuadable physician, 416
The nurse's multiple responsibilities, 417

20 Dealing with our own grief, 420

Corinne Ann Sovik

Introspection—becoming aware of our own feelings, 420
Fears, 421
Fear of causing pain, 422
Fear of causing death, 422
Fear of loss of control, 423
Fear of loss of identity, 425
Fear of loss or lack of support, 425
Separation of our own feelings from the clients', 426
Clinical situations, 426
Perception of time of death, 426
Personality conflicts with clients, 427
Application of theories of Kubler-Ross, 427
Support structures, 429
Conclusion, 429

21 Nurse-coordinated care of the child with advanced cancer, 431

Ida M. Martinson

Identification of need, 431
Hospice concept, 431
Home care for the child with cancer project, 432
Background, 432
Program description, 433
Process of referral, 434
Characteristics of home care nurses, 434
Project objectives, 434
Assessment of needs, 435
Nursing interventions, 437
Findings of project, 438
Appropriateness of nurse-coordinator model, 438
Clinical implications, 439
Change of attitudes on the part of parents, 439
Conclusion, 439

VI
MAJOR CLIENT NEEDS OR HIGH-INCIDENCE PROBLEMS

22 The spectrum of care for clients with cancer, 443

Lisa Begg Marino

Documentation of client and family needs, 443
Importance of nursing care in cancer, 444
Overview of needs, 445
  Unifying needs, 446
  Specific needs, 449
General format for section, 453
Conclusion, 454

23 Children with cancer: a developmental approach, 455

Mary Morrow
Harry L. Wilson

Concepts of therapy, 456
  Surgery, 456
  Chemotherapy, 457
  Radiation therapy, 458
  Modes of therapy, 459
  Process of therapy, 464
  Philosophy of care, 466
Developmental approach, 468
  Overview, 468
  Infant—birth to 1 year, 468
  Toddler—years 1 to 3, 471
  Preschooler—years 3 to 6, 473
  School age—years 6 to 12, 476
  Adolescent—years 12 to 18, 480
Conclusion, 486

24 Morbidity and the quality of life in clients with breast cancer, 488

Lisa Begg Marino

Scope of breast cancer problem, 488
  Incidence, 488
  Risk factors for the development of breast cancer, 488
Overall client needs, 491
  General needs, 491
  Specific needs, 491
Cancer morbidity and its impact on the quality of life, 491
Morbidity associated with breast cancer, 492
  Morbidity resulting from breast cancer surgery, 492
  Morbidity associated with radiation therapy, 497
  Morbidity secondary to cancer chemotherapy for breast cancer, 499
  Morbidity associated with immunotherapy for breast cancer, 501
Morbidity directly related to disease progression, 501
Case study, 502
  Personal history, 502
  Background to illness, 502
  Period of hospitalization, 503
  Posthospital course, 504
Conclusion, 506

25 Nutritional problems in clients having gastrointestinal cancer, 508

Phyllis Palka Cullen

Scope of the gastrointestinal cancers, 508
  Incidence, 508
Phases of care, 509
  Phase I, 509
  Phase II, 509
  Phase III, 509
Nutrition as a functional problem, 511
  Emotional aspects associated with nutrition, 512
  The nurse as the provider, 512
  Review of the nutrition problem in cancer, 513
  Assessment and identification of the nutritional problem, 514
  Guidelines for nursing care, 515
Conclusion, 520
Case history, 520
Summary, 523

26 Infection control in clients with acute leukemia, 524

Mary D. Bates
Mary Beth Orton

Incidence, 524
Pathophysiology of acute leukemia, 524

Clinical presentation, 525
Treatment of acute leukemia, 526
Management of complications of acute leukemia, 527
Anemia, 527
Hemorrhage, 528
Infection, 529
Nursing interventions, 535
Preventive nursing aspects, 535
Specific treatment measures, 538
Sepsis/septic shock, 539
Isolation techniques, 540
Protected environment, 540
Infections in the outpatient leukemia population, 541
Case study, 543
Discussion, 545
Conclusion, 546

27 Female sexuality and gynecologic cancer, 547

Saundra Elaine Saunders

Recognition of a need, 547
The concept of sexuality, 547
Body image, 547
Definition and components of sexuality, 548
Assault to sexuality, 549
The stigma of cancer, 549
Cancer as a chronic illness, 551
Cancer treatment, 552
Sexuality and terminal cancer, 555
Considerations for rehabilitation, 556
Wholeness, 556
Desirability, 557
Individuality, 558
Conclusion, 559

28 Changes in body image associated with head and neck cancer, 560

Mary Jo Dropkin

Characteristics of head and neck cancer, 560
Body image: defining the concept through research, 561
Development of body image, 564
Significance of the head and neck to body image, 565
Significance of body image to nursing care of the head and neck cancer patient, 565
Physiologic alteration: cancer of the larynx, 567
Case history, 571
Diagnosis, 571
Treatment, 572
Complications, 573
Body image alteration: nursing care, 574
Physiologic needs, 574
Self-concept, 576
Role function, 577
Interdependent relations, 578
Conclusion, 579

29 Safety problems encountered by clients with brain tumors, 582

Pearl Moore

Malignant brain tumors, 582
Signs and symptoms, 582
Diagnostic methods, 583
Treatment, 584
Problems encountered by clients with brain tumors, 585
Mental status changes, 585
Motor and sensory function changes, 586
Side-effects and complications of treatment, 586
Appearance changes, 589
Role change, 590
Isolation, 590
Case study, 591
Summary, 594

30 Male sexuality and genitourinary cancer, 595

Gary R. Houston
Dorothy Rodriguez

Overview of incidence, 595
Cancer of the prostate, 595
Symptomatology, 595
Staging of prostate cancer, 596
Treatment, 596
Nursing care, 597

Cancer of the bladder, 598
  Symptoms, 598
  Treatment, 599
  Nursing care, 599
Cancer of the kidney, 600
  Staging, 601
  Treatment, 601
  Nursing care, 601
Cancer of the testes, 602
  Symptoms, 602
  Staging, 602
  Treatment, 603
  Nursing care, 603
Cancer of the penis, 604
  Symptoms, 604
  Treatment, 604
  Nursing care, 604
Male sexuality, 604
  Problems specific to genitourinary cancers, 605
  Nursing approaches, 606
Stomal care, 607
  Case study, 607

VII
CONCLUSION

31 Cancer nursing: current progress and future trends, 617

Lisa Begg Marino

Current progress, 617
  Cancer nursing practice, 617
  Cancer nursing education, 620
  Cancer nursing research, 621
Future trends, 622
  Cancer nursing practice, 622
  Cancer nursing education, 622
  Cancer nursing research, 623
Conclusion, 623

I

OVERVIEW OF CANCER

1

A conceptual framework for cancer nursing

LISA BEGG MARINO

HISTORICAL PERSPECTIVE

Patients are not always told that they have cancer—you may never know what a cancer patient is thinking, fearing, or hoping. Remember that hope is a wonderful prop as you try to understand his hopes, fears, and discomforts. Remember, too, that a terminal illness is difficult for the patient's family; your understanding, attitude, and sympathetic care of the patient will help them through a trying time. Leave any discussion of the progress of the disease to the doctor. Concentrate your efforts on making each day as comfortable as possible for the patient.[17]

This quote gives an indication of the role that nursing played in cancer during the 1950's. At best, the role of the nurse was a limited one. This was primarily due to the fact that cancer was essentially a fatal illness for which there were few interventions. No one, including the physician, had the tools to really help these clients. Those persons who developed cancer were isolated by the numerous social stigmas and fears that were rampant during this time. Those caring for these clients, whether they be physicians, nurses, or other health care providers, were equally isolated and frustrated. This cycle only kept all the parties—the client, the family, and the health care providers—apart.

Fig. 1-1 illustrates the dilemma that was common during this earlier period. It was almost as if all the parties functioned in isolation. Each group was a spectator observing the others with no meaningful communication occurring as to what was really happening. This action, while understandable given the fatalistic climate that permeated this era, only further denied the parties' opportunity to share the stresses and grief together.

The barriers that separated the three parties were basically communicational in nature. The fear of disclosing the diagnosis, the fear of acknowledging that little in the way of therapy could be offered the client, and the social stigmas that abounded regarding cancer all combined to make it very difficult for those involved to acknowledge the reality of the situation. Acknowledging even the first fact—that cancer did exist in this person—meant dealing with the rest. For most people, this acknowledgment was too difficult and was therefore suppressed. Unfortunately, the cancer was still present; there-

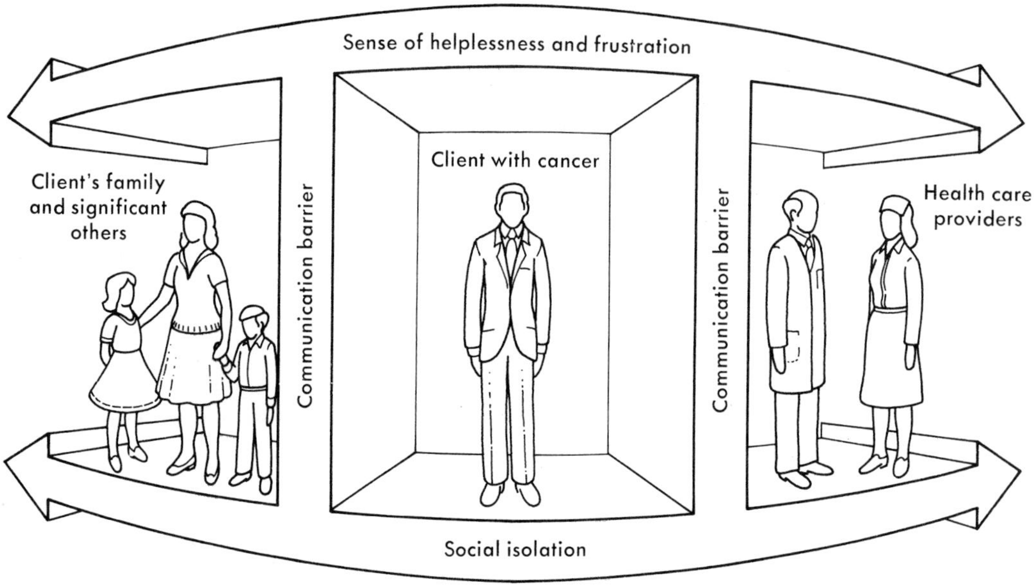

Fig. 1-1. Model of cancer care during earlier era.

fore, only the *adjustment phase* suffered and the problems grew larger as the disease progressed.

Disclosure that the client was going to die from cancer could serve as an example of how these communication barriers separated the parties. The impact of this breakdown was significant. For example, a client who had metastatic colon carcinoma that had spread to his liver can serve as the simulated case study. Mr. G. is 63 years old and normally weighs 160 pounds, but he has lost 40 pounds in the last year. Mr. G. no longer works because of extreme fatigue and limited mobility; he stays in bed most of the time. Additionally, his food and fluid intake is poor because of frequent nausea, vomiting, and pain. Mrs. G., his wife, cares for him most of the time. The illness has been protracted, lasting over 1½ years. Mrs. G. is fatigued herself but spends many hours each day trying to prepare attractive foods for Mr. G. in the hope that he can regain some of the lost weight. Conversations are stunted. Each time Mr. G. comments on how weak he is getting, Mrs. G. quickly changes the subject. Conversations that focus on future events are even more painful, and care is taken to avoid any reference to future times. These two people are avoiding the reality that Mr. G. is dying. Acknowledgement of this fact is admittedly difficult and feelings of grief and loss are overwhelming, but *not* acknowledging the situation only serves to keep this couple apart. Mr. G. is suffering but essentially *alone*. His fears are still there, but there is little chance to express them and work them through. The same can be stated for Mrs. G. The reality is still there, but because it is not being dealt with, support and mutual sharing are not taking place.

CHANGING ATTITUDES

Fortunately, major scientific advances have given the clinician working with clients who have cancer many more therapeutic tools. Likewise, this improved situation has fostered better attitudes on the part of the health care providers and many segments of the population. Cancer is still a feared disease, but more open discussions are taking place so that the sharing of these fears is minimizing the individual burdens.

An example of these changing attitudes is a recent study that demonstrated an almost complete reversal of attitudes between 1961 and 1977 among physicians disclosing a diagnosis of cancer. Specifically, these researchers questioned physicians at Strong Memorial Hospital in Rochester, New York, as to whether they generally told their clients of a confirmed diagnosis of cancer.[10] Of the 40% who responded, 98% indicated that they generally did tell their clients. This study is in sharp contrast to the 1961 study by Oken, which found 90% of those physicians generally withholding disclosure of a diagnosis of cancer.[11]

The 1977 researchers indicate that social factors such as the increase of consumerism, the malpractice issue, and increasing scrutiny of the medical profession by the public may have contributed to this new openness. The improvements in cancer treatment and the discussion of this problem within the medical school curriculum were also cited. Quite interestingly, the physicians questioned in the 1977 study cited *personal* observations as the reason for disclosure and not *scientific* data that more open communication benefited all the parties. The last point illustrates that although attitudes are improving, much more needs to be done to place cancer in the mainstream of health care.

NEW NURSING ROLES IN CANCER

There have not been any attitudinal studies of how nurses currently view cancer, but other activities give an indication. As the scientific advances increase, clients with cancer are experiencing more varied treatments and are living longer. These changes have stimulated increased interest in many nurses as witnessed by the large attendance at national and regional nursing meetings concerned with cancer. Likewise, organizations specifically established around cancer such as the Oncology Nursing Society have been formed. Efforts to identify guidelines for providing nursing care to these clients have been successful with the completion of *Outcome Standards For Cancer Nursing Practice*.[13] These standards, the first attempt to define the scope of cancer nursing practice, were developed by the Oncology Nursing Society and the American Nurses' Association.

Fortunately, for those persons at risk for cancer, or who actually have developed cancer, the emergence of a more active role for nurses is very important. The treatment advances and the great concentration on cancer research have made the delivery of care much more complex. The nursing profession, because of its great numbers and strong theoretical and practical base, can do much to fill existing gaps in care and better coordinate the care being rendered.

A CONCEPTUAL FRAMEWORK FOR CANCER NURSING

Fig. 1-2 (see accompanying boxed material) illustrates the changing picture of cancer within the American health care system and the opportunities where nurses can, or do, impact on client outcomes. This model is being presented to show the integration of cancer and nursing within the health care system. It is also being presented to provide the reader with a framework for intervening with these clients by the identification of needs that are known and to encourage further exploration of possible needs and ways the nurse can expand to further impact

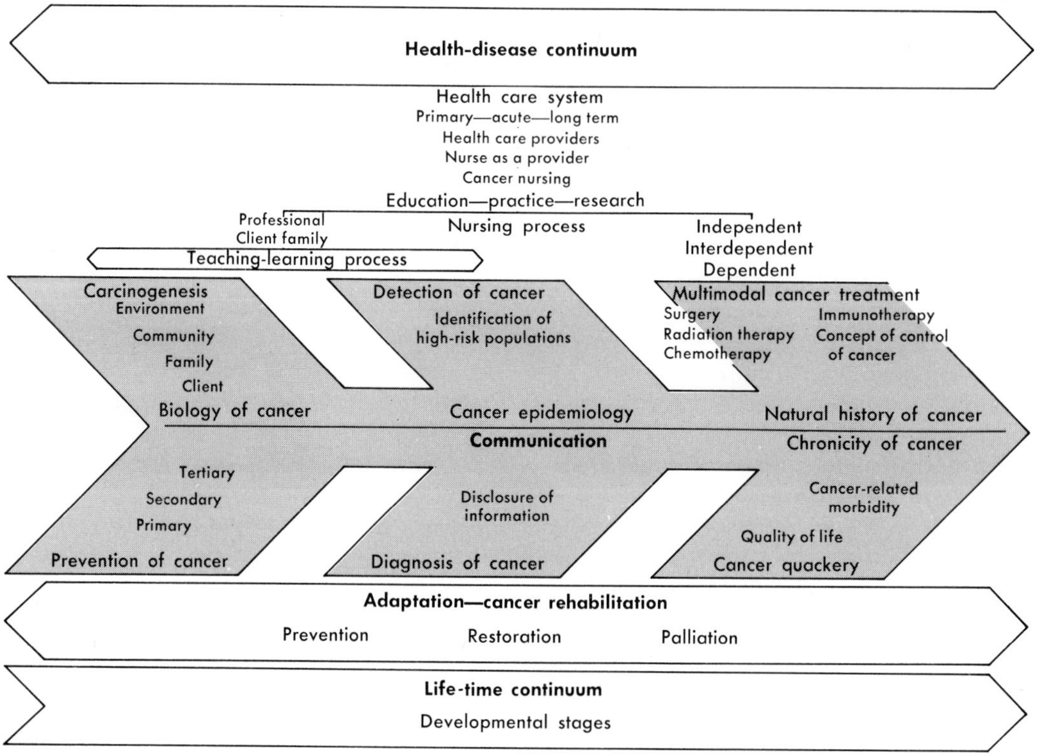

Fig. 1-2. Conceptual framework for cancer nursing.

on care. This model also serves as a guide to content elsewhere in this book, so that after completion of reading this book the nurse will have more information with which to care for this population of clients. Discussion of the major components of the model follows and starts with the health-disease continuum.

Health-disease continuum

The presentation of the concept of a health-disease continuum assists in the identification of issues that impact not only on clients at risk for cancer, or who actually have cancer, but also on the utilization of nurses. Because of the complex needs of this population of clients and the important contributions nurses can make in this area of health and disease, discussion will also cover ways the nurse can minimize impediments to practice.

For example, the health-disease continuum is a dynamic and everchanging state in which the individual moves back and forth almost continuously. This varied movement contrasts with the unrelenting nature of the life-time continuum represented at the bottom of the model. The client simply moves along from birth until death. This movement does impact on the health-disease continuum; however, as age increases, developmental stages are achieved and bodily function degenerates.

In relation to health and disease, most people experience only a few discrete periods of complete health or complete disease.

DEFINITIONS

adaptation—the ability to respond to changes in the client's environment in such a fashion that injury is prevented or damage is repaired[3]

cancer—a group of diseases in which the mechanism within the cell, and in its microenvironment, is responsible for restraint of growth and defects[15]

cancer nursing practice—the roles of professional nursing practice necessary to promote optimal levels of functioning and well-being in health and illness of the cancer client and family[13]

cancer quackery—the intentional misrepresentation and/or deliberate misapplication of diagnostic or treatment measures that impedes or delays the patient's entry into legitimate, constructive forms of cancer treatment[5]

carcinogenesis—the production or origin of cancer[16]

client—any individual or group demonstrating actual or potential needs for heatlh education, health maintenance, or preventive or curative treatment by health care providers[13]

community—social, cultural, political, and economic surroundings of client and family[12]

disease—failures or disturbances in the growth, development, functions, and adjustment of the organism as a whole or of any of its systems[6]

environment—physical surroundings external to the client

family—persons who are directly related to client or who represent a significant support group[13]

health—not a condition of an individual but a state of interaction between self and environment (It is a ceaseless struggle between a basically hostile environment and a series of defenses we are endowed with and that we add to when necessary. The homeostatic balance of forces is our goal and this may be accomplished by decreasing the threat of the environment or by raising the capability of the host to defend himself.)[4]

health care providers—represent all levels of professional and allied health personnel[13]

health care system—availability, access, and utilization of health care settings, health care providers, and resources[12]

morbidity—a negative change in the physical or psychologic functioning of the client that is a direct result of disease or its treatment

multimodal cancer treatment—the combination of any or all of the following modalities—surgery, radiation therapy, chemotherapy, and immunotherapy

natural history of cancer—the course that a particular form of cancer takes from the time of diagnosis to control of the pathologic process or the death of the host (This term implies that no therapeutic interventions are made. This is clearly not the case. The term really reflects the evolution of the disease within the confines of the existing or past society.)

nursing process—an orderly, systematic manner of determining the client's problems, making plans to solve them, initiating the plan or assigning others to implement it, and evaluating the extent to which the plan was effective in resolving the problems identified[19]

rehabilitation—a process of enhancing restoration and maintenance of optimal physical and psychologic functioning[9]

teaching-learning process—a conscious, dynamic process to promote a planned change in attitude, knowledge, or skill in the learner[9]

Rather, it is more descriptive to discuss *levels* of health or disease. Whether or not the individual becomes ill or maintains wellness is largely dependent on the psychologic and physical states at that point in time, the disease in question, the stresses being experienced, and the individual's coping ability. Health and disease are highly individualized within each person. What causes disease in one person may promote greater health in another. Stress is clearly involved with many diseases but, as of yet, is poorly understood on an individual basis.

General application of the health-disease continuum

Acknowledging the concept of the health-disease continuum has important implications for both the specialty of oncology and the nursing profession. Much research into cancer is under way to better identify high-risk populations so that closer and more cost-efficient monitoring can be done. It is widely recognized by cancer experts that most people have some aberrant cell changes within their bodies at frequent intervals. Why those aberrant cells go unchecked in one person so that a clinical cancer develops may involve many factors. One assumption is that this person's immunologic surveillance system is lacking. Yet in another person no cancer ever develops because the body is able to control these cells by some means. Observations have been made, but to date no discrete "cause and effect" relationship can be documented. These problems only point up the complex relationship of biologic and social factors that have an impact on the incidence of cancer.

In nursing, this complexity points up the need for improved observations relating to levels of health or disease as well as general factors that promote the development of cancer. Nurses have the knowledge base and the observational skills that can assist clients to identify potential or real problems at an earlier time. This fact is of great importance since most cancers can be treated at earlier stages or prevention can totally avoid the likelihood of cancer ever developing.

The recognition of this changing concept of a health-disease continuum, coupled with the advances in treating cancer, has yielded a more accurate perception of cancer. No longer is cancer regarded as one disease; it is more accurately described as a *group* of diseases with clinically distinct presentations, and differing biologic behavior and clinical manifestations. Likewise, cancer is no longer a universally fatal disease but rather a *group of chronic diseases* for which *something* can be done. These diseases are still very serious and life-threatening, but the hopelessness that prevailed in earlier periods is not generally evident today. Clients who have been successfully treated for their cancer are essentially healthy and should be regarded as such. However, these people are still at risk for the possible development of a new cancer and should be followed carefully, but they definitely should not be regarded as ill. Likewise, clients who still have some residual cancer that is being treated may not be completely ill. Today, the concept of *levels* of health and disease can be directly applied to cancer. Not only is this change more accurate, but it also provides more resources to the client, family, and health care providers such as nurses. The nurse can do a great deal to instruct others in these changes, so that the client who does have cancer will have resources to draw from.

Continuum applied to the health care system

Our current health care system is geared toward treatment with only a slight emphasis on prevention. This orientation affects cancer negatively because information on carcinogenesis is poorly understood by the public, and available knowledge in preventing cancer is not always fully utilized. Yet, the incidence of cancer is second only to heart disease.[2] Likewise, cancer affects all age groups from infancy to old age. Both sexes are affected as are all settings in which health care is rendered. This includes the community through which private and public health nurses function as primary care providers, acute settings such as hospitals, and long-term facilities such as nursing homes and hospices. All treatment areas such as obstetrics, pediatrics, surgery, medicine, geriatrics, rehabilitation, and even psychiatry see clients with known or suspected cancer. Cancer is clearly a major health care problem that providers such as nurses continually face in practice.

This continual association with these clients does not necessarily mean, however, that the health care system effectively provides services. In addition to the lack of a preventive focus, the general course of cancer does not fit well into the current system of health care delivery. For example, cancer can be characterized as a *group of chronic diseases that require frequent, high-intensity monitoring*. This means that at any point in time the client may need acute care facilities for the high-intensity monitoring but not for the more chronic phases of illness. These needs could be better met if the client progressed in an orderly fashion from acute to chronic, but cancer is not always a predictable problem so the client may go back and forth repeatedly. A good example of this is the child with acute leukemia. In the early stages the child is very seriously ill and needs acute care monitoring. However, treatment is such that many children go into remission, which means their cancer has been arrested. The child may not be completely cured of the leukemia but is basically well enough to lead a reasonably normal life. During the period of remission, less intense monitoring is needed. Most of the time this means that the child is at home with only occasional visits to the physician. This chronic phase can last indefinitely, or the child can develop new problems that are life threatening. If this should happen, the acute care, high-intensity monitoring begins again and the cycle repeats itself. These changes are not always predictable so the health care system is not well equipped to deal with them. Most diseases in this country are *either* acute or long-term rather than a combination that repeats itself. In this sense, cancer is unique. The nurse caring for this population of clients can do a great deal to better coordinate services between the primary, acute, and long-term settings so that the client can obtain care regardless of what phase of the illness is being experienced.

Health care providers defined

Aside from the uniqueness of cancer care within the health-disease continuum and the delivery system, many types of health care providers are involved. This variety can be problematic if no one is *coordinating* the care. For example, diagnosing and evaluating treatment options for the client require many medical specialists from diagnostic radiologists to nuclear medicine specialists to possibly surgeons, radiotherapists, medical oncologists, hematologists, or immunotherapists. Aside from physicians, nurse specialists may be consulted as might dietitians, social workers, or physical therapists. If the client is religious, clergy may be asked to consult. The client is already under considerable stress because of the suspected or confirmed diagnosis of cancer and may be completely overwhelmed by this large number of people "evaluating" the situation. Having someone who understands the overall plan and who can relate to all these professionals and interpret the ongoing activities to the client and family is very helpful. This role of coordinator *over time* provides the client and family with some degree of consistency. It is a role ideally suited for nursing.

The nurse as provider defined

It has now been stated that the nurse is ideally suited to provide care to clients at risk for, or with an actual diagnosis of, cancer. How a nurse relates to this frequent contact can vary with each individual. Unfortunately, many nurses still function in the social vacuum characterized by Fig. 1-1. Neither meaningful communication with the client and family nor coordination of care occurs. All too often, no real communication exists *among* the health care providers either. Whereas the former case involving the client and family may be due to ignorance on the part of the nurse as to available resources, a different basis exists for the latter situation.

The latter case of limited communication among the health care providers caring for these clients demonstrates role conflict. The nurse may not be willing, or able, to assume the full professional role. One mechanism seems predominant. It is a reluctance on the part of the nurse to become involved in resolving the communication problems associated with cancer. The assumption is that the nurse *does not have a right or obligation to resolve conflicts that impede quality of care*. Even today, few people are truly comfortable with cancer so the barriers place the nurse on the defensive to justify intervening. It is more troublesome to intervene than to go along with the closed system. Unfortunately, the closed system does not promote client-family involvement or a high level of care. It would be far better for nurses to assume they have the *right and the obligation* to become involved. This attitude opens up more opportunities than the passive position of allowing the status quo to continue. This posture also provides the client and family with an important professional to assist in information gathering and decision making. Both of these functions are important in such a changing and complex specialty. Likewise, as difficult as it may be to charter a full professional role, the opportunities for satisfaction are great. Open communication among the care providers, client, and family can never be encouraged too much. The nurse, sensitive to both sides of the problem, can do a great deal to provide for more open communication and an improved level of care.

Cancer nursing defined

Cancer nursing possesses the same three components common to all of professional nursing. These components are education, practice, and research. The educational component is based on teaching-learning principles that are applied to clients, their families, and other health care providers. Teaching the client and family is particularly important because of the numerous misconceptions about cancer that persist and cause increased anxiety and interference with the recommended course of action.

Education of health care providers is also crucial. This is particularly true for nursing as it is the largest of the health professions with numerous opportunities to impact on care. Toward this goal, guidelines for educating nurses have been developed that provide for fundamental and advanced educational levels.[12] These guidelines seek to identify behaviors and levels of knowledge necessary to provide proper care for this population of clients. They are intended to complement standards of care for this same population of clients.[13]

These standards form the basis for defining the scope of cancer nursing practice by identifying 10 high-incidence problem areas for clients in any care setting, whether it be primary, acute, or long term. These 10 areas are prevention and early detection, information, coping, comfort, nutrition, protective mechanisms, mobility, elimination, sexuality, and ventilation.[13] Future research will undoubtedly require additions or revisions in these standards, but for the present they serve to target nursing interventions along with providing parameters for evaluation of such action.

The educational and practice components form the basis for cancer nursing research in that levels of expected behavior are identified as are major client needs. The research component is a very broad one because the nurse can function in any of three ways: independently, as when the nurse initiates a research study; interdependently, as when the nurse cooperates with other disciplines in a research study; and dependently, as when the nurse assists other researchers such as physicians conducting therapeutic research. This component is receiving major emphasis in nursing because of the strong research emphasis in cancer. Opportunities to advance the nursing profession are numerous.

Integrating the health-disease continuum, the health care system, and the health care providers including cancer nursing specialists, demonstrates the complexity of the situation. The cancer nurse can easily become overextended in attempting to deal with the multiple issues. For this reason, it is particularly important for the nurse to employ the nursing process as a basis of action. Using this systematic process, the nurse can determine the need, plan a course of action, and initiate and evaluate the efforts. This process utilizes an ethical basis for action and employs all three components of professional nursing.

Integrating adaptation and rehabilitation with cancer nursing model

The principal goal of cancer nursing is to assist the client and family to adjust maximally to their circumstances. In other words, the nurse intervening with these clients seeks to promote adaptation and maximal rehabilitation. This broad orientation permits the nurse wide latitude with these clients so that professional satisfaction can be achieved in most cases. Achieving satisfaction is important if more nurses are to become involved with these clients because feelings of frustration and helplessness affect the nurse as a care provider as much as they do the client and family. Unfortunately, unless these signs are recognized and dealt with successfully, "burnout" or professional distance, as discussed in Chapter 8, develops, which only further isolates the client and family. However, these problems need not develop, since the adaptation-rehabilitation approach provides many opportunities for the nurse.

Preventive cancer rehabilitation nursing. The nurse focusing on rehabilitation can assist the client to avoid many common problems currently seen in cancer. For example, the nurse properly trained in enterostomal therapy can work with the client and surgeon to locate the future stoma in a position that will allow for a minimum of problems postoperatively. In earlier periods, the nurse was not well versed in stomal management and so the client went to surgery with little thought given to the best placement of the stoma. Unfortunately, the client may have been cured of the cancer but became a social recluse for fear of fecal or urinary spillage. Today, it is a well-known fact that the placement of the stoma is of great significance to the successful rehabilitation of the client. The nurse is the key provider in this regard.

Restorative cancer rehabilitation nursing. Relative to restorative rehabilitation, a prime example is the client who is undergoing chemotherapeutic or radiotherapeutic treatments that are interfering with nutritional intake. The treatments must be given, but it is also important to maintain adequate nutrition. The nurse can work with the client and family to identify daily schedules and preferred or tolerated foods and fluids so that a plan can be developed that will permit the needed treatments to continue while promoting an improved nutritional state. The nurse has the knowledge to know whether taste sensations have been altered by the treatments and how to arrange added rest periods. The nurse also has the clinical experience to suggest more frequent, smaller meals and having the client remain out of the kitchen because of increased sensitivity to food odors. Again, it is the *nurse* who possesses the broadest skills to assist the client and family.

Palliative cancer rehabilitation nursing. As for palliative rehabilitation, the client who has metastatic breast cancer to the bone is an ideal candidate for the nurse with skill to plan for limited and safe mobility. Generally, this type of a client would receive palliative radiation therapy to the affected bone or bones to relieve the pain and promote healing. The radiotherapy arrests the cancer in that area. In no way does it cure the client, but significant relief can be achieved by this means. Once the therapy is completed, the nurse can consult with the client's physician to develop a safe, limited plan of mobility. This mobility is important for two reasons. First, the client does have metastatic breast cancer and will probably die eventually, but this form of cancer is relatively slow growing and amenable to treatments so one would expect the client to be able to live fairly comfortably for some time. Mobility prevents further deformity and also enhances the client's quality of life. Second, mobility will generally reduce the likelihood of hypercalcemia developing. Since this problem can be life threatening, prevention is preferable. Again, it is the nurse who can best arrange this care.

The focus in these three areas of adaptation and rehabilitation is on assisting the client and family to live to the maximum while minimizing the existing deficits. The seriousness of cancer is never denied but neither is the opportunity to provide the client, family, nurse, and other health care providers with opportunities to be successful. This focus allows the care providers, particularly the nurse, to be able always to do *something* for the client and family. It minimizes the earlier feelings of helplessness and frustration under which many nurses suffered. It also reflects more accurately the state of knowledge about cancer and the changing dynamics of the physician-nurse relationship. It does not deny the physician a major role to play in cancer but does considerably expand the role of the nurse. Given the complexity of the health care system, the controversy and complexity of cancer care coupled with the gaps in care caused by the rapid advances, the nurse has both the *opportunity* and *responsibility* to participate more fully with this population of clients. To encourage the nurse, discussion will follow that concentrates on three main areas of cancer: prevention and carcinogenesis, cancer detection and diagnosis, and cancer treatment.

Nursing opportunities in cancer prevention and carcinogenesis

The area of cancer prevention and carcinogenesis illustrates the underutilization of nurses. Part of the reason may be due to the limited concentration on prevention within our current health care system. In reality, this is probably only a partial answer, since nurses do not promote themselves as health educators. Unfortunately, cancer health education of the public is what is needed if the confusion and controversies are to be more clearly understood by the public. Likewise, information on cancer prevention is not fully utilized.

For example, some cancers can be prevented but are not being minimized because information is poorly understood. The best example is lung cancer and its association with cigarette smoking. The American Cancer Society's statistics for 1979 indicate that lung cancer will affect over 100,000 people.[2] Adults who have been smoking for some time have an admittedly difficult time stopping, but efforts to discourage teenagers from starting need greater emphasis. School nurses are in an ideal position to influence these adolescents by providing them with correct and complete information on the hazards of smoking.

Also, cigarette smoking in certain occupational groups is highly dangerous. A prime example of this enhanced risk is asbestos workers who smoke. They increase their risk of developing cancer significantly because of the co-carcinogenic effects of cigarettes and asbestos. Occupational health nurses are the target group to help identify high-risk workers and provide them with correct information on the known risks.

Altering self-destructive habits such as smoking is admittedly difficult. Innovative approaches are greatly needed as is a wider distribution of information about known carcinogens. Nurses, because of their visibility and access to the public, can greatly facilitate the transmittal of information relating to cancer.

Likewise, the issues of identifying carcinogenic substances, developing policies to deal with the problem, and the economic and social consequences are not always apparent. Interpretation of the maze of conflicting data that surface almost daily only serves to confuse the public. Many people believe that "everything causes cancer" or "it doesn't matter what I do, I'm going to get cancer." *Neither* of these statements is accurate. Nurses can explain the regulating procedures involved in the determination of carcinogenic substances. Additionally, nurses have the theoretical knowledge to explain the long latency period between exposure and development of cancer, the difficulty in isolating the carcinogen from other possible agents, the wide variation in available testing devices, and the need for careful monitoring of the incidence of certain types of cancer in different populations over a period of time. For example, examination of cancer mortality by county within the United States has revealed patterns of etiologic importance, particularly relating to the incidence of bladder cancer in males working with industrial dyes.

Nurses can support the correct interpretation of such research and monitoring as well as initiate research to minimize self-destructive habits.

Unfortunately, there are no easy solutions to these problems, but the nurse, as an informed health care provider, can do a great deal to alleviate confusion and promote an increased level of understanding in the primary prevention area.

Nursing opportunities in cancer detection and diagnosis

Just as the area of cancer prevention and carcinogenesis is offering the nurse new avenues of involvement, the whole area of secondary prevention of cancer affords the nurse even more opportunities. These opportunities can be divided into six broad categories: promoting better utilization of existing resources to detect cancer at its earliest point, identifying high-risk groups for cancer, offering counsel to high-risk groups, performing examinations and procedures to detect cancer, providing support to the client and family during the detection and diagnostic phases, and assisting the client and family in obtaining information with which to make an informed decision following confirmation of the diagnosis.

Promoting better utilization of existing resources. An example of how a nurse can promote better utilization of existing resources would be the Papanicolaou test of cervical cytology. This test, first introduced in the 1930's, has led to a 70% reduction in cervical cancer mortality.[2] The unfortunate fact, however, is that in spite of this sizable reduction in mortality, many women are still dying from this form of cancer. These deaths are attributed to detecting cervical cancer at more advanced stages when treatment is not as likely to be successful. An American Cancer Society survey[1] has shown only some 30% of adult American women have annual "Pap smears." This fact points up the tragedy as this test done periodically can detect cervical cancer at a very early stage called "in situ," which is universally curable. Nurses could do a great deal in terms of formal and informal public education to promote increased utilization of this valuable test in women who are over 18 years of age or who are sexually active.

Identifying high-risk populations. Because of the growing importance of identifying high-risk groups, this is another ideal area in which nurses can excel. Nurses function in a social system with varied roles: family member, parent, spouse, citizen, and health provider. Contacts with other people, whether of a personal or professional nature, are numerous. Opportunities for case finding are readily available. Likewise, sharing of information on why controversies exist as to what constitutes high risk is also important because the public tends to become discouraged with the apparent inconsistencies. This indifference results in decreased resources.

An example of a population at high risk for cancer that nurses come in contact with are women who have a family history of breast cancer. These family members would need to be sisters, aunts, or the mother to put this individual at a higher risk. If the history taking yields information of this nature, the nurse should make sure the woman knows how to do breast self-examination and sees a physician as to whether any tests should be undertaken.

Likewise, children with mongolism or Down's syndrome have an increased risk of developing acute leukemia. Parents are not always aware of the correlation and should be advised. Colon cancers tend to run in families, so knowledge of colon cancer in family members would alert the members to be on the lookout for any suspicious signs such as a change in bowel habits, unusual bleeding, or tarry stools. The nurse also needs to strongly suggest that a physician be contacted to determine if any tests should be undertaken.

The problem with detecting many cancers early is that people tend to ignore subtle changes. Noticing a changed mole might be very significant in discovering a melanoma early. The nurse can do a great deal as a health educator to reinforce the significant role the *individual* plays in discovering cancer.

Offering counsel to high-risk groups. Once a person is determined to be at higher risk for the development of a form of cancer, the nurse can work with other health care providers to minimize anxiety and maximize sound decision making. A good case in point would be the client who has ulcerative colitis that has been in long-term remission. Recent studies have shown these persons to be at increased risk for the development of colon cancer. This discovery is particularly tragic since many of these people have spent years getting their colitis under control only to find that they now have another battle to wage. Anxiety is also heightened by frequent tests that are needed. Nurses can be very helpful to these clients as they consider whether prophylactic surgery should be done. Significant life-style changes also depend on this decision.

Performing examinations to detect cancer. Another underutilized area for nursing is in performing examinations to detect cancer. Two of the limited examples of nurses being employed to perform detection examinations were the Breast Cancer Detection Centers funded during the 1970's by the National Cancer Institute and the American Cancer Society and the ongoing CANSCREEN program at the Preventive Medicine Institute–Strang Clinic in New York City. To date, no systematic evaluation has been conducted as to the value and proficiency of nurses assuming these roles. An evaluation would be helpful because of the large number of people involved and the physician costs. Moreover, these functions ideally should include a strong client education program that nurses can carry out with proficiency.

Providing support to the client during the diagnostic phase. Some forms of cancer can be diagnosed easily and quickly, while other types of cancer require lengthy and complex procedures. Unfortunately, this period is one of client and family apprehension. A 1973 study demonstrated that the delay in following up on suspicious symptoms remained the same as in a study done in the 1930's. The delay period did not vary significantly with regard to age, sex, or socioeconomic level.[8] This points up the continued fear about cancer that keeps the public from seeking help and the importance of having an informed provider such as a nurse to support the client and family. Anxiety cannot, nor should it, be denied, but neither should the client and family be forced to suffer in isolation during an acknowledged stressful period. Additionally, anxiety may be increased if cancer is suspected in a valued part such as the breast or would require extensive surgery as in the case of head or neck cancers.

Assisting the client and family in obtaining information. The last category where the nurse can participate more fully is in the area of providing the client and family with information once the diagnosis has been confirmed. The starting point is the disclosure of a diagnosis that cancer has been found. As was previously stated, it appears that more physicians are informing their clients if a cancer is found. Unfortunately, no survey can ascertain whether cancer is discussed or whether euphemisms such as "tumor," "growth," or "pathology" are used. Likewise, it is difficult to document *how much* information the client and family receive. What role(s) nurses should play in this area is still unclear, but serious consideration should be given to assisting the client and family to understand the treatments to be employed, their risk versus benefits, and the long-term consequences. It will probably be some time in the future before the public and health groups regard cancer as openly as other diseases. The social fears still exist and can be exemplified by Shand's observation that a diagnosis of cancer is like "an amputation of the future."[14] All health providers, whether they be physicians, nurses, or social workers, are first *private individuals* who are subject to the same social distress about cancer as those individuals in the general population.

Likewise, the dynamics of the physician-nurse relationship are undergoing extensive review by such bodies as the National Joint Practice Commission, various state legislatures, and various political groups. These reviews will undoubtedly increase as health care costs become greater and pressures to find alternative ways of lowering the costs of health care increase. Activities to expand nursing contributions are increasing specifically in regard to cancer. Activities are under way in some well-functioning cancer teams composed of physicians, nurses, social workers, clergy, and other support personnel to see whether the provider with the best rapport should be the one to disclose important information to the client. This change is in sharp contrast to the traditional position that the physician is "captain of the ship" and discloses key points of information. Documentation of the impact of this change still needs to be made as do the adjustments within the legal realm. However, justification for the change is being postulated on the grounds that morally the nurse, like the physician, has the obligation to answer client's questions.[18]

Regardless of whether this innovation becomes widespread, it does point up two areas the nurse should consider. These are: the burden that disclosing information to clients with cancer presents to the physician and the need for a more systematic sharing of information with these clients and their families. In the former case, many nurses choose to criticize the physician for not providing more complete information instead of being more *constructive* in helping the physician perform a very stressful task. The nurse can perform a significant contribution through observing the client's level of understanding, the family's level of understanding, and the family dynamics. These observations are important in developing the disclosure approach. Likewise, the nurse should accompany the physician during these important discussions and validate the level of comprehension. The current confusion in this area does not release the nurse from the responsibility of assisting the client in obtaining information, nor does it allow the nurse to ignore the other health care providers' needs.

Research in the area of client and provider needs is under way, but more research is needed. As the complexity of cancer plans continues and the number of cancer care providers increases, more astute ways to deal with these needs must be made. For example, documentation of how to minimize the stresses associated with diagnosing cancer needs to be made if we ever hope to diminish the delay period. Documentation of how best to utilize health care providers in general needs to be done. If nurses are to be employed for certain functions, documentation of their value needs to be made. Other areas need to be considered, but clearly the nurse has ample room and justification to enter this area of health care.

Further, the strong research orientation in most areas of cancer can increase fears and anxieties on everyone's part, including the health care providers. This stress is not generally acknowledged but does exist. Research implies that answers are *not* known, which is why the experiment is being initiated. There are problems of uncertainty, of therapeutic limitations, of the involvement of humans as study subjects, and of the inability to predict accurately the consequences of clinical actions. These are major problems that must be dealt with if complete disclosure is to take place. The resulting dilemmas that are forced on all the participants are very well discussed in an observational study conducted on clients undergoing metabolic research.[7] Many parallels exist between this type of research and cancer research.

Nursing opportunities in cancer treatment

The same communication network that is evident in the prevention and detection settings carries over into the area of cancer treatment. Here, the nurse can contribute in the following ways: educating the client and family about the treatments and self-care, coordinating care throughout the course of treatment regardless of the setting, aiding the client to minimize treatment-related morbidity so that the quality of life can be enhanced, and assisting the client and family in obtaining information throughout the course of treatment so that informed decisions can be made.

Client-family education. Present-day cancer treatment provides many opportunities for the nurse to educate the client and family. These opportunities are primarily due to the multiple modality treatments that are commonly employed. These combinations are generally complex and usually lengthen the course of treatment. Because of the realization that the best chance to eradicate cancer is the first effort, very careful pretreatment evaluations are also conducted. These evaluations are done to determine as much information as possible about the extent of cancer so that the most appropriate form or forms of treatment can be employed. An example of this extensive pretreatment evaluation is that done for Hodgkin's disease. The evaluation includes numerous radiographic examinations, blood tests, and general surgical staging laparotomy. The client is carefully screened so that if the disease is discovered at an early stage, curative radiation therapy can be given, and if more extensive disease is found, the client can be put on combination chemotherapy. The period of time needed to completely evaluate the client may be weeks, and the nurse can do a great deal in terms of teaching and providing support during this period.

The treatments generally employed in cancer are usually quite sophisticated and toxic. The client and family need to understand what they can do to help themselves as well as the health care providers. This teaching is especially important because so much of cancer treatment is given outside acute care settings. Ordinarily, close monitoring would be readily available, but when the client is being managed with only periodic visits to the physician's office, having information as to just what is important cannot be stressed too much.

Coordinating care. Coordination of care during the phases of treatment is another important nursing function. The importance of this role results primarily because of the sophistication of the treatments and the chronicity of cancer. Treatments such as surgery and chemotherapy are employed for a wide variety of cancers. The head and neck cancers are treated by surgery, radiotherapy, and chemotherapy. These treatments can extend over the period of a year, utilizing the hospital and outpatient settings a number of times. Maintaining communication with the large number of providers in these settings is both important and time consuming. Additionally, the client and family need reassurance that they are carrying out their obligations so the nurse spends a great deal of time in this area.

This coordination continues regardless of whether the client responds well to the treatments. In fact, much of the nurse's time is spent evaluating the client for *long-term needs* should there be a recurrence. If the client does prove to be refractive to treatment so that a recurrence of cancer develops, these early assessments will be very important to better meet identified needs and services.

Minimizing treatment-related morbidity to enhance the quality of life. Minimizing the morbidities commonly seen with cancer treatment has taken on new importance as clients live longer. For example, most cancer chemotherapeutic agents cause nausea or vomiting, myelosuppression, and sometimes alopecia. These effects, although transient, do impact on the quality of the client's life. The deleterious effects can be minimized by alerting the client that more frequent rest periods may be needed and that a wig will probably be necessary and should be obtained before hair loss occurs. Diets can be modified to promote needed nutrition during acute treatment periods. Nurses can perform these functions because they possess the necessary theoretical background, an understanding of the overall goals of treatment, the ability to coordinate the required adjustments with the other providers, and the ability to help the client or family to help themselves.

Obtaining information about treatment. Information sharing during cancer treatment centers on that information needed before treatment is initiated as well as periodic updates during the course of treatment. Since so much cancer treatment is conducted in a research setting, legal statutes also come into consideration but so does the morally grounded premise that clients should be aware of all options, risks, or potential benefits as well as long-term consequences. Aside from these aspects, information will help the client and family participate more fully and understand why interventions are made and how best to help the health providers achieve success. Since this is an anxious time, before appointments or key testing periods, the nurse can be of great value by consistent attention to assisting and validating the client's and family's understanding; information may need to be repeated *over time*. Again, these activities are well suited to the nurse.

Lastly, more nursing research in the area of cancer treatment is needed. Some efforts are currently under way in the area of client retention of information, documentation of treatment-related morbidity, and methods to reduce such untoward effects. Nurses are also assisting therapeutic research efforts and devising questions for study that complement those of medical research. However, more research needs to be undertaken.

CONCLUSION

In conclusion, a conceptual framework for nursing within the specialty of cancer was presented. Its overall place within the health-disease continuum, health care system, and overall nursing demonstrates how integration can be accomplished. This latter point needs to be stressed because cancer nurses *do not* function in a vacuum but rather within a large and dynamic system. If nurses are to impact on the care of clients with cancer and their families, then they need to understand not only the cancer-related areas but also the *larger issues that can inhibit successful professional functioning*.

This model was also presented to provide the nurse with a framework for intervening with this population of clients and their families and to promote further participation and exploration of important issues. I strongly believe that cancer nursing is the *ideal* area for nursing to expand its contributions, and I encourage the reader to promote such expansion for both the benefit of the client and family and for the nursing profession as a whole.

REFERENCES

1. American Cancer Society: 1978 facts and figures, New York, 1978, American Cancer Society, Inc.
2. American Cancer Society: 1979 facts and figures, New York, 1979, American Cancer Society, Inc.
3. Beland, I. L.: Clinical nursing—pathophysiological and psychosocial approaches, ed. 2, New York, 1970, MacMillan Inc.
4. Besson, G.: The health-illness spectrum, Am. J. Public Health **57**:57, 1967.
5. Burkhalter, P. K.: Cancer quackery—what you need to know. In Burkhalter, P. K., and Donley, D. C., editors: Dynamics of oncology nursing, New York, 1978, McGraw-Hill Book Co.
6. Engel, G. L.: A unified concept of health and disease, Perspect. Biol. Med. **3**:459, 1960.

7. Fox, R. C.: Experiment perilous, Philadelphia, 1959, University of Pennsylvania Press.
8. Hackett, T. P., Cassem, N. H., and Raker, J. W.: Patient delay in cancer, N. Engl. J. Med. **289**(1):14, 1973.
9. Madden, B. W.: Rehabilitation—principles, philosophy, practices. Proceedings of the National Conference on Cancer Nursing, New York, 1973, American Cancer Society, Inc.
10. Novack, D. H., et al.: Changes in physician's attitudes toward telling the cancer patient, J.A.M.A. **241**(9):877, 1979.
11. Oken, D.: What to tell cancer patients, J.A.M.A. **175**(13):86, 1961.
12. Oncology Nursing Society: Core educational guidelines, Pittsburgh, Pennsylvania, 1979, Oncology Nursing Society, Inc.
13. Oncology Nursing Society: Outcome standards for cancer nursing practice, Kansas City, Missouri, 1979, American Nurse's Association, Inc.
14. Shand, H. C.: The informational impact of cancer on the structure of the human personality, Ann. N. Y. Acad. Sci. **125**:883, 1966.
15. Sprout, E. E.: Pathology. In Hulland, J. F., and Frei, E., editors: Cancer medicine, Philadelphia, 1973, Lea & Febiger.
16. Taber, C.: Taber's cyclopedia medical dictionary, ed. 10, Philadelphia, 1970, F. A. Davis Co.
17. Thompson, E. M., and LeBanon, M.: Simplified nursing—the essentials of practical nursing, ed. 7, Philadelphia, 1960, J. B. Lippincott Co.
18. Yarling, R. R.: Ethical analysis of a nursing problem—the scope of nursing practice in disclosing the truth to terminal patients, Part II, Sup. Nurse **9**:29, 1978.
19. Yura, H., and Walsh, M. B.: The nursing process, ed. 3, New York, 1978, Appleton-Century-Crofts.

2

The nature and scope of the cancer problem

LISA BEGG MARINO

Now that a model for nursing in cancer has been presented, discussion will focus on those areas specific to cancer that influence nursing's role in the care of these clients. Major areas are the theoretical basis for defining what cancer is, incidence and survival patterns, and the economics of cancer.

DEFINING CANCER

Definition of cancer

The definitions of the diseases commonly referred to as "cancer" are numerous. Each definition, from the very simple to the complex, varies somewhat from the other definitions largely because the exact biologic mechanisms of cancer are not known and many controversial areas still exist. It is for this reason that the issues relating to carcinogenesis will be discussed in detail in Chapter 9; this section will concentrate on *defining* cancer.

Even the *terms* used to describe the cancerous state vary; the terms frequently used are *tumor, malignancies, neoplasms, oncology,* and *growth* in addition to *cancer*. Some of these terms are more accurate or descriptive than others. For example, the term "neoplasm" really means "new growth"; this new growth can be characterized as benign or malignant in nature. To be completely accurate, the term "malignant neoplasm" would need to be used to be synonymous with cancer. Likewise, the term "oncology" means the study of tumors, which makes it synonymous with neoplasm.

Thus the most accurate terms are malignancy and cancer. *Malignancy* is a Latin term meaning "engendering harm" because malignant cells have the propensity for invasion and distant spread. *Cancer,* another Latin term, means crab or ulcer. However, for purposes of discussion, a more comprehensive and updated definition will be employed: cancer is a *group of diseases* in which the mechanism within the cell and in its microenvironment responsible for restraint of growth is *defective*.[9] This definition implies only that the constraints under which normal cells replicate is damaged, and therefore the cancer cells reproduce without regard for *need*.

Differentiating normal and malignant cells

Beyond the characteristic of *constraint of growth,* it is difficult to characterize cancer cells from normal cells or from neoplastic cells because these are all *relative* states. For example, definitions state that cancer is "rapid growth" when in fact there are a number of *normal* cells that have higher mitotic indices than many cancer cells. Mitotic indices mean the proportion of cells in active mitoses. Normal cells such as those found in the bone marrow and intestinal epithelium effectively replace themselves every few days by continual renewal. This rate is faster than many cancer cell populations. Therefore, although these bone marrow and intestinal epithelial cells are perfectly normal, they have high rates of mitoses. In contrast, other normal cells such as the neurons or cells in striated muscle tissue are stable throughout the individual's life, except during the embryonic or early postnatal periods. These normal cell populations do not need to replace their numbers and, unless altered by some action, will not replicate. The chief difference, then, is that the normal cells achieve a *balance* between cell production and cell loss. In the normal cells, *the restraint of growth* remains intact so that replication occurs *only* if the cells are stressed or injured, both of which are perfectly normal features.

Degree of differentiation. Degree of differentiation is a relative state in that cancer cells can run the gamut of well to poorly differentiated in character as can similarly "normal" cells and benign neoplasms. In fact, some cancer cells are so well differentiated that only a *minor* imbalance between cell production and cell loss is evident so that the growth rate is slow. In contrast, other cancer cells are so poorly differentiated that identifying their tissue of origin is impossible. These types of tumor cells are referred to as "anaplastic," which means they have highly irregular structural features that serve no useful purpose; they also tend to be large and bulky with a necrotic center. This type of disorganization occurs because the tumor is so inefficient that nutrients cannot reach many of the cells, thus death occurs to the innermost cells.

Rate of tumor growth. Although degree of differentiation has lost some importance in the definition of cancer, it serves as an important indicator as to the rate of tumor growth. Rate is important because it can give the clinician an indicator of how sensitive a particular type of cancer will be to treatment. This is crucial information, since one type of cancer may be treated quite differently than another type because of the *degree of sensitivity or refractiveness* that is exhibited. For example, a form of cancer that is very sensitive to chemotherapy is acute leukemia. Acute leukemia cells are rapidly dividing and therefore have a high rate of growth. Conversely, most forms of malignant brain tumors such as the gliomas have much slower cell turnovers or rates of growth. These cells are much more likely to be refractive to therapy. Additionally, these brain tumors are protected by the blood-brain barrier so that chemotherapy drugs have difficulty penetrating the brain cavity. This is just another example of how important it is to know exactly which tumor type is present and what rate of growth is being exhibited prior to deciding on what form of cancer treatment to administer.

Likewise, the rate of cell growth *in general* is important in cancer treatment because of the toxicities that are common to many of the treatment modalities. Toxicity is defined as any untoward effect exhibited on the host. Because any form of cancer treatment must weigh the potential risks versus the potential benefits, toxicity must be carefully balanced with therapeutic effect. A good example is the myelosuppression, diarrhea, nausea, or alopecia commonly seen with many chemotherapeutic agents. All these consequences are considered toxicities directly resulting from some type of cancer chemotherapy. These toxicities result because the cells that comprise the *normal* bone marrow, gastrointestinal mucosa, and hair follicles all have high rates of growth and are thus adversely affected by the chemotherapeutic agents. These agents not only affect *cancer* cells; they also affect normal cells that have higher rates of growth. This important balance of tolerable toxicity of normal cell populations is generally required in order to obtain sufficient antitumor effect.

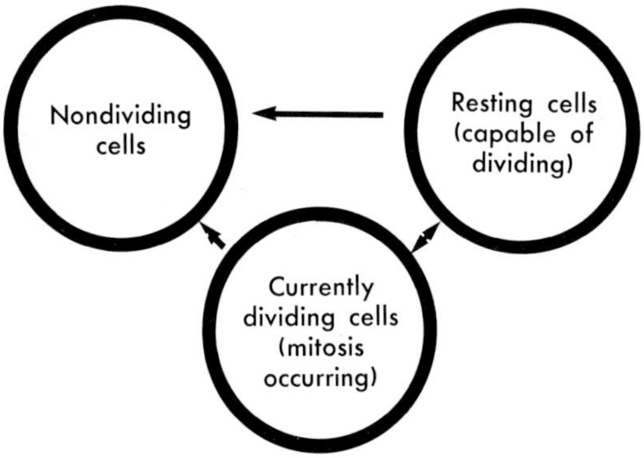

Fig. 2-1. Cancer cell subpopulation.

Heterogeneity of cell populations. In addition to the variations in growth rates that exist between and among normal and malignant cell populations, the rate of growth *within* a discrete population of cells often varies. This can be best exemplified within a primary tumor site where *some* cells have a higher rate of growth than the majority of the other cells in the same tumor. Cell populations are rarely homogeneous. This fact partially explains how different cells can exist in a tumor; it is often seen with some sarcomas. Additionally, growth can be enhanced or retarded by *extracellular* factors such as hormonal or immunologic mechanisms. These limits on growth are often incomplete or inefficient but many times succeed in limiting the tumor's size.

These constraints on growth may limit the tumor somewhat but are often ineffective in the long term because of cancer's inherent property to metastasize. If left unchecked, these metastases will cause death of the client. Fortunately, many of the recent advances in cancer treatment have been suc-

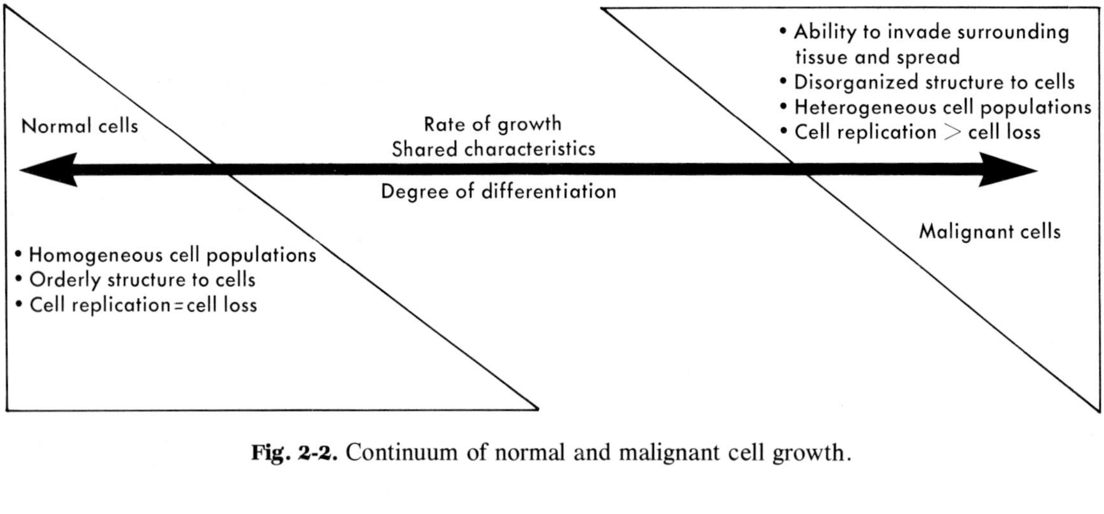

Fig. 2-2. Continuum of normal and malignant cell growth.

cessful even after metastases occur so the client's cancer can be controlled to a great extent.

These various advances have complicated the study of malignant growth to such a degree that scientists now believe the only accurate time to observe cell changes is *early* in the tumor formation period.

Cell subpopulation. Most cancer cell populations have varied proliferation activity. Fig. 2-1 illustrates this concept. The tumor is composed of cells in three different proliferative states: actively dividing cells, resting cells that are capable of dividing but are not, and nondividing cells that will eventually die. The percentage in each of these categories will determine the size of the tumor as a whole as well as its responsiveness to the various forms of cancer treatment. Fig. 2-2 illustrates the continuum on which many characteristics are *shared* by both normal and malignant cells along with *either* normal or malignant cells.

Because of the subtleties associated with defining malignant growth as opposed to normal or benign growth, histologic examination of the cells is mandatory. The principle reasons for this strong statement are twofold. First, cancer is a serious and life-threatening illness for which equally serious treatments are employed. Realistically and ethically, these treatments should only be rendered on clients who have *confirmed* diagnoses of cancer. Second, the *first* attempt to eradicate or control the cancer is also the *best* opportunity to do so. Sec-

Table 2-1. Frequency distribution of histologic types in some major sites of cancer: United States, 1969-1971 (Third National Cancer Survey, microscopically proven cases only)*

Site	Histologic type	% within site
Lung, bronchus, and trachea (20,255 cases)	Epidermoid carcinoma	34.7
	Adenocarcinoma	16.5
	Oat cell carcinoma	13.4
	Bronchiolar carcinoma	3.2
	Other and unspecified carcinomas	29.9
	Sarcomas and lymphomas	0.4
	Other and unspecified cancer	1.8
Breast (23,630 cases)	Duct carcinoma and Paget's disease	51.0
	Adenocarcinomas	38.6
	Medullary carcinoma	3.5
	Lobular carcinoma	2.8
	Colloid carcinoma	2.2
	Other specific carcinomas	1.3
	Stromal sarcomas and lymphomas	0.4
	Other and unspecified cancer	0.2

*From Levin, D. L., Devesa, S. S., Godwin, J. D., and Silverman, D. T.: Cancer rates and risks, ed. 2, Bethesda, Md., 1974, U.S. Department of Health, Education and Welfare.

Continued.

Table 2-1. Frequency distribution of histologic types in some major sites of cancer: United States, 1969-1971 (Third National Cancer Survey, microscopically proven cases only)—cont'd

Site	Histologic type	% within site
Colon and rectum (24,430 cases)	Adenocarcinomas	87.0
	Colloid carcinomas	7.8
	Papillary carcinoma	2.2
	Squamous cell carcinomas	1.6
	Other specific carcinomas	0.1
	Malignant carcinoids	0.5
	Sarcomas and lymphomas	0.4
	Other and unspecified cancer	0.4
Stomach (5,085 cases)	Adenocarcinomas	70.9
	Mucinous carcinomas	6.6
	Signet ring carcinomas	1.3
	Other and unspecified carcinomas	12.8
	Leiomyosarcoma	1.9
	Lymphosarcoma	1.9
	Reticulum cell sarcoma	2.5
	Other and unspecified lymphomas	1.0
	Other and unspecified cancer	0.9
Prostate (13,306 cases)	Adenocarcinomas	98.6
	Medullary carcinoma	0.3
	Transitional and/or squamous cell	0.3
	Clear cell carcinoma	0.2
	Other specific carcinomas	0.4
	Sarcomas and lymphomas	0.1
	Other and unspecified cancer	0.2
Uterine cervix (5,169 cases)	Epidermoid carcinoma	84.1
	Adenocarcinoma	6.1
	Other and unspecified carcinomas	9.1
	Sarcomas	0.7
Uterine corpus (6,593 cases)	Adenocarcinomas	79.5
	Papillary adenocarcinoma	6.4
	Adenocanthomas	7.6
	Other and unspecified carcinomas	2.9
	Mixed müllerian tumors	1.5
	Leiomyosarcoma	0.9
	Stromal sarcoma	0.7
	Other sarcomas	0.5
	Unspecified cancer	0.2

ondary treatments for cancer after the initial efforts have failed or been poorly chosen are just not as effective. To best serve the client and family, very careful evaluation of the particular type of cancer present as well as its full extent needs to be determined accurately *before* treatment is begun.

Classifying cancer. Histologically, there are two broad categories of cancers—carcinomas and sarcomas. Carcinomas, the most common histologic category, originate from epithelial tissue that makes up the body's internal and external surfaces. For example, adenocarcinoma arises from the glandular structure as found in the prostate, breast, and bowel. Squamous carcinoma arises from the skin and other nonglandular surfaces such as in the lung.

Sarcomas are much less common but more troublesome because of their refractiveness to treatment and their propensity for hematogenous spread. These cancers are mesodermal in origin and are seen in such connective tissues as striated muscle, cartilage, and bone.

Table 2-1 provides evidence of the frequency of the histologic types of cancer in major sites as well as their frequency *within* each cancer site.

CANCER INCIDENCE

In 1979, 765,000 people were expected to be diagnosed with some form of cancer. Nineteen sites accounted for 95% of these new cases. The sites range from the most common cancers such as the lung cancers, colorectal cancers, and breast cancers with 112,000, 112,000, and 107,000 new cases, respectively, to the less common sites such as thyroid cancer with 9,000 new cases.[1] This wide range reinforces the random nature of cancer in that not all persons found to be at "high risk" for the development of cancer actually succumb to cancer. Likewise, some of those persons who are considered "low risk" for cancer do, in fact, develop cancer.

The statistics that follow have been taken from a number of sources and include both mortality or cause-of-death statistics as well as incidence statistics.

Mortality or cause-of-death statistics

Mortality or cause-of-death statistics relate to the principal or underlying cause of death in the client. These are useful statistics because many countries file such information on each citizen within their country. Unfortunately, many countries file only the principal cause of death and so further analysis is limited except where further validation of the death certificate is made. Likewise, it is generally conceded that mortality statistics *underestimate* the occurrence of the particular disease being studied. Specific to cancer, this distortion can be readily seen in those cancers that have a *high* incidence but *low* mortality, as in the nonmelanomous skin cancers. To minimize this distortion, most analyses will list both incidence and mortality statistics to give a more complete accounting.

Incidence statistics

Incidence statistics report the number of *new* cases of a disease that occur in a well-defined population, such as those residing within a region or country. Incidence statistics concentrate on two areas, demographic and medical. The former category consists of such information as the sex of the person, age, marital status, and usual residence. The medical category includes information such as the onset of illness, location of the tumor, clinical stage, and histology of the tumor. This information is more helpful and detailed than the death certificate previously mentioned and has been useful in documenting changing incidence and survival patterns when coupled with mortality statistics. Examples of programs that detail incidence statistics are the registries in the states of Connecticut and Iowa, along with such ad hoc projects as the Third National Cancer Survey conducted from 1969 to 1971.

Relative to the incidence of cancer, the truly unfortunate fact is that 80% to 90% of *all* cancers are preventable. This figure is computed by ascertaining the highest incidence as well as the lowest incidence of a particular form of cancer. For example, colon cancer is a leading cancer site in virtually every industrialized country in the world but is only occasionally seen in the African countries. This variance gives strong support to the assumption that colon cancer is preventable if the environmental factor or factors could be identified. Extreme variance from one country to another is seen for many forms of cancer and provides valuable information as to the possible causative relationships that exist within the environment.

Table 2-2. Leading cancer sites*

Site	Estimated incidence for 1979
Lung	112,000
Colon-rectum	112,000
Breast	107,000
Prostate	64,000
Uterus†	53,000
Lymphomas‡	38,500
Bladder	35,000
Head and neck§	24,400
Stomach	23,000
Pancreas	23,000
Leukemias	21,500
Bone and connective tissue	20,000
Ovary	17,000
Kidney	16,200
Skin‖	13,600
Liver and biliary passages	11,600
Brain and CNS	11,600
Larynx	10,400
Thyroid	9,000

*From 1978 National Cancer Institute Fact Book, National Cancer Program, Publication No. 79-512, Bethesda, Md., 1978, U.S. Department of Health, Education and Welfare.

†Includes invasive cervical cancer and endometrial cancer.

‡Includes Hodgkin's disease, non-Hodgkin's lymphomas, and multiple myeloma.

§Includes lip, tongue, mouth, pharynx, and salivary gland.

‖Melanoma only; nonmelanomous skin cancers exceed 300,000 new cases each year.

Types of cancers

As Table 2-2 demonstrates, the variety of cancers that develop in humans is quite limitless. Cancer can develop in such diverse organs as the liver and ovaries or in the entire systems such as the lymphatic system. Likewise, the distribution of cancer can vary with different races as exemplified in Table 2-3. In this table, it can be shown that the incidence of cancer of the female breast accounted for a higher proportion of cancer among whites than among blacks. In contrast, cancers of the lung and bronchus represented a higher proportion of cases in blacks. However, both were major sites in both races, accounting for fully one fourth of *all* cancers in both races. Aside from the proportion of cases, there are differences in the types of cancers seen as well as markedly different proportions. For example, cancers of the esophagus and pancreas appeared more often in blacks than whites; cancers of the urinary bladder and brain appeared more often in whites than blacks. Cancer of the cervix, while common in both groups, was much more common in blacks than whites.

Characteristics of population affected

Just as the histologic variations are extensive, the population groups affected with cancer vary greatly.

Age. Cancer incidence relative to age shows an increasing rate as age increases.

Table 2-3. Distribution for the 10 leading cancer sites in the survival series by race (1960-1973)*

	White		Black	
Rank	**Site**	**%**	**Site**	**%**
1	Female breast	12.9	Lung and bronchus	13.5
2	Lung and bronchus	12.2	Female breast	11.2
3	Colon	9.0	Prostate	9.0
4	Prostate	6.6	Cervix	9.0
5	Rectum	4.8	Colon	6.3
6	Bladder	4.8	Stomach	5.1
7	Corpus	3.8	Rectum	3.4
8	Stomach	3.6	Esophagus	3.3
9	Cervix	3.6	Pancreas	3.2
10	Brain	2.6	Corpus	3.1

*From Cancer patient survival, Report No. 5, Publication No. 77-992, Bethesda, Md., 1976, U.S. Department of Health, Education and Welfare.

The one exception is during childhood, when cancer leads all other diseases in incidence. The predominant site during these early years is in the bone marrow areas, which are identified as the leukemias. With most other cancers, however, the incidence will correspond with the percentage of older people within the population. In the case of the United States, the incidence of cancer continues to slowly rise because improved life expectancy is increasing the percentage of older people in the general population. For example, the 1978 estimate for new cases of breast cancer was 91,000; the 1979 estimate for this same group of cancers was 108,000.[1] These figures may appear to indicate an increase in breast cancer incidence, but in fact this is not the case. The difference is attributable to the population increase (1970 census versus 1978 census figures) and the increased percentage of women over the age of 50 in whom 60% of all cases of breast cancer occur. This variance in total incidence could have been misinterpreted if the basis from which the statistics were taken was not ascertained.

Age is also significant with regard to the *type* of cancer that develops. Generally speaking, most forms of cancer become more common as age of the client increases. However, there are some major exceptions. These exceptions can be classified into two main age groups: cancers that are prevalent early in life over a restricted age range and cancers that occur somewhat later in life but peak quickly and maintain that level during adult life. Cancers that show a steady increase in risk from early adulthood through old age are the most common pattern seen today.

Examples of cancers that occur early in life are the nephroblastomas or Wilm's tumors, which have their peak incidence at 2 years of age; acute childhood leukemia, which has a peak incidence at 4 to 5 years of age; and the remaining childhood cancers, 50% of which occur prior to age 7. While the cause(s) is not totally known, many cancer researchers believe that exposure to a powerful carcinogen, perhaps even in fetal life, causes the later development of cancer.[4]

The second pattern in which the cancers

peak during early adult life and continue at that rate can be best exemplified by cancer of the cervix uteri. It has been suggested that the carcinogen surfaces in the client's youth and then disappears or loses its potency.[4]

The last category of increasing risk can be seen in the patterns of stomach cancer for certain European countries. The increasing risk for this cancer is thought to occur because of a continuous exposure to some carcinogen.

Sex. Considering all forms of cancer and all age groups, the incidence of cancer is greater in men than in women. Comparison of incidence and mortality rates for a 25-year period, 1949 to 1974 and 1951 to 1976, indicates that both figures are increasing in men, while both figures are decreasing in women. The *overall* incidence, however, has increased slightly in this same period.[2]

The reasons for these changes center on the increased incidence of lung cancer in men followed by smaller increases for cancers of the colon, prostate, pancreas, and bladder.

When age is related to sex, cancer in women between the ages of 20 to 40 is three times as common as cancer found in men of these ages. However, cancer appears more commonly in men between the ages of 50 and 80. Breast cancer is the principal reason for the preponderance of cases in women, and cancers of the lung, prostate, and bladder account for the cases in older men.[3]

In contrast to men, the overall incidence in women has decreased largely because of decreases in cancers of the bladder, stomach, and cervix, along with no change in colorectal cancer incidence. This pattern may change if the incidence of lung cancer in women continues to increase.

Likewise, the mortality figures coincide with the pattern of incidence. More men die from some form of cancer than do women. In a recent comparison of two different 25-year periods, 1949 to 1974 and 1951 to 1976, the age-adjusted cancer mortality rate per 100,000 population showed that for *all* cancer sites the male rate went from 130 to 161.5. This represents a 24% increase. For women, the figures went from 117.8 down to 108, an 8.5% decrease. The large increase for men was attributed to deaths associated with lung cancer.[1]

Place of residence. Even after adjustments for self-selection and errors in adjusting for a client's place of residence, there remains higher mortality rates for many causes of death including cancer. This excess risk may be related to life-style, in that urban dwellers use more tobacco and alcohol; to occupation, because urban dwellers work more with industrial pollutants; and to the environment of the cities themselves.[3]

COMPARISON WITH OTHER DISEASES

Cancer remains second in overall mortality to cardiovascular diseases. Based on 1976 statistics, cardiovascular diseases took 723,729 lives, while cancer took 377,312 lives. These figures represent 38% and 20%, respectively, of all deaths in the United States.[7]

SURVIVAL FOLLOWING DIAGNOSIS OF CANCER

The major source of statistics on the changing rates of survival for clients with cancer is the End Results program of the National Cancer Institute, National Institutes of Health. This federally funded program was established in the 1950's to provide detailed information on the major trends or changes in cancer mortality. The program is now known as the Cancer Surveillance, Epidemiology, and End Results Program (SEER).

The latest report available was published in 1976 and indicates that while cancer had a

20% overall survival rate in 1930, it increased to 33% in 1955 and 41% in 1976. Survival is defined as being alive without any evidence of disease 5 years after diagnosis.[2] Tables 2-4 and 2-5 show the gains registered during the 23-year period of 1950 to 1973.

Trends in survival data

Both tables present the data in terms of *relative survival rate,* which is defined as mortality that has been adjusted for differences in age and sex, so that comparison can be made and "normal" mortality can thus be adjusted.[3] Table 2-4 represents data on all cancer patients, while Table 2-5 represents the *leading* cancer sites, accounting for 63% and 65% of all cancers among whites and blacks, respectively. Review of the figures in the latter table indicates that with the exception of cervical cancer in white women, improvements have been demonstrated. Sites showing the greatest improvements are cancers of the breast, prostate, bladder, and rectum in blacks and cancers of the bladder and prostate in whites. The differences in the survival of whites and blacks has been attributed to socioeconomic levels as opposed to genetic or other factors.

These improvements appear to be firm and not just artifact from earlier detection efforts, since the *percentage* of cancers diagnosed at localized stages or those cancers limited to the site of origin remained fairly constant. Thus, improvements in the relative survival rate would appear to be a direct result of improved management of these clients. For example, cancer of the prostate in white males rose from 47% in the 1950's to 53% in the 1960's to 59% in the 1970's. These increases occurred even though the percent of localized cancer changed from 52% to 62% and remained at that level for the last 6-year period. This improved management is due largely to earlier gains in surgical and radiotherapeutic techniques and the more recent successes within the drug development program.

Survival relative to tumor site. In addition to advances in cancer management and the extent of the cancer at the time of diagnosis, the site of the tumor is extremely important to survival. Review of Table 2-5 demonstrates ranges of survival in whites during the 1967 to 1973 period of 79% for uterine cancer down to 14% for cancer of the pancreas.

Survival relative to sex of client. When sex of the client is considered, females generally have a markedly higher survival rate than do males. This difference in survival can be attributed to the differences in the primary cancer site distribution between females and males. For example, the four leading cancer sites in white males are lung, prostate, colon, and bladder. Their 5-year relative survival rates are 8%, 51%, 43%, and 56%, respectively. In contrast, the four leading sites for white females are breast, colon, uterine, cervix, and uterine corpus

Table 2-4. Relative survival rates (%) for all cancer patients combined (1950-1973)*

Relative survival rate (years)	Year of diagnosis		
	1950-1959	1960-1966	1967-1973
Whites			
1	60	61	64
3	44	45	47
5	39	40	41†
Blacks			
1	51	50	54
3	34	33	37
5	29	28	32†

*From Cancer patient survival, Report No. 5, Publication No. 77-992, Bethesda, Md., 1976, U.S. Department of Health, Education and Welfare.

†Complete 5-year follow-up is not available for cases diagnosed in 1970 or later.

Table 2-5. Trends in 5-year relative survival rates for the leading cancer sites by race (1950-1973)*

Cancer site	Race	Localized cancers (%)			All cancers (%)		
		1950-1959	1960-1966	1967-1973	1950-1959	1960-1966	1967-1973
Corpus	White	71	79	79	3.8	3.6	4.0
	Black	51	52	51	3.5	3.3	2.9
Breast	White	43	48	48	13.0	12.7	13.0
	Black	30	31	32	11.6	11.1	11.4
Cervix	White	53	52	44	5.4	4.0	3.1
	Black	32	41	39	15.7	10.5	7.7
Bladder	White	69	79	77	4.9	5.1	4.6
	Black	44	51	53	3.5	3.0	2.6
Prostate	White	52	62	62	6.8	6.8	6.5
	Black	43	52	54	9.4	9.2	8.8
Colon	White	39	42	41	9.5	9.3	8.8
	Black	27	32	31	5.7	6.2	6.4
Rectum	White	44	47	47	6.2	5.0	4.5
	Black	30	33	34	4.3	3.6	3.3
Stomach	White	17	20	18	5.7	4.2	3.1
	Black	9	12	17	8.5	6.0	4.3
Lung	White	17	19	17	8.4	11.0	13.3
	Black	12	17	16	8.3	11.9	15.0
Pancreas	White	14	16	14	2.5	2.5	2.5
	Black	13	10	10	3.6	3.4	3.0

*From Cancer patient survival, Report No. 5, Publication No. 77-992, Bethesda, Md., 1976, U.S. Department of Health, Education and Welfare.

with survival rates of 62%, 48%, 60%, and 72%, respectively. Even when males and females are compared for individual cancer sites, females do consistently better than males.[3]

Survival relative to age of client. Cancer is generally considered a disease of old age and the statistics generally support this. Fully 75% of all cancers in men and 63% of all cancers in women in the United States are diagnosed at age 55 or over. Generally, the outlook for survival decreases with age, particularly if the general state of the client's health is not good. On the average, the life expectancy of persons with cancer is reduced approximately 16 years as a direct result of their disease. This average reduction is less for older clients and greater for young clients.[3]

Applying these factors to the 1977 data indicates that two thirds of the total new cases of 700,000 had local or regional stages of cancer that were amenable to surgery and radiotherapy. Unfortunately, the remaining 200,000 cases had widespread or metastatic cancers for which more limited treatment options were available. About one half of this latter group, 92,000, can benefit from existing chemotherapy with 60,000 of them enjoying significant prolongation of life.[2]

For the initial group of 500,000 clients with local or regional cancers, more than one half of them will be successfully treated by surgery or radiotherapy. However, the remaining group of approximately 220,000 clients will develop recurrence of their cancer because of apparent microscopic foci. This biologic discovery had led to therapy initiated early in the course of the cancer, called adjuvant therapy. This innovation in cancer treatment is significant and will be closely followed in terms of continued improvements in survival.

COSTS OF CANCER

Calculating the costs associated with cancer is a complex endeavor because of the different categories of costs, the varied and often chronic course of cancer, the degree of sophistication applied to diagnosing and treating cancer, and the incalculable costs associated with the suffering and inconveniences of the client and family. However, difficult as the task may be, a discussion will follow so that the nurse-teacher will more completely understand these aspects and be better equipped to assist the client and family to minimize the expenses and maximize the utilization of resources.

Major categories of costs associated with cancer

Schottenfeld[8] is one of the few authors to examine the specific costs associated with cancer. He has offered three major categories of costs: the direct costs, the indirect costs, and the economic costs.

Direct costs. Direct costs of cancer are those expenditures for hospital and nursing home care, medical and nursing services, drugs, medical research and training of health personnel, construction of facilities for these clients, the net costs of insurance, and miscellaneous expenditures such as for public education.[8,10]

Indirect costs. Indirect costs are defined as losses incurred in output owing to time lost from work because of cancer morbidity, disability, and mortality.[8,10]

Economic costs. Economic costs are calculated as the losses borne by the individual with cancer, the larger community, and society, and for which quantification in monetary terms can be made. Unfortunately, not all costs can be calculated because data are not available for such noneconomic costs as the pain, suffering, and inconveniences related to cancer.[8]

Calculation of direct costs associated with cancer

Hospital care. Most hospitals that admit and care for cancer clients are community-level facilities. These hospitals accounted for 82% of *all* hospitals in the United States and 92% of all admissions in 1970. Of these admissions, 1.2 million cancer clients required almost 8.8 million days of care at an average stay of 15.2 days per client. The cost of this hospital care alone was $1.6 billion. In 1976, the figure increased to $3.5 billion.[10] These figures closely parallel a study conducted by the National Cancer Institute in which 3,151 cancer clients were followed for a 2-year period. The data indicated that for these clients, 61% of them required only one hospital admission during this period, with the average number of admissions being 1.7 per client. The typical in-hospital stay lasted an average of 16 days and cost $1,400. Assuming there are 1.3 million cancer clients under hospital care each year in the United States, $1.8 billion would be expended solely for this service.[6]

The cancer sites that comprised the group ranged from cancer of the bronchus and lung, with 10.3% of the cases averaging 16.4 days, to cancer of the cervix, with 7.7% of the total sample remaining in the hospital an average of 8.8 days. Interestingly, the average length of hospital stay did not vary appreciably from one cancer site to the other nor with the age of the client. However, 78% of *all* admissions in this study were for persons 50 years of age and over.[8] In another study, Cancer Care, Inc., an agency specializing in providing support and counseling to advanced cancer clients and their families, studied 115 such client families during 1971 and 1972 to determine costs. The responses ranged from hospital bills of $800 to more than $50,000, with the median cost being $19,054. Seventy-five percent of these families paid more than $5,000 and one half of the families' hospital bills exceeded $10,000.[10]

Physician services. The figures for physician services are based on the estimates from the National Disease and Therapeutic Index of the number of visits for cancer treatment to physicians in private practice in 1970. This index indicated that cancer clients accounted for 2% of all visits to physicians, amounting to 29.6 million visits in 1970, an increase of 45% over the previous study done in 1962. The estimated expenditures for medical services totaled $551.9 million, an increase of 220% over expenditures in 1962. These increased costs were largely due to the 45% increase in client visits and fee increases, which ranged from 263% for specialists' office visits to 68.4% for specialists' hospital visits.[8]

Cancer research and cancer control. For the fiscal year 1978, the total national resources for cancer research and cancer control totaled $1,401,369,000. Fig. 2-3 illustrates the breakdown of these funds, with the National Cancer Institute contributing 62.3% of the funds and non-NCI sources contributing 37.7% of the funds. The latter source of funds ranges from industrial contributions of nearly $200 million a year to private institutions contributing $32 million a year. The cumulative appropriations to the National Cancer Institute from its inception in 1937 until 1978 totaled $7 billion.[7]

Training. In fiscal year 1978, the National Cancer Institute, the largest contributor to the training of health personnel, spent more than $34 million to advance this goal.[7]

Construction. Construction costs totaled over $212 million in 1970.[8]

Expenses for prepayment and administration. The subcategory of expenses for prepayment and administration is also called the net cost of insurance and represents the difference between earned premiums or subscription income and benefit expenditures or claims expenses of health insurance organizations. This amount consists of operating expenses, additions to reserves, and profits. Expenses for administration refer to the federally financed health programs such as Medicare, Medicaid, and the Veterans Administration. For these programs, the 1970 total national expenses for prepayment and administration were $2.97 billion, $1.44 billion being expenses for prepayment on the net cost of private health insurance.[8]

Expenses attributable to cancer are calculated by assuming the same proportion of total expenses for prepayment and administration as the ratio of expenditures on short-term hospital care and physician services for cancer clients to total expenditures for the health services. In 1970, the net total revenue in community hospitals was $19.93 billion and the national expenditures for physician services were $13.6 billion. Thus, the 1970 expenses for prepayment and administration associated with cancer are estimated to be $134.9 million.[8] Data from 1975 indicate that more than 165 million people under the age of 65 were covered by private health insurance. Twelve and a half million of this group *also* received Medicare

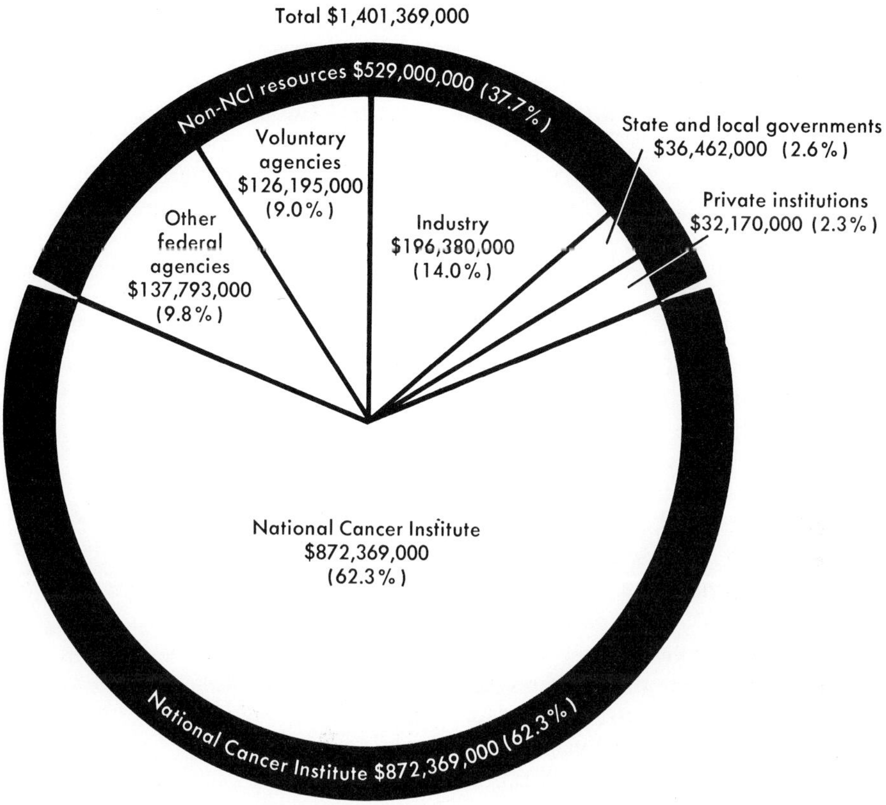

Fig. 2-3. Total national resources for cancer research and cancer control—fiscal year, 1978. (From 1978 National Cancer Institute Fact Book, National Cancer Program, Publication No. 79-512, Bethesda, Md., 1978, U.S. Department of Health, Education and Welfare.)

coverage. The *type* of coverage is also important because of the catastrophic nature of cancer. Approximately 143 million persons were covered by extended catastrophic insurance coverage. Unfortunately, most extended policies are limited to $10,000 maximum, so if treatment was extended over time and sophisticated diagnostic tests were run, the maximum could easily be exceeded, with the family forced to pay the remainder.[10]

Other health and medical services. This subcategory consists of such things as public information and education, which amounted to $28.8 million in 1970.[8]

Drugs, nursing services, and nursing home care. Drugs used for treating cancer clients amounted to $52 million in 1970. Nursing services, which are defined as private duty and professional nursing in the hospital and home, visiting nurses associations, and homemaker services, amounted to $42.4 million. Additionally, home care for cancer clients totaled $108.7 million in 1970.[8]

These subcategories of direct costs total $3.38 billion, with the largest percentage coming from hospital care at 56.6%, physician services at 16.3%, and research at 8%.

Calculation of indirect costs associated with cancer

Indirect costs are defined as losses sustained as a result of cancer in the areas of work and home because of disability, morbidity, or mortality.

Cancer morbidity. For men, the person-years lost and the costs of male deaths steadily increase with the age of the client. For women, the total person-years lost and the costs of female deaths were found to be stable for the ages 15 to 34 and increased for the ages 35 and over.[8]

Cancer mortality. To calculate the cancer mortality subcategory of indirect costs, person-years lost were estimated by including labor force participation, employment, housekeeping rates, and average annual earnings after adjustment for wage supplements. The age distribution employed in the analysis consisted of 5-year intervals from ages 15 to 64 and then 65 or over. Given that there were 330,840 deaths caused by cancer in 1970, the cost of these deaths came to $708.4 million, $432 million of which represents loss of male earning power.

A second approach that can be employed to measure the impact of cancer mortality if a reduction in loss of life was possible is to examine the gain in work-years. Assuming that a person's working life is between 20 and 65 years of age, approximately 1.8 million work-years would be gained each year. The number of work-years would vary with the various cancers.[3]

Additionally, the total economic cost of cancer including direct expenditure, indirect cost of morbidity, and the value of lifetime earnings is estimated at $18.9 billion each year.[3]

SUMMARY

The diseases that are commonly referred to as cancer are complex and varied in their origin, widespread in their occurrence, and expensive in terms of human suffering and loss. As the major group of health professionals who care for these clients and their families, nurses can do much to help clarify the numerous misconceptions about cancer causes, their patterns of incidence, and ways to minimize the losses associated with these types of illnesses.

REFERENCES

1. American Cancer Society: 1979 cancer facts and figures, New York, 1978, American Cancer Society, Inc.
2. Cancer patient survival, Report No. 5, Publication No. 77-992, Bethesda, Md., 1976, U.S. Department of Health, Education and Welfare.
3. Levin, D. L., Devesa, S. S., Godwin, J. D., and Silverman, D. T.: Cancer rates and risks, ed. 2, Bethesda, Md., 1974, U.S. Department of Health, Education and Welfare.
4. Muir, C. S., and Peron, Y.: Special demographic situations, Semin. Oncology, **III**(1):35, 1976.
5. National Cancer Institute Third National Cancer Survey, NCI Monograph No. 41, Washington, D.C., 1975, U.S. Government Printing Office.
6. National Cancer Institute Third National Cancer Survey, Publication No. 76-1094, Bethesda, Md., 1976, U.S. Department of Health, Education and Welfare.
7. 1978 National Cancer Institute Fact Book, National Cancer Program, Publication No. 79-512, Bethesda, Md., 1978, U.S. Department of Health, Education and Welfare.
8. Schottenfeld, D.: Cancer epidemology and prevention: current concepts, Springfield, Ill., 1975, Charles C Thomas, Publisher.
9. Sproul, E.: Pathogenesis of cancer. In Holland, J. F., and Frei, E., editors: Cancer medicine, Philadelphia, 1973, Lea & Febiger.
10. Breast cancer digest, a guide to medical care, emotional support, educational programs and resources, Publication No. 79-1691, Bethesda, Md., 1979, U.S. Department of Health, Education and Welfare.

3

The organizational structure of cancer health care

LISA BEGG MARINO

Given that an overview of the scope of the cancer problem has been presented, along with discussion of a conceptual framework for cancer nursing, attention will now focus on those agencies and organizations that impact on the delivery of cancer services. These agencies include such large federal efforts as the National Cancer Program administered by the National Cancer Institute as well as large voluntary agencies such as the American Cancer Society. Along with these rather obvious choices go such agencies as the Food and Drug Administration, the Office for Protection from Research Risks, and the professional societies representing the major health disciplines. Not to be negated is the impact the United States Congress has on both the funding and the overseeing of much of cancer health care.

Reasons for including this type of a chapter in a clinical nursing book are twofold. First, to perform at a professional level, nurses need this information so that they can be a resource to clients and families. Second, most of these agencies have little nursing input, which removes a key health professional's input to promote an improved level of care. This lack of involvement may have been justified in past years because few nurses were involved in cancer care and research on any substantive level. However, the current situation is far different. For example, there are a large number of nurses participating as full partners on cancer care teams as well as a growing number of nurses contributing to sophisticated nursing research. It is for these reasons that nurses have both the talent and the obligation to become more involved in the policymaking that affects cancer health care.

UNITED STATES GOVERNMENT AGENCIES AND BRANCHES

The following discussion highlights the major units within the United States government that conduct research, regulate, or perform both functions in relationship to the cancer problem. The units, representing entire institutions or agencies, are numerous and complex in their organization and functioning. However, the nurse working with persons at potential or actual risk for cancer, in addition to those persons undergoing cancer treatment, needs to have this knowledge to provide information and potential resources to clients and families. Additionally, the nurse can perform a valuable function in increasing the public's understanding of the complexity of the federal programs that impact on cancer.

National Cancer Institute

The National Cancer Institute (NCI) was the first of the National Institutes of Health to be established by Congress in 1937. Its major purpose was to "provide for, foster, and aid in coordinating research relating to cancer."[6] An initial appropriation of $700,000 was made to establish the necessary research programs. The level of funding rose to nearly $1 billion by 1979 with a cumulative amount totaling $7 billion, most of which came after 1971. In fact, the early years of the institute show the intramural research program being quietly established in 1947, a full-scale clinical research program in 1953, along with the extramural Cancer Chemotherapy National Service Center being established in 1955. This last creation was to serve as a highly visible program to the NCI through the participation of the major university research centers cooperating in multi-institutional cancer research clinical trials for clients with advanced cancer. A great deal of information was identified by studying these clients, and many of these discoveries were able to benefit clients in earlier stages of cancer.

Program expansion. The NCI efforts were given a major boost when President Richard M. Nixon signed into law the "National Cancer Act of 1971." With further amendments in 1974, the National Cancer Program (NCP) was established to expand efforts toward eradicating cancer. The NCI director, with the advice of the National Cancer Advisory Board, was mandated to "plan and develop an expanded, intensified and coordinated cancer research program encompassing the programs of the NCI, related programs of the other research institutes and other federal and non-federal programs."[8] This major expansion of efforts was also symbolic in promoting greater cooperation among, and between, the federal and nonfederal programs directed at cancer. From 1971 to 1979 alone, federal appropriations rose from $230,383,000 to $937,129,000. These large increases in funding have not been without their detractors.

Many people from the scientific, public, and political areas have criticized the recent efforts to eradicate cancer as being unsuccessful in curing these diseases. Interestingly, a recent report indicates that a "cure for cancer" would have little impact on the average human life span. In fact, if there were *no* cancer, the life expectancy for 65-year-olds would increase only 1.4 years. Two and one-half years would be added to the average life expectancy for 35-year-olds. This small gain is based on the discovery that removing cancer as a cause of death would only allow more people to die from cardiac conditions or strokes.[10]

The fact that cancer has received the public attention and the congressional and presidential support that it has in spite of the gains that are possible only reinforces how feared a group of diseases it is. The morbidity as well as the mortality are substantial with cancer. The public recognizes this fact, as do the public officials they have elected. It is for this reason that future federal appropriations will probably remain substantial, and emphasis on minimizing cancer will continue.

Despite the common belief that cancer research efforts will continue to receive extraordinary support, intense debate has and will continue to take place. For example, the National Cancer Act was renewed in 1978 but not without a major change in its mandate. The 1978 amendment redefined the NCP and stated that "the NCP shall consist of an expanded, intensified and coordinated cancer research program encompassing the research programs conducted and supported by the Institute and the related research programs of the other research institutes and including an expanded and intensified research program for the prevention of cancer caused by occupational or environmental exposure to carcinogens."[6]

Structure of the NCI. To achieve these goals, the NCP has three major program components: research, control, and support. The first two components have the greatest effect on nursing and will be discussed in detail as they pertain to the scientific and technical activities. The last component includes activities such as construction and manpower development.

Relative to scientific and technical activities, Fig. 3-1 details the organizational arrangement of the major units within the NCI, the agency that administers the NCP. These units set the policy and administer all programs developed to achieve the overall goals. Under the law, the NCI director is charged with coordinating all of the activities of the National Institutes of Health relating to cancer with the NCI.

National Cancer Advisory Board. To develop the policies necessary to carry out its mandate, the law established a National Cancer Advisory Board so that the NCI director could "consult with, obtain advice from, or secure the approval of projects, programs or other activities to be undertaken without delay in order to gain maximum benefit from a new scientific or technical finding."[7] This board is comprised of 23 members: 18 members appointed by the

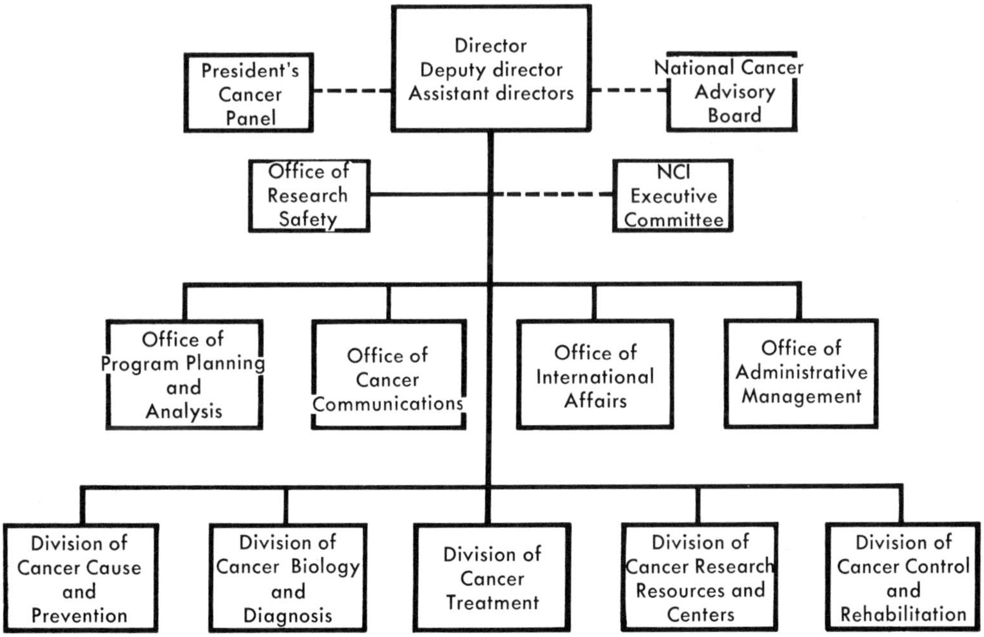

Fig. 3-1. Organizational structure of the National Cancer Institute. (From 1978 National Cancer Institute Fact Book, National Cancer Program, Publication No. 79-512, Bethesda, Md., 1978, U.S. Department of Health, Education and Welfare.)

president and five ex officio members, including the Secretary of Health and Human Services (formerly Health, Education and Welfare) and the Director of the National Institutes of Health. Of the 18 appointed members, not more than 12 can be scientists or physicians and not more than eight can be representatives of the general public. No specific mention was made of nurse representatives, and in fact, the scientific and medical authorities had to have outstanding records in the "study, diagnosis or therapy of cancer or in fields related thereto."[7] By virtue of its mandate, this board plays a major policymaking role for the entire NCP.

President's Cancer Panel. Overseeing the work of the NCI director and the National Cancer Advisory Board is a presidentially-appointed committee called the President's Cancer Panel. Three members, two of whom must be exceptionally distinguished scientists or physicians, compose this committee, which is charged with monitoring the development and execution of the NCP. They report directly to the president with the exception of the ex officio National Cancer Advisory Board members, because both of these committees are composed of nongovernmental authorities. However, the remaining units in Fig. 3-1 are all staffed by governmental workers except for the Boards of Scientific Counselors, which advise each of the divisional units of the NCI. These boards are also staffed by nongovernmental scientists.

From a nursing perspective, the five divisional units along with the Office of Cancer Communications are the most applicable. The five divisions are the Divisions of Cancer Cause and Prevention, Cancer Biology and Diagnosis, Cancer Treatment, Cancer Research Resources and Centers, and Cancer Control and Rehabilitation. Each of these units will be discussed in detail.

Office of Cancer Communications. The Office of Cancer Communications (OCC) reports directly to the NCI director who is responsible for the development and management of program communications activities of the NCI and NCP. Within this overall focus, the OCC responds to public inquiries through its Cancer Information Clearinghouse. The clearinghouse collects and disseminates information on materials, programs, and resources related to public, client, and professional education. Documents collected are abstracted, indexed, and stored. Bibliographic information is made available on request in areas of screening and detection, cause and prevention, diagnosis and treatment, and rehabilitation and behavioral aspects. The clearinghouse offers a variety of services for organizations that are engaged in cancer education, including routine information searches, referral services, special information packets, and topical bibliographies.

Additionally, there also exists the International Cancer Research Data Bank (ICRDB), which actively promotes and facilitates, on a worldwide basis, the exchange of information between cancer scientists and the dissemination of information to all physicians for the public good. The ICRDB's mandate was contained in the original National Cancer Act of 1971. This data bank became operational in 1974. CANCERLINE is the computer-based system of abstracts from published results of cancer research, along with descriptions of ongoing cancer research centers.

Division of Cancer Cause and Prevention. The Division of Cancer Cause and Prevention plans and directs a program of laboratory, field, and demographic research on the cause and natural history of cancer. This effort includes such intramural programs as carcinogenesis research, whether it be biologic, chemical, or physical in nature. Additionally, this division provides the statistical services for all of the NCP research programs.

Division of Cancer Biology and Diagnosis. The Division of Cancer Biology and Diagnosis plans and directs the NCP's general laboratory and clinical research activities and serves as the national focal point for programs to improve the detection and diagnosis of human cancers. This division also plans and manages collaborative programs in tumor immunology.

Division of Cancer Treatment. The Division of Cancer Treatment plans, directs, and coordinates an integrated program of cancer treatment activities directed toward curing or controlling human cancers. These efforts utilize combination modalities including chemical, surgical, radiologic, and certain immunologic techniques, along with administering a total drug development program. To carry out these activities there are four major programs: cancer therapy evaluation, clinical oncology, developmental therapeutics, and the Baltimore Cancer Research Center.

Within the Cancer Therapy Evaluation Program, the key branches to which nursing most relates are the Investigational Drug Branch and the Clinical Investigations Branch. The former branch oversees all of the testing of investigational new cancer agents and as such regulates their use. Many of the phase 1, 2, and 3 agents that are used in research centers are provided by this branch. A further description of their activities is detailed in Chapter 14. The Clinical Investigations Branch administers the Cooperative Cancer Programs in which many nurses participate. This cooperative program evolved from the Cancer Chemotherapy National Service Center, which was established in 1955. Currently, there are 15 multi-institutional cooperative groups studying such cancers as early stage breast and colorectal cancers, pediatric tumors, gynecologic cancers, and many of the advanced stage cancers and the various modalities such as radiation oncology.

The other important program is the Developmental Therapeutics Program, which houses the Pharmaceutical Resources Branch. This branch has information on all of the investigational agents being tested so that a nurse who is unfamiliar or unsure of how to proceed can contact this branch for further information.

Division of Cancer Research Resources and Centers. The Division of Cancer Research Resources and Centers is undergoing a major change and will probably be renamed the Division of Extramural Activities. Its focus has undergone some refinement and is now primarily centered on the review of all contracts and grant proposals submitted to, or requested by, the NCI. This function makes the approval and awarding of funds solely the division's responsibility with the scientific monitoring of each award continued by the appropriate division.

Division of Cancer Control and Rehabilitation. The Division of Cancer Control and Rehabilitation is also undergoing change and will probably be renamed the Division of Cancer Resources, Centers, and Community Programs. With its new name, its responsibilities have been expanded to include the Cancer Centers Program, which administers funds to the Comprehensive Cancer Centers established in many of the leading United States universities, in addition to the previous control and rehabilitation programs. These latter efforts identified, tested, evaluated, demonstrated, and promoted the widespread application of available and new methods of reducing the incidence, morbidity, and mortality of cancer. Along with the research units of the NCI, this division administers such efforts as the Breast Cancer Detection Demonstration Programs, the community programs, and programs in the area of continuing care such as hospices.

The NCI, because of its congressional mandate and substantial funding, is one of the leading international agencies in cancer. It is a valuable resource to nurses working to aid clients and their families and can serve as a highly visible forum for advancing the profession of nursing.

Food and Drug Administration

The Food and Drug Administration (FDA), a federal agency totally separate from the NCI, interfaces with the cancer program in two main areas. The first area is regulation of all drugs, including anticancer agents, prior to allowing them on the commercial market. The second major area is that of judging the safety of food and color additives.

Regulation of new agents. Activity and procedures relative to regulation and the approval of all investigational new drugs require the FDA to work closely with a number of units within the NCI. Chief among these is the Investigational Drug Branch of the Division of Cancer Treatment. The NCI units approve and monitor institutions involved in investigational cancer research. Reports of therapeutic results as well as documentation of toxicities are carefully monitored by the NCI and forwarded on to the FDA. Likewise, commercial pharmaceutical companies that develop new cancer agents must prove their safety and efficacy before the FDA will allow them to be marketed.

There are discrete phases each agent must go through prior to its approval. These phases are discussed in detail in Chapter 14. Briefly, there are four phases: one for preclinical testing and the last three for testing of human use to determine dose ranges, toxicities, and antitumor activity along with widespread testing as a last test before approval.

Judging the safety of food and color additives. The Delaney Clause, a 1958 amendment to the Federal Food, Drug, and Cosmetic Act, requires the FDA to ban the use of a food additive when "it is found to induce cancer when ingested by man or animal, or if it is found, after tests which are appropriate for the evaluation of the safety of food additives, to induce cancer in man or animal."[11]

This act was further amended in 1960 and again in 1962, extending the authority of the FDA under the Delaney Clause to color additives used in foods, drugs, or cosmetics as well as allowing carcinogenic chemicals to be used in animal feeds *only* if no residue was detectable in the food or caused harm to the animal.

The Delaney Clause has been controversial for some time because the technology to detect increasingly smaller quantities of cancer-causing agents is now available as well as the fact that the language only addresses the issue of *presumed risk* and does not consider *potential or real benefits* to society.

A good example of how inflexible the Delaney Clause can be is best exemplified by presenting the recent data on saccharin. In 1976, a Canadian study revealed that ingesting saccharin caused bladder cancer. By virtue of its mandate, the FDA was required to review these data and make a decision on whether to ban the use of this artificial sweetener. The FDA decided that the data were sufficiently strong to warrant a ban. The resulting public outcry was substantial. Millions of diabetics rely on saccharin as do many weight-conscious Americans. The Congress was inundated with negative responses and held a series of congressional hearings on saccharin, which resulted in an 18-month moratorium initiated to reevaluate the data before a ban would be allowed to take effect. During this period, the original Canadian study and other relevant material were reviewed with the assistance of NCI staff; no further substantiation of a link between bladder cancer has been found to date.

Although this particular controversy was resolved, it does point up the different perspectives that can be generated in this area. Segments of the scientific community felt there was sufficient evidence to confirm that saccharin was a health hazard. In contrast, the public perceived saccharin as a beneficial agent. The Congress was ambivalent, having first passed the inflexible Delaney Amendment and then essentially voiding it by prohibiting the FDA from carrying out its mandate. The Delaney Amendment and the regulatory function of the FDA are still being discussed, but it appears certain that the controversy as to what is harmful to the public will continue to engender dispute and ambivalence for some time to come. It behooves nursing to strive to understand both the significance and controversy surrounding the functioning of the FDA so that correct and meaningful information can be provided to the public as well as to clients being treated for cancer.

The legislative branch of the United States government

The United States Congress has a major role to play in cancer health care because of its role in appropriating funds and monitoring the progress of the NCI. Involved in these roles are both the Senate and the House of Representatives through their separate committees.

In the Senate, the Finance Committee oversees Medicare activities as well as home visits through its Subcommittee on Health. Both of these programs are utilized extensively by cancer clients and their families. In the House, the full committee is called the Ways and Means Committee and its Subcommittee on Health.

Appropriations of operating funds for the NCI are controlled by separate committees, namely the Senate Appropriations Committee and the House Appropriations Committee. Both of these full committees have Subcommittees on Labor and Health, Education and Welfare. It is these subcommittees that eventually determine the level of funds actually appropriated.

As for reviewing the progress of the National Cancer Program, the Senate's full committee is called the Labor and Human Resources Committee, which has a Subcommittee on Health and Scientific Research. In the House, the Interstate and Foreign Commerce's Subcommittee on Health and the Environment overviews the cancer program.

Overall review of the cancer program takes place at the renewal of the National Cancer Act. This was done in 1974, 1978, and again in 1979. The length of renewal that is granted appears to be directly related to the degree of congressional satisfaction with the progress being made. Increasingly, it is being recognized that advances in the complex diseases called cancer will come piecemeal with many years required to make significant across-the-board improvements in client survival. Unfortunately, the pressures to produce major improvements burden both the Congress and the National Cancer Program.

Environmental Protection Agency

The Environmental Protection Agency (EPA) established in 1970 is responsible for clean air and water and safe pesticides. Together with the FDA, they jointly sponsor the National Center for Toxicological Research to study the biologic effects of potentially toxic environmental chemicals. The principal goal of the center is to develop better methods to evaluate the degree of toxicity of chemicals.

Additionally, the EPA, through the authority vested in it by the Federal Insecticide, Fungicide and Rodenticide Act, requires manufacturers to prove the safety of their products to the EPA before they can sell them. The major concern is that if a pesticide remains in a food product, a tolerance level has to be set by the EPA. If the pesticide is a carcinogen, the EPA must set a tolerance level or exempt it from this requirement.

Likewise, the EPA has authority over the quality of drinking water, clean air, and the protection of people from radioactive materials through the Nuclear Regulatory Commission and the Energy Research and Development Administration.[11]

Consumer Product Safety Commission

The Consumer Product Safety Commission, created by the Consumer Product Safety Act of 1972, is an independent regulatory agency that has the responsibility of reducing the unreasonable risk of injury associated with consumer products. This authority was exercised when data indicated that flame-retardant substances mandated for children's pajamas were carcinogenic.

The supreme irony appears, however, when it is discovered that one of the major consumer items, cigarettes and other tobacco products, is specifically excluded from this act. Tobacco products are proven carcinogens that have been linked with many cancers but are allowed on the market because no real health regulation exists to deal with them.[11]

National Institute of Occupational Safety and Health

The National Institute of Occupational Safety and Health (NIOSH) was created by the Occupational Safety and Health Act of 1970 to conduct and sponsor research and reviews so that criteria to protect workers could be developed. NIOSH serves as initiator of documents and supporting data for the Occupational Safety and Health Administration.[11] Increased emphasis on research in the area of occupational carcinogenesis has occurred in the last 5 years.

Occupational Safety and Health Administration

The Occupational Safety and Health Administration (OSHA) sets and enforces occupational safety and health standards that pertain to many areas such as farm vehicles and exposure of chemical workers to a carcinogen. OSHA cannot ban production or use of hazardous chemicals, but it can protect a worker from exposure to them.[11] This is accomplished by the Secretary of Labor restraining employers from exposing employees to imminent dangers. A court order, requested by the Department of Labor, is required to enforce this regulation.

National Institute of Environmental Health Sciences

The National Institute of Environmental Health Sciences plays a lesser role in the study of cancer-causing substances in the environment because of the concentrated effort of the NCI, its sister institute. However, it is charged with identifying factors, be they chemical, physical, or biologic, that adversely affect people. It also contributes the scientific rationale to regulations designed to minimize the public's risk.

Office for Protection from Research Risks

The Office for Protection from Research Risks (OPRR) is a federal agency entirely separate from the NCI but heavily influences the institute's activities. OPRR is charged with assuring that research subjects' rights are not compromised during federally sponsored research efforts. It is this agency that enforces the regulation that "informed consent" be obtained prior to the client entering into a research trial. Likewise, the principal investigator responsible for the conduct of the specific research must explain both the potential risks and the possible benefits, informing clients that they can withdraw from the research trial at any time without jeopardy and that if scientific information is discovered that could affect their therapy, it will be shared with them and their treatment adjusted accordingly.

To control the conduct of research done at the sponsored institutions, OPRR requires that certain criteria be met prior to the actual monetary award being made. This approval is called an "assurance" and implies that the institutions receiving the funds have an unbiased operative institutional review board that monitors the research in question at the local level. The committee's monitoring consists of studying the research procedures for protecting the rights of the human subjects who will participate in the trial. Additionally, certain reporting requirements and the composition of the committee are mandated by the regulations that OPRR enforces. It is of note that no professional nurse is required on these committees. The regulations that govern the OPRR were developed by the National Commission for the Protection of Human Subjects of Biomedical and Behavioral Research, created by Congress in the National Research Act of 1974. The commission, composed of individuals from multiple disciplines with the majority being nonresearchers, was mandated to recommend guidelines to the Secretary of the Department of Health and Human Services for research involving human subjects until its demise in 1978. Additionally, the commission was charged with recommending proposals to Congress for regulating non–Department of Health and Human Services funded research and to consider whether or not various guidelines developed by the commission should be extended to federally funded health care delivery efforts.[3]

The recommendations generated by this commission have undergone substantial review and refinements during the last 5 years because of the ethical questions raised by the conduct of research involving such populations as the mentally infirm, the unconscious client, and the unborn child.

Given the discovery of these earlier problems and the current climate in this country, it seems unlikely that the ethical conduct associated with cancer research will become less important in the near future. This fact, coupled with the important role nursing plays in representing the client and family, can only serve to encourage more nurses to become involved on the local as well as national policymaking levels pertaining to research conduct involving human subjects.

It should now be apparent to the reader that the federal efforts directed toward cancer's causes, treatment, and rehabilitation are complex, with many areas potentially or actually overlapping in their mandates. Billions of dollars are spent each year on research relative to cancer, with billions more at stake in terms of disruption of major industries. The nurse can do much to translate the information being generated to better use by the community as well as identifying gaps that exist.

CANCER ORGANIZATIONS

Voluntary agencies such as the American Cancer Society

Major purposes. The American Cancer Society (ACS) is one of the largest and oldest voluntary health agencies in the United States.[4] It was originally established in 1913 under the name American Society for the Control of Cancer to "disseminate knowledge concerning the symptoms, treatment and prevention of cancer, to investigate conditions under which cancer is found and to compile statistics in regard thereto."[4] These goals were implemented through close cooperation with state and local medical societies, health departments, and the creation of affiliates in the various states.

In its earliest years, the society was the principal organization concentrating public interest in cancer and as such supplied the medical and statistical information to Congress. This information served as the basis for action in establishing the National Cancer Institute as the first of the National Institutes of Health in 1937. Activities continued to increase until a reorganization was completed in 1945, along with a name change to the American Cancer Society. The board of directors was enlarged to include an equal number of members of the medical and scientific professions along with representatives from business, financial, public informational, and educational fields. The society's fund raising, educational, and service programs were greatly expanded so that a broad voluntary cancer research program could be undertaken. Four million dollars were raised in 1945, with this sum in 1978 totaling nearly $130 million.[2]

The restructured ACS involved separate incorporations for each of the affiliated divisions that had annual charters extended to them. These divisions are further divided into units that are organized on a county basis and branches that represent various communities within the unit.

Governance. Policy is made in the House of Delegates; the delegates are elected from each of the divisions. Approximately one half of the delegates represents the medical and dental professions, and the other half represents the laity. In the medical group, there must be two members with either a doctor of philosophy in the biologic sciences or a doctor of science. Within the lay group, two members must have doctorates in a field relating to lay programs in cancer control.

The society is guided by its board of directors, which is composed of one-half medical or dental representatives and one-half laity. The same board composition is seen within the individual divisions and units.

Both the board and the house are geographically representative of the country and the divisions so that broad national policies that will guide the society can be realized. Fig. 3-2 illustrates the organizational framework of the ACS.

There are some 65,000 physicians, dentists, other health professionals, and lay vol-

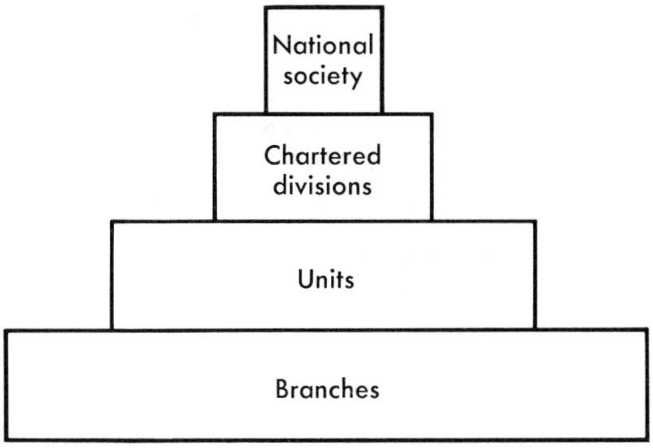

Fig. 3-2. Organizational structure of the American Cancer Society. (From Holleb, A. I.: The American Cancer Society: a voluntary health agency. In Ariel, I. M., editor: Progress in clinical cancer, vol. VII, New York, 1978, Grune & Stratton, Inc. By permission.)

unteers throughout the nation who serve on the society's national, divisional, and unit levels; Board of Directors; and committees. There are 3,000 salaried staff and over 2 million volunteers.

Major activities. The major activities of the ACS are research, professional and public education, service, and rehabilitation. The research efforts involve four main areas: clinical investigational grants, institutional research grants, training and research personnel support grants, and research development grants. The mechanism of review is first to the specific advisory committee and, if approved, onto the Council on Research and Clinical Investigations and finally the National Board of Directors. Of the $130,000,000 that was raised during the 1978 fiscal year (ending August 31, 1978), approximately 29%, 27%, and 22% went to support research, education, and services, respectively. Fig. 3-3 details the total expenditures.

Self-help organizations within the ACS. Within the service and rehabilitation area, the national ACS serves as an umbrella for many self-help groups such as the laryngectomee rehabilitation program, which was founded in 1952; the mastectomy rehabilitation program called Reach to Recovery; and the ostomy rehabilitation program. These programs have a high degree of visibility and do appear to be helpful to the client. For example, the laryngectomee rehabilitation program concentrates on postlaryngectomy speech training, aiding laryngectomees to return to their former work, or when this is not possible, helping them to obtain training and employment in a suitable position. These former clients also visit the client preoperatively and postoperatively.

Professional societies

There are a multitude of professional organizations that have been formed to provide continuing education to their members.

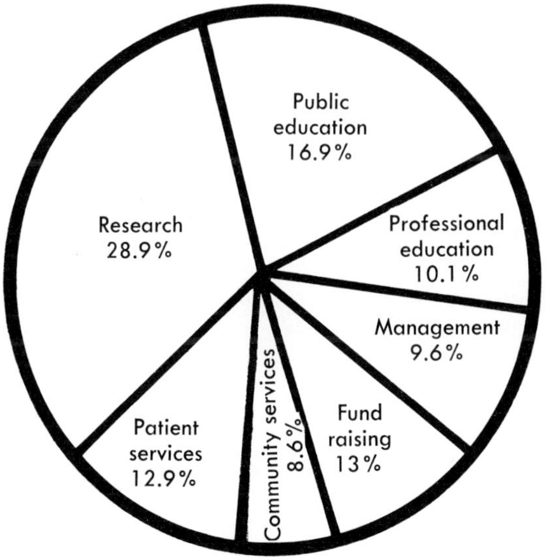

Fig. 3-3. How American Cancer Society funds are spent. (Reprinted with permission of the American Cancer Society, 1978 Annual Report.)

Table 3-1. Professional organizations in cancer

Physician-oriented	Multidisciplinary	Nurse-oriented
Society of Surgical Oncology	Association of Community Cancer Centers*	Oncology Nursing Society
American Society of Therapeutic Radiologists	American Society of Clinical Oncology	International Association of Enterostomal Therapists
American Association for Cancer Research	American Association for Cancer Education	Association of Pediatric Oncology Nurses
American Radium Society	National Hospice Organization	
American College of Surgeons	American Society of Preventive Oncology	
Society of Head and Neck Surgeons	International Study Group for the Detection and Prevention of Cancer	
American Society of Hematology		
American College of Radiology		

*Permits institutional membership as well.

Table 3-1 lists the major groups and delineates those that have predominantly physician members, nurse members, or multiple disciplines. Most of the organizations are physician oriented, since this discipline recognized cancer as a specialty area many years ago. Most of the physician groups have as their principal activity their annual scientific meeting. However, in the last several years, many of these groups have established committees to develop position papers aimed at expanding research programs, training programs, or identifying problem areas in client care. Many of these documents have been presented to the National Cancer Institute and the American Cancer Society. Some papers, however, have been put before other organizations as in the case of the American Society of Clinical Oncology's study of outpatient chemotherapy costs sent to a major insurer for consideration.

Nursing organizations are beginning to move in this direction as well. For example, the Oncology Nursing Society developed *Outcome Standards For Cancer Nursing Practice*[9] as a mechanism to identify the scope of cancer nursing practice and to provide guidelines to nurses caring for these clients.

Other guidelines have been developed by such multidisciplinary organizations as the Association of Community Cancer Centers that concentrate on establishing cancer units in community hospitals.

All of these efforts are attempting to improve the science of cancer or the services rendered to clients as well as the individual skills of its members. Increasingly, these organizations are being recognized as valuable resources and as a feedback function by the cancer policymakers.

Institutional and national organizations

Just as the professional societies are having an impact on the policymaking and conduct relative to cancer care and research, so are other agencies listed in Table 3-2. They represent cancer facilities and international cancer activities that influence cancer health care. One of the largest such organizations is

Table 3-2. Other cancer-related organizations

Membership based on country of origin or major organization/agency	Institutionally based membership	Lay membership or voluntary health agencies
International Union Against Cancer (UICC)	American Association of Cancer Institutes	Candlelighters
International Agency for Research on Cancer		Make Today Count
		Reach to Recovery*
		United Ostomy Association*
		International Association of Laryngectomees*
		American Cancer Society
		Leukemia Society of America
		American Lung Association

*Unit within the American Cancer Society.

the International Union Against Cancer, commonly referred to as the UICC.

The UICC is a nongovernmental, voluntary organization devoted solely to promoting the campaign against cancer in the world through its research, therapy, and prevention programs. The UICC has developed into a worldwide association with member organizations in 78 countries. The UICC works toward achieving its goals by facilitating the exchange of information between national cancer organizations and conducting international cancer congresses, conferences, and symposia. Additionally, committees are continually at work reviewing published research reports to promote greater standardization of the nomenclature and classifications.[12]

Also on the international level is the International Agency for Research on Cancer (IARC), which was established in 1965 by the World Health Organization (WHO). IARC functions as an independently financed organization within the overall structure of WHO, conducting predominantly epidemiologic research, education, and training of personnel for cancer research.

Within the United States, the American Association of Cancer Institutes represents virtually all of the major American Cancer Care and Research facilities. This organization provides the National Cancer Institute with valuable feedback relative to policies set forth by that agency.

Self-help groups. Self-help groups are those organizations that evolve out of largely unmet needs identified by specific groups of clients or families. An example of one such group is the Reach to Recovery Program, which was independently founded by Terese Lasser during the 1950's following her own mastectomy. Ms. Lasser's stated purpose for establishing this group was to provide information and support to women undergoing surgery for breast cancer by utilizing volunteers who had had successful operations for this cancer. The organization grew to be very successful and during the 1970's joined with the American Cancer Society. This group, and others of its type, provides a mechanism to help the client and family cope with the changes required by illness and promotes increased understanding about the illness as well as specific information on rehabilitation. These functions tend to reduce anxiety experienced by the client and family as well as correcting misconceptions they may have.[1]

LOCAL CANCER EFFORTS

At the local or community level, there exists a number of agencies and programs that influence the level of cancer health care that is delivered.

Hospital Cancer Program of the American College of Surgeons

The American College of Surgeons, to be referred to as the college, has been involved in efforts to improve the level of cancer health care since 1913. The college periodically conducts surveys designed specifically to improve the care of cancer clients on the local level through established guidelines of organization, facilities, and personnel. The desired goal is that more effective cancer care will become available. One of the major mechanisms for promoting this goal is through the Hospital Cancer Program administered by the Commission on Cancer of the college.

For an institution to be approved in this program, it must meet four basic requirements: be accredited by the Joint Commission on Accreditation of Hospitals or its equivalent; have an operational cancer committee, which is responsible for a functioning Cancer Registry, conduct multidisciplinary educational cancer conferences; have a consultational service for cancer clients; and have a system for quality-of-care evaluation with criteria concerning diagnostic, therapeutic, and rehabilitational guidelines monitored by the cancer committee. If an institution meets these criteria, it is approved as having the capability to provide the best cancer care possible within its specific designations. A list of all approved institutions along with a survey of their cancer facilities is published in the approved cancer programs publication.[5]

Institutional review boards

All institutions receiving funding from the federal government for research involving humans must meet certain requirements relative to the approval and monitoring of research projects within their institution. These requirements were discussed earlier in this chapter, but suffice it to say that these committees promote compliance regarding the obtaining of informed consent of the client. The requirement that the client is given a written explanation of the aims of the research, the potential risks as well as the benefits, along with a description of what the research will entail makes for a more informed judgment on whether to participate. This mechanism also promotes the sharing of information. Unfortunately, most committees have no nurse representatives but rely on medical-legal-lay representatives. Since most of cancer involves research undertakings, these committees could provide the nurse with an opportunity to impact on care within the entire institution.

CONCLUSION

The focus of this chapter has been on those organizations and agencies having a substantial impact on cancer health care. These agencies range from professional societies for cancer specialists to major international agencies such as the World Health Organization. While numerous examples were cited, the discussion was not exhaustive. It could not be because cancer care and research do not occur in a vacuum. Physicians, nurses, and the other health professionals relate to their discipline *before* they can relate to their specialty of choice. Hospitals must adhere to many regulations, not just those set forth by the cancer agencies. Therefore, such important organizations as the American Medical Association (AMA), the American Nurses' Association (ANA), and the American Hospital Association (AHA) have not been discussed. Likewise,

ANA's code of ethics was not cited nor was discussion of AHA's "Statement on a Patient's Bill of Rights" or the Professional Standards Review Organizations. It has been assumed that the reader is familiar with all these important areas, and the discussion has concentrated only on agencies having an exclusive or major impact on cancer.

It is hoped that by providing an overview of these cancer organizations the nurse reader will become more involved in their activities. To date, nursing has had little or no impact into the policies evolving from these many agencies. This fact is both tragic and increasingly avoidable, for nurses *do* have the knowledge and skills with which to compete for positions of power in this area. Nurses have the obligation to more completely utilize their knowledge and skills to identify client needs and strive toward an improved level of care for this special population of clients and families.

REFERENCES

1. Adams, J.: Mutual-help groups: enhancing the coping ability of oncology clients, Cancer Nurs. **2**(2):95, 1979.
2. Breslow, D. M., editor: Where does your ACS dollar go, UCLA Cancer Cent. Bull. **6**(1):11, January/February, Los Angeles, 1979, Jonsson Comprehensive Cancer Center.
3. Davis, A. J., and Aroskar, M. A.: Ethical dilemmas and nursing practice, New York, 1978, Appleton-Century-Crofts.
4. Holleb, A. I.: The American Cancer Society: a voluntary health agency. In Ariel, I. M., editor: Progress in clinical cancer, vol. VII, New York, 1978, Grune & Stratton, Inc.
5. 1974 cancer program manual, American College of Surgeons Commission on Cancer, Chicago, Ill., 1974.
6. 1978 National Cancer Institute Fact Book, National Cancer Program, Publication No. 79-512, Bethesda, Md., 1978, U.S. Department of Health, Education and Welfare.
7. National Cancer Act of 1971 with changes made by the National Cancer Act Amendments of 1974, Appendix A, National Cancer Institute, **59**(2): (Suppl.), August, 1977.
8. Newell, G. R.: The national cancer program, 1971-1976. In Piel, I. M., editor: Progress in clinical cancer, vol. II, New York, 1978, Grune and Straten, Inc.
9. Outcome standards for cancer nursing practice of the Oncology Nursing Society and the American Nurses' Association, Kansas City, Mo., 1979, American Nurses' Association.
10. Report says cancer cure would lengthen life little, The Nation's Health, May, 1979.
11. Report to the Congress by the Controller General of the United States: Federal efforts to protect the public from cancer-causing chemicals are not very successful, Publication No. MWD-76-59, June, 1976.
12. Wakefield, J., editor: Public education about cancer, vol. 34, UICC Technical Report Series, Geneva, Switzerland, 1976.

II

ISSUES IMPORTANT TO THE NURSE

4

The psychosocial care of cancer clients and their families: periods of high risk

LISA BEGG MARINO and JUDITH A. KOOSER

The subject of psychosocial care of persons with cancer is one that is both over- and underdiscussed. This apparent paradox is evident in the following examples. Consider on one hand the frequent, stereotypic association of cancer with death and dying versus the rare discussion of the significance that hospital discharge has for clients' perception of their disease state.

While no one would deny the life-threatening nature of cancer, it is an oversimplification to categorize clients with cancer as dying persons. The universal fact is that all persons begin the dying process the moment they are born. It is true that some cancer clients can be more sure than most people of when they will die, but not all clients can be that sure. Even for those clients who will die from their cancer, they will *continue to function* within a social network until their death. Cancer is not only a biologic phenomenon, it is a social one as well. Clients with cancer, regardless of the ultimate outcome of their disease state, still relate to, and interact with, other people. These people may be from within their family unit, their work or social environments, or even the hospital network. Clients still communicate with these other people, so labeling them as "dying persons" or "terminal clients" only serves to further stigmatize them. The labels create more distance among family and health care provider groups and further isolate the client at a time when support should be given. It would be far more constructive and accurate to view these persons as *living with a potentially fatal illness*. This reorientation not only provides the client with more resources but also allows the health care provider more opportunities to intervene.

Likewise, the fact that these clients are living for longer periods of time is leading to the identification of additional needs. One of these needs, recognition of the importance of major landmarks such as initial hospital discharge, has been identified. This event is now considered to be a period of "high risk" for the client, requiring additional interventions on the part of the health care provider. The initial hospital discharge is stressful because the security and attention available within the hospital setting cannot readily be duplicated at home. The home may be perceived as "warm and friendly," but since the client may worry about problems developing, the need for appropriate resources becomes paramount. Once thought of as "routine" office visits and test periods are no longer considered as such because we now recognize that the client and family perceive these events as potentially identifying a recurrence of cancer. The stress level of the client and family increases before and during office visits and test periods.

NEED FOR INCREASED NURSING INVOLVEMENT

The reexamination of these high-risk periods and additional needs are common today because the very nature of cancer is changing. More and more, cancer is being characterized as *a group of long-term illnesses that have both acute and chronic episodes.* Unfortunately, this more enlightened attitude about the disease state has not totally removed the stigma of cancer that affects the clients, their families, and the health care providers. This fact is the primary reason for the inclusion of this chapter. Another reason is that most of the literature relating to psychosocial aspects of cancer is anecdotal. There is a definite need to chronicle the needs of clients and families over time and to indicate the broadness of these needs as well as the interventions that are appropriate to them. With this information, we hope that more nurses will intervene on behalf of the client and family to promote more open and effective communication so that the isolation engendered by societal stigmas can be diminished. Moreover, nurses through their large numbers and highly visible day-to-day charge of these clients, can do much to promote more secure and honest care. Therefore, this chapter will identify why nurses should intervene and give suggestions for how they can effectively aid cancer clients and their families.

CONCEPT OF NORMALITY

There has been, and continues to be, discussion as to the presence of a "cancer personality." Simonton and Simonton[7] are some of the more outspoken researchers in this area, observing four personality characteristics. They state that cancer clients have a great tendency to hold resentment and exhibit a marked inability to forgive; a tendency toward self-pity; a poor ability to develop and maintain meaningful, long-term relationships; and a very poor self-image.[7] These personality traits may, or may not, become accepted as valid. Even if it is shown to be correct through research, it has little significance to the health care provider. This is because the presence or absence of these traits has not precluded the social functioning of these persons or their participation in treatment. These clients are functional in a psychologic sense so interventions should be directed toward those events that are problematic to the client and family, namely their cancerous condition. Therefore, the attitude of the authors is that cancer clients are normal persons under severe stress.[2]

This concept, labeled normality by the authors, forces changes in nurses' behaviors. For example, the argument that nurses need to have special training to effectively intervene with these clients is dispelled. An empathetic approach and a commitment to continue to assist the client and family regardless of what happens to them are what is needed. Likewise, the concept of normality implies that these clients can exert control over their lives and can adjust to the circumstances of their diseased state. The client has a past history that required decisions and adjustments to be made. The individual was capable of accomplishing these life events and is now capable of decision making in regard to the discovery of cancer, treatment options, and required alterations in life-style. Unfortunately, the typical approach of most health care providers is to protect the client and family from the decision making that would allow them to experience the losses and grief that are inherent with any serious illness. In this way adaptation is hindered because to integrate these experiences successfully requires the individual to be aware or to acknowledge the loss and decide how to continue to live with the new reality of a diminished life span, altered body image, or recurrence of disease. Decision making is essential to the successful adjustment to a diagnosis of cancer, and the nurse can do a great deal to assist the client and family to obtain adequate information so that informed decisions are possible. The nurse can also create a climate of respect for the client and family so that the other health care providers will interact in a more enlightened manner. Coordination of care will also maximize communication and provide for more orderly care.

THE FAMILY AS THE UNIT OF CARE

Cancer is a life-threatening illness requiring major adjustments on the part of the client and is inherently a family experience.[3] This orientation does not negate the nurse's obligation to the client but extends interventions to the family members. We have found that utilizing the family as the unit of care minimizes the stresses through mutual sharing. Moreover, the discovery of the cancer is but one event in the life of the client, and health care providers must realize that clients will continue to function in their social network. The chronic nature of cancer involves many people and events. It is fatiguing to care for ill persons over time, therefore, dividing that effort among a number of people limits the individual efforts.

Basing care on the family also encourages authentic communication among the members. All too often, the client's experiences of reality are separate from the family's, with a conspiracy of silence pervading all interactions. This results in the most superficial communication so that no one is upset by discussing the true situation. The presence of a sympathetic health care provider can do much to aid the family to identify explicit facts that have been kept from surfacing within the unit as a whole. These exchanges facilitate the necessary grieving process, which helps to avoid the destructive consequences of intense, hidden, and unresolved grief. Dealing more constructively with these problems enhances the intrinsic strengths often present in these families and increases their cohesiveness.[11]

A discrete problem that is family centered but different occurs when the client is a child. Caring for a child with cancer is one of the most difficult areas in which a health care provider must intervene. The fears and discomfort evoked by caring for adults with cancer are further heightened with children because of increased feelings of vulnerability and injustice. Society, as a whole, is ill prepared to deal with life-threatening illnesses in children, so the health care provider lacks structure in this area. There are no easy answers to this unique problem, but two different approaches are offered in Chapters 21 and 23.

RISKS TO THE NURSE

Cancer care is acknowledged as a difficult specialty for nursing. The entire health care system is geared toward cure, a goal not generally obtainable with the current level of knowledge about cancer. Furthermore, the strong research orientation of cancer care produces additional stresses because outcomes are not assured and untoward consequences can occur, however well-intentioned the health care provider may be. The constantly expanding knowledge gained from research requires the professional roles to change. Personal involvement with clients who are seriously ill can cause "professional burnout," a phenomenon discussed in Chapter 8. All together, cancer care may appear to offer few opportunities for professional satisfaction, but fortunately, this is not the case. Cancer must be acknowledged as a high-risk specialty, but supports can be established that will allow the health care provider, particularly the nurse, to continue to function at a professional level. These supports can include regular sessions and informal encounters with psychiatric nurses and involvement with clients who have less serious illnesses or require less acute cancer care. Maintaining contact with cancer clients over time permits the nurse to see people who are leading relatively normal lives by continuing with work and family responsibilities. Generally, nurses working in hospitals only see cancer clients when the diagnosis is made, when an acute problem develops, or when they are dying. All these situations are stressful. It is easy to see why nurses might become frustrated in trying to have satisfying professional experiences. In contrast, administering chemotherapy to clients who are on their way to work or vacation gives an entirely different perspective.

Because cancer is statistically a major health care problem, it is difficult for nurses to avoid professional contact with these clients. We acknowledge that the nurse will not always be able to intervene with these clients for reasons ranging from personal difficulties to professional overload. When these clients' needs cannot be met, the nurse still has the responsibility to arrange for alternative resources. Many times nurses can, and should, influence the overall delivery of cancer health care. Interventions with other health care providers on behalf of clients or manipulation of the multiple systems affecting care must be viewed as legitimate professional actions. Awareness of these actions provides additional and vital sources of satisfaction for nurses.

HIGH-RISK PERIODS FOR THE CLIENT AND FAMILY

There is general agreement that cancer places the client and family under enormous stress. If this isn't enough of a burden, research has further identified events of even greater stress. These events are labeled "landmarks" because they represent significant junctions in the client's physiologic or psychologic state.

There are four major periods: prediagnostic, diagnostic, treatment, and end of life. Two of the four periods have subsections within them because discrete phases that require different intervention strategies can be identified. The following is a list of these periods as well as the subsections.

1. Prediagnostic
2. Diagnostic
   a. Intradiagnostic
   b. Immediately postconfirmation
3. Treatment
   a. Definitive therapy
   b. Initial hospital discharge
   c. Adjuvant treatment
   d. Time of first tumor recurrence
   e. Advanced disease state
4. End of life

Each of these periods will be discussed in detail so that the nurse can see areas of need as well as strategies for interventions. Before the specific phases are addressed, a few general comments will be made to put them in perspective.

The diagnosis of cancer is very disruptive to the client and family, so the overall nursing goal should be to counter the emotional disorganization experienced. A client's silence in the face of such disruption should not be equated with acceptance or denial of the situation. Adjustment to cancer is more complex than that, therefore, the silence may only mean the client is sensing the nurse's discomfort and waiting for sanction to discuss feelings and fears. It has also been discovered through interviewing many clients that patterns of communication can be identified that closely parallel the stage of the client's cancer. This finding will become more evident as the discussion progresses,

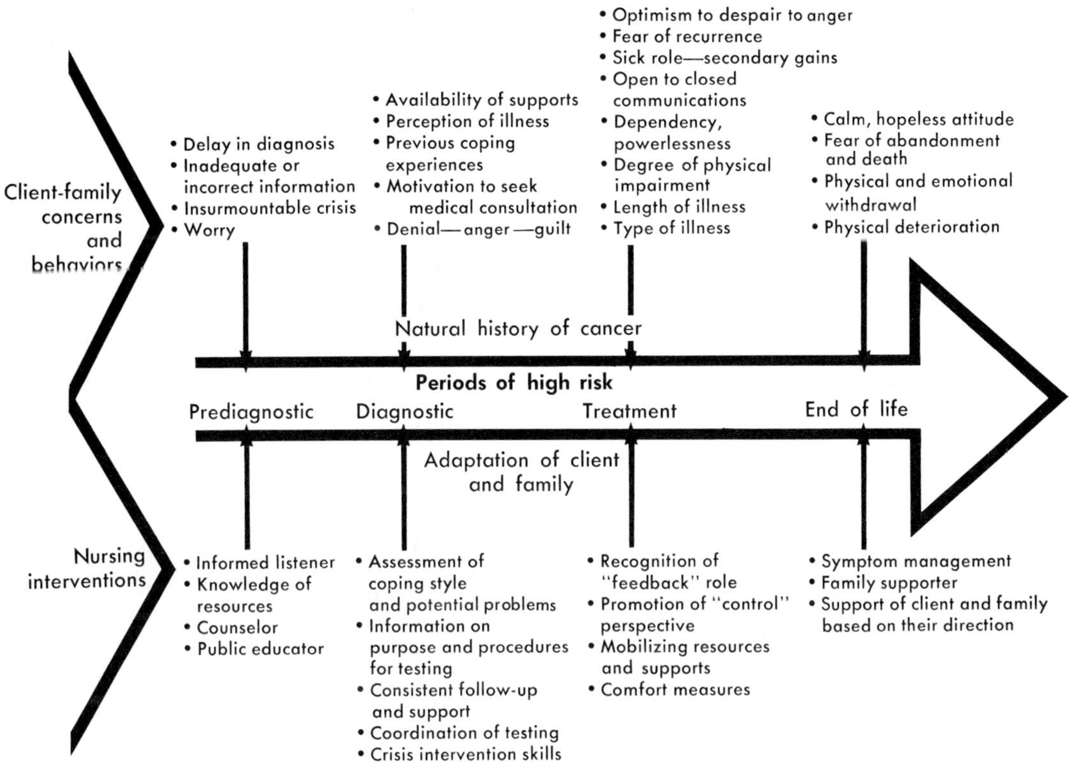

Fig. 4-1. Dynamics of psychosocial cancer care.

but it can be exemplified by the open communication evident during definitive treatment, which becomes more closed as recurrence of the disease is discovered.[1]

The model in Fig. 4-1 shows the interplay of forces and complex patterns of communications and therapeutic interventions. Central to the psychosocial care of these clients is the state of their cancer. Natural history is the term used in the model to connote the evolution of the disease state, taking into consideration the fact that therapeutic interventions will be made. Adaptation on the part of the client and family will occur regardless of interventions. However, more *successful* adaptation can be influenced by the nursing interventions shown in the lower half of the model. These interventions are in anticipation of, or in response to, the behaviors exhibited by the client and family and are shown at the top of the model. The arrows connote a dynamic and fluid state.

Prediagnostic period

The period preceding a diagnosis of cancer is crucial in determining the stage at which the cancer will eventually be detected as well as in providing information about the coping style of the client.

Delay in diagnosis. Hackett, in a study of delay in diagnosis, compared the results of a survey done in the late 1960's with one done 30 years earlier. He found the delay period, defined as the time from the client's first awareness of symptoms or signs to the first consultation with a physician, to be the same in both studies. Only 29.4% of the earlier group and 33.7% of the latter group consulted a physician within the first month of awareness. In the latter group, two-thirds waited more than a month to seek medical assistance, with 15% waiting more than a year to act on their suspicions.[4]

Pursuing the reasons why people did eventually seek medical assistance, Hackett found five major reasons as shown below.

Worry	37%
Pain	33%
Incapacity	8%
Advice of a friend	13%
Annual physical	7%
Other	2%

Most striking was the finding that 33% of the study group acted only after pain developed. Pain is generally a late symptom of cancer. Even more surprising, 8% did not act until they became incapacitated by their cancer. A significant number of these persons were found to be "worriers," and worriers tended to delay action for longer periods of time than did nonworriers. Worry was related to a lack of information and decreased when correct and complete information was given.[4]

Site of the cancer also influenced the delay period. Breast cancer shortened the delay and rectal cancer lengthened it substantially. Higher socioeconomic class shortened the delay period, perhaps because these individuals knew more about cancer and had more resources to consult.[4]

What is alarming about this study is that fully 78% of these people were motivated to act on purely negative grounds such as worry, pain, and incapacity. For a person to wait until pain or incapacity develops only serves to demonstrate the fearsome perception most people have of cancer, as well as the difficulty they have in coping. Shand,[6] in discussing the informational impact of the diagnosis of cancer, labels the period as being an informational crisis. Crisis has many definitions, but for purposes of discussion here it is defined as "a situation which the individual considers to be hazardous."[5] Crisis develops because the individual's normal, stable state is disrupted through internal disorganization, disrupted expectations, and the threat to well-being. At the time when the first symptoms are realized, clients generally begin to anticipate what they think will happen to them during treatment. They grow apprehensive based on the variety of stories, some of which are distorted, of what has happened to other people the client knows who have undergone cancer treatment.

Intervention strategies. In terms of interventions, most of these persons will remain outside the mainstream of health care until they decide to act on their suspicions. This fact might seem to preclude any responsibility on the part of the health care providers; however, we disagree. Health care providers, particularly nurses, should intervene wherever they can to minimize the crises these individuals experience. This can be done in a number of ways. Anxious people may be eager to talk with helpful persons with little prompting necessary. Nurses, because of their frequent contact with the public, are readily available resources who are perceived as less threatening to the client than physicians. Since these encounters have serious implications to the client, nurses have the responsibility to take advantage of this aspect of the role and serve as valuable resources.

Cancer is perceived differently by different people and has widely varying implications to them. Providing these individuals with an informed listener can be helpful to them as they work to integrate this massive threat to their sense of well-being. Correcting misconceptions about cancer, identifying potential resources, and encouraging action are the essence of professional activities during this period.

The general approach during this period is to compartmentalize the crisis by having the person consider one step at a time. First, find out if a cancer exists and then determine what course to pursue. For example, the traditional way most American surgeons deal with a woman referred to them for evaluation of a breast mass is to perform procedures such as mammography and breast biopsy in addition to physical examination. If the physical examination and mammography are inconclusive, a biopsy is required to determine the presence or absence of a cancer. Most surgeons still do what is called a "one-step" procedure, consisting of an excisional biopsy and mastectomy if the frozen section demonstrates a cancer. This technique forces the woman to simultaneously deal with two very stressful events, the question of whether or not a cancer is present and the possible loss of her breast. It would seem a more humane way could be found, and in fact there is the "two-step" procedure that many surgeons have adopted. Nurses, through their counseling role, can make women aware of this option. This approach entails an excisional biopsy or needle biopsy done initially so that tissue can be examined histologically. If a cancer is confirmed, the woman is informed and discussion follows as to the available options. This allows the woman to take one step at a time, thus making the crisis more manageable. No study has been done on the traumas associated with the "one-step" procedure, but with the advent of an alternative plan the woman can decide which course she wishes to pursue. Nurses, because of their knowledge of the medical community, can serve as resources to enable the client to seek the preferred plan of action.

Diagnostic period

Once clients decide to act on their suspicions by consulting a physician, the period of diagnosis is said to begin. There are two discrete subsections to this period: the intradiagnostic phase and the phase immediately following the confirmation that a cancer exists.

Characteristics of the intradiagnostic phase. The intradiagnostic phase extends from the initial consultation with a physician to the actual confirmation that a cancer exists. The period can range from one office visit to a period of several weeks until tests and procedures can be completed. Moreover, the clients' psychologic state can vary depending on the reasons for seeking medical consultation. These reasons can range from prompting by family members to the serendipitous discovery during a routine health examination. The presenting symptom can also influence the psychologic state of the client; a symptom such as hematuria will elicit more alarm than constipation and back pain. The former example may only serve to confirm a terrifying fact already considered, while the latter example may catch the client totally unaware.

Intervention strategies. It is appropriate during this period to discuss with clients their perceptions of what is happening and the significance the events have for them, as well as providing them with information and resources if desired. In addition to exchanging information, these discussions permit the nurse to assess the coping style and capacity of the client and family. As stated previously, individuals have the capacity to cope and successfully adapt to this threat. However, supportive intervention on the part of the health care providers such as nurses can facilitate the client's adaptation.

For example, there is generally a whole battery of tests and procedures that are done to confirm whether or not a cancer exists and, if so, its extent. These tests can be done on an outpatient or hospital basis. Regardless of the setting, clients would have to make adjustments in their daily schedule to complete the tests. Making these adjustments, particularly if they infringe on work time, requires the client to offer explanations of what is happening. This may increase the stress because clients may not want their employer to be aware of their potential problem. Considering the discrimination experienced by cancer clients, this may be an understandable attitude. Less understandable are clients who do not want their families informed of the possibility that a cancer may be found, again under the misconception of protecting them from unpleasant news. Closed communication only increases the burdens each member will experience, so the health care provider should try to persuade and aid the client to disclose this information.

Because anxiety is generally high during this period, the client may not hear what the physician says, therefore, consistent follow-up to validate the client's perceptions is helpful. Likewise, informing the client as to the diagnostic plan, the day-to-day time frame for conducting the tests, and what the client can do to ensure successful completion of the tests is an appropriate nursing function. A barium enema that has to be repeated because of inadequate bowel preparation may seem a minor irritation to the nurse but can be a source of great tension to the client. Confirmation of the existence of a cancer may be delayed until completion of this test. Nurses can help clients to help themselves as well as to participate more fully in their care by informing them of what needs to be done and why and the procedures that need to be followed. This will better ensure the successful completion of the necessary tests and thereby reduce the uncertain and stressful interval.

Characteristics of the immediate post-confirmation phase. Once the diagnosis has been confirmed, the anticipatory fear ceases and the crisis begins at an even higher level than during the prediagnostic phase. Shand's description of the diagnosis of cancer as an "amputation of the future" graphically describes the situation.[6] Clients recounting this terrifying period frequently comment that their whole life passed before them.

Self-questioning is very common during this period as clients ask, "Why me?" "What did I do to cause this to happen?" Many times bitterness over a perceived shortened life is directed at others or projected inward to the client. The reaction of clients very much depends on their life experiences, their feelings about themselves, and the kinds of expectations they have about relationships with others.

Intervention strategies. It is important to find out what the illness means to the client. For some, it may represent a threat to livelihood, to their family's economic security, to self-respect as a productive member of society, or to valued roles such as parent. For others, worries about the continuance of valued social relationships, recreational activities, or sexual attractiveness may be significant.[10] Secondary gains from illness may also influence clients' reactions. The diagnosis of cancer may represent a right to demand special attention, sanction to act out, or a way out of displeasing situations or relationships. Great preoccupation occurs as well as feelings of anger, denial, or guilt.

Denial in itself is not bad, particularly if the client is able and willing to participate in the decision making relative to treatment options. Interestingly, Waxenberg[10] discovered that a low rank in postoperative psychogenic invalidism was directly proportional to a high level of denial that cancer ever existed. In contrast, those women who answered yes, thus indicating they deemed their illness important, critical, and damaging to their lives, were more likely to experience some degree of invalidism.

Anger in the client is more difficult to deal

with because it inhibits the exchange of information and support. Health care providers need to keep in perspective that the anger is not directed at them per se but is more a reflection of what they represent to the client. For example, the meaning of a hospitalization can be very negative to many clients. Other times, anger may be expressed at the staff as opposed to the intended person, the physician. This occurrence happens a great deal in cancer because the client is afraid of losing the physician and so will not jeopardize their relationship. Dependency is a very real problem with cancer clients. It is important that the nurse encourage independence as well as continue to supply information and support as needed.

Guilt often surfaces because many people associate cancer with the "unclean." Families often feel guilty because they think they could have encouraged the client to seek aid earlier. These feelings are very evident if the cancer is diagnosed in an advanced stage.

Clients exhibit guilt through attributing the cancer to something they did or did not do. Because nothing good can come from clients' or families' guilt, it is important that the nurse discourage such feelings and reinforce the perspective of the situation.

Likewise, allowing the client and family the opportunity to discuss their fears about mutilation and death is extremely important. The nurse should not give false hope but rather reinforce the chronicity of cancer.

The last aspect of this period is to determine how best to proceed. The nurse can be helpful in identifying resources as well as aiding the client and family in information gathering.

Period of treatment

Once the diagnosis of cancer has been confirmed and the client agrees to undergo treatment, a new period begins. As in the diagnostic period, discrete phases occur that require different interventions. These five phases are: definitive therapy, initial hospital discharge, adjuvant therapy, time of first tumor recurrence, and the advanced disease state.

Changes in communication are very evident during this period and range from open and hopeful communication to stilted when the client reaches the advanced stages. It should be kept in mind that the comments can only be general in that some clients will be in the treatment phase only a short period of time, while others may be under treatment for years. Moreover, some clients will be cured of their cancer and therefore never progress beyond the second subphase. Given the projections, however, it is more likely that two thirds of the more than 700,000 new cancer cases will have residual or recurrent disease. Because this group is so large, it is doubly important that nurses appreciate the dynamics of the situation.

Definitive therapy phase. The definitive therapy phase generally occurs in hospital settings and evokes a wide range of emotions. On the one hand is the hospital admission, which confirms the anticipatory fears encountered during the prediagnostic period. Feelings of helplessness, dependency, and powerlessness are common. The day of admission is extremely stressful because the client must deal with the reality of having cancer and the plan to undergo treatment. Sleep and eating habits may be disturbed. In contrast, a high level of activity is present as everyone strives to cure the client. Optimism predominates because of the hope that therapy will be successful. No one wants to dwell on the prospect that treatment will be unsuccessful. Hope prevails and the nurse should not feel any reluctance for this is important to the client's and family's mental state. Hope can be fostered by the nurse entering into a contract with the client and family to assist them through the course of disease. The nurse can specifically address the importance of information gathering and offer a commitment to assist the client and family to obtain needed information on which to base decisions.

Information gathering is important in the definitive therapy phase because of the controversies that exist as to the best treatments for a number of cancers. Such examples as the debate over which mastectomy, standard radical, modified radical, or others, should be employed in which type of client continues. Radiation therapy has also been suggested as an alternative to surgery for certain stages of breast cancer. The great research orientation to most areas of cancer therapy emphasizes the importance of information so that clients and their families can assess the potential risks versus the potential benefits of the proposed therapy. They must understand that research cannot predict all outcomes and must be assured that withdrawal from the research project without jeopardy to further treatment is allowed.

Preparing the client for treatment is difficult, particularly if extensive surgery is required. Preoperative teaching is common today, but it should be pointed out that because of the high anxiety, clients may not completely absorb all of the information. Short sessions lasting no more than 20 minutes are best; repeated sessions are also advisable.

Acute undeniable grief is commonly seen in clients waiting for the initiation of treatment. Signing the informed consent, which signifies agreement to the proposed procedure, can trigger an acute reaction as the realization that they do have cancer requiring certain interventions is forced into their consciousness. The more extensive the procedure, the greater the adjustment required of the client. Likewise, obvious signs of disease, such as amputations, require more adjustment on the part of the client than do lesser procedures.

In general, this acute phase offers both hope to the client and family as well as major adjustments. Initially, the health care providers serve an important feedback function as the clients observe how other people react to them in their new state. For example, the nurse who utilizes rubber gloves when caring for the client with a new colostomy will indicate to the client a more negative reaction than the nurse who does not use gloves. Clients generally have a diminished self-concept during these acute phases of illness, and so it is important that the health care providers do all they can to support them, not further stress them. The key actions during this period are to listen, watch, and act on the client's indications of what is necessary to preserve and foster a functional state.

Initial hospital discharge. There are a wide range of client reactions to the seemingly happy event of the initial hospital discharge that may go unnoticed by many health care providers. The client may have been in the hospital a period of weeks and moved from the acute illness state to convalescence and preparation for discharge. During this period, the client has received a great deal of attention from the various health care providers. As unhomelike as the hospital is, it is secure. If something goes wrong, the client can obtain help with the push of the call light. The client is well aware of the importance of these resources. The discharge marks a "landmark" in terms of the secondary gains associated with the sick role. During the definitive therapy phase, the client is acutely ill and thus unable to participate in work or family obligations. However, when the client is well enough to be discharged, the general perception is that the client has recovered substantially. The courtesies, the special attention from family and friends, and the exemption from responsibility extended to the client during hospitalization are withdrawn. The client is normal. Depression occurs at the time of discharge in many people, but for the cancer client who may not be cured or who will have to undergo additional treatment, the reaction may be more severe. Others perceive them as well when in fact they are not well.

The hospital can represent many things to clients. Many clients regard the hospital as possessing the capacity for cure or at least having a major impact on illness. Thus, a discharge may inadvertently indicate that "nothing more can be done for me." Depression is a common reaction. It is, therefore, important for the nurse to determine how the client feels about the expected discharge and what it means personally to the client. This provides the nurse with an opportunity to reinforce the long-term commitment the health care provider has to the client and family as well as correcting any misconceptions about the purpose of the discharge.

Discharge from the hospital may also cause anxiety because the client realizes that explanations about the illness may have to be given to family members, particularly children, friends, and employers. Moreover, being at home may mean the client is faced with such anxiety-provoking experiences as engaging in intimate relations, which may focus the attention of both partners on physical appearances or exposure of the affected part. Nurses can be particularly helpful to clients by exploring with them just how they intend to deal with these encounters. Encouraging clients to confront these issues can provide them with some "advance" time to prepare for these experiences. If these issues are not dealt with directly, the client may become a social recluse or have limited encounters with family members.

Adjuvant therapy. Adjuvant therapy, defined as therapy given after definitive treatment to kill any microscopic remnants of cancer in clients deemed at high risk for recurrence, is a relatively new concept in terms of its widespread application. During the 1960's, adjuvant therapy was employed for Wilms' tumor, a childhood solid cancer, and in limited settings for breast cancer. It was not until the 1970's, however, that adjuvant therapy was extended to such cancers as osteogenic sarcomas, colorectal cancers, breast cancers, head and neck cancers, and lung cancers. The specifics of this form of therapy are discussed in Chapters 11, 14, and 24, but in terms of psychologic needs, adjuvant therapy occupies a major area.

Adjuvant therapy is a stressful interval for clients because it labels them as high-risk candidates for tumor recurrence. Scientifically, this is the only justification for administering adjuvant therapy. For example, cancers that are determined to have spread to the nearby lymph nodes in such cancers as colon, rectum, and breast can lead to tumor recurrence and possibly death. This fact may be difficult for the client and family to recognize because initially no symptoms or disability is present. Moreover, the possibility of recurrence is continually reinforced to the client during the treatment visits and testing periods. Denial, a valid protective mechanism, is difficult to maintain over this period. From a psychologic perspective, the period is analogous with follow-up. While no treatment is given in follow-up, the reminder that cancer did occur and could recur is reinforced by the periodic examinations and tests.

Interventions in this phase center on correcting misconceptions about what "high risk" really means. Office visits and testing periods should see the nurse spending more time with the client and family so that necessary support to diminish anxiety can be given. Diversionary activities during these stressful events are helpful. Helping to minimize the disruptions associated with cancer treatments should be emphasized so that losses from the work and home environments can be lessened. The nurse can also stress the concept of tumor control so that the client and family understand that something can be done if, and when, there is a recurrence. Reinforcing the client's sense of personal control can be done by stressing the importance of maintaining the therapy plan, completing all required tests, and reporting any unusual symptoms. This helps to identify the client and family as partners in the treatment plan. Because the client can suffer a relapse, it is important that assessment be made of resources within the family and their community so that they can be mobilized later if necessary.

Time of first tumor recurrence. The time of the first tumor recurrence confirms the worst fears of the client and family. All the hopes raised during the earlier periods and all the work that went into minimizing the likelihood of recurrence have now ended in failure. Recurrence of the original cancer has been documented. No real victory, only the avoidance of defeat, is now achievable.

This recognition is more devastating than even the shock of the initial diagnosis because denial and hope were strong then. Now the recognition of the refractiveness to therapy is undeniable since the cancer was not contained. The threat of death that surfaced earlier is more difficult to ignore during this phase, and the client demonstrates a deep concern about dying. Death seems much more likely now. Communication is more difficult now. Client-to-family and client-to-staff communications are more superficial. It is not just the client who failed; it is also the staff. The sense of failure lowers defenses. The realization that progressive weakness and immobility are likely to occur heightens fears of dependency.

Chief among the client's many fears is the fear of becoming an intolerable burden on the family members. These fears are not unfounded as a serious illness such as cancer forces the client to place extraordinary demands on the other family members. The clients fear that those closest to them will abandon them and disappear. This response may be a metaphoric expression of the client's own fears of oblivion or dying.[11] Glaser and Strauss[8] have labeled this period as being one of "interactional awkwardness" because the social relationships become disrupted, falter, or worse still, disintegrate.

Interventions in this phase are based on minimizing the crisis that developed at the time recurrence was documented. The client and family must grieve here because of the significance first recurrence has to the natural history of cancer. The reality of this fact should not be hidden from clients because they are losing an immense amount and so grief is inevitable. Supporting the client and encouraging the family to discuss their feelings, assisting the client to continue with needed treatments and tests when the client feels like giving up, and mobilizing the previously identified resources are important nursing responsibilities during this phase. The last function becomes very important in lessening the client's worry and guilt feelings about burdening the family.

Advanced disease state. The advanced disease state is characterized by the documented presence of metastases that are being treated with the aim of retarding the future spread of cancer. Cure or even significant control is no longer possible. Symptom control and treatment regimens take up an increasing amount of the client's and family's time. This leaves only limited time and lessened energy to complete the unfinished business of living before the inevitable pulling out. Clients frequently describe themselves as being "out of it" as family and friends absorb more of their obligations.

Social arrangements become less stable as the disease state progresses and the client continues to deteriorate. Interactions may be further distorted by alterations in the client's physiologic and psychologic state. The use of steroids, which is common during this phase, can cause significant mood swings.

Operations such as oophorectomy and adrenalectomy can cause major changes in physiologic as well as psychologic states. Client and spouse may have difficulty discussing their fears during this phase because of concern with increasing the other person's anxiety or heightening the other person's grief. Sadly, this only leads to estrangement as the high level of anxiety continues. If care requires a great deal of effort, the client may actually promote abandonment for the good of the other family members.

Interactions with the staff are also affected because the client and family don't know how to get started in talking over their fears. Isolation within the family, and family to staff, continues to build. Clients may begin to express anger toward the physician because unconsciously they equated compliance with expected cure. Now that it is obvious that a cure will not occur, the client begins to express the anger and frustration that has been building up over time.

Interventions during this phase are concentrated on comfort measures, maintaining contact, facilitating communication, and support. A nonjudgmental attitude is important to assure the client and family that their outbursts are permissible and will not jeopardize care. Special attention or planning may be needed to assist the client in accomplishing some remaining important tasks of personal life as time and energy run short. The nurse's supportive behavior should also extend to other health care providers in light of the stress they too are experiencing so that care continues to be given in the face of advancing disease.

End of life

The last period, end of life, is the time when death is fast approaching. All pretenses at curing or significantly controlling the cancer have ended. The client is in a very weakened physical condition, so weakened that continuation of valued activities is impossible, leaving the mother who cannot "do," the father who cannot "support" his family, and the child who cannot "play."

The psychologic state of the client is muted. Calm, hopeless expressions are commonly observed. Other reactions will vary depending on the differing perceptions of social death. For some clients and families, death is perceived as a punishment or disgrace. For others, death may be perceived as a time of peace because of a belief in the union with God that follows.

Some clients fear death itself, the ordeal of dying, the fear of losing touch with reality, the fear of dependency, or the tremendous fear of abandonment. During this period, it is important to be available to the client and family but also to provide them privacy as they deal with the approaching death.[9]

For some clients, resolution occurs so that "loose ends" are tied up, goodbyes are said, and there is a quiet awareness of their fate. In some cases, psychologic withdrawal may occur so that the client is observed to "withdraw from living." With these clients, few interactions occur with either staff or family. Here, the health care provider should concentrate on supporting the family as they experience the anticipatory grief and deal with the withdrawal of the client from interactions with them.

The nurse must show respect for clients and let them set the pace in what they wish to discuss and what they need in order to cope. Clients sick enough to die do not need to be told what is happening to them. They may need the consolation of knowing another person shares this awareness. They know what is happening—the client is dying.

CONCLUSION

This chapter has presented an overview of the psychosocial needs of clients and their families. Four periods determined to be high risk were discussed together with suggestions for intervening with these persons.

Communication is considered the central core of this care. Chapters 7 and 19 offer two examples involving nursing interventions in this area of cancer communication.

Four factors affecting the level of psychosocial care for clients with cancer are: the type of illness, the length of illness, the degree of physical dependency imposed on the client, and the number and type of support people available.[3]

The nurse intervening with these clients is involved in six important functions: counseling the client and family, managing symptoms, instructing the family in direct client care, helping them to locate other resources, working with the other health care professionals and agencies, and providing support and comfort.[3]

Nursing has made substantial contributions to the psychosocial care of clients and their families. Research is under way to better document additional needs. Nurses will have greater opportunities for developing more effective points of interventions as they clarify their understanding of the natural history of cancer, the periods of increased risks, and the attendant needs.

REFERENCES

1. Abrams, R. D.: The patient with cancer: his changing pattern of communication, N. Engl. J. Med. **274**:317, 1966.
2. Bard, M.: The price of survival for cancer victims, Transaction **3**(2):10, 1966.
3. Benoliel, J. Q., and McCorkle, R.: A holistic approach to terminal illness, Cancer Nurs. **1**:143, 1978.
4. Hackett, T. P., Cassem, N. H., and Raker, J. W.: Patient delay in cancer, N. Engl. J. Med. **289**(1):14, 1973.
5. Rapoport, L.: The state of crisis: some theoretical considerations. In Parad, H. J., editor: Crisis intervention: selected readings, New York, 1965, Family Service Association of America.
6. Shands, H. C.: The informational impact of cancer on the structure of the human personality, Ann. N. Y. Acad. Sci. **125**:883, 1966.
7. Simonton, D. C., and Simonton, S. S.: Belief systems and management of the emotional aspects of malignancy. In Kruse, L. C., Reese, J. L., and Hart, L. K., editors: Cancer: pathophysiology, etiology, and management—selected readings, St. Louis, 1979, The C. V. Mosby Co.
8. Strauss, A. L., and Glaser, B. G.: Chronic illness and the quality of life, St. Louis, 1975, The C. V. Mosby Co.
9. The International Work Group on Death, Dying, and Bereavement: Assumptions and perceptions underlying standards for terminal care. Am. J. Nurs., vol. 79, February, 1979.
10. Waxenberg, S. E.: The importance of the communication of feelings about cancer, Ann. N. Y. Acad. Sci. **125**:1000, 1966.
11. Worby, C. M., and Babineau, R.: The family interview: helping patient and family cope with metastatic disease, Geriatrics **29**:83, 1974.

5

An ethical basis for cancer nursing practice

JEANNE QUINT BENOLIEL

This chapter is based on an assumption that nursing practice in its essence is a moral art and not a set of scientific and pragmatic techniques. As an art, it draws on knowledge from the arts and the humanities as well as science and technology to be used in the best interests of the consumers of nursing services. It also requires the practitioner to make choices among alternative courses of action that affect the recipient of services in diverse ways but may be highly variable in their support of basic human rights and personal integrity. On a day-to-day basis, cancer nursing practice means frequent choices relative to the personhood and the clienthood of the individual who happens to have cancer. An ethical basis for cancer nursing practice sees attention to personhood—the unique human goals and needs of individuals who happen to be clients—as having top priority in these decisions.

RATIONALE FOR NURSING PRACTICE AS A MORAL ART

Fundamental goals of nursing

According to Curtin,[7] the ethical dimension of nursing practice derives from nursing's historical concern with the welfare of human beings and the special vulnerability of those who are sick. In her view, nurses occupy a unique position among all health professionals to attend to the human needs of those who happen to be clients and to counteract the impingements of disease processes and treatments on loss of independence, loss of freedom of action, and interference with ability to make choices.[9] Such a position sees protection of the humanity of the individual as a primary moral obligation of the nurse.

In recent years, much has been written about the physician's moral obligation to be respectful of the human rights of clients and to avoid exploitation of the vulnerable. Concerning the relationship of medical goals to the personal integrity of clients, Fried[12] described the physician's prime function as not so much the prevention of death as the preservation of life capacities permitting realization of a reasonable life plan. Fried's orientation to personal integrity of recipients of medical care implies four basic rights: lucidity—the right to know all relevant details about one's situation; autonomy—the right to be free from fraud, force, and violence including treatment imposed against the person's wishes: fidelity—the right to expect faithfulness in living up to explicit and implicit expectations in the physician-client relationship; and humanity—the right to have one's particular humanity taken into account.

Given the nature and characteristics of the nurse-client relationship, these concepts are equally relevant to nursing practice, which, perhaps more so than medical practice, influences the social environment in which client care takes place. In Curtin's[9] perspective, nurses can and do control the environments of the institutions in which they work, and they have great power to contribute to the humanizing of these environments. From a moral perspective, nurses as a collectivity have an obligation to create and foster social environments that are responsive to the human concerns of people who are giving and receiving health care services.

Given nursing's historical concern with the care and comfort of those unable to be self-sustaining, nurses can also be viewed as having a moral obligation to implement the principle of distributive justice through equitable allocation of available nursing resources. According to Frankena's[11] usage, distributive justice does not equate equality of treatment with identical treatment. Rather it means providing resources that make the same relative contribution to the goodness of people's lives—in other words, help according to need. Chinn[6] believes that one of the key factors contributing to inadequate infant care in the United States is an underdeveloped use of nursing care resources, and she makes a case that the nursing profession has a moral responsibility to improve the quality of newborn care by more equitable distribution of nursing services among the population. This position subscribes to a moral value of ensuring help to those who are powerless to help themselves. It also implies a moral obligation to protect those who are vulnerable to exploitation from being used in inhuman ways by ruthless or unthinking people.

Vulnerability of people with cancer

Another reason for nursing's concern with ethical matters comes from the reality that nurses' work brings them into frequent contact with people at times of crisis and change. There can be little doubt that living with the various crises associated with cancer is a stressful human experience as has been described in recent writings by Abrams[1] and Weisman.[21] People living in circumstances of crisis and change are highly vulnerable to paternalistic practices by families as well as health care providers, and the nursing literature is full of tales about cancer clients whose right to be informed about their illness was violated by other people.

Given cancer's associations with basic existential concerns, people diagnosed with the disease can be viewed as extremely vulnerable to the power of the medical expert because of their deep-seated wishes to have the cancer cured. The vulnerability of captive populations (such as prisoners or institutionalized clients with mental illness) to uninformed or coerced participation in biomedical experimentation led to federal guidelines governing procedures for informed consent in research involving human subjects.[23] The essence of these guidelines is protection of the individual's right to participate in research only under conditions of informed consent and to withdraw from participation at any time without personal jeopardy.

The special concerns expressed about the use of captive populations in biologic experiments are based on an assumption that people under such circumstances can easily be coerced into giving up their basic human rights to information and choice. The position taken here is that people with cancer comprise another captive population whose captivity rests in their extreme dependency on physicians for information and decisions bearing directly on their personal choices and existential concerns. As Benoliel and McCorkle[4] have shown, captivity for people with cancer can become extreme in terminal illness.

Nursing and nurses occupy powerful positions for fostering an atmosphere in health care that is respectful of human rights and responsive to the human needs of individuals and families faced with disturbing and difficult transitions of which cancer is certainly one. To do so they must confront the reality that nursing work involves two major goals that may not always be congruent.

Conflicts between care and cure

Physicians and nurses have always been caught between two somewhat conflicting goals of practice: to do everything possible to foster and maintain life but to do nothing to prolong pain and suffering needlessly. The cure goal is concerned with clienthood and lifesaving activity. The care goal is concerned with personhood and the quality of human existence. Analytically, the goals of care and cure can be shown to have differences in their origins, major objectives, focal concerns, and modes of intervention as has been outlined in Table 5-1.

A growing problem in nursing practice today is the achievement of a balance between the goals of care and cure. In great measure, the difficulty rests with a health care industry dominated by the biomedical model of disease and institutionalized around the primacy of the lifesaving ethic.[5] The acceleration of advanced medical therapies for cancer, for instance, places pressure on nurses to support and facilitate the goals of medical practice even though these may be at variance with the wishes of some clients.

Finding a balance between care and cure is not simply a matter of choice between one or the other goal. Rather, finding a balance requires an approach for analyzing and understanding clinical situations in which the goals of care and cure come into conflict and create moral problems in which human rights are at risk.[3] Learning to differentiate between moral problems and technical problems in cancer nursing practice requires an understanding of the difference between a nurse's moral obligations and the technical obligations associated with professional expertise.

Moral basis of nursing

In common with all professionals offering services of a health care nature, the nurse has general obligations based on the established moral principles of truth telling, promise keeping, nonharm to clients, and

Table 5-1. Differences in goals of care and cure

Elements	Care	Cure
Origins	Humanities, arts	Science, technology
Major objective	Welfare and well-being of the person	Diagnosis and treatment of disease/illness
Focus of concern	Subjective meanings of disease/treatment experience	Objective aspects of the case
Intervention modes	"Doing with"	"Doing to"

protection of the vulnerable. In addition, the nurse has particular moral obligations rising out of the nurse-client relationship and the client's vulnerability owing to inequality in power. This state of inequality places a special burden on the professional practitioner to protect and facilitate what Pellegrino[19] calls the moral agency of the client and Fried[12] describes as personal integrity. It also makes technical competence a moral obligation on the part of the practitioner as a necessary condition to fulfill the professional contract with clients, whether the contract is explicitly or implicitly stated.

Until recently, very little has been published about the moral dilemmas faced by nurses and the moral obligations carried by them as professional providers. Rather, some writers, such as Gustafson,[13] have referred to nurses as instruments of medical orders with no rights of conscientious objection in morally problematic situations created by physicians. Curtin[7] argues that this denial of the rights of nurses to conscientious objection is not in keeping with the basic tenets of most ethical theories and treats nurses as nonprofessional workers without access to moral autonomy in decision making. One of her concerns is the willingness of society to recognize the importance of the nurse's role in health care delivery and to support the ethical commitments of nurses in their efforts to provide personalized services to their clients. At the same time many nurses, as Langham[15] observed, respond to moral issues encountered in their work by falling back on their established personal belief systems without critical analysis of the moral basis for the position they have taken. Neither the position of no moral rights for nurses nor excessive reliance on unquestioned personal values as a basis for decision making in practice can serve as a moral basis for nursing.

CONDITIONS THAT INHIBIT ETHICAL NURSING PRACTICE

It seems clear that the majority of nurses have not been educated to apply ethical concepts to decision making in practice. Nurses who have had courses in ethics have most likely been introduced to a specific moral doctrine rather than a rational approach for weighing moral and nonmoral elements in particular clinical problems. Thus, among the circumstances that inhibit ethical nursing practice is inadequate education of nurses for the moral nature of their work.

Value conflicts in the work context

Despite inadequate preparation of nurses for responding to moral problems in practice, the nurse-client relationship typically occurs in a context in which conflicts in values, beliefs, and goals are commonplace. The very nature of nursing work brings nurses into frequent confrontation with conflicts regarding life-and-death situations, drugs and behavior control, truth telling versus withholding of information, and the application of triage to the allocation of health care resources. Although triage is generally associated with emergencies, the practical realities are that nurses make triage decisions every day about the distribution of nursing services among their clients.

Murphy[16] believes that the nurse's role in an institutional setting involves inherent conflict between two normative components: an obligation to the rights of the client as an individual and an obligation to uphold and support the goals of the institution. The latter is likely to be utilitarian in nature, meaning the greatest good for the greatest number; nurses are often forced to choose for the institution instead of the individual client. Murphy argues further that the centrality of decision-making practices in hospitals and other health care agencies effectively controls the communication systems in these institutions and prevents practicing nurses from exercising their moral autonomy as professional providers. In other words, the organized system of bureaucratic communication operates to impinge on the nurse's freedom of choice and action in a moral sense. This impingement is reinforced by the problematic nature of coping simultaneously with two chains of command—administrators and physicians. Working in an environment that denigrates the human rights of nurses as well as clients cannot help but affect nurses' attitudes, work habits, and expectations about themselves as health care providers.

Sexist stereotypes of nurses

The fact that nursing is composed primarily of women also functions as an inhibitor of ethical nursing practices. As women, nurses suffer from a sexist stereotype that defines them as passive followers and not as professional providers with rights to stand up for their own autonomy. This image of the nurse is closely related to the traditional feminine role of dependence on the male and limited responsibility for major decisions. Furthermore, there is evidence to suggest that educational environments for nurses have fostered and encouraged the traditional values of subservience and obedience instead of facilitating the development of independent action and autonomous reasoning.[17] In a sense, nurses have been educated for a form of moral reasoning that is oriented to the maintenance of social order and existing rules rather than the human rights of individuals, including themselves. Nursing as a profession suffers from the heritage of the traditional socialization of men and women into restricted roles. These sex-role stereotypes for nurses and physicians are reinforced by the organization of the health care business around professional dominance by physicians.[16]

Confusion between nonmedical questions and medical expertise

A condition deriving directly from professional medical dominance is the health care system's reliance on the physician as expert even though the problem at issue may not appropriately be solved by medical expertise. Yarling[24] makes the point that there are profound differences between a decision to intubate a client and a decision about the disclosure of diagnostic and prognostic information to a terminal client. The former involves a problem that clearly depends on professional technical expertise. The latter is a problem that is moral in nature and should be resolved on the basis of moral considerations. In Yarling's view:

> . . . denying a terminal patient information about his condition is equivalent to denying that person the freedom of self-determination with respect to a fully informed encounter with the ultimate and final experience of human existence.[25]

Yarling[25] notes further that there are serious moral considerations in the physician's order that nurses not disclose diagnostic and prognostic information to a terminal client who asks for it because this action places nurses in triple jeopardy on moral grounds. The argument that withholding such information is in the best interests of the client is based on an assumption that the individual is not capable of dealing with freedom of self-determination (a position originally used as a justification for slavery). A physician who takes such action places the nurse in the position of having to lie to the client on grounds that may not be acceptable to the nurse and also to lie for the physician out of loyalty or deference. In addition, this action creates the problem of the benevolent lie, which undermines trust in the nurse-client relationship and asks the nurse to serve as executor of a policy that lacks ethical standards.

The solution of nonmedical questions in client care by medical expertise and power has serious moral implications not solely for the consumers of services but also for other health care providers. Nurses who are asked to support policies and practices that deny their basic human rights work in a context that lacks institutional justice and fair play. The development of personalized services for clients has limited chance for success when nurses and other health care providers are treated as instruments instead of as human beings with professional and personal rights. The creation of environments conducive to personalized services requires changes in the moral climate of health care institutions and changes in the education of nurses and other providers.[16]

A CONCEPTUAL FRAMEWORK FOR CANCER NURSING PRACTICE

An ethical basis for cancer nursing practice requires a conceptual framework that combines moral and clinical knowledge and skill into a coherent whole. Such a framework makes explicit the values of nursing in statements that clarify the nurse's primary obligation to the client. It offers a methodology for incorporating ethical standards and practices into clinical problem-solving on an ongoing basis.

Protection of self-care agency

According to Orem,[18] the primary focus of nursing practice is the maintenance of self-care activities by individuals to sustain life and health, recover from disease and injury, and cope with the effects of incapacitation and change. In society nurses are called on to implement systems of therapeutic self-care for individuals and families when there are deficits in their abilities to provide for themselves. Curtin[9] believes that nurses by virtue of the unique circumstances of their contacts with clients have a special responsibility to protect the unity of the person and to serve as human advocates for the uniqueness of the individual. Given this orientation, cancer nursing practice carries a primary obligation to assist the person with cancer in coping with the personal meanings that clienthood has brought about and in supporting freedom of choice and direct involvement in decision making about present and future life.

Problem analysis in clinical situations

Cancer nursing practice requires a problem-solving approach that amalgamates knowledge and skills of several kinds into a conceptual framework that makes logical sense and encompasses the context as well as the focus of work. The knowledge base for cancer nursing comes from a range of sources and includes the following: malignant disease, its manifestations and modes of medical treatment[14]; personal responses to adversity and coping strategies[21]; family dynamics, adaptations, and coping modes[22]; direct care activities including comfort measures[10]; information exchange and evaluation of outcomes[3]; communication strategies and evaluation of outcomes[3]; and crisis theory and support systems.[22] To these should be added two relevant domains of knowledge: (1) analysis of social systems, identification of points of influence, and evaluation of interventions in the system and (2) moral philosophy with an emphasis on normative ethics.

Knowledge for knowledge's sake is not enough for cancer nursing practice. Clinical knowledge and skills are essential for understanding the impact of clienthood on the person and for taking action to protect and facilitate self-care agency. As Welch[22] has noted, assessment of the impact of cancer and cancer treatment involves not just the client and family but also the nurse. She identified four areas of concern in planning interventions involving the person with cancer: information giving, client education, direct client care, and communication skills. Four additional areas of concern were related to dealing with the families of clients: assessment of family resources and adaptations, family education, direct family intervention, and emotional support and communication skills.

The art of cancer nursing practice means using these several skills in deliberate ways to assist the client and family in coping with the impact of cancer on their lives. This process of making choices and decisions in clinical situations depends on more than knowledge in isolation. It requires conceptual understanding and the application of logical reasoning to problems encountered in the field. It is facilitated by a capacity to differentiate between science and practice in terms of primary goals, major values, and expected outcomes. It is an area in which many nurses have had limited opportunities for personal development.

A decision-making model to guide choice of action

Assuming that protection of personal integrity in the nurse-client relationship is a central commitment in cancer nursing practice, responsible ethical choice becomes an imperative. Sigman[20] describes the derivation of responsible ethical choice in nursing and examines how such choice involves the concepts of responsibility, accountability, risk, commitment, and justice. In her view, nurses are faced daily with decisions involving moral and ethical choices and could profit from knowledge about normative ethics and its application. More than that, Sigman[20] makes a case that each individual nurse needs to develop a personal ethical system as a basis for taking reasoned and deliberate action in situations involving moral principles and true choices between alternative courses of action.

The development of a personal ethical system is not a trivial matter. Ethics is concerned with the values of human life—what is good and what is right—organized in a systematic manner. Ethics is simultaneously concerned with definitions of duty in the moral sense. Tied together the two theories of value and obligation provide a framework for a particular ethical system that can guide the individual nurse in making responsible ethical choices. As Sigman[20] has made clear, every ethical problem faced by a nurse is a combination of *choice* between what "ought to" be done (duty) and *judgment* about the value (moral rightness) of a chosen action.

The establishment of a knowledge base in normative ethics requires an understanding of basic human rights and the meaning of moral conduct in human interactions and transactions. Bandman[2] makes the point that for any human right of importance three conditions must be met: the equal right of all persons to be free; rights imply achievable obligations to others; and conditions of justice and equality must exist. Bandman also notes that although clients have a right and a choice with regard to participating in a prescribed treatment, health care providers have a duty and no choice. Duty as a professional obligation is not a right in the human rights sense of the word. It is a special responsibility to the client based on professional expertise, but its exercise is a privilege requiring the consent of the person being served.

One function of a personal ethical system is to provide direction for the establishment of priorities in cancer nursing practice. The application of critical ethical analysis to concrete situations can be used to differentiate between moral problems and profes-

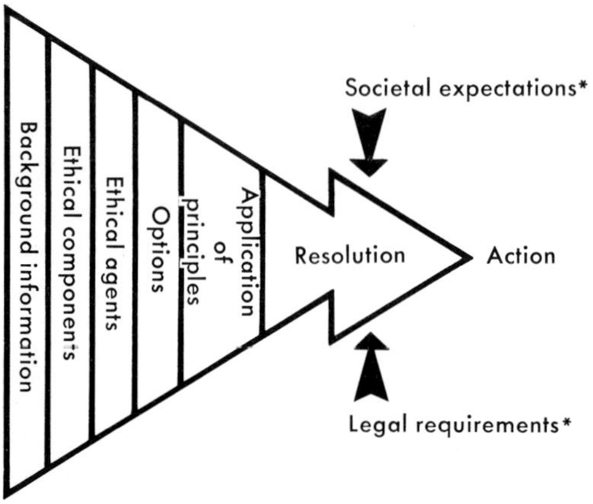

Fig. 5-1. Schematic of proposed decision-making model. *"These extrinsic factors may sway the resolution of the conflict one way or another. But one must not confuse the notions of what is legal (or expected) with what is good, right or proper—they may or may not coincide." (From Curtin, L. L.: Nurs. Forum **XVII**(1):17, 1978.)

A PROPOSED MODEL FOR CRITICAL ETHICAL ANALYSIS*

A method or model for ethical decision making ought to have incorporated all the following factors:

Background information. Not every factor in a situation will have relevance, but quite frequently we cannot fully understand or correctly appraise the "rightness or wrongness" of a given action without first knowing as much about the circumstances as possible. Those factors having direct bearing on the decision at hand must be identified and organized so that we can get as clear a picture as possible of what precisely *is* the problem.

Identification of ethical components. Once we have clarified the problem, we must identify its ethical components; very few dilemmas are purely ethical. Examples of such components would be: freedom vs. authority; truth telling vs. withholding the truth; treating or letting die; alleviation of pain vs. the preservation of life; and conflicts of rights.

Ethical agents. Ethical agents are all those persons who are involved in the decision making. In the health care context this would first and foremost involve the patient. Other persons involved would (or could) be the patient's family, physician, nurse, institution, clergyman, social worker, physical therapist, various consultants, and perhaps even the courts. The rights, duties, and responsibilities of each must be clarified and analyzed. One might also consider various situational factors that could limit the freedom of each to engage in rational decision making and/or to implement action. All the persons engaged in the decision making may or more likely may not agree, but the scope of their rights, duties, and authority can be identified and clarified.

*From Curtin, L. L.: Nurs. Forum **XVII**(1):13, 1978.

A PROPOSED MODEL FOR CRITICAL ETHICAL ANALYSIS—cont'd

Identification of options. All possible options must be explored in light of the duties and responsibilities of those involved and accepted or rejected according to actual or potential results each action could (would) produce. This process will most likely limit the number of acceptable options. Those situations in which our duties conflict with the results of our actions form the most difficult subject matter of ethics. A common example of this conflict would be that of a soldier captured by the enemy who is given the choice between becoming a traitor (duty to country) and being tortured, mutilated, and/or killed (undesirable outcome).

Application of principles. Generally ethicists hold that ethics is not concerned with human behavior per se, but rather with *human acts;* i.e., those actions that are intentional and freely chosen. Only human acts are held to have ethical import. An adequate approach must take into account: 1) what sort of human beings we are or ought to be; 2) the extent to which the human being is free rather than determined; and 3) the way in which the human person carries on the processes of ethical deliberation and decision making. Some theories hold certain actions to be wrong in themselves because they either debase the human being or frustrate his/her nature; others to be right in themselves because they enhance human nature. Other theories may hold that actions contrary to the dignity and freedom of individuals are wrong in themselves, and those that promote freedom and dignity are right in themselves. Those ethical theorists who espouse an appeal to authority in the form of the sacred Scriptures would also preclude certain human acts as wrong in themselves or include others that are right in themselves (e.g., the Ten Commandments). It would always be wrong to murder, to steal, and so on—and it would always be right to worship God, honor your parents, be faithful to one's spouse, and so on. If an act is judged to be wrong in itself (depending upon the general principles applied), it would be eliminated from the remaining options.

Resolution and ethical ideals. Normative ethical theorists have always sought for principles or guides by which to judge acts and situations. Identifying the principles relied upon in this particular situation will help: 1) to clarify the meaning and application of the general principles; 2) to clarify for the individuals involved the reasons for which a particular decision is made (as such it will not guarantee agreement, but certainly will promote understanding); and 3) will also help in future decision making regarding similar situations.

After examining the relevant data, rights, duties, consequences and ethical principles involved in a specific situation, one will be as prepared as possible to determine a course of action.

Perhaps this proposed model, or some other model, may offer some assistance to those in the health professions who must make difficult decisions—particularly when they may be deciding what is "good" for someone else. Obviously one of the major duties of nurses, physicians, and others must be to refrain from making decisions for patients/clients insofar as possible and do all in their power to facilitate (not manipulate) decision making on the part of patients/clients and their families. However, there will always be the patient who is unable to make a decision and who may not have a surrogate or advocate. For this reason alone, courses in ethics emphasizing and developing skill in critical ethical analysis should be a priority for all those in the health professions.

sional problems in the clinical world and to facilitate choice of action appropriate to the problem at issue. Fig. 5-1 and the accompanying boxed material contain a schematic of a proposed decision-making model developed by Curtin[8] as a guide for critical analysis of problems with ethical components. Her original description of the factors comprising the model are listed within the model.

ORGANIZATIONS CONDUCIVE TO ETHICAL DECISION MAKING

The daily work of nurses offering services to people with cancer involves them in complex clinical problems with professional, moral, and legal implications of various kinds. Yet few have been prepared for giving serious attention to the ethics of health care practice, and the system through which these services are delivered can scarcely be characterized as equitable and just in the balance of attention given to care and cure. Increased consideration of the moral dimensions of these services requires health care providers oriented to the ethical problems they face, social contexts that promote moral decisions, and public policy that demands moral accountability.

Practitioners educated for accountable nursing practice

Murphy[16] believes that accountable nursing practice requires nurses who have learned to engage in moral reasoning that is separate from institutional norms and authority. Such learning can probably only come about when schools of nursing create learning environments that recognize the rights and dignity of the learner and promote institutional justice through fairness and democratic processes. Nursing assignments that perpetuate unquestioning obedience and lack of responsibility for the consequences of actions taken need to give way to assignments that introduce conflict and contradiction as real life situations to be confronted through dialogue and exchange of ideas with the faculty.[16]

Nurses educated to be held accountable for ethical decisions would need to have developed a reflective understanding of basic human rights and the concomitant obligations implied by those rights. Such nurses would have developed an ability to weigh various alternatives and to estimate the consequences of one action over another. These nurses would have learned to give consideration to situational factors including the rights of all participants in the decision-making process. These nurses would be capable of differentiating among professional, legal, and moral obligations and of taking action appropriate to the situation. In a collective way, these nurses would be capable of effective collaboration in practice and responsible for the services they offer together.

A context that promotes moral decisions

Just as the learning of moral reasoning requires an educational setting that is equitable and just in its treatment of the student and the faculty, so also the offering of health care services geared to basic human rights requires a social structure respectful of both the recipients and the deliverers of services. Such a context cannot thrive in an atmosphere of professional dominance but requires the development of social mechanisms that safeguard the professional prerogatives and moral autonomy of all health care providers involved and promotes collaborative working arrangements among them. Special social mechanisms are needed for responding to difficult moral problems in which the best interests of highly vulnerable clients are at stake. These special arrangements should provide for membership and representation from all concerned parties as well as methodologies for dealing with differences of opinion in an equitable manner.

A context that promotes moral decisions in practice does more than simply provide for the protection of vulnerable people. It is organized to promote the enhancement of the autonomy of all persons involved, recipient and deliverer of services alike. Such a context for practice would be based on an overall ethic of health care in which moral considerations in the delivery of services to the public—in this case, people with cancer and their families—would depend on three interrelated elements: ethically oriented practitioners in all of the health care disciplines, mutually accepted and understood standards and norms governing interdisciplinary as well as individual decisions in practice, and societal policies and practices that allocate available resources in terms of equitable cost/benefit determinations and that safeguard the interests of future as well as present generations.[4] A context promoting ethical decision making in practice would clearly need a well-developed ethic of collaboration.

Public policy and moral accountability

Ultimate public policy in a democratic society determines the extent to which organizations that deliver human services and the people who provide them will be held accountable for their moral responsibilities to individuals and to society. As citizens, nurses need to be aware of the importance of consumer involvement and active participation in the determination of policies governing the allocation of resources for care and cure and the protection of vulnerable people from conditions of exploitation. As professional providers long concerned with the human side of practice, nurses as a collectivity have an unusual opportunity to influence the direction of health care in the future through political action as informed consumers. Curtin[7] believes that nurses have a moral obligation to support their professional associations as a means of working together toward the goal of quality nursing care for the citizens of society.

REFERENCES

1. Abrams, R. D.: Not alone with cancer, Springfield, Ill., 1974, Charles C Thomas, Publisher.
2. Bandman, B.: The human rights of patients, nurses, and other health professionals. In Bandman, E. L., and Bandman, B., editors: Bioethics and human rights, Boston, 1978, Little, Brown & Co.
3. Benoliel, J. Q.: Overview: care, cure and the challenge of choice. In Earle, A. M., Argondizzo, N. T., and Kutscher, A. H., editors: The nurse as caregiver for the terminal patient and his family, New York, 1976, Columbia University Press.
4. Benoliel, J. Q., and McCorkle, R.: Ethical issues in treatment. In Proceedings of the Second National Conference on Cancer Nursing, New York, 1977, American Cancer Society, Inc.
5. Benoliel, J. Q.: The changing social context of life and death decisions, Essence **2**(2):5, 1978.
6. Chinn, P. L.: Issues in lowering infant mortality: a call for ethical action, Adv. Nurs. Sci. **1**:63, 1979.
7. Curtin, L. L.: Nursing ethics: theories and pragmatics, Nurs. Forum **XVII**(1):4, 1978.
8. Curtin, L. L.:A proposed model for critical ethical analysis, Nurs. Forum **XVII**(1):12, 1978.
9. Curtin, L. L.: The nurse as advocate: a philosophical foundation for nursing, Adv. Nurs. Sci. **1**:1, 1979.
10. Donovan, M., and Pierce, S.; Cancer care nursing, New York, 1976, Appleton-Century-Crofts.
11. Frankena, W. K.: Ethics, ed. 2, Englewood Cliffs, N.J., 1973, Prentice-Hall, Inc.
12. Fried, C.: Medical experimentation: personal integrity and social policy, New York, 1974, American Elsevier, p. 94.
13. Gustafson, J. M.: Mongolism, parental desires and the right to life, Perspect. Biol. Med. **16**:529, 1973.
14. Kruse, L. C., Reese, J. L., and Hart, L. K.: Cancer: pathophysiology, etiology, and management, St. Louis, 1979, The C. V. Mosby Co.
15. Langham, P.: Open forum: on teaching ethics to nurses, Nurs. Forum **XVI**(3 and 4):220, 1977.
16. Murphy, C. P.: The moral situation in nursing. In Bandman, E. L., and Bandman, B., editors: Bioethics and human rights, Boston, 1978, Little, Brown & Co.

17. Olesen, V. L., and Whittaker, E. W.: The silent dialogue, San Francisco, 1968, Jossey-Bass, Inc., Publishers.
18. Orem, D. E.: Nursing: concepts of practice, New York, 1971, McGraw-Hill Book Co.
19. Pellegrino, E. D.: Toward a reconstruction of medical morality: the primacy of the act of profession and the fact of illness, J. Med. Philos. **4**:32, 1979.
20. Sigman, P.: Ethical choice in nursing, Adv. Nurs. Sci. **1**:37, 1979.
21. Weisman, A.: Coping with cancer, New York, 1979, McGraw-Hill Book Co.
22. Welch, D.: Assessing psychosocial needs involved in cancer patient care during treatment, Oncology Nurs. Forum **6**:12, 1979.
23. Wojcik, J.: Muted consent, West Lafayette, Indiana, 1978, Purdue University Press, p. 7.
24. Yarling, R. R.: Ethical analysis of a nursing problem: the scope of nursing practice in disclosing the truth to terminal patients, Part I, Supervisor Nurse **9**:40, 1978.
25. Yarling, R. R.: Ethical analysis of a nursing problem: the scope of nursing practice in disclosing the truth to terminal patients, Part II, Supervisor Nurse **9**:29, 1978.

6

Client education: an integral part of cancer nursing

JUDITH BOND JOHNSON and MARY H. GREEN

Any chronic disease requires active client participation for it is the *client rather than the health care provider* who must live with the disease day after day. This fact is no less true of cancer. With over 700,000 newly diagnosed cancer patients annually, increased attention is being given to not only how *long* people can live with cancer but also to how *well* they might live within the constraints of their illness. Client education programs can contribute much to providing quality of life for persons with cancer.

OVERVIEW AND BACKGROUND OF CLIENT EDUCATION

Changing concepts

Client education is not a new concept in the health care system. In the past decade, however, the concept of client education has changed substantially. There has been a shift from primarily unplanned, fragmented, and incidental experiences to programs that are purposefully designed, systematically applied, and comprehensive in scope.[7]

Today, client education is designed for inpatients and outpatients; implemented on a one-to-one basis or in groups; delivered in a variety of settings; and conducted by physicians, nurses, social workers, or by people specifically designated as client educators.[6] The one element central to all client education programs is the necessity of gearing it to the *specific needs* of the persons or the group for whom it is intended.[39]

Numerous factors in recent years have provided the rationale for, and contributed to, a growing emphasis on client education. These factors will most likely influence the future direction of client education as well.

Aging of the population

As the population of elderly persons in the country increases, so also will the number of individuals increase who have chronic diseases and disabilities. The identification of chronic illnesses as major health problems has provided considerable stimulus for the development of client education services.[37] Herein lies a challenge for cancer nurses who need to find a means of assisting chronically ill persons with cancer to care for themselves.

The consumers' rights movement

The consumers' rights movement also impacts on the development of client education. "A Patient's Bill of Rights," adopted by the American Hospital Association, outlines the client's right to know. It states that "the patient [client] has the right to obtain from the physician complete current information concerning his diagnosis, treatment, and prognosis in terms he can be reasonably expected to understand . . . ." and that "the patient [client] has the right to refuse treatment to the extent permitted by law and to be informed of the medical consequences of his action . . . ."[2]

Changes in the delivery of health care

Medical practice itself is changing. Prepaid health care plans, offered to people in various forms, are on the increase. National health insurance is being proposed by the federal government. There is nationwide concern with health care delivery, its quality and its cost.[40]

Increasing accountability of the health care provider

A further element that has set the stage for expansion of client education has been legal actions and judicial decisions. The policies of "informed consent" and "informed discharge" are altering the health care system. Health care institutions have a responsibility for determining the quality of care that is provided to clients. Client education is considered one component of quality of care. Auditing medical and nursing records is now part of hospital regulations.

RATIONALE FOR CLIENT EDUCATION WITHIN CANCER NURSING PRACTICE

Client education has increasingly become a recognizable component of cancer nursing practice. The document, *Outcome Standards for Cancer Nursing Practice,* coauthored by the Oncology Nursing Society and the American Nurses' Association, provides a set of standards and criteria for the practice of cancer nursing. Client education is distinctly identified as outcome criteria for the majority of the 12 standards. In addition, one standard is set aside *specifically* for client education. It reads:

> The client and family possess knowledge about the disease and therapy in order to attain self-management, participation in therapy, optimal living, and peaceful death.[29]

The rationale for this standard is:

> The client and family have a right to accurate information about the disease, options for treatment, consequences of treatment, potential oncologic emergencies, alternative care settings, and resources.[29]

Thus, client education is clearly identified by the authors of these standards as an essential component of cancer nursing practice.

When cancer is viewed as a group of chronic illnesses, the concept of rehabilitation becomes a necessary element of the health care plan for persons with cancer. Rehabilitation emphasizes the restoration of individuals to optimal function and performance in the face of a chronic disease and the reintegration of the individuals into the affairs of daily living and society commensurate with the limitation imposed by the disease process.[25] A significant component of rehabilitation is the modification and adaptation of behavior to adjust to the disease. This usually requires the learning of new behavior on the part of the clients. Educational programs that help clients learn these new behaviors are an appropriate part of the rehabilitation process of a person with cancer. The process of rehabilitation can be accelerated by increasing clients' knowledge of the latest health care practices encompassing cancer.

JUSTIFICATION FOR CLIENT EDUCATION: STUDIES RELATED TO ADAPTING TO CHRONIC ILLNESS

Cancer makes demands on clients and family members because of the illusive nature of the disease and the resultant stresses.[26] This usually requires the development of new coping strategies that will facilitate adaptation to the disease. The way in which clients adapt to their chronic disease often determines the difference between optimum recovery or psychologic invalidism.[23]

Goals and objectives for client education embrace a number of significant factors directed at successful adaptation. It is difficult to attribute program success to one of these factors as they are closely interrelated within the person's whole being. The following studies demonstrate the necessity for providing educational opportunities if, indeed, clients are to be considered active participants in their own adaptation process.

Providing information

Information giving is frequently cited as the major goal of client education programs. Clients who are expected to participate actively in their own treatment need information about their illnesses and their related treatments. The problem that exists is that much information is not understood by the client, nor is instruction necessarily followed by the client.[17] Research has shown that physicians generally underrate clients as to what health information they possess, so they therefore tend to be too elementary in their explanations.[32] Another study demonstrated that half of the clients discharged from hospitals had unanswered questions at the time of discharge. The problem of noncompliance with medical regimens was substantiated by Steward and Cluff[38] who reported that 30% to 50% of clients fail to take their drugs properly. Simmonds summarized a number of other studies by saying that it appears that today's clients do not comply with at least one half to two thirds of the recommendations made by their physicians.[37]

When client education is properly related to other components of health care services, there is clear potential for impact on improved health behaviors of people with diagnosed illnesses. For example, a program of information to diabetic clients in a county hospital setting reduced the annual rate of readmissions to approximately one in five. Emergency room visits were reduced by 50% and a potential cost savings of between $1.7 million and $3.4 million was projected.[14] Other studies indicated that when clients are adequately informed regarding their treatment and care, they adhere to prescribed diets, follow physicians' instructions, have fewer hospital admissions, and have shorter hospital stays.[3,34] Hendin[15] found significant changes in a program of self-infusion for hemophiliac clients. Hospital days were cut from 432 to 42 and outpatient visits decreased per client from 23 to 5. This alteration in health behavior directly affected the survival rate for these people.

Numerous studies indicate that when clients receive instruction directed at helping them understand the nature of their illness and the specific role they are expected to play in their own rehabilitation program, there is less need for hospitalization and greater adherence to medication, rest, diet, and exercise regimens.[17] Thus, health educators have reason to develop programs of education that facilitate people learning how to exercise their responsibility for taking care of themselves to the maximum extent possible.

In addition to people's physical problems, there are also emotional responses to chronic illness. These reactions influence how people proceed toward adapting to their illness. The quality and speed with which learning takes place will also be affected.[27]

Reducing anxiety

Anxiety is probably the most common emotional reaction people experience when becoming ill. This reaction may be manifested in many ways and may vary in degree, but it frequently leads to confusion and limits a person's coping ability.[24] Educational programs have been shown to assist people in recognizing their anxiety and in developing strategies for dealing with the underlying causes of their anxiety.

Information about aspects of diseases and their medical treatment has been shown to reduce clients' anxiety levels. In some cases it made the difference between a client seeking treatment or not.[13] DiBartalo[9] concluded from his study that anxiety level and body image perception were significant factors for success in the rehabilitative program of persons with cancer of head and neck. Other studies suggested that people who have adequate means for discharge of their tension and anxiety may have a more favorable later course with cancer than those without such adaptive opportunities.[22] Holland[16] researched women's psychologic adjustment to radiotherapy for the treatment of breast cancer. She reported that diffuse anxiety decreased significantly in the group of women who were informed and prepared emotionally for their treatment. In a study done by Johnson,[19] clients' anxiety levels were significantly reduced following their participation in a 12-hour educational course about cancer and related concerns.

Minimizing the sense of helplessness

Cancer may also elicit a sense of helplessness in clients. The onset of this chronic disease may require them to alter their lifestyle. This, in turn, modifies or causes loss of the sense of meaning and purpose that has been their source of identity and the mainspring of their energy in the past. Cancer also forces people to relinquish control of their lives, at least temporarily, to their physicians. Feelings of powerlessness and frustration are caused by loss of control over such things as medical procedures, appointments, and hospital routines. A lack of knowledge about the disease further heightens people's fears relative to loss of power and personal control over what is happening to their bodies and to their lives.[18]

Fostering hope

It is most vital to foster hope in clients. Coping, as a goal-directed process, allows people to define problems. It brings relief, reward, and equilibrium.[21] The following studies give evidence to support the notion that a sense of meaning in life appears to be related to how a person adapts in the face of illness.

Both Seligman[36] and O'Neill[30] found that feelings of helplessness and loss of control were very real for persons dealing with a life-threatening disease. Another study showed that clients who held a strong negative feeling about their illness had less hope, were more anxious, and had little faith in the competence of their physician.[35] In a study by Johnson,[19] participation in a client education course was found to have a significant effect on cancer clients' self-reported sense of meaning in life. Crumbaugh[8] reported that when people must yield to an altered lifestyle, they experience a loss in sense of meaning and purpose in life, which in turn affects their sense of actualization and source of energy. New values and reasons for living must be explored, otherwise people will lapse into a state of hopelessness and despair.

This review of studies in the field of client education justifies the necessity for providing educational opportunities for persons who must learn to adapt to chronic illnesses, particularly ones that are as serious as cancer. The available data show that educational programming can offer clients assistance in redefining their life goals and expectations, in learning new health behaviors, and in supporting them in becoming active participants in their own health care.

The demonstrated impact of client education and its natural applicability to nursing mandates a discussion of ways nurses can increase their participation in this area of health care. Therefore, the remainder of this chapter will be directed at providing practical step-by-step guidelines for developing, implementing, and evaluating client education programs.

STEP-BY-STEP DEVELOPMENT OF CANCER CLIENT EDUCATION

Education may be thought of as involving two types of knowledge—*content knowledge,* which is theory, facts, principles, and protocols, and *process knowledge,* which is the practical application of content knowledge and all that is learned by individual experience. The purpose of this discussion is to provide some of the *content knowledge* in client education; the *process knowledge* can then be developed by the nurse based on individual practice settings.

The methods presented here are widely used in client education, and the references cited here have been found to be germane to all phases of client education. Encouragement is given to obtain and utilize these resources as the essential "how to" tools they are.

The following two publications are available; they describe in detail the steps of client education as discussed in this chapter:

Deliberations of the Cancer Patient Education Workshop, January 30-31, 1979
U.S. Department of Health, Education and Welfare
Public Health Service
National Institutes of Health
Order from: Office of Cancer Communications
National Cancer Institute
Building 31, Room 10A18
9000 Rockville Pike
Bethesda, Maryland 20205
Cost: Free

A Model for Planning Patient Education—An Essential Component of Health Care, Publication No. 76-4028
Report of the Committee on Educational Tasks in Chronic Illness, Public Health Education Section, American Public Health Association (APHA)
Order from: NTIS, Operations Division
U.S. Department of Commerce
5285 Port Royal Road
Springfield, Virginia 22161
OR
Superintendent of Documents
U.S. Government Printing Office
Washington, D.C. 20402
Cost: Free

The five steps described in the APHA model will serve as a framework for the remainder of this chapter. These steps are sequential and dependent on previous steps but are not isolated one from another. In actual practice, the steps generally interrelate and overlap.

Step I. Identify the educational needs of client and family

As in the nursing process, assessment or identification of needs is the first step in client education. Assessment involves a careful, methodical, time-consuming gathering of information that "seeks the counsel of many." Adequate assessment is *essential* if effective education is the goal.

It is difficult, if not impossible, to make

meaningful observations based on planned activity. It is generally through casual observation that the beginning point for assessment is started. This is a process whereby impressions are formulated, broad areas of concern are identified, or general problems become apparent. This type of observation should be approached with as few preconceived ideas or biases as possible. Casual observation helps the observer begin to define what *should* be observed in a more systematic way with more specific goals or questions. Beyond the casual observations a variety of more specific assessment methods are useful for different settings including:

- The one-to-one interview that has a structured or nonstructured format and is done in person or by telephone
- The group interview that can have a structured or nonstructured format
- The survey or questionnaire
- The computer library search such as ERIC or MEDLINE

Assessment of the client can be accomplished by using at least *two* different methods to obtain information from at least *two* different sources. Table 6-1 provides a list of potential sources of information to be used for assessment. Resources such as time and money, type of institution, and experience of the assessor will influence the various methods and sources to be used. However, clients should always be included as one major source of information during the assessment stage. Utilizing multiple methods and sources provides more objective verification of actual needs.

For example, casual observation during nursing rounds may help the nurse-teacher formulate the *subjective* opinion that clients repeatedly ask questions about skin reactions after radiation therapy. The observation that these questions signify unmet needs should then be *objectively* verified. This verification may involve a survey of clients and health care team members to identify what is *being* taught and what *should* be taught. Surveying both these groups identifies discrepancies and omissions by comparing answers from both sources.

It should be reinforced that the ability to ask questions in a manner that elicits meaningful answers is a skill that can be learned. Table 6-1 lists the type of information most often derived from each source. Knowing or anticipating the kinds of information that can be expected from potential assessment sources helps to formulate meaningful questions. Numerous texts on interviewing techniques are also helpful in learning how to ask meaningful questions. Help in learning how to write good test and survey questions is available in a booklet:

Instructions for the Construction of Test Items in Health Fields
Professional Examination Service
475 Riverside Drive
New York, New York 10027
Copyright 1972

Other valuable resources for developing assessment questions and surveys are nurses in nursing education or inservice departments in hospitals and schools of nursing educators or instructors in education departments in community colleges.

Step II. Establish educational goals for client and family

Step II in the client education planning process should ideally read "establish educational goals *with* client and family." The establishment of goals should involve the client–family learner rather than be mandated solely by the nurse-teacher. Likewise, goals should be written so that the desired results can be measured.

A learning goal or educational objective is a statement of desired changes in the

Table 6-1. Potential sources of assessment information and types of information expected

Potential sources of information	Types of information
Clients; family members/friends	Identification of psychosocial needs; unique perception of cancer's impact on their lives; regrets—what they wish they had done, known, or been told; advice for others—ways to cope, solutions to problems
Health care professional, for example, nurse, physician, dietitian, social worker, dentist, dental hygienist, physical and occupational therapists, chaplain, and so forth	Opinions of common problems and solutions; perception of unmet needs; opinions on what clients need to know—life alterations, expectations, treatment—disease effects, self-care measures, new skills
Medical and nursing records/ audit	Statistics identifying common client care problems, some of which may be amenable to educational intervention; areas of omission or increased liability
Morbidity/mortality statistics—institutional, community, state, national	Statistics identifying incidence of various diagnoses, treatment and diagnostic procedures, utilization of services, causes of death, causes of disease complications; areas of high risk such as environmental and/or occupational
Professional literature	Verification of commonality of needs; suggestions or solutions to similar problems; lack of evidence in literature may also strongly support need to define and solve newly identified problem
Lay literature	Topics of interest to public; evidence of incorrect or misleading news articles, especially in tabloids; insight into what clients may understand and read
Nursing and physician grand rounds, conferences, and tumor boards	Casual observation of common needs and problems; incidence statistics of causes of morbidity and mortality
Service organizations, for example, American Cancer Society, Leukemia Society, United Ostomy Association	Availability of resources, services, and teaching materials; statistics on use of resources indicates some degree of need or interest and evaluation of service or teaching material; opinions on unmet areas of need
Professional resources, for example, Oncology Nursing Society, Office of Cancer Communications and Cancer Information Clearinghouse of National Cancer Institute, American Society of Clinical Oncology	Identification of unmet needs; information on availability of resources for solutions to problems, teaching materials, client education programs, pertinent research studies

Table 6-2. Some verbs for use in stating behavioral objectives*

Indicates ability to recall knowledge	Indicates understanding	Indicates transfer of knowledge
Define	Restate	Translate
Memorize	Discuss	Interpret
Repeat	Describe	Apply
Record	Recognize	Employ
List	Explain	Use
Recall	Express	Demonstrate
Name	Identify	Dramatize
Relate	Locate	Practice
Underline	Report	Illustrate
	Review	Operate
	Tell	Schedule
		Shop
		Sketch

*From Bloom, B. S., editor: Taxonomy of educational objectives: handbook I—cognitive domain, New York, 1956, David McKay Co.

learner's behavior as a result of learning. The desired behavioral change may involve differences in knowledge, attitudes, or skills on the part of the learner. Nevertheless, well-formulated learning objectives have four components:

who—who is the learner?
task statement—desired change in behavior or result
criteria—standard utilized to measure success in achieving the desired change in behavior
conditions—provisions that describe optimal circumstances for a performance

Table 6-2 lists action verbs that are useful in developing behaviorial objectives. The following examples of educational objectives utilize some of these verbs with the four components indicated in parentheses for each example.

- After viewing leukemia A-V program (*condition*), client (*who*) will define leukemia (*task statement*) as a cancer of the bone marrow, not as disease of the blood (*criteria*).
- Client (*who*) will restate (*task statement*) four of six signs of infection to report to local physician (*criteria*) as listed in "Chemotherapy Teaching Plan" before hospital discharge (*condition*).
- Client (*who*) will list (*task statement*) all the colostomy supplies his wife should purchase for home use (*task statement*) by July 10 (*criteria*).
- Client's children (*who*) will begin (*criteria*) to express their feelings about the changes in their mother's appearance (*task statement*).

These four components were developed by Jones and Oertel[20] and are an excellent resource for learning to formulate educational objectives:

Developing Patient Teaching Objectives and Techniques: A Self-Instructional Program
Nursing Resources, Inc.
Box J-77
607 North Avenue
Wakefield, Maine 01880

Step III. Select appropriate educational methods

The choice of the actual teaching-learning method to be employed depends on a combination of factors such as the number of clients with identified learning needs, the nature of learning objectives, the availability and experience of the teacher(s), the availability of teaching materials, and the learning style of the clients.

Individuals do have learning styles or ways in which they learn most effectively. Some people need the support of a group for learning while others prefer to study independently. It is generally acknowledged that most people do not know how they learn best, possibly because they have never thought about it. Therefore, accurate tools to assess learning styles and associated personality factors that affect learning can be useful in selecting the most efficacious educational methods.

Table 6-3. Methods of teaching/learning and possible teaching tools

Teaching/learning methods	Teaching tools and materials
One to one	Films/video tape
Discussion	Slides
Interview	Filmstrips
Questioning	Slides or filmstrips with audio tape/audio record
Role modeling	Tours or field trips
Demonstration	Transparencies
Recitation	Pamphlets
Behavior modification and contracting	Handouts
Independent study	Flip charts/posters
Programmed learning	Talking books
Computer assisted	Chalk boards
Autotutorial	Flannel boards
Correspondence course	Models
Telelecture	Textbooks
Creative writing or artwork	Computer audio and/or video
Group	Tape recordings
Discussion	Drawing or coloring materials (such as coloring books)
Lecture	Written materials
Recitation	
Role playing	
Demonstration	
Simulation games	

Table 6-3 provides a list of various teaching-learning methods and subsequent teaching tools from which to choose. The choice of the best method or tool is generally based on knowledge of the factors just listed. There is no magic formula for deciding which method or tool is best. What the nurse thinks will work best for the client population is a most significant factor. For example, learning stoma self-care can generally be learned more efficiently and effectively when the learner is involved in an actual demonstration of care rather than by a group discussion or lecture.

Because of the recent intensive activity in client education, many teaching aids and complete client education programs have already been developed. In terms of cancer education, one of the best resources is the Cancer Information Clearinghouse, located in the Office of Cancer Communications of the National Cancer Institute, National Institute of Health. Adapting available programs to the individual setting and client population is generally more economical than attempting to produce all the client teaching programs within your institution.

If new materials are needed, an essential step in developing these materials as well as utilizing those produced elsewhere is the comparison of the reading level of the client and that of the instructional messages. Much of what has been intended as information for *clients* is not easily understood by them because the terminology is too technical. Drug package inserts are prime examples of this. The National Cancer Institute[28] has developed a helpful pamphlet with easy to apply formulas for evaluating client education materials:

Readability testing in cancer communication methods, examples and resources for improving the readability of cancer messages and materials, Publication No. 79-1689
Office of Cancer Communications
National Cancer Institute
Building 31, Room 10A18
9000 Rockville Pike
Bethesda, Maryland 20205

Step IV. Carry out the educational program

The implementation step is simply putting into action the educational program that has been developed. In addition, other elements exist that, if they have not already been dealt with previously, must be addressed during this step. Failure to tend to these elements can generally inhibit an otherwise worthwhile client education endeavor.

Topping the list of these elements is communication, preferably in writing, with everyone who needs to know about a planned client education intervention. Practically speaking, "everyone" means all those who have anything to do with the client. It is far better to overcommunicate, if that is possible, than to err in the direction of forgetting someone whose interest or job responsibilities may be affected by an educational program. The entire planning process should involve key people from the beginning, so this last minute communication is a key technique to assure more complete communication. However, it is *not* for the purpose of asking permission; it *is* a demonstration of consideration for co-workers to alert them to the plans. Even if client education efforts are limited to one client, most likely several people need to know.

Documentation is another major element. What to document and how are universal dilemmas in client education. If documentation is a problem, two questions need to be asked:

- What are the reasons for documentation?
- What will the nurse do with the information that is documented?

Some of the answers may be to serve as communication with other caregivers for promoting continuity of care, as a record for clients of what they have learned and what needs to be learned, to indicate the need for information, to record informed consent, and to record the need for and utilization of client education services.

Flow sheets, checklists, and short answer forms are widely used to document the education of individual clients because of their ease of completion. On the other hand, documentation of the use of programs or learning tools may simply involve keeping a record of the number of participants or the items utilized. This type of record, while helpful, is of no value in documenting what learning has occurred but may be an indication of need or interest for further programming. Figs. 6-1 and 6-2 are examples of some short-answer documentation forms currently being utilized.

Other activities associated with implementation are of the "housekeeping" variety but are equally important. The following checklist serves as a sample reminder of possible activities in this area.

- Is there an adequate supply of teaching materials?
- Is there someone available to operate the audiovisual equipment?
- Are there spare light bulbs or batteries for audiovisual equipment and extension cords for such equipment?
- Is there more than one teacher available and prepared to present the class(es) in case of illness or vacations?
- Is the room large enough to comfortably accommodate the expected number?

- Is the room free from noise and traffic distractions?
- Are the chairs and the room temperature comfortable?
- Are the lights adequate, and are there sufficient restrooms?
- Have announcements or advertisements been provided to notify clients and families of the available client education programs?
- How will clients and families be transported to the program?

Type of stoma ______________________________

Ileal conduit or ileostomy checklist

	Date	Nurse
Instruction booklet		
Preoperative teaching		
Family present		
Mark stoma site		
Stoma care		
Client observed		
Family observed		
Client performed		
Family performed		
Measurement of stoma		
Appliance*		
Client observed		
Family observed		
Client performed		
Family performed		
Seen by volunteer		

	Date	Nurse
Equipment		
Permanent name		
Temporary name		
Procurement of supplies*		
Care of equipment		
Night drainage		
Miscellaneous		
Ostomy hygiene		
Follow-up care (clinic)		
Home care or other referral		
Diet		
Discuss client		
Discuss family		
Odor control		

Discussion pointers

1. Travel and travel kit.
2. Discuss skin problems and their management (redness, excoriation, and so on).
3. Discuss appliance and measurement of stoma.
4. Discuss activities permitted or prohibited.
5. Discuss underwear and wardrobe.
6. Discuss resumption of social activities (sexual if applicable).
7. Discuss with client his thoughts and feelings about his changed body image.
8. Discuss odor control.
9. Discuss emergency situations.
10. Discuss maintenance of good hydration to prevent crystals and stones.
11. Availability of hospital personnel to help with problems arising after discharge from the hospital (emergencies and phone numbers).
12. Discuss return to work and what to tell family and friends.
13. Discuss the ostomy procedure generally.
14. Discuss the need for privacy during appliance change.
15. Discuss cost, insurance aid, Medicare, and so on.
16. Discuss precautions--no enemas or rectal temperatures.

*Instruction sheet given.

Fig. 6-1. Ileal conduit or ileostomy checklist documentation. (Modified from the North Memorial Medical Center, Minneapolis, Minnesota.)

Vital sign range: BP___/ - /___ P______
R__________ T____________
(If febrile, notify Dr.)

Skin color:
- WNL
- Pale __________
- Cyanotic ________
- Flushed ________
- Other ________

Skin condition:
- WNL
- Edema--site ________
- Bruises--site ______
- Decubitus--site_____
- Other ____________

Stocking measurement: size ordered_____
Calf______________
Thigh______________
Length______________

Date surgery scheduled:______________
Time:______________

Mental status:
- WNL
- Disoriented to person, place, time

Motor ability:
- WNL
- Weakness/paralysis: site________

Speech:
- WNL
- Slurred, hoarse, other__________

Vision:
- WNL
- Glasses, reading only__________
- Contacts, prosthesis__________

Pupils:
- Equal, unequal, explain__________
- React to light R-L __________
- Nonreactive R-L __________

Hearing:
- WNL
- Deaf, partially deaf __________
- R-L R-L

Learning:

	Date	Instructed by:	Review needed?	A-V aid used?	Comments (review done, S.O. taught, problems)
1. Client is able to briefly define surgery (what is going to be done).			Yes No		
2. Client is able to briefly explain why surgery is being done.			Yes No		
3. Client is able to demonstrate to nurse the ability to perform coughing, deep-breathing, and leg exercises.			Yes No		
4. Client is able to restate what tubes or drains may be present postoperatively and their purpose.			Yes No		
5. Client is able to explain purpose of ICU if indicated.			Yes No		
6. Other __________			Yes No		

Concerns, fear, or anxieties expressed by client ______________________

Does client wish to see religious advisor? No_____ Yes_____ Notified__________

Other pertinent information ______________________

Signature ______________________ Date __________ Time __________

Fig. 6-2. Preoperative assessment and learning record. (Modified from the Ellis Fischel State Cancer Hospital, Columbia, Mo.)

Step V. Evaluate client and family education

The final step in the process of client education programming is the evaluation or reassessment to see if learning goals were met. Evaluation techniques are essentially the same as the assessment techniques originally employed to define client needs. It is most useful for evaluation to be based on the behavioral objectives that were determined in Step II, but the documentation forms as determined in Step IV may also be utilized. The two major aspects that occur in the evaluation step are the evaluation of the learner and the evaluation of the actual program.

Evaluation of the learner may be accomplished in several ways. One way is to ob-

To the nurse: Please date and initial the kinds of instruction the client has received up to now. Make a carbon copy to give client, original to stay in chart.

None ______
Sound-slide chemotherapy program ______
Chemotherapy pamphlet ______
Drug sheet(s) ______
Explanation by physician(s) ______
Explanation by nurse(s) ______
Chemotherapy class--outpatient clinic ______
Other (please describe) ______

To the client: These are questions we hope you will answer. Your answers will help us to know what concerns you may have about your treatment and what information you may want about caring for yourself at home. Please answer all questions by either filling in the blank space or by circling the answer you choose. Your nurse will go over your answers with you.

1. What is chemotherapy?
   a. Chemotherapy is a test done to determine the best treatment for cancer.
   b. Chemotherapy refers to the combination of surgical and radiation treatment.
   c. Chemotherapy is a form of treatment with drugs for cancer.
   d. Chemotherapy refers to tests used for discovering or diagnosing the presence of cancer.

2. Why are you receiving (or going to receive) chemotherapy?

3. What does the term "side-effects" mean to you?

4. What does the term "bone marrow suppression" mean to you?

5. Which is most important to remember about dental care?
   a. Regular visits to the dentist are not necessary if you wear dentures.
   b. Daily brushing and flossing of teeth and gums will help prevent infections.
   c. Chemotherapy will help fight infections in your mouth.
   d. Mouthwash is the most effective way to destroy germs in the mouth.

6. Infections of the urinary bladder:
   a. Can often be prevented by using douches or hygiene spray.
   b. Cause chemotherapy patients to become sterile.
   c. Are not common problems for chemotherapy patients.
   d. Can often be prevented by proper use of toilet tissue.

Continued.

Fig. 6-3. Chemotherapy teaching-learning form. (Modified from the Ellis Fischel State Cancer Hospital, Columbia, Mo.)

7. Chemotherapy clients should:
   a. Try to avoid infections because antibiotics will interfere with chemotherapy.
   b. Not worry about getting infections because antibiotics will protect against infection.
   c. Try to avoid infections because chemotherapy may interfere with defense against infection.
   d. Not worry about getting infections because chemotherapy will protect the body against infection.

8. If your platelet count is low:
   a. You should not be concerned about hemmorrhoids.
   b. You should be careful not to cut or injure yourself.
   c. You should not use an electric razor.
   d. You should clean your teeth with dental floss.

9. If your body does not have enough white blood cells, its ability to:
   a. Fight infection is decreased.
   b. Clot blood is decreased.
   c. Carry food to cells is decreased.
   d. Remove wastes from the cells is decreased.

10. Which is true about chemotherapy side-effects?
    a. The drugs work on normal cells as well as cancer cells.
    b. The different side-effects you have indicate how effective the drugs are.
    c. If you don't experience any side-effects, your drugs are not strong enough.
    d. Every client receiving the same drugs should have the same side-effects.

11. What are the signs of infection you should watch for while at home?

12. What are the signs of anemia you should watch for while at home?

13. What are some signs of bleeding you should watch for while at home?

14. What questions do you have?

Your physician here should be notified if you notice any of the signs of infection, anemia, or bleeding. Please ask your nurse or physician any questions you may have.

Nurse's signature after reviewing questions and answers with client: ____________ Date:________

Fig. 6-3, cont'd. Chemotherapy teaching-learning form.

serve the behaviors set forth in the learning objectives. This method is probably most objective but is not always possible because the desired behavior may not *occur* within the proximity of the nurse-teacher or may occur over a long period of time. Ways to observe and evaluate such behaviors include videotapes of the client(s) or completion of checklists when the identified tasks have been satisfactorily completed. This latter method is especially useful when standardized procedures such as self-injection, colostomy irrigation, or tube feedings are to be learned.

When direct observation of the desired behavior is not possible, questioning the learner will provide an indication of accomplishment of the desired behavior. A series

The purpose of this exercise is to help you see yourself and decide what you need help on during the "I CAN COPE" classes.

There are no right or wrong answers. Please place an "X" in the space that is closest to your feelings today. Do not dwell on a particular question.

	Dissatisfies me greatly 1	Dissatisfies me somewhat 2	Neither satisfies nor dissatisfies me 3	Satisfies me somewhat 4	Satisfies me greatly 5
1. The image I have of myself					
2. The goals I have set for myself					
3. My ability to find meaning and purpose in life					
4. My sense of control of my life					
5. My ability to deal with fears					
6. My ability to deal with feelings					
7. My physical fitness					
8. My closeness with my immediate family					
9. My relationship with my children					
10. My ability to talk with my family about my disease					
11. My ability to get help when I need it					
12. My spiritual needs being met					
13. The knowledge I have of my disease					
14. My ability to talk with my physician					
15. My ability to talk with health resource people					

Fig. 6-4. Exercise sheet—life satisfaction. (Reproduced courtesy of the American Cancer Society, Inc., Minnesota Division.)

of questions based on the learning objectives may be asked either verbally or in written form. Questions may be true-false, multiple choice, short answer or essay, but they need to measure knowledge, attitude, or self-report of behavioral changes. Fig. 6-3 is an example of knowledge evaluation about a chemotherapy program. This form can also be utilized as a method of documenting client teaching-learning or as an assessment tool or a teaching tool. Fig. 6-4 can be utilized as a pre- and post-intervention measurement to evaluate changes in attitude. The exact relationship between knowledge, attitudes, and behavioral changes is not clear; however, it may be useful to keep in mind that knowledge and attitudinal measurements may not necessarily *predict* the desired behavioral changes.

Evaluation of the educational program it-

1. How would you rank the information you heard about today? (Circle one)

   Not helpful 0 1 2 3 4 Helpful

   Comments:

2. What did you learn new today?

3. How did you like the speaker? (Circle one)

   Poor 0 1 2 3 4 Helpful

   Comments:

4. How did you like the teaching aids used today? (Circle one)

   Poor 0 1 2 3 4 Helpful

   Comments:

5. How do you think you might use the information you heard about today?

Fig. 6-5. Program evaluation form. (Reproduced courtesy of the American Cancer Society, Inc., Minnesota Division.)

self is often based on utilization statistics and comments of the learners. Learner satisfaction, while not objective, is certainly valid as an evaluation measure, since positive feelings are often associated with greater learning. Evaluation measurement should include measurement of the teaching methods employed, including the speakers, teaching tools, and materials (Table 6-3). Fig. 6-5 is an example of a program evaluation form.

PRINCIPLES OF CLIENT EDUCATION

The following educational principles are intended to serve as both a summary of the client educational process and an indication of how integral this process is to cancer nursing practice.

Principle 1. *Learning is more effective when it is in response to a felt need of the learner.*[10]

CLIENT EXAMPLE: A premenopausal client with a suspicious breast lesion is likely to learn alternative methods of contraception when the use of the birth control pill must be discontinued because of her cancerous condition.

Principle 2. *Active participation on the part of the learner is essential if learning is to take place.*[10]

CLIENT EXAMPLE: Giving a client a pamphlet to read places the responsibility on the client to read it, especially if the client expects to be questioned about the material later.

Principle 3. *Learning is made easier when material to be learned is related to what the learner already knows.*[10]

CLIENT EXAMPLE: Teaching a breast client that hormones affect breast tissue is easier when the woman already has the perceptual knowledge of what constitutes premenstrual breast changes.

Principle 4. *Learning is facilitated when the materials to be learned are meaningful to the learner.*[10]

CLIENT EXAMPLE: Materials that reflect similar ethnic and social values and are easily understood are usually more effective. Gourmet recipes using exotic and expensive seafoods may not be useful for an anorexic elderly farmer accustomed to simply prepared food.

Principle 5. *Learning is retained longer when it is put into immediate use than when its application is delayed, or stated another way, learning should be arranged or scheduled so that it may be applied immediately.*[10]

CLIENT EXAMPLE: Instruction to the client in preparation for x-ray studies to be done should immediately precede the procedure rather than being given at the time the appointment is made several months in advance.

Principle 6. *Periodic plateaus occur in learning.*[10]

CLIENT EXAMPLE: Learning plateaus may not be evident or identifiable as such to the nurse-teacher but often occur in clients because of other factors such as the stage of disease, the phase of acceptance in the client, or during a period of wellness when information may not be perceived as necessary by the client. It is generally acknowledged that learning does not occur at a steady rate.

Principle 7. *Learning must be reinforced.*[10]

CLIENT EXAMPLE: A woman diagnosed with cervical cancer who has had a postradiation implant is instructed and questioned during each checkup about use of her vaginal dilator. The client is able to gauge the importance of the vaginal dilation because the information is repeated at each visit.

Principle 8. *Learning is made easier when the learner is aware of the progress being made.*[10]

CLIENT EXAMPLE: Postmastectomy exercise records indicate the week-to-week increments in the amount of exercises and increase in range of motion allowable to the client.

Principle 9. *Control of the environment is an aspect of teaching.*[31]

CLIENT EXAMPLE: It is important to instruct the staff not to interrupt their teaching sessions except for emergencies and to schedule teaching sessions in relationship to the client's comfort measures, meals, and visiting hours.

While the preceding examples are generally recognized as important to successful learning, they may not be applicable to the individual nurse's setting. It is helpful, however, for the nurse to think of ways to apply each principle for each client education effort attempted.

CONCLUSION

Cancer clients are telling the health professionals that they need to have opportunities for learning about their cancer and its ramifications. The following are excerpts paraphrased from speeches that were given by clients at professional conferences. They tell us of the relative importance of client education within the total cancer care program.

From Lynn Ringer, CanSurmount Coordinator, Denver, Colorado:

> It's wonderful when professional folks tell us of ways to help us cope with our disease. Not just about surgery, radiation, and chemotherapy; I'm thinking of such things as learning how to relax, eating better, and the benefits of exercise. These and other kinds of approaches may not help everyone but they do help many. Offer us the TOOLS and let us choose the options. We can feel more in control then.[33]

From Neil Fiore, Psychologist, Kaiser Clinic, Oakland, California:

> We patients need to take responsibility and participate in our own health care. We must be equipped with coping mechanisms for improving the quality of our lives if we are to be unambivalent about returning to health. This means learning how to express feelings and to communicate, how to make decisions about changes in careers or life roles, how to deal with financial burdens of cancer, how to relax about the worry of recurrence, and how to cope with a number of issues of guilt, depressions, and family discord.[11]

From Mara Flaherty, Porter, Novelli & Associates, Inc., contractor to the Office of

Cancer Communications, National Cancer Institute:

I need to have control over my body and over my life. Beyond imparting information, offer me options, choices, and specific suggestions for self-care. Then I can decide to not only do something about an aspect of my health but also have some choice as to how to do it. Offer us (patients) your respect—give us the right to have a say in our own health care. Be willing to teach us—not just tell us.[12]

From Carie Becker, a 19-year-old student from Elk River, Minnesota, who shared this poem with nurses working with her:

Who Am I?

I am a person, a human,
I need knowledge, compassion and a friend.
Who am I,
If I do not know what's coming?
I am faced with a forked road, one going left, one right.
Who am I?
But a person facing reality in the face of illness.
Only I can choose the road to travel,
But only you can put the signposts up.
I may take a road you would not have taken.
But with the knowledge you gave me,
I will take the road I feel is right for me.[4]

The most desirable outcome of any client education program is a client who is aware of the alternatives and their potential effects and who chooses voluntarily and intelligently whether or not to follow medical advice. Cancer nurses might well be challenged by the goal of the Task Force on Patient Education for the President's Committee on Health Education:

The ultimate goal of organized, planned patient education programs is to help individuals acquire new or modify existing knowledge, attitudes and behavior that will promote their ability to care for themselves more adequately; maintain a positive state of health; and prevent possible recurrences when feasible.[3]

REFERENCES

1. Alt, R. E.: Patient education program answers many unanswered questions: readings in health education, Chicago, 1969, American Hospital Association.
2. American Hospital Association: Statement on Patients' Bill of Rights, Health Educ. p. 23, July-August, 1976.
3. Avery, C., Green, L. W., and Kreider, S.: Report on President's Committee on Health Education, Regional Hearings, Pittsburgh, January, 1972.
4. Becker, C.: Who Am I? Unpublished poetry from private collection, Minneapolis, 1979.
5. Bloom, B. S., editor: Taxonomy of educational objectives: handbook I—cognitive domain, New York, 1956, David McKay Co.
6. Breckon, D.: Highlights in the evolution of hospital-based patient education program, J. Allied Health **3:**35, 1976.
7. Brown, A. J.: Patient education: a comparison of viewpoints, Health Educ. **7:**19, 1976.
8. Crumbaugh, J. C.: Everything to gain, Chicago, 1973, Nelson-Hall Co.
9. DiBartolo, R.: Self concept and attainment of esophageal speech, Microfilms No. 69-20, 576, 1969.
10. DuGas, B.: Introduction to patient care, ed. 2, Philadelphia, 1972, W. B. Saunders Co.
11. Fiore, N.: Presentation at Second National Patient Education Symposium, San Francisco, September, 1978.
12. Flaherty, M.: Presentation at Fourth Annual Oncology Nursing Society Congress, New Orleans, May, 1979.
13. Gillum, R. F.: Patient education, J. Nat. Med. Assoc. **66:**156, 1974.
14. Goldstein, T., and Miller, L.: More efficient care of diabetic patients in a county hospital setting, N. Engl. J. Med. **286:**1388, 1972.
15. Hendin, D.: Failure to use health knowledge creates wastes, Rocky Mountain News, Denver, October 29, 1974.
16. Holland, J.: Psychological management of cancer patients and their families, Prac. Psychol. Phys., p. 14, October, 1977.
17. Jernigan, A. K.: Discharge diets versus patient education, Hospitals **45:**100, 1968.
18. Johnson, D. E.: Powerlessness: a significant determinant in patient behavior? J. Nurs. Educ. **6:**39, April, 1967.
19. Johnson, J. L.: The effects of a patient-centered educational program on persons' adaptability to

live with a chronic disease, doctoral dissertation, University of Minnesota, Microfilm, 1979.
20. Jones, P., and Oertel, W.: Developing patient teaching objectives and techniques: a self-instructional program. Reprinted from Nurse Educ. **2**(5), Sept.-Oct., 1977.
21. Lazarus, R.: Psychological stress and coping in adaptation and illness, Int. J. Psychiatry Med. **5**(4):321, 1974.
22. LeShan, L.: An emotional life-history pattern associated with neoplastic disease, Ann. N. Y. Acad. Sci. **125:**780, 1966.
23. Lipowski, Z. J.: Physical illness, the individual and the coping processes, Psychiatry Med. vol. 1, 1970.
24. Litin, E.: Emotional aspects of chronic physical disability, Arch. Phys. Med. Rehabil. **38:**139, 1957.
25. Madden, B.: Rehabilitation: principles; philosophy; practice, Nurs. Dig. **5**(2):297, 1977.
26. Miller, M., and Nygren, C.: Living with cancer coping behaviors, Cancer Nurs. **1**(4):302, August, 1978.
27. Mowrer, O. H.: Learning theory and personality dynamics, New Haven, Conn., 1950, Yale University Press.
28. National Cancer Institute: Readability testing in cancer communication methods, examples and resources for improving the readability of cancer messages and materials, Publication No. 79-1689, Washington, D.C., 1979, U.S. Department of Health, Education and Welfare.
29. Oncology Nursing Society and American Nurses' Association: Outcome standards for cancer nursing practice, Kansas City, Kansas, 1979.
30. O'Neill, M.: Psychological aspects of cancer recovery, Cancer **36:**271, 1975.
31. Pohl, M.: The teaching function of the nursing practitioner, ed. 2, Philadelphia, 1968, W. C. Brown Co.
32. Reed, E.: Obligation to teach as well as to treat, J. Fla. Med. Assoc. **51:**292, May, 1964.
33. Ringer, L.: Presentation at American Cancer Society Human Values Conference, Chicago, September, 1977.
34. Rosenberg, S.: Patient education leads to better care for health patients, Health Rep. **86:**703, 1971.
35. Schwab, J. J., Clemmons, R. S., and Marder, L.: The self concept: psychosomatic applications, Psychosomatics **7:**1, 1966.
36. Seligman, M. E.: Depression and learned helplessness in man, J. Abnorm. Psychol. vol. 84, 1975.
37. Simonds, S.: Current issues in patient education, New York, 1974, Care Communications in Health, Inc.
38. Stewart, R. B., and Cluft, L. E.: A review of medication errors and compliance in ambulant patients, Clin. Pharmacol. Ther. **13:**463, 1972.
39. Ulrich, M.: How hospitals evaluate patient education programs. Reprint of speech presented at the National Conference on Hospital Based Patient Education, August, 1976, Atlanta, Georgia. U.S. Department of Health, Education and Welfare, 1976.
40. Wolle, J.; Multidisciplinary team develops programming for patient education, Health Serv. Rep. **89:**8, 1974.

ADDITIONAL READING

Benjamin, A.: The helping interview, ed. 2, Boston, 1974, Houghton Mifflin Co.

Fourth Annual Oncology Nursing Society Congress: Instructional session: patient education tapes, New Orleans, May, 1979.

Kidd, J. R.: How adults learn, New York, 1975, Associated Press.

Knox, A. B.: Adult development and learning, San Francisco, 1977, Jossey-Bass, Inc., Publishers.

Lazes, P.: The handbook of health education, Maryland, 1979, Aspen Systems Corp.

National Cancer Institute, Office of Cancer Communications: Coping with cancer, Washington, D.C., 1978, Porter, Novelli & Associates, Inc.

National Cancer Institute, Office of Cancer Communication: Deliberations of the cancer patient education workshop, U.S. Department of Health, Education and Welfare, January, 1979.

Redman, B. K.: The process of patient teaching in nursing, ed. 3, St. Louis, 1976, The C. V. Mosby Co.

U.S. Department of Health, Education and Welfare in cooperation with American Hospital Association: Media handbook, Chicago, 1979, American Hospital Association.

U.S. Department of Health, Education and Welfare in cooperation with American Hospital Association: Implementing patient education in the hospital, Chicago, 1979, American Hospital Association.

7

Nursing research applied to cancer nursing practice

MARY G. MacVICAR

There was a time in the not too distant past when cancer and cancer nursing were synonymous with death and care of the dying client. Fortunately, the myths about cancer and the stereotyping of cancer clients and cancer nurses are being challenged on several fronts. Intensive medical and technologic research have produced a variety of therapeutic modalities that have enhanced survival for many individuals with cancer. Indeed, the prospects for cure or control have become a reality for many people. At the same time, the single criterion of increased survival rates cannot be accepted as the only measure of success in the treatment of cancer clients. The care of individuals and their families throughout the illness trajectory still presents many unknowns. Of increasing concern is the "quality" of client survival, involving such issues as the emotional, physical, and economic impact of cancer on family systems; how families and clients cope with remissions; and, perhaps the most difficult problem confronting individuals with cancer or a history of cancer, vocational rehabilitation and job placement.[3] Clearly, many of these aspects of the cancer problem are within the province of cancer and cancer nursing research.

As a result of rapid medical advances in medical science, nurses are faced with the unprecedented need to modify or develop new nursing techniques and skills used in the care of cancer clients and their families. In the absence of systematic research studies, nursing interventions will evolve from trial and error, a costly process for the clients, families, and the health care system in general. Emphasizing the need for cancer nursing research is the increasing responsibilities nurses are assuming for client-family management in both institutional and home environments. In spite of all that is written, very little is known about the continuity of care between agencies delivering acute care, clinics that are responsible for long-term therapeutic management, and supportive maintenance of clients in their homes.

Therefore, the thrust of this chapter is on the research process as it applies to cancer nursing practice. Following a brief discussion concerning the relevance of research for continued professional development, the steps of the research process will be reviewed. A study of the impact of cancer on the family will be used to illustrate the kinds of decisions and problems confronting the clinical investigator in development of a research project in the specialty of cancer nursing.

RATIONALE FOR RESEARCH

The reasons for pursuing research are as diverse as the individuals engaged in research projects. Often the impetus for initiating a study is to solve a problem that could not be resolved by knowledge and techniques based on traditional assumptions, practice, or past experience. For example, the problem of pain control in individuals with cancer has not been solved using traditional techniques and methods. This has led to a myriad of studies in several disciplines including nursing. Such investigational efforts not only attempt to solve the problem of pain control but also to contribute new knowledge to one or several disciplines.

Another extremely important reason for investigational studies is consumer activism. The doctrine of client-consumer rights; the new role of the family as primary caretaker of the client, particularly in the home; and the subsequent impact of this role on the family clearly intensify the need for research on the client-family system. Further, studies concerning the role of nurses as client-family therapists will facilitate the expansion of nursing's role by identifying the parameters of this new dimension of professional practice.

Finally, perhaps the most important reason for nursing research is to distinguish between the beliefs and knowledge accumulated from early training and experience and those scientific facts established by systematic investigation. Scientific study takes a phenomenon beyond the realm of opinion, personal values, and beliefs. Objectivity is what makes the scientific method superior over other means of obtaining knowledge.[6] This does not mean, however, that the individuals involved in research should be, or could be, devoid of personal values and beliefs. Indeed, these personal attributes may constitute the foundation of the investigator's area of interest. But research is anchored as much as possible in the reality existing outside the individual investigator's value system.

The nursing profession is challenged as never before to be accountable for the effectiveness of its interventions, efficiency, cost-effectiveness, and humaneness.[17] The hard reality confronting nursing is that either nurses become involved in research relevant to the nursing process and client care or it will be done for them by professionals outside the field of nursing. In which case, the results may not be in the best interest of the clients, their families, or nursing.

RESEARCH DEFINED

Research covers a broad range of activities from the study and authentication of historic documents, development of theoretical models, and technical inventions to evaluative studies of social programs.[8] The common theme throughout all these investigative efforts is the acquisition of knowledge based on objective study of the phenomenon. It is very evident that any definition of research is linked to the individual scientist's discipline and background. Therefore, only a few definitions of research are reviewed here.

In a strict sense, research can be defined as the collection of data in a rigorously controlled situation for the purpose of prediction and explanation.[13] Abdellah[1] conceives of research as an activity that is directed to questions that would provide new knowledge. Others view research as a scientific process that begins with theory and feeds back into theory.[8] On the other hand,

French[4] defines research as a problem-solving process, intensive and systematic study directed toward increased scientific knowledge of the subject. In reviewing the various conceptions of research, it is apparent that research activity has a twofold purpose: to search for new facts and to fit the facts into a meaningful pattern.[2,10]

It is worth noting at this point that although the research process and problem solving may appear to be similar, they should not be viewed as synonymous. Problem solving typically is directed toward a specific situation or condition. When a solution is defined, the problem solving process is usually terminated. Further, the problem solving process may or may not be based on objective collection of data, depending on the individuals involved and the nature of the problem. Finally, those involved in resolving a problem do not develop the elaborate procedures inherent in a research design. A research project, on the other hand, is a very tightly constructed study that may solve a problem but also adds to, or refines, the theoretical knowledge base of a discipline.[15]

RESEARCH PROCESS

The single most important aspect of doing research is in planning the project. Each step of the research process must be addressed with the greatest attention to detail. During the planning phase, the investigator attempts to clarify major concepts, reviews relevant literature, and evaluates data collection techniques. It should be emphasized that the initial review of the literature during this planning stage is a preliminary review. It is anticipated that the investigator will return to the literature time and again throughout development of the project.

The research process generally involves 10 basic steps, each of which is extremely important. Ambiguity in any of the steps will take the researcher off course with potentially disastrous results. Each of the following steps in the research process will be discussed in greater detail in the following section:

1. Statement of the problem
2. Review of the literature
3. Formulation of the objectives and hypothesis
4. Formulation of the theoretical framework
5. Description of the research design
6. Selection of variables
7. Operationalizing the variables
8. Identification of the target population
9. Selection or development of methodological procedures
10. Determination of data analysis techniques

DEVELOPMENT OF A RESEARCH PROPOSAL: IMPACT OF CANCER ON THE FAMILY

Interest in family response to cancer developed from observations of cancer clients and their families in hospital units and chemotherapy clinics. The questions raised by family members, including the afflicted member, revolved around how the family could manage the tasks necessary for continuity of family life and at the same time assume responsibility for the care of the sick member. It was observed that although many concerns raised by these families were similar, there was considerable variation in the ways families coped with their problems. Some families managed the multiple demands of daily living and care of the sick member very well, while others demonstrated rapid disintegration as a family system. The research problem was twofold: first, identification of problems experienced by families when confronted with a long-term, life-threatening illness and, second, identification of factors associated with the family system that were conducive to group survival. It was reasoned that if specific problems could be identified, nursing interventions could be directed toward prevention of the occurrence of problems through more intensive planning, counseling, and teaching families about the illness and treatment regimen earlier in the illness trajectory. Further, development of family profiles would assist in identifying families "at risk."

Statement of the problem

A statement of the research problem is a specific declaration of the topic area and indicates the parameters of the problem.

The impact of cancer on the family would appear to be a reasonably well-defined problem statement. But the phrase "impact of cancer on the family" reflects one of the common errors many researchers make—the problem statement is much too broad. Numerous issues can be identified that, if left unresolved, would compromise all subsequent steps in the research process. For example, such factors as family size, number of dependent children living in the home, client's disability status, and family role occupied by the client would all have a bearing on the conduct of the investigation. In general, the problem statement should be as specific as possible. With regard to studying the impact of cancer on the family, the problem statement was narrowed down to, "the impact of cancer in the male spouse on the family with dependent children."

Review of the literature

The literature review provides the investigator with an opportunity to evaluate many different approaches to the problem. First, it is necessary to obtain the most current facts relevant to the problem. Second, a thorough literature review will assist the researcher with the selection or development of the theoretical and methodological approaches to the problem.

Although there was a wealth of literature on the family, there were no studies examining the impact of cancer on the family that could be located. The majority of research in this area focused on the terminal phase of cancer. While these investigative efforts provided insight into the crisis nature of cancer primarily for the afflicted individual, the basic thrust of the proposed study was on how families and clients live with the disease.

The literature review was expanded to include the more general concepts of chronic illness, disability and rehabilitation, and family crisis. These areas of theory and research provided numerous accounts of the impact of long-term illness on the family. Further, the studies provided a variety of theoretical and methodological approaches that could be adapted to the study of families and cancer. Specific variables related to the family's coping ability were identified. These included family resources, hardships defined by the family, disability status, and a number of demographic factors such as occupation and education.

Based on findings from the literature search, specific objectives of the study could be formulated. It should be emphasized that the objectives and the hypothesis must be congruent with the statement of the problem.

Formulation of the objectives and hypothesis

The objectives of a study are a set of statements concerning what the investigator wants to learn about the problem. A hypothesis, on the other hand, is a conjectural statement of relationship between two or more variables. An example of the former would be "to describe the disabilities associated with lung cancer." A hypothesis could be stated "there is a relationship between the disabilities associated with lung cancer and client's knowledge of the disease and treatment."

A study may have either, or both, objectives and a hypothesis. In the study under review, only objectives were developed because, other than terminal aspects of cancer, very little was known in regard to how families adapted to the illness event. The objectives, as stated, reflected broad categories of variables found to be significant to family adaptation in very general terms but appeared applicable to the study of the impact of cancer on the family. The four objectives of the study were:

1. To describe the disabilities associated with cancer
2. To identify available family resources
3. To describe family hardships associated with the illness event
4. To describe patterns of family coping

The objectives serve to identify the major analytic areas. In this study these areas included patient disability, family resources, family hardships, and family coping. The next task involves development of a theoretical framework that would articulate these major concepts and provide the rationale for the study. It should become apparent that if the problem statement is too broad or the objectives and hypothesis are ambiguous, the formulation of a theoretical framework and a sound rationale for the study will be difficult at best.

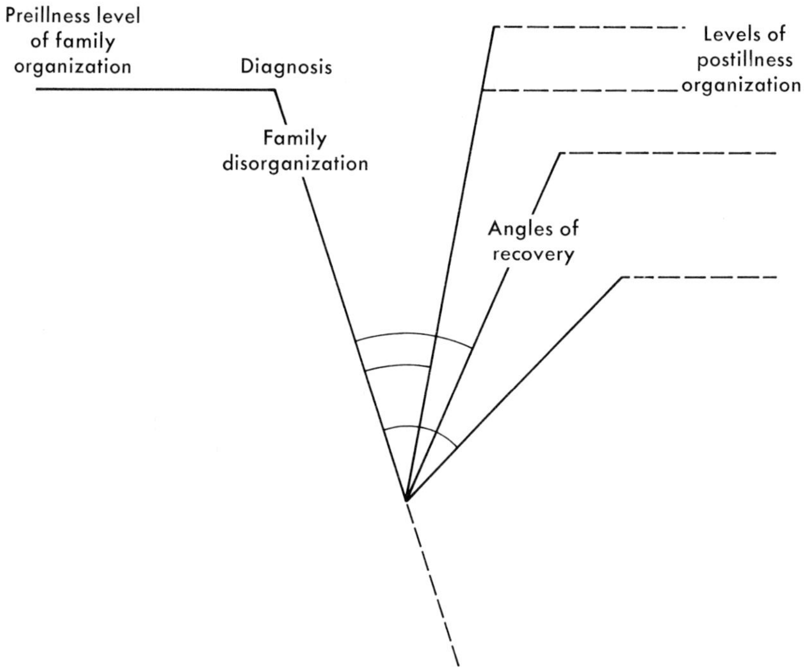

Fig. 7-1. Family crisis framework. (Adapted and modified with permission from Hansen, D.A., and Hill, R.: Families under stress. In Christensen, H. T., editor: Handbook of marriage and the family, Chicago, 1964, Rand McNally, p. 782.

Formulation of the theoretical framework

Theory is defined as a "set of interrelated principles and definitions that serve conceptually to organize selected aspects of the empirical world in a systematic way."[13] Further, research is not simply the search for, and documentation of, facts but the search for order within the facts.[2] Essentially, theory serves to link research findings to a broader, more abstract body of knowledge. On the other hand, research contributes to the development, refinement, or reformulation of theory by testing it in the world of reality.

The theoretical approach selected for this family cancer study was based on Hansen and Hill's conceptual framework of family crisis.[5] Their theoretical formulation of family crisis, in particular the crisis process, included the major analytic areas outlined in the study's objectives as well as accommodating the concept of coping. Adaptation of the family crisis model to the study of the impact of cancer in the male spouse on the family with dependent children is presented in Fig. 7-1.

This particular approach provided the opportunity to study pre- and postillness family patterns, specifically in relation to the major study objectives. It was assumed that a diagnosis of cancer would constitute a crisis for most families and that a period of family disorganization occurs subsequent to the diagnosis. The *angles of recovery* represent the family's attempts toward coping with the illness event by way of reorganizing family roles, tasks, and resources necessary to maintain the family system. The angles of recovery also reflect a time dimension, that is, how long it takes the family to reorganize. Levels of postillness organization indicate whether the family system is functioning in a positive or negative direction relative to preillness organizational patterns. It should be evident that this is a situational approach and does not take into account many psychologic variables.

The next step in the research process is to outline the basic protocol or research design. This is more or less a blueprint indicating the overall conduct of the study.

Description of the research design

A research design can be either experimental or nonexperimental. In both cases, the investigator attempts to control as many relevant variables as possible. However, if the researcher intends to manipulate variables as well, then the experimental design is appropriate. Classical experimental protocols are more typical of laboratory studies where rigorous control of critical variables is more feasible.

In nonexperimental research, the investigator does not attempt to manipulate variables but does attempt to account for as many variables as possible. In other words, if the investigator wishes to observe how A affects B, other factors that could affect B must be identified and controlled within practical limits of the study.

The family cancer study would be defined as a descriptive, nonexperimental design. The selection of this type of format was based on the fact that it was an exploratory effort to examine relationships between variables. Further, only three conditions could be controlled: the disease category, since only families of men diagnosed with cancer were included; broad disease parameters, such as those clients in the diagnostic phase and clients in the terminal stage of disease being excluded; and family composition, consisting of families in which there were both spouses and dependent children present. Tighter control of more variables would have enhanced the overall design and outcome of the study; however, there were numerous logistic problems. For example, cancer is more typically a disease of the older population age groups, but the older age group is less likely to have dependent children living at home. Therefore, control over disease category and staging was sacrificed to gain more control over family variables. This is an illustration of the kind of procedural problems confronting most investigators throughout the research process. So long as decisions are based on a logical rationale and limitations are carefully noted, the investigator is on relatively safe ground.

Selection of variables

A variable can be defined as the "characteristic, property, trait, or attribute of the person or thing observed in a study."[1] The variables should be selected on the basis of the problem statement, theoretical framework, and objectives as well as the research protocol or design.

In studies where the investigator attempts to examine the relationship(s) among variables, it is necessary to specify the independent and dependent variables. The independent variables can be those that exist in a natural state or that are manipulated by the investigator. Dependent variables are those conditions or attributes that are observed to change in some way in response to the independent variables. For example, it was reasoned that there would be a differential impact of cancer on the family depending on the severity of the disease and availability of family resources. Therefore, the independent variables were defined as the illness and family resources, and the constellation of dependent variables consisted of family hardships and coping. It should be obvious that a thorough literature search is essential to establish a logical rationale for designation of variables as dependent or independent and facilitates the "operationalizing" process reviewed in the next step.

Operationalizing the variables

The term "operationalizing" refers to measurement procedures. It is the statement that identifies observable actions or things that can be observed and verified by others.[11] This process is often the most frustrating step in the research process. The selection of variables used as indicators must be based on a sound rationale and be consistent with what is being measured and the objectives of the study. To illustrate, indicators of family hardship included family health status. This variable was measured by documenting the number of illnesses or disabling conditions of family members other than the male spouse. Other indicators of family hardship included employment status of family members, monthly financial obligations, and decreased social participation in the community. The other class of dependent variables was related to family coping and included such measures as wives' request for information concerning their husbands' illnesses and application for medical or social welfare agency assistance.

Operational equivalents of the independent variables were specific to the cancer event and family resources. The indicators used to measure the illness were diagnosis, disability status, maintenance of daily living activities, length of illness and wives' definitions of their husbands' prognoses. Family resources included the variables of level of family monthly income, major source of income, home assistance, and past experience with serious illness. The constellation of variables just outlined was selected on the basis of findings in the literature and related back to the problem statement and objectives. In other words, variables used to measure a phenomenon must be consistent with the theoretical framework of the study and be capable of empirical testing.

Identification of the target population

If the preceding steps of a research project are reasonably well defined, development of criteria for inclusion of subjects is not difficult. The population for this study was families where the male spouse was diagnosed with cancer and there were dependent children living in the home. However, to gain greater control over the stage of illness, two other criteria were imposed: only clients where the diagnosis was already established and those who were not defined as "terminally ill" were included. This narrowed the population considerably.

Selection or development of methodological procedures

Selection of the sample involved a number of issues that had to be resolved. First, if the disease category were limited to one kind of cancer pathology such as lung or colon cancer, the population and subsequent sample would be extremely small. Certainly, it would be easier to assess disability status if the client sample were homogeneous in regard to the pathology. But a larger sample, even with diverse cancer pathology, would provide greater insight into family events. Thus, disease category was sacrificed to enhance observation of family variables. The decision was not an easy one but was forced by practical considerations. The sample size was set at 100 families to facilitate statistical analysis. Time and cost were serious constraints. Based on the criteria of family selection, the population was already limited to a relatively young age group in which cancers are not typically found. Therefore, the sample would be increasingly difficult to obtain.

The second basic issue involving sample selection was a technical one, but one directly related to the ability to generalize to the population. Ideally, a random sample of families should be selected, whereby each family has an equal probability of being included. This would enhance the representativeness of the sample, on the one hand, but would take considerably longer, on the other hand. Again, the limitations of time and money led to the decision to use a nonrandom, prospective sample. Briefly, this meant that all families meeting the criteria and agreeing to participate in the study were included. The limitations of this type of sampling include a nonrepresentative sample, biased estimators of the variables, and findings that cannot be generalized to the population. Nevertheless, a study with limitations is better than no study at all.

Selection of data analysis techniques

The selection of data analysis techniques should be determined by the kind of data, how the variables are measured, and the sampling method. Generally, it is helpful to seek consultation concerning the alternative statistical techniques appropriate to the study, the objectives/hypothesis, and the level of data collected. It would make a great deal of difference if data represented simple dichotomous categories such as "yes" or "no" and "female" or "male," or if it fitted more discrete categories. Often, a variety of data analysis techniques can be used. The reason statistical analysis is necessary is to determine whether the differences occurring between subgroups or categories are true population characteristics or occurred by chance.

RESEARCH FINDINGS

The final step for all research efforts is the preparation of the report in which the findings of the study are presented. Data can be presented in the form of graphs, tables, or a combination of techniques that will illustrate and clarify the results of the research.

However, the real challenge is in the ability to exercise logical reasoning, creative insight, and intellectual sensitivity when interpreting the results. Numbers after all are only numbers. Statistical findings must be interpreted in light of the study's problem statement, objectives, and hypothesis being tested, as well as the theoretical framework. Further, analysis and interpretation of the study's findings should be related to the broader base of related theory and research to add to the existing knowledge of the topic. Finally, limitations of both theoretical concepts and methodology should be noted.

In the following discussion, the major findings related to the investigative areas in the family cancer study are summarized. In general, data tended to support the framework of family crisis and disability used in the study. It was assumed that although the presence of a potentially fatal illness such as cancer is a stress-inducing force in the life process of a family, the impact of the event could be assessed on the basis of factors other than the disease. In keeping with the conceptual framework derived from studies of family crises, the impact of cancer was measured in terms of the nature of the impairments associated with the disease and the resources used by the family as it attempted to cope with the hardships imposed by the illness.

Two constellations of variables were effective in assessing the impact on the family of cancer in the male spouse. The nature of the impairment was measured by diagnosis, physical limitations, maintenance of daily living activities, length of illness, and wives' definition of the prognosis. Family resources included postillness monthly income, major source of income, home assistance, and previous experience with serious illness.

Specifically, hardships associated with cancer in the male spouse were more likely to occur in families under the following conditions:

1. Male spouse was in his 30's or 40's
2. Within the first 2 years of illness
3. Male spouse employed in labor or craft occupations
4. Physical disabilities existed that made the male spouse dependent on others for activities of daily living
5. Previous experience with serious illness
6. Low educational attainment of the male spouse

Family coping included the wives' requests for information concerning their husbands' illness and application for agency assistance. Requests for information tended to fall into two categories: concern regarding the husbands' "change in behavior" and "illness management problems." Wives inclined toward behavioral concerns tended to be those in families in which the male spouse:

1. Was in his 30's or 40's
2. Had low educational attainment
3. Was employed in labor or craft occupations
4. Demonstrated no physical limitation and was independent in activities
5. Was unemployed after onset of illness
6. Demonstrated declining income after onset of illness

Illness priorities were more characteristic among women whose husbands reflected the following:

1. In the 20- and 30-year age categories
2. Had high educational attainment
3. Employed in sales or management position
4. Remained employed after onset of illness
5. Physically disabled and dependent on others
6. Families with high postillness income

The other indicator of family coping was application for agency assistance. This tended to be more typical of families in which the male spouse:

1. Was in his 20's or 30's
2. Had low educational attainment
3. Was employed in labor or craft occupations
4. Was unemployed after onset of illness
5. Had been ill less than 2 years
6. Was physically disabled and dependent on others
7. Came from a family without previous experience with serious illness

Although space does not permit an extensive discussion of every finding, it can be seen that the preillness status of the family, along with select demographic factors such as age, income, and occupation, was at least as influential as the pathology in terms of family coping. In essence, the impact of cancer in the male spouse on the family with dependent children is shaped by the nature of the pathology in terms of disability as well as the resources used by the family as it copes with the hardships associated with a degenerative, progressive condition.

Although the study provides some insight into the impact of cancer on the family, several limitations should be noted. First, the sample does not represent a random selection of families. Therefore, the findings cannot be generalized to the population of families in which the male spouse has been diagnosed with cancer. Further, a selection bias exists in that only families willing to be interviewed participated in the study. This gives rise to possible differences between participating and nonparticipating families.

Second, the problems reviewed in this study existed in the families at the time of data collection. The conditions existing prior to illness are known only through recall of the respondents. In other words, there is no way of determining the preillness stability or integration of these families except through the respondent's reports. A longitudinal study in which repeated measurement of the same families over time occurred would contribute more insight into this area. Finally, in regard to the coping process, considerably more information is needed concerning the process by which families reorganize and identify priorities.

IMPLICATIONS FOR CLINICAL PRACTICE

General implications

From the standpoint of clinical practice, the result of this study highlights the need for expansion of the cancer nurse's role, particularly in the area of independent functions. These include continuous family assessment, family education and counseling, and assuming the responsibility of family advocate as the need arises.

The findings from the project clearly portray the differential impact of cancer on the family. Response variability can be attributed, in part, to select sociodemographic factors that must be included in the family assessment process. At the same time, family assessment and the development of family profiles can lead to stereotyping of clients and their families. If the family system is conceived to be an open system capable of change, the dangers inherent in rigid classification of families will be minimized.

More specific assessment criteria

The goal of family assessment should be twofold: to identify existing problems and to identify factors that could either exacerbate current problems or generate further crisis within the family. For example, the restructuring of roles, role conflict, or ambiguity of roles tends to increase tension, particularly in families adhering to traditional patterns of family structure. Assessment in this area would include such factors as former patterns of decision making, occupational and home-care tasks, and childrearing practices. If the stricken member can no longer perform his or her role, how will the associated tasks be allocated and to whom? In essence, family assessment is the first prerequisite to effective intervention. Not all aspects of family assessment, however, can be or should be accomplished in a single interview. Assessment is a *process* occurring over time and represents the accumulation of data that the nurse and other members of the health care team will use in establishing the parameters of care and services needed by the client and family. Specific items that proved reasonably successful in assessing families in this study are listed below.

Illness related

1. Pathology, staging, system(s) affected
2. Disability status
3. Treatment and side-effects (if any)
4. Supportive drugs, therapies
5. Areas of potential rehabilitation
6. Family's definition of the illness and therapy

Resources

1. Occupations of all family members
2. General income level, insurance, sources of support income
3. Community groups, agencies, social support groups

Past experience with serious illness or crisis situations

1. Past crisis experienced by family, significant losses, changes in life-style
2. Individuals identified by the family as those who assisted in past crises
3. Previous experience with community agencies

Priorities

1. What do family members perceive to be the most serious problem?
2. What additional problems are identified by the family and how would they rank these in order of priority?

Family assessment tools can be succinct and functional. As stated earlier, not all information can or should be collected at the same time. As the family changes and adapts to the exigencies of the illness, the data obtained from the assessment form will reflect these changes.

Importance of client-family education

Client-family education is another function of the cancer nurse that is increasingly important. The complexity of cancer care requires a more knowledgeable consumer if treatment is to be effective. Our scientific jargon is complex and mysterious to the client and family. It cannot be assumed that information directed to the family is interpreted accurately or remembered within the proper context. The majority of the families in this study could state the diagnosis and define the prescribed therapy, particularly in light of numerous side-effects that tended to make the client "sick." Understanding dietary principles was virtually nonexistent. The subjects in this study indicated they were told to eat what they could and to exercise when they felt up to it. Further, few families had any knowledge concerning drug interactions and therefore did not understand why "home remedies" could not be taken in conjunction with the prescribed medical therapy.

Client-family teaching must be timely, based on the need to learn, and facts must be relevant to the current situation and presented in nontechnical terms.[7] In addition, there must be an opportunity for an evaluation of client-family learning or a feedback process from clients and families that would allow correction of misinterpretation and translation of cancer "information" publicized by the media.

Impediments to successful learning

It is important to remember when working with cancer clients and their families that all members of the family are experiencing some degree of stress. Under these conditions, client-family education must be planned, repetitive, and presented in terms congruent with the families' ability to understand the facts. Do not presume that the educational level achieved by clients is necessarily indicative of their ability to understand scientific medical terms. In this study, an economics professor was not familiar with the concept "metastasis." The staff assumed the client had a much higher level of general conceptual understanding of his disease than he actually possessed. As could be expected, there was a serious breakdown in communication. The client, too embarrassed to pursue the meaning of the medical terms, became withdrawn and increasingly hostile. It was his wife who asked for clarification and made the staff realize that she and her husband needed pertinent facts expressed in plain English.

Minimum content of educational program

Based on the findings of this study, educational components of cancer care should include:

1. Differences between normal and malignant cells
2. Why a cancer cell is destructive
3. How cancer cells are destroyed by chemotherapy or radiation therapy
4. A nutrition program
5. An exercise program within parameters of the client's disability
6. Instructions on self-care, such as drug interactions or where to call to obtain the information; temperature; personal habits, such as smoking or alcohol that may be contraindicated

As with family assessment, client-family education is continuous and requires some method of evaluating what the client is learning and how the information is being used.

Client-family counseling

The data from this study suggest a distinct need for client-family counseling. Counseling has become a "catchall" term for anything from listening to giving the client instruction on medications. True counseling, however, is a much more complex process. Counseling is defined as a systematic procedure designed to help clients and their families accomplish specific changes in their perceptions and behaviors and to increase their understanding of family dynamics.[14] Inherent in the counseling process is a thorough understanding of communication theory.

General findings

A problem common to most families in this study was the difficulty the parents experienced in providing information to the children in an accurate but nonthreatening manner. Generally, it was found that children under 12 years of age were rarely told anything that resembled the truth, while those over 12 years of age tended to be "overloaded" with detail. Furthermore, teenagers were often expected to contribute to the father's care and assume roles for which they had little preparation. Concomitantly, the mothers reported regressive behavior in young children and failing grades and delinquency in the teenage group.

Intensive counseling early on, preferably within the first 3 to 6 months of illness, may have provided valuable guidance and insight into family problems for the ill parent and spouse. Thus, many of the difficulties experienced by the family system, particularly the children, could have been avoided. The tendency to protect children was strong in many families. There was a groping for the "right" words to explain the seriousness of the father's illness. Individual family members tended to retreat from the reality of the illness and rationalize the problems according to individual interpretation. Unfortunately, this often led to "scapegoating," blaming others in the family, even the client, for the growing family turmoil.

Counseling is indicated not only to assist in the restructuring of family relationships, roles, and communication patterns, but it can also be beneficial in dealing with anticipatory grief. The expectation of loss by the client or members of the family can result in a myriad of feelings and behaviors such as guilt, withdrawal, and anger. Studies have shown that early counseling efforts facilitate adjustment to death of the family member and result in reduced morbidity in survivors.[9,16]

Finally, counseling should be an added dimension of care for clients in remission. Although there is little research in this area, many clients and their families verbalize their continuing fear of recurrence of the disease. Although the progression of the disease may be halted or a cure has been achieved, such individuals still face numerous problems in community reentry. It stands to reason that counseling would be beneficial in facilitating the resumption of their lives.

Situations benefiting from counseling

Data from this project indicate counseling would be appropriate in the following areas:

1. Coping with fear of the disease and the connotation that cancer is synonymous with death
2. Restructuring roles as needed based on individual capabilities to assume such roles or ability to "learn" the roles
3. Role flexibility—the ability to relinquish roles when the client is capable of resuming and desires to assume former role(s)
4. Communication patterns—between spouses and between parents and children, as well as communication with individuals external to the family
5. Communication techniques with health care professionals
6. Bereavement counseling
7. Counseling for community reentry

Client-family advocate

The last area of independent function of the cancer nurse to be discussed is that of client-family advocate. Family needs during prolonged illness will vary both quantitatively and qualitatively. Although many families in the study attempted to seek assistance within the community, discouragement was their usual reward. The structure of our health and social welfare system is a labyrinth of specialized agencies, regulations, and qualifying criteria for assistance of any kind. The younger subjects in this study tended to be more assertive and persevered for longer periods of time in seeking aid. But all families expressed despair and frustration in dealing with various community agencies. Even families with strong church affiliation cited the lack of aid and interest from institutional officials. Older women were more reluctant to seek agency assistance. They tended to view community aid as welfare and rarely pursued the matter beyond one or two phone calls.

As client-family advocate, the nurse is in a unique position to assess and match the family's needs to available agencies. However, skills in advocacy require more than informing the family of what agencies are available or "going to bat" for the family. Families should be taught *strategies* in dealing with agencies, such as how to evaluate criteria for acceptance, how to interpret administrative policies, and so on. Furthermore, the cancer nurse has the opportunity and challenge to educate community agencies concerning the kinds of problems cancer clients and their families experience. Most agencies can be enticed to examine the issue more closely when the potential for expanding their services and clientele is pointed out. These requests for additional services are interpreted as a justification for increased funding. At the very least, data need to be documented concerning the inequities and inadequacies of service for cancer clients and their families.

SUMMARY

The study of the impact of cancer in the male spouse on the family suggests four areas of independent nursing functions relevant to the care of cancer clients and their families. Based on the data of this project, these areas of nursing intervention include family assessment, family education, counseling, and client-family advocacy. The broad goal of these activities is to strengthen the family as a unit and restore control of the family to the family. Families not receiving these interventions, which admittedly go beyond the conventional medically prescribed protocol, will succumb to the hopelessness-helplessness syndrome that characterized the majority of families in this study. When families can achieve a level of self-determination so that they become their own advocates and participate more fully in their care, health care professionals and consumers will have achieved a collaborative relationship. Only then can we anticipate an end to the superior-subordinate flavor that dominates current transactions between clients, their families, and health professionals.

Logically, family involvement in the care of members stricken by cancer will increase dramatically in the next few years. The growing emphasis on home care programs and the rights of clients and families to share in the decision-making process concerning therapy mandates an expansion of the roles of all health professionals. The cancer nurse remains in a unique "gatekeeper" position by virtue of frequent and prolonged contact with these clients. In the final analysis, it is the *cancer nurse* who sets the standards and level of care received by clients and their families throughout the illness trajectory. There is both challenge and opportunity for the cancer nurse in this important area of health care.

CONCLUSIONS

This discussion focused on the research process and the development of the study of the impact of cancer on families. The project was essentially a nonexperimental, descriptive study examining the relationships between the cancer event and family resources as well as the hardships experienced by the families and their attempts toward coping. The theoretical framework was adapted from studies of family crisis and included concepts drawn from the literature on disability and rehabilitation. The objectives outlined the major analytic issues and guided the development of methodological tools. Sample size was based on statistical considerations as well as population estimates and practical concerns of time and cost of the study. Findings of the study indicated that there is a differential impact of cancer on the family as well as highlighting areas of further study.

The development of this project and subsequent commitment to research evolved slowly. There was the typical frustration and episodic despair born of inexperience. However, the findings of this preliminary effort to study the impact of cancer on families confronted the investigator with the complexity of care of cancer clients and their families. Cancer nursing care must include both traditional skills, interventions, and techniques as well as explaining new areas of care. Nursing research provides the opportunity to increase knowledge concerning the effectiveness of nursing interventions, to expand the conceptual basis for nursing practice, and to identify new directions for professional development.

REFERENCES

1. Abdellah, F. G., and Levine, E.: Better patient care through nursing research, New York, 1965, Macmillan, Inc., p. 712.
2. Brownowski, J.: The common sense of science, New York, 1968, Vintage Books, p. 129.
3. Cobb, B. A.: Medical and psychological problems in the rehabilitation of the cancer patient. In Cobb, B. A., editor: Special problems in rehabilitation, Springfield, Ill., 1974, Charles C Thomas, Publisher, p. 111.
4. French, R.: The dynamics of health care, New York, 1968, McGraw-Hill Book Co., p. 111.
5. Hansen, D. A., and Hill, R.: Families under stress. In Christensen, H. T., editor: Handbook of marriage and the family, Chicago, 1964, Rand McNally, p. 782.
6. Kerlinger, F. N.: Foundations in behavioral research, ed. 2, New York, 1973, Holt, Rinehart & Winston, Inc., p. 6.
7. Nagi, S. A.: Disability and rehabilitation: legal, clinical and self concepts, and measurement, Columbus, 1969, Ohio State University Press, p. 18.
8. Nagi, S. A., and Corwin, R. G.: The research enterprise: an overview. In Nagi, S. A., and Corwin, R. G., editors: The social contexts of research, New York, 1972, Wiley-InterScience, p. 1.
9. Parkes, C. M.: Bereavement: studies of grief in adult life, New York, 1973, International Universities Press, Inc., p. 118.
10. Plutchik, R.: Foundations of experimental research, New York, 1968, Harper & Row, Publishers, p. XI.
11. Polit, D., and Hungler, B.: Nursing research: principles and methods, New York, 1978, J. B. Lippincott Co., p. 36.
12. Some conceptual issues in disability and rehabilitation. In Sussman, M. B., editor: Sociology and rehabilitation, Cleveland, 1965, The American Sociological Association, p. 100.
13. Theodorson, G. A., and Theodorson, A. G.: Modern dictionary of sociology, New York, 1969, Thomas Y. Crowell, p. 347.
14. Thorisen, C. E., and Anton, J. L.: Intensive counseling. In Peters, H. J., and Aubrey, R. F., editors: Guidance: strategies and techniques, Denver, 1975, Love Publishing Co., p. 322.
15. Treece, L. W., and Treece, J. S.: Elements of research in nursing, St. Louis, 1973, The C. V. Mosby Co., p. 38.
16. Weisman, A. D.: Coping with cancer, New York, 1979, McGraw-Hill Book Co., p. 94.
17. Wooldridge, P. J., Leonard, R. C., and Skipper, J. K.: Methods of clinical experimentation to improve patient care, St. Louis, 1978, The C. V. Mosby Co., p. VII.

ADDITIONAL READING

Campbell, D. T., and Stanley, J. C.: Experimental and quasi-experimental designs for research, Chicago, 1963, Rand McNally.

Oberst, M. T.: Priorities in nursing research, Cancer Nurs. **1**(4):281, 1978.

Polit, D., and Hungler, B.: Nursing research: principles and methods, New York, 1978, J. B. Lippincott Co.

8

Burnout: antecedents, manifestations, and self-care strategies for the nurse

PAMELA K. S. PATRICK

Ms. C. has been a registered nurse for 3 years. Lately she's felt less and less enthusiastic about her work; she often finds herself resisting the idea of getting ready to go to the hospital. The cancer clients have been posing so many problems that she's reluctant to go into certain rooms. Over the past week, what would ordinarily have been a transitory upper respiratory infection has turned into a nagging cold that she just can't seem to shake. Perhaps, she thinks, it's time to change hospitals.

The above fictional account of an R.N.'s feelings and thoughts about caring for cancer clients can probably be matched *in fact* by many nurses who have felt or thought similarly. Ms. C. is experiencing a phenomenon called the *burnout syndrome* (BOS). It occurs every day in nurses who become emotionally exhausted as a consequence of work-related stress. In this chapter, the burnout syndrome will be defined, described, and analyzed. With an understanding of the parameters of this pervasive experience, prevention and intervention strategies will be considered. The context for this discussion is cancer nursing, that is, the situations in which the nurse's professional attention is devoted to caring for persons of any age who have a form of cancer and who receive medical and/or surgical treatment. How the nurse manages stress and feelings of burnout directly affects cancer clients in terms of nursing care delivered and interactions that take place. It, therefore, is imperative that cancer nurses not only examine the burnout phenomenon but assume an active role in its prevention and management. Much of this chapter's content may be applicable to many other specialty areas of nursing practice. My purpose, however, is to concentrate on the unique aspects of cancer nursing that contribute to a higher potential risk of burnout.

DEFINITION OF BURNOUT

An extremely vivid description of burnout is used with some frequency in many of the helping professions: "If so-and-so doesn't slow down, he/she is going up in flames." Although this is merely an expression, it accurately depicts the symbolic essence of burnout—helpers who *burn out* have a sense of being consumed, of losing a crucial aspect of identity or satisfaction, or of having a part of themselves changed, submerged, or emptied.

Definitions of burnout vary according to the setting in which it occurs. In the context of cancer nursing, burnout is here defined as: the feeling of emotional exhaustion [15,16] and depletion occurring in nurses who have intimate, intense, and continuous contact with cancer clients. This feeling is reflected by attitude shifts and behavior changes toward care recipients. While the burnout syndrome is multifaceted, the *feeling* of burnout resides within each affected nurse. Burnout occurs as a consequence of stress. In this chapter no attempt will be made to present an essay on the phenomenon of stress—such a task would, at best, be exceedingly lengthy and not entirely relevant to the identified topic. The emphasis here, then, is on a specific consequence of stress as it is seen in the context of cancer nursing. "Stress" refers to the nurse's *response* to stressors (causative elements). Burnout occurs in response to stress. Hence, the following sequence depicts the relationship between these terms:

Stressor → Stress → Burnout

ANTECEDENTS OF BURNOUT: FACTORS THAT INCREASE BURNOUT RISK

Burnout does not occur suddenly; the nurse does not wake up one morning and acquire a "case of burnout." It is an *evolutionary* process occurring over time and in relation to identifiable antecedents. Events, settings, demands, and a host of other complex elements set the stage for burnout to develop. Each person's stress response style determines vulnerability to the occurrence of burnout. When placed in similarly stressful circumstances, one nurse may thrive while another may become emotionally exhausted. This difference in who becomes affected and how and why some seem to be "immune" is currently under empirical investigation. The material presented here, therefore, is based on my personal experience as well as empirical data contained in currently available descriptive research.

Nature of cancer nursing

Nurses who interact with and care for cancer clients have chosen a dynamic and stimulating area of practice.[4] At the same time, the very nature of cancer care may increase the nurse's susceptibility to burnout. Factors that influence the nurse and may contribute to emotional exhaustion include cancer complexities, physical care requirements, and technologic developments.

Cancer complexities. Although over 3 million Americans[2] are living following cancer treatment, thousands die each year from the ravages of the illness. This fact is disturbing to those who seek to treat the cancer client. Many clients will die despite all the care administered. Cancer occurs in approximately 100 different forms. Such complexity and the demands it places on the nurse's knowledge and caregiving resources can be tremendous sources of stress.

The continuing, mysterious etiology of cancer adds an element of elusiveness to the cancer nurse's grasp of the client's disease. Not knowing adds to one's sense of lack of mastery or control over highly threatening experiences. As the nurse continuously views and is involved in the care of cancer clients, questions of "why," "how," and "what for" may arise. Over time, unanswered and unanswerable questions can become vaguely nagging sources of intellectual discomfort.

The manifestations of cancer are extremely varied. The disease occurs in all age, ethnic, and socioeconomic groups. It recognizes no boundaries in who it recruits. Nurses interacting with cancer clients over long periods are impressed by this *variability* in appearance as well as by each person's *vulnerability* to its occurrence. No matter how well one cares for oneself, it is still possible to become a cancer client. Cutting down on the odds via responsible self-care seems to be the best that can be done. The threat to the nurse's physical integrity and health posed by cancer is reinforced on a daily basis as cancer clients are cared for; that is, the nurse *also* is a potential cancer client candidate.

Physical care requirements. As with many areas of nursing practice, cancer clients require varying degrees of physical care. These physical care requirements can range from intravenous fluid administration to heavy lifting and turning of severely debilitated persons. Many cancer clients become so weakened that the nurse must frequently reposition or transfer them from one location to another without their assistance. The client's dependence on caregivers for total physical care can lead to physical stress on the nurse. Although utilization of body mechanics is repeatedly emphasized, the cancer nurse faced with the care of several dependent clients may not adhere to these self-care measures. This continuous physical stress can increase the nurse's chance of becoming a burnout candidate.

Technologic developments. Over the past decade, cancer care has been revolutionized by numerous technologic developments ranging from laminar airflow rooms to intra-arterial hepatic infusions. The knowledge and technical skill *currently* required to accurately use and monitor this highly complex technology may become a source of stress. At the same time, ongoing demands for the nurse to keep abreast of *new* developments in cancer diagnostic and therapeutic technology require attention to continuing education and in-service education activities—both require an investment of time that the nurse may feel has already been committed. While realizing the necessity and value of such activities, this potential conflict in time use may be associated with increased burnout risk.

Technology allows the nurse to provide a degree of comprehensive care that can enhance the client's quality *and* quantity of life. On the other hand, highly stressed nurses who are exhibiting signs and symptoms of burnout may use this technology as a barrier to interpersonal intensity; that is, machines, not clients, become the object of care.

The nature of cancer nursing may inherently increase the nurse's risk of burnout. In addition to these general factors, a number of others significantly add to the probability of burnout.

Environmental factors: the setting for care

The process of delivering intimate, painful, or rigorous nursing care to the cancer client can be positively or negatively influenced by surrounding environmental factors. Noise levels, the amount of space in which care is administered, and the availability of privacy can either enhance or inhibit caregiving activities. When there is insufficient room to accommodate equipment, visitors, or personal belongings, the overall comfort of the client may be reduced. At the same time, the nurse may have difficulty gaining access to the client in emergency or acute care situations. The nurse can experience increased stress levels when nursing care must be given in cramped, confined quarters. (Obviously, the client also may experience adverse consequences as a result of limited environmental space.)

Creating a sense of privacy and quietness is frequently necessary when the nurse seeks to provide psychologic support to the cancer client. If this setting is impinged on by noise or interruptions, the nurse may find it necessary to expend larger portions of energy to maintain the interpersonal contact and process. This additional expenditure may result in increased stress for the nurse if it occurs repeatedly because of chronic problems with environmental factors.

The setting in which the nurse works can become a dominant source of sensory monotony. Seldom are changes made in how the nursing unit looks, sounds, or feels. The piped-in music does not vary in quality; walls, counters, floors, ceilings, desks, charts, windows (or the lack thereof), and so on all keep the same colors and textures unless renovation is necessary or new products in these categories are purchased. This sensory monotony can increase the nurse's experience of routineness, "being in a rut," or a general sense of boredom. *Where* one works, *what* it looks and sounds like, and *how* it affects the nurse can be important contributory factors to burnout—or its prevention. The environment can be a primary supportive element to delivery of high-quality cancer nursing care, or it can increase the amount of stress one experiences, thereby adversely affecting the caregiver's enthusiasm. To ignore the impact of environmental factors on the nurse's performance and reactions is to court premature burnout.

Psychologic and social factors: demands versus limits

In this section, major psychologic and social factors that foster emotional exhaustion or burnout for nurses are outlined. These factors are described in general terms with full acknowledgment that each nurse's psychologic experience is colored by individual beliefs, values, and life history.

Life-threatening illness: daily confrontations. To care for someone who has a life-threatening illness such as cancer is to continually confront issues of living and dying, of success and failure, of control and loss of control, of freedom and dependence. Cancer clients are people . . . they are mirrors of what may or can happen to the caregivers . . . also people. Giving of oneself, as the cancer client is cared for, provides the nurse with an opportunity to become intensely aware of personal fears, hopes, fantasies, and goals.

Repeated or continuous contact with life-threatened persons requires activation of psychologic coping mechanisms. These emotional protections make it possible for the nurse to initiate and maintain meaningful relationships with cancer clients. The coping, or defense, mechanisms that may be used include rationalization, projection, denial, displacement, and isolation. (The manner in which excessive use of these psychologic mechanisms results in signs and symptoms of nurse burnout is discussed in a later section.) While each of these coping strategies helps the nurse manage feelings related to client care situations, their implementation and maintenance require steady output of emotional energy. The nurse who continually expends this energy experiences emotional drain. As resources are depleted on the job, the impact may be felt in the nurse's personal life—there is less to give to family, friends, or self. Although "recharging" should occur during rest and recreation time away from client care settings, this does not always occur. The result can be emotional exhaustion in which the nurse begins to realize that a chronic state of "low energy reserves" exists.

Hurting and helping: paradox of cancer care. A second major psychologic antecedent to nurse burnout is represented by the following paradox: "In order to help you, sometimes I have to hurt you." This is such a simple statement; yet it is so potentially stressful for the nurse *and* client.

Cancer treatment generally requires implementation of surgical, radiologic, chemotherapeutic, and/or immunotherapeutic intervention. The impact of these interventions can be overwhelming to both recipient and caregiver. For example, the nurse who administers highly toxic chemicals to retard or halt malignant cell growth both helps and hurts the client: helping occurs with remission, increased freedom of movement, pain control, or increased longevity. At the same time, the side-effects of such drugs may cause severe physical discomfort, changes in body appearance and functioning, or emotional dysfunction. Foreknowledge of the potential adverse effects can prepare the nurse and client for their appearance, but it may not prepare the nurse for the client's individualized physical or emotional reaction.

For each client, the experience of radical surgery, radiation therapy, chemotherapy, immunotherapy, or a combination of these modalities is unique. As the nurse cares for many cancer clients and participates in their treatment process, it may become emotionally stressful to observe the often dramatic adverse changes that occur—the hurting part must precede the realization of help. It is generally a difficult task to observe the pain or discomfort of another. Because the frequency of "hurting/helping" in cancer nursing is often high, the nurse may become adversely affected in terms of emotional response. This element of stress, when combined with others, can increase the nurse's burnout risk.

Dying and death: depleting emotional resources. Cancer nursing focuses on a disease entity and client population for which the inability to attain cure is devastatingly common. Many clients have forms of cancer that are resistant to the treatments currently available, and for this reason, the nurse frequently must shift the emphasis of nursing care from cure to palliation. The dying cancer client is as much a part of cancer nursing as are cancer clients who achieve long-term survival. Yet, these dying people and their feelings of pain, anguish, and fear require a degree of human-to-human giving and involvement that may be emotionally draining for the nurse.

When the hope for cure must be abandoned, the nurse as well as other health team members may react with feelings of frustration, futility, anger, and sadness. These natural responses to anticipated loss or personal judgment of failure, when combined with the desire to support the client emotionally, can lead to a chronic state of exhaustion. While provision of nursing care for the dying cancer client is an integral part of cancer nursing, it must be recognized that the stress placed on emotional reserves can be severe. Over time, if precautions and preventive measures are not taken, the cancer nurse may find it necessary to withdraw from this area of practice. A primary reason given by some nurses in this specialty for such withdrawal is the continuous need for emotionally intense care that leaves the nurse exhausted and depleted.

Emotional exhaustion, or burnout, may also be related to the characteristics of the dying person. For some, it may be more stressful to care for (1) the dying child; (2) the parents of a dying child; (3) the dying person who is similar to the nurse in age, life-style, or personal history; (4) family members of a dying person, for example, interacting with the husband of a dying wife when school-aged children are involved; (5) an acquaintance, friend, or family member who is dying of cancer; or (6) the dying cancer client who continues a destructive behavior thought to be the cause of the disease, for example, the cigarette smoker with lung cancer. These and many other situations may be especially difficult to manage emotionally. If the nurse continues to care for clients under these circumstances, the risk of burnout can increase.

When a client dies, the cancer nurse must deal with another set of potentially draining circumstances. Postmortem care must be given, which in itself may be difficult to manage if frequency of death is high among the clients cared for. The family of the deceased often requires and strongly benefits from nursing support and caring during the most acute phases of grief. Assisting survivors with funeral arrangements and planning for departure from the hospital is mandatory and, at the same time, is stressful for the caregiver. Viewing and sharing in the emotionally painful and wrenching first hours of grief may deplete the nurse for the remainder of the work shift. As this is repeated over time and different situations, the burnout syndrome gains support.

System support: restrictive or enhancing. Because cancer nursing requires such tremendous outpourings of skill, knowledge, emotional investment, and philosophic commitment, it is reasonable to hypothesize that in order to do the work, support is required. "Support" may consist of (1) development and reliance on a peer network; (2) administrative backup in terms of staffing, facilities, pay, and other benefits; (3) a pronursing medical staff; (4) an understanding family; (5) reasonable work loads; (6) a degree of self-awareness that allows the nurse to seek help when needed. These supportive elements may or may not be present for each nurse caring for cancer clients.

The nurse who is highly stressed because of any one or more of the previously mentioned burnout antecedents may not realize the need to actively seek support. Thus, if support is not built into the care system, the nurse's burnout risk may be sharply increased. On the other hand, the nurse may actively seek support only to find that it is difficult to attain or is not available.

In cancer nursing as in other specialty areas of practice and occupations, nurses are expected to perform with expertise. Unfortunately, many health care institutions either are not aware of or are unwilling to provide the supportive elements that will allow the nurse to meet these expectations without incurring a high burnout risk. Other institutions purposefully design cancer care programs that achieve varying degrees of success in preventing burnout via implementation of supportive elements. Perhaps as health care systems become more sensitive to and aware of the burnout phenomenon, efforts will be made to provide support in a purposeful manner.

Personal life factors: stress external to nursing. The antecedents of burnout previously discussed are confined to nursing practice as it relates to cancer care. However, burnout may be exacerbated by stresses occurring in the nurse's personal life. Problems with family or social relationships place additional stress on the nurse, which may draw on emotional reserves previously devoted to client care situations. The reverse, of course, is also possible; that is, the nurse who experiences varying degrees of job-related burnout may have less to give to family and social relationships. The nurse who is experiencing personal life problems may be more susceptible to the stresses associated with burnout risk. As more physical or emotional energy is invested in resolution of personal problems, vulnerability to burnout antecedents may heighten.

The described antecedents of burnout represent major factors that increase the risk for development of signs and symptoms of emotional exhaustion. As previously noted, not every cancer nurse burns out. One's individual susceptibility varies across time and

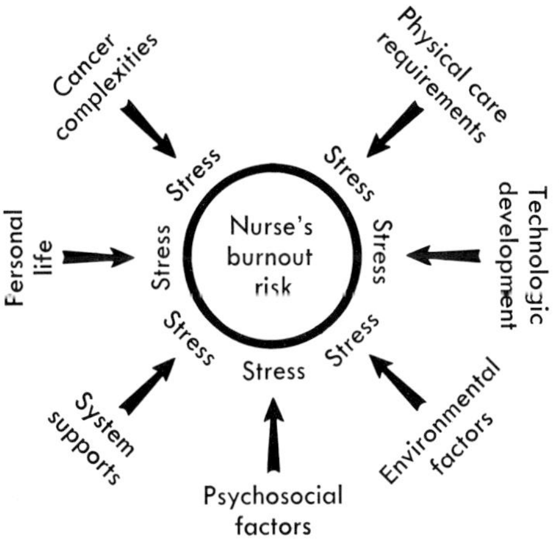

Fig. 8-1. Burnout, stress, and the nurse's risk of burnout.

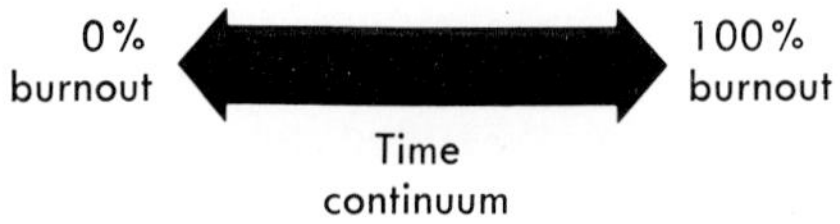

Fig. 8-2. Nurse's feeling of emotional exhaustion can range from 0% to 100%.

circumstance. In Fig. 8-1 the relationship of antecedents to burnout risk is depicted. These antecedents can result in increased stress levels, which in turn can increase the nurse's risk of experiencing a degree of burnout. It is important to emphasize that the burnout phenomenon is also a *process* occurring on a continuum of time (see Fig. 8-2). The nurse may feel more or less emotionally exhausted, according to current resources for coping. How the burnout syndrome manifests is the subject of the following section.

MANIFESTATIONS OF BURNOUT

The signs and symptoms of burnout can be easily identified in retrospect. However, the nurse who is *in the midst* of experiencing varying degrees of emotional exhaustion may not be aware of (1) the causes for these unsettling feelings, (2) the appearance of burnout behaviors or attitudes, or (3) the relationship of these signs and symptoms to client care. Feelings of burnout can have an adverse impact on the quantity and quality of client care given. Despite this potential adverse effect, it is vitally important for the nurse to refrain from self-condemnation and "blaming." The major goal of this chapter is to encourage the nurse to become keenly aware of the causes and manifestations of burnout. With this self-understanding well in hand, interventive and preventive strategies have a greater probability for success.

Psychologic and behavioral signs and symptoms

The observable and self-reported manifestations of burnout discussed here are representative of *major* changes that *may* occur with nurses who care for cancer clients. Obviously, not all cancer nurses burn out. For those who do, the following information can serve as self-assessment guidelines.

Shift in attitudes. In studies of the burnout syndrome, a primary finding has been a shift in attitudes on the part of caregivers toward clients.[9,15,17] Clients may be viewed as "difficult," "a problem," "not cooperative," or "always complaining." The underlying reason for such a shift from positive to negative attitudes is directly related to the caregiver's feeling of frustration, disapproval, or disappointment about client behavior or response to treatment. For example, the cancer client on chemotherapy refuses to eat despite all efforts to find appealing foods and preferences. The nurse who is experiencing a degree of burnout is more likely to (1) have a lower tolerance for the client's refusals, (2) be less understanding of the client's reasons for not eating, (3) reduce repeated attempts to follow up on nutritional needs, (4) convey disapproval to the client about not cooperating, and/or (5) evaluate the client as not worthy of care efforts. This client may be labeled a "problem" and, as a consequence, will be responded to in a more defensive manner by other caregivers. If this nurse were not experiencing burnout, it is likely that the client's refusal might be reassessed and relabeled as (1) an inability to eat because of continuing side-effects of chemotherapy administration, (2) fear of nausea and vomiting discomfort after appetite has returned, or (3) emotional adjustment problems related to treatment and prognosis. Emotional exhaustion, or burnout, *distorts* the nurse's ability to consistently assess, intervene, and evaluate in client care situations.

Shifts in attitudes may occur in relation to some clients and not others. In addition, attitude shifts may not be evidenced in a concrete fashion; that is, some nurses continue to provide comprehensive client care in a consistent . . . yet *distant* manner. In these cases, nurses emotionally distance themselves from interpersonal contact with the client or family—"efficiency" and "professionalism" are emphasized.

Attitudes toward co-workers, the institution, or hospital management may also shift from positive to negative. For instance, as the nurse continually cares for cancer clients over time, the caregiver's individualized need for emotional support increases. If peers or hospital management is not aware of the burnout risk, supportive services may not be provided. In turn, the nurse can begin to feel isolated and, in a sense, abandoned. One response to this sense of isolation can be anger directed toward these sources and/or the client.

The nurse may not be aware of a shift in attitudes, and in many cases, it is not identified until the caregiver terminates employment or seeks a transfer to a less stressful unit. Perhaps the most obvious example of gradual attitude shift is that which occurs with the newly graduated registered nurse—the "new grad syndrome." On graduation, the nurse is enthusiastic, innovative, and generally seeking an opportunity to practice nursing using these abilities. Soon, however, the new graduate may find that the social system of the unit does not necessarily place an equal value on enthusiasm and innovation. Over time, the graduate nurse assimilates to the mores and values of the nursing unit, that is, "the way things are done here." For many newly graduated nurses, this experience is discouraging and frustrating. A shift in attitude has occurred from positive enthusiasm to, hopefully, positive conformity. The risk in this situation has to do with setting the stage for burnout: If the new graduate's enthusiasm and innovation are severely stifled, the risk of rapid burnout increases. Of course, not all newly graduated nurses experience a muffling of motivation; however, in a highly stressful setting coupled with the social pressures to conform to usual standards of behavior, the new graduate may have an increased susceptibility to the antecedents of burnout.

Attitude shifts, therefore, can have an adverse influence on the care received by the cancer client. *Awareness* of this change from positive to neutral to negative client attitudes is dependent on (1) the degree of one's sensitivity to inner feelings, (2) the willingness to identify self-changes, (3) the amount of information received from the surrounding environment, and (4) the rapidity or slowness of burnout onset. The experience of emotional exhaustion is usually insidious. For this reason, continuous self-monitoring of attitudinal and emotional states is necessary. A hallmark of incipient or actual burnout often is a conscious reluctance to want to go to work. This resistance is not unusual in itself, yet when combined with other signs and symptoms of burnout, it is significant and noteworthy.

Defense mechanisms intensify. Psychologic defense mechanisms allow one to defend against anxiety.[10] In highly stressful and chronically stressful work situations, anxiety is continually activated. In response to the stress and related anxiety that are often associated with cancer care, the cancer nurse may intensify the unconscious use of these emotional coping devices. Evidence that intensified use of defense mechanisms has occurred is generated by (1) statements made about clients, families, or peers; (2) changes in approach and avoidance behaviors toward clients; and (3) the less tangible personal sense of dissatisfaction with one's performance. Certain defense mechanisms influence the nurse and, consequently, client care.

Rationalization. As a temporary anxiety reduction measure, rationalization allows the nurse to logically explain feelings or behavior that produces an inner sense of uncertainty or guilt. For example, the nurse passes by Mr. K.'s room although he has requested information on an upcoming diagnostic test. The nurse has the information but with use of rationalization has devised several logical reasons for not conveying it to Mr. K. For the nurse who is feeling burned out, these reasons might include: "I don't have the time," "He wouldn't understand," "That's really the physician's responsibility anyway." A reason is given for not doing what the nurse, under less stressful circumstances, would do. On a temporary basis, this reasoning may reduce anxiety related to nonperformance of the task.

Displacement. By discharging emotions, feelings, or ideas onto a person other than the one(s) to which they should be directed, the nurse does not risk the consequences of an emotional discharge that might be unacceptable. One example of displacement used by the nurse in a cancer care context is as follows: After a frustrating hour of trying to teach colostomy care to Mrs. L., the nurse, Ms. J., has just enough time to take a quick coffee break before medications must be passed. During the rest break, another nurse accidentally tips over a cup of coffee. Ms. J. sharply criticizes this nurse and abruptly leaves the lounge. In this case, Ms. J.'s feelings of anger, frustration, or failure regarding the client teaching episode were displaced onto a co-worker. Nurses who are experiencing increasing degrees of burnout may displace feelings generated in client care situations onto co-workers. The emotional discharge must occur somewhere, and in most cases, the nurse is not aware of ways to express nonpositive personal feelings with clients. In some cases, the buildup of emotional tension caused by burnout may be displaced in a more concrete manner by expressing feelings in a supportive group setting.

Projection. Attribution of personally unacceptable feelings or thoughts onto another or the environment is termed projection. Monotonous and stressful client care contexts may be associated with the cancer nurse's use of this emotional coping mechanism. A limited number of examples will be cited here although the reader may readily identify numerous situations in which projection is used in the daily practice of nursing: "I could do that wound irrigation if the client wasn't so nervous," "Mr. M. gets so upset and irritable whenever he talks about his cancer," or "There must be something wrong with Mr. K.; he never asks for analgesics." Each statement reflects a projection of the nurse's feelings or thoughts onto the client; that is, "*I* get nervous doing that irrigation," "*I* feel upset and irritated when Mr. M. brings up the subject of his illness," or "*I* sure would want analgesics if I were in his place." Use of projection, per se, is not abnormal. However, when the nurse intensifies its use in client care situations and peer interactions, it may indicate a buildup of emotional exhaustion with a concurrent inability to express the feelings in a more supportive manner.

Denial. Cancer nurses usually can accurately assess the the use of denial by clients. Yet, this defense mechanism may become a major means of refusing to acknowledge intense feelings of emotional exhaustion or burnout. To acknowledge this stressful sensation may imply a personal sense of (1) loss of control over one's emotions, (2) having failed to be a "good" nurse, or (3) threat to one's employment security. In this situation, the cancer nurse may openly deny any changes in feelings toward clients or the quality of care given. Excessive denial can be extremely detrimental in the burnout context. It may preclude an open awareness of a need for support with the ultimate result being (1) resignation, (2) termination of employment, (3) transfer to another position, or (4) physical illness onset.

Isolation/withdrawal. To continue to care for cancer clients when emotional exhaustion is increasing, the nurse may find it necessary to emotionally pull away from the client. This withdrawal or isolation results in less human-to-human contact and interpersonal involvement with clients or peers. If a supportive structure is not made available to the nurse at high risk for burnout, withdrawal becomes an emotional necessity. At the same time, the nurse may feel less satisfied with client care activity because of the reduction or elimination of emotional involvement. Withdrawal from emotional intensity is best exemplified by the "foot of the bed technique." Here, the nurse greets the client, interacts, and determines recovery status or care needs while standing at the foot of the client's bed. The physical distance is antagonistic to emotional intimacy or contact and, therefore, is less threatening for the nurse.

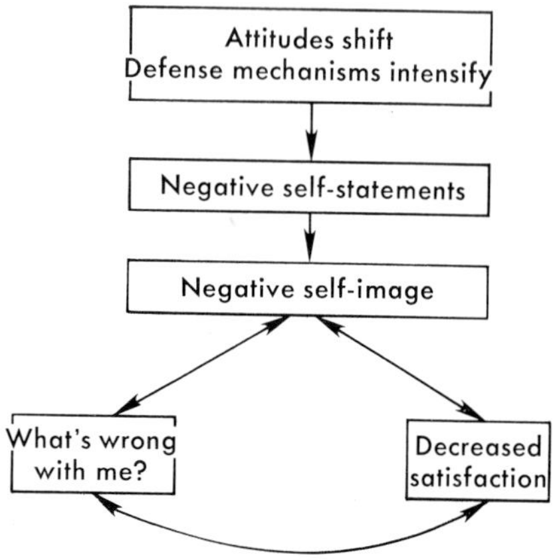

Fig. 8-3. A self-perpetuating negative cycle can develop when the nurse's self-image is affected by burnout.

Activation and intensification of emotional coping mechanisms provide significant clues to the existence of the burnout process. The nurse is not conscious of engaging in projection, denial, and so forth and, thus, need not be harshly or negatively judged when their use becomes apparent. As *clues* to burnout, however, the nurse *can* become more self-aware and sensitive to the onset of increased use of defensive maneuvers. With increased awareness, it is possible to engage in preventive and interventive strategies.

Self-image declines. One's self-image is influenced by thoughts, feelings, and evaluations about personal behavior and interactions with others. When attitudes shift regarding clients or peers and the use of defense mechanisms increases, the nurse may begin to feel less positive about the self. Questions may arise such as, "I just don't seem to care about my work," "I do the client care but don't feel committed anymore," "I used to feel so enthusiastic; where did it all go?" These self-statements reflect negative self-evaluations without a corresponding understanding of the antecedents of the changed image.

An acceptable or positive self-image supports the nurse in continuing to engage in satisfying client care activities. Conversely, if the self-image is negative or damaged, there is less motivation to continue to engage in activities that result in negative self-image evaluations. A self-perpetuating negative cycle may result as shown in Fig. 8-3. If this cycle is not disrupted by specific interventions, the nurse may continue to self-blame, which can perpetuate a downward spiral toward eventual withdrawal from the stressful situation or onset of illness.

Flexibility decreases. As the nurse engages in the burnout process, tolerance for ambiguity declines. It becomes more difficult and unacceptable to operate in unclear or multiple option situations. The person seeks to reduce choices by polarizing options. For example, the nurse who is becoming emotionally exhausted may begin to strictly enforce visiting rules that previously were evaluated on a case-by-case basis. Adherence to policy and rules allows the stressed nurse a degree of freedom from individualized decision making as well as a distancing from personal involvement. Relationships with peers also may be influenced by reduction in flexibility. The nurse may be less willing to alter work schedules or assignments as was previously customary on the unit. By referring to "policy and rules," the nurse may feel less responsible for the criticism received as a result of increasing personal rigidity.

Of course, not all nurses who "go by the book" are burned out, nor is adherence to established policy always inappropriate. When the quality of cancer care becomes more and more dehumanized as a result of strict rule obedience, however, it is necessary to assess the reasons for the change. For instance, the 24-year-old father dying from malignant melanoma may desperately wish to spend private and intimate time with his wife and two preschool-age children. If the nurse is caught up in personal feelings of exhaustion, the request may be denied citing visit or age limitations as the rationale. If this case had arisen at a time when the nurse was energized and sensitive to the client's need, the visiting rule most likely would have been reevaluated.

Emotions change. Many nurses who are burned out first become aware of the process when feelings of depression or anger begin to surface. The emotional depression may be associated with low self-image, dissatisfaction with performance, or the impact of burnout on personal relationships. These feelings of sadness, loss, isolation, and fatigue often are reflected by reduction in verbal social interaction with peers, chronic complaints of fatigue, low energy levels, accomplishing minimal work requirements, or alterations in physical appearance. The depression referred to here generally does not reach pathologic proportions, but it does detract from the nurse's quality of living and working and is highly indicative of the burnout process.

Each person's emotions change according to current mood or situational demands. While change in emotions is not in itself detrimental to one's well-being, prolonged periods of depression or sustained anger can be generalized to one's life situation. When the nurse feels depressed and personal relationships and life-style have *not* contributed to this emotional state, it is imperative that assessment of burnout be undertaken. *Work-related* stress may be the causative factor.

Physical signs and symptoms

Because each person is an interacting and interdependent *system,* change in one element affects all others to some degree. As a consequence, the burnout process may be evidenced by a variety of physical illnesses or dysfunctions. Empirical support for this assertion is provided by the preponderance of research findings relating various illnesses to long-term stressful environments and life events.[5,6,12,18] Correlational research clearly demonstrates a relationship between stressful life-style and illnesses such as cardiovascular disease, migraine headache, and increased susceptibility to cancer, arthritis, and respiratory disease.[3,18,25,26] The nurse experiencing burnout, therefore, *may* have an *increased susceptibility* or *risk* for a number of illnesses and health dysfunctions. In addition, physical signs and symptoms of burnout may manifest as disruptions in various aspects of body functioning.

Lowering of illness resistance. As the burnout process continues, the physical and emotional fatigue that becomes apparent may reduce the body's ability to resist upper respiratory infections (for example, colds or "flu"). When physical resources are utilized excessively in highly stressful nursing care environments, there may be fewer immunologic resources to draw on when such viruses are around. Nurses who otherwise would have a stable cardiovascular system may experience hypertensive episodes of increasing frequency when burnout stresses are of chronic proportions. Long-term emotional exhaustion may also be identified via onset of migraine headaches, various musculoskeletal problems (back pain, chronic muscle tension), or reduced tolerance to painful stimulation. If the nurse continues to work while ill, the recovery period may be prolonged. As with other members of the general population, the highly stressed cancer nurse may become more susceptible to onset of serious dysfunctions, for example, myocardial infarction. The nurse's status as a health professional carries no immunity to such diseases, and when a burnout process is underway, it *may* actually increase susceptibility.

Disturbances in living habits. Prolonged stress and associated burnout are also correlated with disturbances in major living patterns. Table 8-1 summarizes the possible changes in living habits that may occur when the nurse enters into the burnout process. Each of these changes is interdependent. For example, the physically and emotionally fatigued nurse has little energy with which to engage in sexually fulfilling activities or to participate in previously enjoyed recreational programs. Continued sleep disturbances further reduce energy resources and exacerbate fatigue. How disturbances in living habits manifest during burnout will, of course, vary according to the individual's response style. Of importance is the nurse's recognition that emotional exhaustion *can* have adverse impact on nonwork-related areas of life functioning.

Table 8-1. Disturbances in living habits: burning out

Habit	Disturbance
Sleep	Early rising Difficulty falling asleep Disrupted sleep Difficulty remaining asleep
Eating	Overeating Weight gain (nondesired) Loss of appetite Weight loss (nondesired) Change in foods eaten
Sexual	Changes in frequency (nondesired) Loss of interest Reduced satisfaction Sexual dysfunctions
Activity	Low energy levels Cessation of exercise program Loss of interest

The potential manifestations of burnout are numerous and varied. Most signs and symptoms produce observable behavior changes and, hence, allow the nurse who is experiencing burnout to be identified and supported. Burnout is not a mysterious phenomenon. Each nurse caring for clients in an cancer care setting can probably identify colleagues, or oneself, as either burnout candidates or as progressively burning out. No attempt has been made to be all inclusive of every psychologic, behavioral, or physical expression of burnout. The material presented serves as a guideline for self-assessment and intervention strategy planning—the topic of the next section.

STRATEGIES FOR BURNOUT PREVENTION AND INTERRUPTION

The burnout syndrome occurs over time and can, therefore, be conceptualized as a process. It is possible to alter the course of the burnout process in two ways as shown in Fig. 8-4. The interventions, or strategies, presented here are applicable to prevention *and* interruption of burnout. Ideally, the nurse can learn to recognize the antecedents of burnout and institute preventive measures, thereby avoiding the experience of emotional exhaustion. It is of equal importance that the nurse knows *how* to interrupt the process. Third, nurses who feel that emotional exhaustion has reached chronic proportions *can* learn how to *regain* a sense of emotional and physical well-being.

The discussion of strategies presented here is designed to act as a stimulus to the nurse for further study and consideration. Descriptions of specific interventions are brief and should be viewed as *initial* sources to assist in the development of individual self-care plans.

The first step: looking inward

Before one can decide where, how, when, or why behavior should be changed, it is necessary to engage in inward self-examination. The person who is burning out generally is not overtly aware of the nature of the process; that is, being in the midst of emotional exhaustion may preclude identification of the phenomenon. For this reason, the first step in preventing or interrupting burnout is to look inward and to examine awareness, sensitivity, responsibility, and commitment to oneself.

Self-assessment and sensitivity. As burnout begins and progresses, one becomes more and more "out of step" with personal feelings, wants, and goals. Daily work demands require inordinate amounts of energy expenditure leaving little to draw on for other purposes. For these reasons, the nurse must learn to apply a systematic assessment

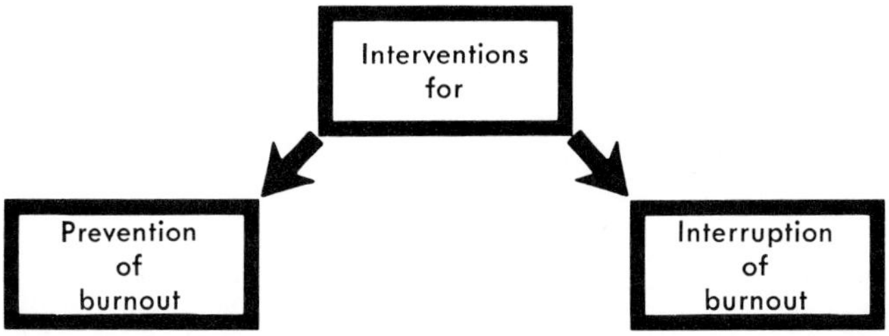

Fig. 8-4. Goals of preventing *and* interrupting burnout can be accomplished.

procedure to the *self*. In order to become more self-aware and sensitive to one's emotional exhaustion status, it may be helpful to consider the following questions and suggestions:

1. On a 10-point scale, how would you rate your *attitude* toward clients, peers, and the work environment? (Use *1* as the poorest and *10* as the best attitude.) If these ratings are below 5, how long have you felt this way? Can you think of any precipitating events or experiences that might explain these attitudes?
2. Rate your attitude toward nursing and cancer nursing (a) at time of graduation from nurses' training, (b) 1 year ago, (c) 6 months ago, and (d) now. How do these compare? Have there been changes in a positive direction or in a negative direction?
3. How many of your clients are "problems," "difficult to manage," "always complaining"? Do other nurses you work with feel the same way about these clients? What, exactly, makes these clients so different?
4. If you had the freedom to do so, would you remain on your present nursing unit or transfer? What factors would influence your decision? Have you always felt this way about your work place? If not, when did things begin to change?
5. Keep a journal or diary for a week. At the beginning and end of each day, rate (using a 5-point scale from high to low) your: (a) energy level, (b) happiness or depression, (c) quality and quantity of sleep and eating, (d) quality of recreation, and (e) amount of work satisfaction and fulfillment. At the end of the week, compare the ratings for each day. Pay particular attention to differences at the beginning and end of each day. Are there sudden changes in ratings? What are they caused by? Are energy ratings very similar regardless of when measured? If so, fatigue may not be decreasing. Are sleep and eating patterns stable and satisfying?
6. Are you feeling muscular tension anywhere in your body? Where? Can you relax it? How long does the relaxation last before the muscles tense again? Were you aware of this tension *prior* to focusing your full attention on it? Keep a record of muscle tension and note specific events that are associated with increases in muscular tightness. Use this information to increase your sensitivity to events that cause you to become tense.
7. What does your work environment look like? How would you rate it: good, fair, dull? In what ways could it be changed or improved? How do you *feel* about your work environment?
8. Where do you get emotional support? Who, at work, knows you most intimately? Can you share inner feelings about client care with someone who will listen? How do you *seek* emotional support? Do you allow clients to give support when you're feeling sad or fatigued? Why or why not?
9. Do you feel enthusiastic about your work? Do you view new client care assignments as challenges or burdens? Rate your enthusiasm for work over a week's time. What influenced changes in your enthusiasm?
10. Over the course of your next working period, self-monitor pulse, respiratory rate, fatigue, and level of job satisfaction three times. Do this two more shifts and compare the results. Notice patterns in these readings and recollect events that may have coincided with these sensations.

Each of these self-assessment items can assist the nurse in evaluating stress levels and, hence, burnout potential or status. Because self-assessment is individualized, the nurse may find that responses to these items foster consideration of other attitudes, beliefs, or values. As one increases inner awareness and sensitivity to the self, it is then possible to assume personal responsibility for a commitment to actively prevent or interrupt the burnout process.

Responsibility and commitment. For the nurse to prevent burnout, and in most cases to interrupt the process, it is essential that the affected person assume responsibility for intervention. One may waste time and energy waiting for an external source (for example, "they") to intervene. This does not imply that one may not *seek* assistance or support from sources external to the self.

Responsibility refers to the nurse's acceptance of an active role in achieving and maintaining optimal levels of self-care. For example, Ms. S. has become aware that she feels unusually tired, has become irritable with her peers and friends, and has minimal environmental stimulation at her work place. Although there is no stress management or burnout treatment program in the hospital, Ms. S. decides to seek emotional support. She discusses the idea of several nurses getting together on a regular basis to discuss emotional issues and feelings. The first meeting takes place and a number of the nurses find that they share similar feelings. Ms. S. and the other nurses feel less isolated and discouraged. Each has taken an active role in altering the burnout process. Nurses in similar or different circumstances might have decided to focus on environmental changes, communication skills, or one-to-one discussions. The important point is that the nurse *can* be effective in managing burnout when the responsibility for achieving a desired outcome is assumed.

A second aspect of personal involvement in one's self-care maintenance is *commitment*. The nurse needs to evaluate personal levels of commitment to self-care. As obvious as the last statement would appear, most nurses work in health care institutions that focus on externally delivered medical treatment for tangible illnesses. This traditional medical model places responsibility for health care on the *system* (for example, physicians, nurses, hospital) and not on the *consumer*. To achieve the goal of optimal self-care with concurrent avoidance or disruption of burnout, the nurse needs to shift to a holistic model of health care. By viewing oneself as composed of many interdependent elements (social, physical, psychologic, spiritual), the nurse can use personal resources as well as those associated with the traditional health care system. The key to the holistic approach is a firm commitment by the nurse to *participation* in self-care activities. In terms of preventing and interrupting the burnout process, a deep feeling of personal commitment to wellness is essential.

The success of the burnout intervention strategies to be discussed is dependent on the nurse's assumption of responsibility for and commitment to maintenance of self-care. Belief that one *can* have an impact on health, as well as illness, provides the nurse with an opportunity to avoid emotional exhaustion and, hence, to achieve a continuing sense of satisfaction in caring for cancer clients.

TAKING ACTION: IMPLEMENTING INDIVIDUALIZED INTERVENTIONS

As the cancer nurse assumes responsibility for prevention or disruption of the burnout syndrome, it is possible to devise an individualized intervention plan to achieve the desired goal: maintenance of wellness. The nurse is a model for self-care by virtue of the designation of health care professional. As such, clients, peers, families, and friends observe how the nurse behaves, what attitudes are projected, and the manner in which self-care activities are undertaken. Some nurses prefer not to be viewed as a health care model for others, and yet, this cannot completely be avoided—the nurse is on the "front line" of the health care delivery system and *will be* viewed as an example of self-care behavior by the nonprofessional.

The amount of responsibility inherent in the status of role model can be tremendous when considered as an external phenomenon. However, if this responsibility can be redefined as an opportunity to focus a portion of one's energies on self-care and wellness, the nurse can achieve optimal benefits such as increased job satisfaction, avoidance of burnout, and heightened sensitivity to the needs of oncology clients. The strategies described here are representative of activities the nurse can evaluate, investigate, and implement on an individualized basis. Each person's plan for preventing or interrupting burnout will be different; there is no "recipe" or "one right way" to maintain wellness.

Review cognitive basis for client care

Review of and attention to one's thought processes and perceptions regarding client care can result in stress reduction and, consequently, lowering of burnout risk.

Values clarification. Central to a program of self-care is values clarification. Each nurse can benefit greatly by reviewing values related to nursing, cancer nursing, and cancer clients. The cognitive-based clarifying process encourages the nurse to identify a value (for example, cancer clients benefit greatly from interpersonal contact with the nurse) and then to consider seven criteria of valuing.[20] After a review, the individual is able to redefine the value in clearer terms, thereby gaining a more intense understanding of an aspect of behavior. Because values are communicated verbally and nonverbally, clarification of how they influence nursing practice and personal goals *can* result in improved communication, reduction in self-blaming/guilt, and a renewed commitment to quality client care. Seven criteria for values clarification are:

1. *Free choice:* A value that has been chosen without coercion or social pressure is a genuine value for that person.
2. *Consideration of alternatives:* A value can only be defined as such if it is chosen after consideration of two or more alternatives. If a choice is not involved, a value does not result.
3. *Reflection on alternatives:* Careful cognitive weighing of alternatives and the consequences of each allows one to make an informed value choice.
4. *Respect, cherish, and prize:* For a value to be retained and used as a guide to nursing practice, it must be positively viewed, cherished, respected, and prized.
5. *Affirmation of choice:* A choice that one is willing to publicly affirm, or even champion, is a value.
6. *Action based on choices:* Values serve as guides for living and, for the nurse, for nursing practice. If a value is held and respected, it is reflected by one's actions.
7. *Repeat of choice:* Over time, a guiding value is repeated. If it is not repeated, the entity is not truly a value.

The values clarification process can be applied to any value. In nursing, it has particular relevance when the nurse becomes aware of feelings of emotional exhaustion. A planned reappraisal of one's values toward a particular situation can foster reduction in confusion and dissatisfaction.

In addition to values clarification, the nurse can reevaluate several cognitive functions that have direct impact on emotional and physical self-care.

Decision making. Review how decisions about nursing care are made: Is there a logical progression, that is, identifying topic, gathering information, identifying alternatives, evaluating alternatives, selecting a solution, implementing, and reassessing. If not, the nurse can reinstitute the decision-making process or seek to revise how the process is carried out. As nurses actively participate in decisions that influence them, there can be a reduction in stress and hence burnout potential.

Goal setting. When caring for cancer clients, it is crucial to establish realistic goals for care. Although nurses understand this principle, over time in highly stressful environments it can be overlooked. A review of how one sets goals and acts on them can result in renewed enthusiasm and a more positive attitude toward nursing, clients, peers, and oneself. Realistic goals may seem insignificant at times, yet for a specific client, in specific circumstances, with specific resources, accomplishment of a "mini-goal" may result in a significant sense of satisfaction for the client, family, and nurse.

Priority and limit setting. Once a burnout process has begun, the nurse is less able to adhere to limits related to energy expenditure. In addition, it can become increasingly difficult to establish priorities and adhere to them. By focusing attention on limit and priority setting, the nurse can become aware of the manner in which these cognitive activities have been neglected. One must *consciously* attend to personal limit and priority setting; failure to do so can support burnout. The nurse can consider the following: Do I allow myself to miss rest breaks repeatedly, accept requests for overtime, or "do it myself" rather than seek assistance with a difficult task? How do I arrange my work: to suit the system or the client? Can I reprioritize my caseload?

The cognitive self-care strategies presented here are not all-inclusive of the areas that the nurse can consider. Other areas might include perception and assumption assessment, alteration, and/or problem-solving strategies.

Review of the cognitive basis for client care is an *ongoing* activity that can be successful only when the nurse assumes continuing responsibility for the process.

Revamp communication styles

One *cannot not* communicate.[10] Communication is the vehicle by which each person interacts with the environment and all that it contains. In high stress contexts, how one communicates can enhance or inhibit the burnout process. While it is not feasible to include a treatise on communication styles here, it is possible to briefly outline areas that the nurse can "tune in to" with respect to clients, peers, and family.

Clarity and specificity of messages. Consider the way in which one makes requests of peers or clients. Are these messages clear and specific? Is there more than one message being conveyed: for example, the obviously rushed nurse asks the client if he wants a back rub. The message here might really be: "I'm asking this question, but I really don't have time to fulfill it." The client will probably get the underlying message and reply, "No, thank you."

A second area involving specificity of communication concerns *expectations.* Nurses, as well as other people, establish expectations of what is wanted from coworkers, clients, clients' families, and health care institutions. If these expectations are not *communicated,* a number of consequences may ensue: (1) disappointment when another person does not do what one expected; (2) anger directed toward a client or peer who failed to comply with an expectation; (3) frustration with another's apparent failure to be sensitive, caring, or to complete a task; and (4) feeling rejected or not respected by client, peer, or family may develop.

Failure to clearly and specifically communicate expectations results in a *message trap.* For example, the nurse expects the client to do a specific task. The client, however, does not know what the expectation is and thinks the nurse will complete the task. When the client does not meet the expectation, the nurse may feel angry and frustrated and may communicate this to the client. Future interactions between this nurse and the client can be adversely influenced by message traps.

The nurse can avoid message traps by (1) becoming aware of unspoken expectations, (2) understanding that others cannot "read your mind," and (3) clearly communicating an expectation to a target person(s). In this way, each party to a communication knows what the expectation is and can respond accordingly.

Verbal and nonverbal messages. For the nurse to improve communication and hence avoid mixed, confusing messages that can drain one's energy, attention to the nature of verbal and nonverbal messages is necessary. It is not difficult to focus on verbal messages. Nonverbal messages require a more concentrated form of self-awareness. For example, ask questions such as: Where do I position myself when I'm with a client or peer—what is the distance between each person? When interacting with a client or family, are my arms crossed? Does the body communicate openness or closedness? Are verbal and nonverbal messages *congruent?* Careful review of the nonverbal messages conveyed to the nurse *by others* can help to increase awareness of the impact of unspoken communication and what these signals mean.

Once the nurse has increased awareness of how nonverbal communication is perceived, it is possible to self-monitor the congruence or matching of verbal and nonverbal messages. Clarity and matching of both levels of communication reduce the recipient's confusion regarding the meaning of messages. Each person is then free to respond to a clear message.

Awareness of the impact or meaning of verbal and nonverbal messages can only be maintained by continued, periodic self-monitoring. Failure to attend to this vital aspect of communication style can increase the overall amount of energy required to interact; that is, when the nurse repeats a message, revises it, or begins to feel frustrated when requests or comments are not responded to as anticipated, energy resources can be inordinately depleted. Conversely, alteration of communication styles can increase the total amount of energy available to the nurse and, therefore, reduce burnout risk.

Assertiveness and message impact. Implementation of an assertive approach to interaction allows the nurse to maintain consistency, intention, and clarity of communication with other people. Being assertive reduces feelings of helplessness and dependence in high-stress environments. In addition, an assertive communication style may decrease the frequency of physical dysfunctions; for example, asthma, general fatigue, or headaches.[1,23] Assertion of one's legitimate rights includes genuine concern for the feelings, wants, and goals of others. Without sensitivity to the rights of those with whom the nurse interacts, communication is characterized more by aggressiveness than by assertiveness.

An assertive communication style supports the nurse's professional contribution to client care. Examples of assertiveness in the cancer care context include: (1) making specific suggestions for client care to co-workers or physicians, (2) client advocacy, (3) initiating client care conferences, (4) establishing staff and/or client support groups, (5) actively offering emotional support to co-workers, and (6) seeking emotional support when awareness of burnout occurs.

Individualized assertive communication of skills can be acquired in structured classes, seminars, conferences, or via self-instruction using available published materials.[1,23]

Revamping communication styles and reviewing the cognitive basis for client care are mutually supportive activities. As the nurse purposefully assesses and continues to self-monitor each element, a feeling of regaining control over essential aspects of life's quality can be achieved. Improvements in self-image, attitudes, and satisfaction have an opportunity to blossom in such a self-nurturing atmosphere.

Recreate and relax for wellness

Some of the most immediately accessible and productive self-care strategies are those that support recreation and relaxation. These two vital aspects of qualitative living, however, are largely taken for granted. As the nurse continues to work in highly stressful client care environments, the ability to truly *recreate* and *relax* becomes impaired if awareness is not focused on the activities in a conscious manner.

Recreation. The purpose of recreational or leisure activity is to *re*create physical, emotional, social, and spiritual capacities. Unfortunately, many of the activities that are labeled "recreation" are characterized by interpersonal intensity (competition) and/or excessive energy expenditure. When participation in a chosen recreational activity results in a feeling of relaxation and an increase in energy level, recreation has occurred. The nurse can increase awareness of the value of recreational activities by completing the exercise that is shown below.

On an 8½ inch × 11 inch sheet of paper, place the following headings along the top of the page:

Activity	Ranked importance	$	Last done	Restfulness

List all leisure time activities that are of value under *activity*. Rank this list as to most important (No. 1), next most important (No. 2), and so forth. Then place an estimated cost ($) for each activity in the next column. Under the fourth heading, rate when each activity was last engaged in. Finally, evaluate how restful each activity is using a 3-point scale: 1=very restful, 2=occasionally restful, and 3=tiring.

Carefully examine the information on the completed sheet. For example, note which activities are *highly* ranked (that is, valued), are of *low* cost, have *not* been done recently, and are *most* restful. This information and the concurrent awareness it produces serve as guides to the revision of recreational activities and goals. With alteration of the nature and frequency of recreational activities, the nurse can increase the quality of restfulness and thus promote a higher level of wellness—burnout is therefore avoided.

Relaxation. It is generally assumed that by lying down, reading a book, watching TV, or not being overtly active one is relaxing. True relaxation involves more than a cessation of physical activity; it consists of a deep sense of restfulness and a slowing of heart rate, respiration, and brain wave activity. To achieve deep relaxation, one must engage in a progressive retraining of the body. Purposeful relaxation prevents and disrupts stress responding, thereby inhibiting burnout. There are numerous ways to learn how to truly relax: (1) participation in relaxation training programs/classes, (2) self-instruction, and (3) individualized training. Two successful relaxation methods are outlined below. The nurse who wishes to learn how to attain deep muscle relaxation should investigate hospital, community, mental health clinic, or published resources for detailed instructions and guidelines.

1. Alternately tighten and relax major muscle groups, starting with hands, arms, and shoulders and slowly progressing to all

parts of the body. This method teaches the person the difference between tension and relaxation and develops control of the relaxation response.

2. Visualize a wave of relaxation slowly traveling throughout the muscles of the body starting with the toes, foot, ankle, calf, and so forth. Each body part is attended to separately until the entire body has been deeply relaxed.

Each method requires approximately 30 minutes to complete in the beginning phase of training. As the nurse becomes more skilled at teaching the body to relax, the amount of time required to achieve deep muscle relaxation is reduced. With continued practice, the nurse can learn to relax the body in a few minutes. In stressful work settings, the ability to relax the body while maintaining mental alertness can be done several times during a work shift; for example, during rest breaks or by sitting quietly and consciously relaxing the body at the nurse's station.

Meditation. The practice of meditation, much like deep relaxation, is counter to maintenance of physiologic stress arousal, specifically arousal of the sympathetic nervous system. The continued popularity of meditation suggests that many people regularly engage in and derive benefit from this self-care activity.

Meditation is an *experiential* activity of attention focusing.[14,18,24] It can either be a disciplining of the mind on single thoughts with a concurrent filtering out of extraneous stimuli (for example, Rinzai Zen, transcendental meditation) or an opening of the mind to undistracted receptivity (for example, Zen or Soto Zen meditation). For the nurse under consistent work-related stress, meditation offers an opportunity for calming the mind and body as well as a growth of inner awareness.

No attempt will be made here to teach the fundamentals of meditation. The benefit of identifying meditation as a valid self-care strategy can only be realized when the nurse actively seeks out a meditation program, class, or teacher and makes a commitment *to the self* to integrate the activity into a long-term, self-care plan.

The self-care strategies presented in this section promote an enhanced feeling of wellness *and* control over one's affective status. Active participation in wellness-promoting activities prohibits burnout; self-care and burnout are mutually exclusive.

Restore physical capacities

A major aspect of self-care maintenance and the prevention of burnout is restoration of physical capacities, which includes the following components: (1) exercise and (2) habit review and revision.

Aerobic exercise. Consistent participation in an individualized aerobic exercise program gradually improves the body's capacity to (1) efficiently utilize calories, (2) strengthen heart, lungs, and muscles via enhanced circulation, (3) absorb and use food, (4) sleep restfully, and (5) avoid psychologic tension.[25] Examples of aerobic exercises are running, jogging, bicycling, swimming, and vigorous walking. The nurse who decides to participate in an exercise program will do so in a gradual fashion, allowing time for heart and muscle conditioning to take place.

Prior to initiating an aerobic exercise program, the nurse should undergo a physical examination and electrocardiogram. To adhere to a graduated exercise program, it is recommended that the nurse (1) participate in a designated physical fitness program, (2) seek advice on how to start a program from a qualified physician, (3) read about the purpose, goals, and philosophy of aerobics,[6,7] and/or (4) find an "exercise buddy" who will also participate in the program. A planned approach to initiation and continuation of a physical fitness program eliminates "false starts"; for example, doing calisthenics vigorously for a few weeks and then stopping altogether.

The nurse who begins and sticks with an aerobic exercise program can increase cardiac and respiratory effectiveness and efficiency. In addition, a greater sense of well-being and relaxation can be achieved. Both of these positive consequences of exercise are antagonistic to a feeling of emotional exhaustion. The increased energy level that can result from exercise allows the nurse to manage work-related stress more easily and at the same time reduces susceptibility to stress-related dysfunctions.

Habit review. One's habits of daily living can either support or inhibit burnout. The nurse who is at high risk for burnout needs to revise major life habits and determine how they impact on physical, emotional, and social spheres of functioning. The following briefly outlines major life habits deserving careful scrutiny.

Eating. Review the kinds, quality, and quantity of foods commonly eaten. What is the nutritional value of these foods? How could dietary changes be made? What changes should be made? Are nutritional supplements used or needed? Is dieting a problem? Why? What would it take to make eating less of a problem?

Smoking. Is cigarette smoking of high value? Why? Can personal responsibility for wellness coincide with a cigarette habit? If not, how and when will this habit be changed?

Using drugs. What quantity and type of drugs are being used? Why? What changes are necessary if a commitment to wellness is made? How does use of drugs (including alcohol and caffeine) support the burnout process? Is use of drugs truly essential?

• • •

Each of these habits has an adverse impact on the nurse, which in turn fosters susceptibility to the burnout process. Self-care involves an acute awareness of the influence of habits on physical, emotional, and social well-being. The nurse who becomes aware of the threat of burnout *must* be willing to actively reverse the process. Maintaining potentially harmful life habits is contradictory to the concept of wellness and prevention of burnout.

Revitalize the work environment

To prevent and disrupt burnout, it is often extremely helpful to seek ways to revitalize the nurse's work environment. Three strategies are presented here.

Support group. By expressing feelings of frustration, fatigue, and emotional overload with co-workers, the nurse learns that others share similar experiences—the nurse is no longer alone and isolated with these feelings. The support group establishes the context for this self-help and self-care.[9,13,15,16]

A support group can be initiated by one or more nurses who wish to reduce interpersonal tensions, as well as discuss issues related to client care, for example, death, dying, cure, and palliation. Giving and receiving emotional support is the strength of this strategy. The group may become an ongoing resource for emotional support and caring.

Individualized support. At times, the nurse may find it necessary to *actively seek* emotional support from peers, friends, family, or professional counselors. Giving oneself the *permission* to seek support is often extremely difficult for the nurse who generally is viewed as the caregiver, not the care receiver. It is important to remember that "the caregiver also needs a caregiver." This does not imply weakness, "mental illness," or an inability to manage one's life. It does imply that the nurse can recognize and make use of a valid self-care alternative instead of assuming, "I can take care of myself at all times, under any circumstances, indefinitely."

Sharing one's feelings with a person who can listen, provide emotional support, and promote self-understanding reduces isolation. In addition, the sharing process promotes development of self-awareness and hence a greater degree of involvement in one's self-care.

Staff development. Regular or periodic educational programs that focus on new cancer information, treatments, and nursing practices can serve as "booster" sessions in high burnout risk contexts. Attendance at such offerings allows the nurse to share ideas, explore new concepts, and renew enthusiasm. The stimulation experienced at a conference or seminar can be brought back to the nursing unit, resulting in positive input for co-workers and clients.

Environmental change. The characteristics of where one works, as previously stated, can influence susceptibility to burnout. The nurse can institute changes in the work environment that may inhibit boredom or dissatisfaction with surroundings. Different work places require individualized alterations. For example, the nurse may want to consider reorganization of supplies, introduction of colorful posters on certain walls, listening to music when on rest breaks, or personalizing the work space. Limits to environmental change must be considered prior to implementation, for example, institutional restrictions and impact on coworkers.

Miscellaneous essentials

Self-care also includes such things as (1) taking rest breaks regardless of a feeling of "I'm not tired," (2) taking meal breaks, preferably in a quiet environment, (3) arranging vacation time in "mini vacation" blocks, and (4) requesting periodic "mental health days" when stress levels reach excessively high levels. As logical as these "essentials" sound, many burned-out nurses state that they terminated these activities as they felt more and more emotionally exhausted. Prevention implies a reduction in the possibility of an occurrence. With burnout risk, engaging consistently in these restful activities can be supportive of burnout prevention.

SUMMARY

This chapter has presented initial information on the antecedents and manifestations of burnout. With an understanding of the dynamics of burnout, the cancer nurse is in a position to assume responsibility for a commitment to prevention of emotional exhaustion. The self-care strategies discussed focused primarily on interventions the nurse can implement. It must be acknowledged, however, that the work setting (that is, institution or hospital) has an equal responsibility to actively support the nurse's self-care activities and institute complementary supportive programs.

Research on the causes, consequences, and interventions appropriate to burnout will provide empirical guidelines for future program development. Nurses can greatly benefit from participation in such research and the self-care programs (that is, organized and individualized) emerging from empirical data. Burnout risk would appear to be inherent in the highly stressful area of cancer nursing. Continued practice of self-care strategies can prevent and disrupt this potentially devastating process. The ultimate outcome is twofold: nurses can experience personal growth and satisfaction, and clients can receive creative, high-quality care.

REFERENCES

1. Alberti, R. E., and Emmons, M. L.: Your perfect right, San Luis Obispo, Calif., 1970, Impact Publishers, Inc.
2. American Cancer Society: 1979 facts and figures, New York, 1978, American Cancer Society, Inc.
3. American Hospital Association: Stress! Chicago, 1977, American Hospital Association.
4. Burkhalter, P. K., and Donley, D. L.: Dynamics of oncology nursing, New York, 1978, McGraw-Hill Book Co.
5. Cohen, H. A., and Orlinsky, N.: Work stress on critical care units, Emergency Medical Services **6**:27, 1977.
6. Cooper, C. L., and Marshall, J.: Occupational sources of stress: a review of the literature relating to coronary heart disease and mental ill health, J. Occup. Psychol. **49**:11, 1976.
7. Cooper, K. H.: The new aerobics, New York, 1977, Bantam Books, Inc.
8. Cooper, M., and Cooper, K. H.: Aerobics for women, New York, 1977, Bantam Books, Inc.
9. Freudenberger, H. J.: Staff burn-out, J. Soc. Issues **30**(1):159, 1974.
10. Gilmore, S. K.: The counselor-in-training, Englewood Cliffs, N.J., 1973, Prentice-Hall, Inc.
11. Haber, J., Leach, A. M., Schudy, S. M., and Sideleau, B. F.: Comprehensive psychiatric nursing, New York, 1978, McGraw-Hill Book Co.
12. Ilfeld, F. W., Jr.: Current social stressors and symptoms of depression, Am. J. Psychiatry **134**(2): 161, 1977.
13. Kahn, R.: Job burnout: prevention and remedies, Public Welfare, p. 61, Spring, 1978.
14. LeShan, L.: How to meditate, New York, 1974, Bantam Books, Inc.
15. Maslach, C.: Burned-out, Hum. Behav. **5**:16, 1976.
16. Maslach, C.: Burn-out: a social psychological analysis, Paper presented at the American Psychological Association, San Francisco, August, 1977.
17. Maslach, C.: Job burnout: how people cope, Public Welfare, p. 56, Spring, 1978.
18. Pelletier, K. R.: Mind as healer: mind as slayer, New York, 1977, Delta.
19. Pines, A., and Maslach, C.: Characteristics of staff burnout in mental health settings, Hosp. Community Psychiatry **29**(4):233, 1978.
20. Raths, L. E., Harmin, M., and Simon, S. B.: Values and teaching, Columbus, 1966, Charles E. Merrill Publishing Co.
21. Selye, H.: The stress of life, New York, 1956, McGraw-Hill Book Co.
22. Shubin, S.: Burnout: the professional hazard you face in nursing, Nursing 78 **8**(7):22, 1978.
23. Smith, M. J.: When I say no, I feel guilty, New York, 1975, Bantam Books, Inc.
24. Suzuki, S.: Zen mind, beginner's mind, New York, 1975, John Weatherhill, Inc.
25. Travis, J. W.: Wellness workbook for health professionals, Mill Valley, Calif., 1977, Wellness Resource Center, Inc.
26. Williams, R. B., Jr., and Gentry, W. D., editors: Behavioral approaches to medical treatment, Cambridge, 1977, Ballinger Publishing Co.

III

CANCER CAUSES, PREVENTION, AND EARLY DETECTION

9

Epidemiology and the study of cancer

NANCY FUGATE WOODS and JAMES S. WOODS

CONCEPTS OF EPIDEMIOLOGY

Concepts of epidemiology have changed markedly over time to reflect the major health concerns and problems of the day, as well as the level of sophistication of scientists' and practitioners' conceptions of health and disease. The initial use of the term "epidemiology" referred to the study of epidemics, and during the era in which the discipline was christened, the major health problems of the world were outbreaks of infectious diseases. As the kinds of major health problems have changed, so have the concerns of epidemiologists. Although the subject matter of journals of epidemiology currently includes studies of infectious disease, these journals also chronicle epidemiologists' interests in chronic illnesses such as cardiovascular disease, cancer, metabolic disorders, nutritional problems, occupational health problems, accidents, and even homicide. Epidemiologists' interests have clearly transcended the boundaries of disease and include such concerns as population dynamics, health and illness behavior, and health program evaluation.[40]

Despite the wide-ranging interests of the discipline, there are some commonly accepted definitions of epidemiology. The word "epidemiology" is literally translated as the study of what comes upon people: *epi* = upon, *demos* = people, *logos* = study. Omran[40] defines epidemiology as the "study of the occurrence and distribution of health conditions and disease and population change, as well as their determinants and consequences in population groups." This definition is sufficiently broad to encompass the spectrum of cancer epidemiology of interest to nurses whose concerns are not only with the etiology of cancer and its prevention but also with the consequences of the disease and related therapy for the quality of life. Other epidemiologists would specify that the assessment of outcomes of therapy, its human and economic costs as well as its utility, is an appropriate challenge for the discipline.

Scope of epidemiology

The scope of epidemiology includes the study of a variety of health-related phenomena and the people affected by these phenomena. The phenomena of interest include health and physiologic states, disease and death, health-related behavior and population dynamics, as well as the determinants of and intervention programs for each of these. The characteristics of people studied might include group characteristics such as age and sex, behavioral characteristics, risk factors in certain population groups, and environmental settings of the people. While the scope of epidemiology is similar to that of some other disciplines, there are three principal traits that are specific to the way epidemiologists study phenomena:

1. The epidemiologist's primary concern is with a population or an aggregate of people rather than with individuals from that population.
2. Epidemiologists are concerned with comparisons between groups or populations.
3. Epidemiologists are interested not only in asking the question, "Why do those people having a certain condition have it?" but also "Why were the people who do not have the condition spared?"[40]

Strategies used in epidemiologic investigations

Epidemiology as a discipline contributes to the *description* and *analysis* of health-related conditions. One common focus of epidemiologists is the description of the natural history of disease, how the course differs in people having different characteristics or environments, and how the disease course may be altered in response to prevention or therapy. Another focus includes the description of patterns of health and disease in communities, often referred to as "community diagnosis." Commonly used descriptive measures of health status are the incidence or prevalence rates of a disease or the mortality rates associated with it. Description of population dynamics is another important concern of epidemiologists, as is the development of descriptive indices such as the rates and ratios used in describing morbidity and mortality.

Epidemiology has contributed significantly to the understanding of the etiology of disease. These contributions have included the documentation of causal relationships between factors and disease as well as the study of epidemics to identify their origin.

Increasingly, epidemiologic methods are used in experimentation, such as in the clinical trials of new therapies or preventive measures and even experiments with animal models. Studies of program acceptance and evaluation of health programs are commonly using epidemiologic methods.

With this overview in mind, we shall explore in more detail the descriptive, analytic, and experimental approaches to epidemiology and their application to the study of cancer.

EPIDEMIOLOGY AND THE STUDY OF CANCER

While the development of cancer epidemiology as a specific focus of the discipline is relatively recent, observation of the incidence and determinants of cancer has a long tradition. As early as 1700, there was speculation about the risk factors involved in breast cancer. Ramazzini of Padua's *Treatise on the Disease of Tradesmen* noted that breast cancer was found more frequently among nuns than among other women; he initially speculated that the risk might be related to celibacy and later attributed it to childlessness. Pott's 1775 description of cancer of the scrotum among chimney sweeps hinted at the carcinogenic effects of chronic exposure to soot.[43] Throughout modern history there are accounts by clinicians, statisticians, and epidemiologists of trends in the incidence of cancers as well as speculation about correlates of the disease.

The current study of cancer epidemiology is concerned not only with describing the incidence of cancer but also with the elucidation of its etiology and the description of causal models. In addition, cancer epidemiologists are frequently involved in the conduct of clinical trials to evaluate various therapies and preventive actions.

Descriptive approaches to the epidemiology of cancer

Descriptive epidemiologic approaches have yielded important information concerning the etiology of various cancers. The traditional descriptive variables explored by epidemiologists are person, place, and time. By studying the amount or distribution of various cancers within a population according to these three variables, epidemiologists have been able to generate hypotheses to guide more focused investigations of cancer etiology.

Person. Although there are numerous characteristics of individuals that may be explored, it is customary for epidemiologists to explore the frequency of cancers for various age, sex, and ethnic or racial groups. In addition, such variables as religion, social class, occupation, income, education, marital status, family variables (for example, family size and type, birth order, parental characteristics), and the individual's general health status are explored.

Table 9-1 illustrates the relationship between several "person" variables and the incidence of breast cancer. Investigation of the frequency with which certain cancers are seen among populations with varying personal characteristics is important for several reasons. First, high-risk groups can be identified, and close surveillance can be planned so that cancers can be detected and treated early in their course. Second, trends in cancer incidence and mortality among high-risk groups can be systematically studied. Third, identification of characteristics associated with cancer can provide a basis for the generation of hypotheses regarding their etiology and further etiologic studies.

Place. The frequency of occurrence of various cancers can be related to the geographic area in which they occur. Place can be described in terms of natural boundaries, political subdivisions, or international or rural versus urban comparisons. In addition, the comparison of cancer rates for people who migrate from one area to another is of assistance in separating the role of genetic from environmental factors in disease incidence. One example in which location has

Table 9-1. Examples of personal risk factors for breast cancer in females*

Factor	High risk	Low risk
Age	Old age	Young age
Socioeconomic class	Upper	Lower
Marital status	Never married	Ever married
Race	White	Black
Age at first birth	Older than 30	Younger than 20
Body build	Obese	Thin
Age at menarche	Early	Late
Age at menopause	Late	Early
History of fibrocystic disease	Yes	No

*Data adapted from Kelsey, J.: A review of the epidemiology of human breast cancer. In Sartwell, P., editor: Epidemiologic reviews, vol. 1, Baltimore, 1979, School of Hygiene and Public Health, Johns Hopkins University.

been shown to be closely associated with the occurrence of cancer is the case of Burkitt's lymphoma, a common cancer in African children. Burkitt's lymphoma has been found to be most prevalent in an area now known as the African lymphoma belt (see map, Fig. 9-1). Burkitt's exploration of the climatic factors that contributed to the development of the tumor revealed that the distribution of the tumor conformed to the geographic distribution of malaria. Further work has elucidated the multistep pathogenesis of Burkitt's lymphoma: it has since been suggested that the persistent immunologic stimulation caused by heavy malaria burdens might be a critical factor in promoting Burkitt's lymphoma, perhaps by increasing the size of the pool of lymphoid cells that will give rise to a clone of tumor cells. (Chromosomal anomalies are also implicated as another factor in the development of Burkitt's lymphoma.)[8]

Frequently, mapping techniques are employed in studying the geographic distribution of cancer. Maps such as those prepared by the National Cancer Institute (NCI)[33] in their *Atlas of Cancer Mortality for U.S. Counties: 1950-1969* have proved to be particularly useful in this respect. The atlas shows geographic variation of cancer death rates across the United States for 35 anatomic sites of cancer and therefore provides clues as to the geographic location of environmental factors that may be important in cancer etiology. For example, the use of the atlas to identify high rates of lung cancer among male residents of southern United States coastal counties led to studies showing a correlation between lung cancer mortality and the heavy industrial characteristics of those counties (see Fig. 9-2).

Time. Epidemiologists are concerned not only with the occurrence of cancer but also with changes in its patterns of occurrence over time. Time variations can be described several ways. First, one can differentiate *endemic* and *epidemic* disease. Endemic conditions are always present in an area in some form, whereas an epidemic is a temporary rise in the incidence of a disease to a level greater than that usually expected. For example, Burkitt's lymphoma is said to be endemic in the area known as the African lymphoma belt. Second, one can examine the *periodicity of a disease* to determine if it is seasonal or cyclic. Seasonal variation in the incidence of Burkitt's lymphoma has been described, with the greater incidence occurring during the second part of the year.

Third, *secular trends* in disease or mortality can be described. Such a trend has been noted in the incidence of lung cancer among women, and examination of secular trends in the incidence of smoking among women has suggested a relationship between smoking and lung cancer (see Fig. 9-3). In addition,

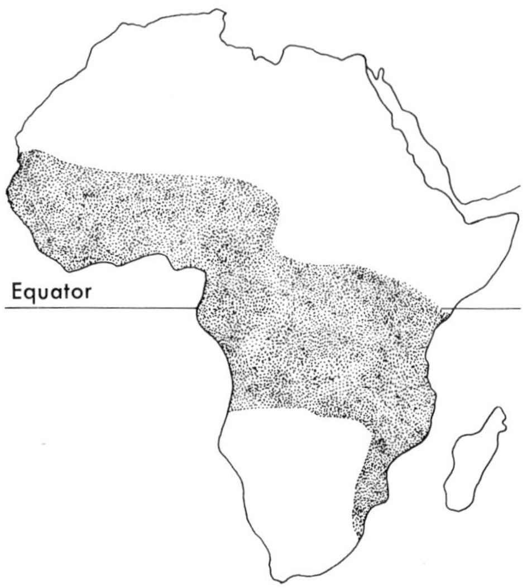

Fig. 9-1. Burkitt's lymphoma: geographic distribution. (From Kelsey, J.: A review of the epidemiology of human breast cancer. In Sartwell, P., editor: Epidemiologic reviews, vol. 1, Baltimore, 1979, School of Hygiene and Public Health, Johns Hopkins University.)

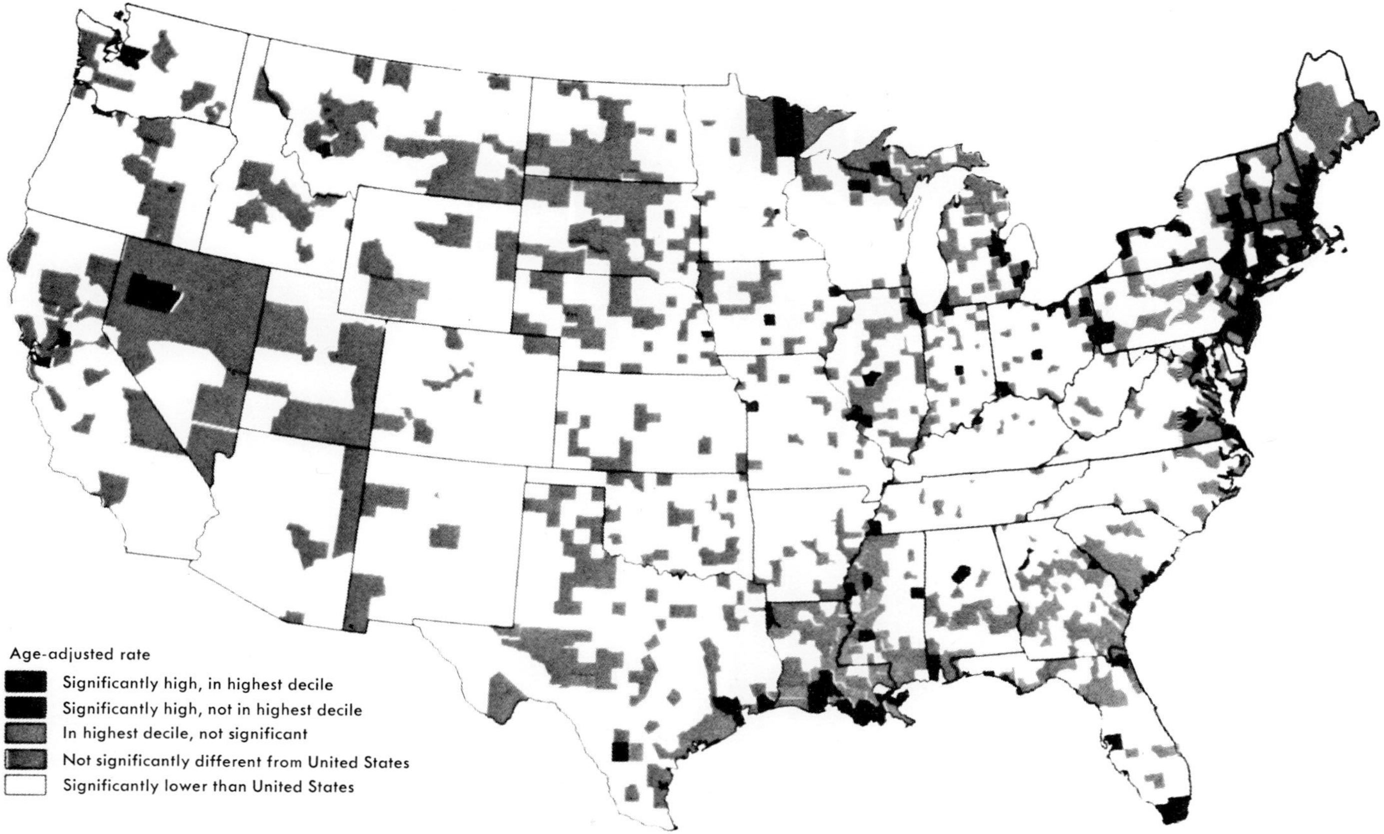

Fig. 9-2. Mapping of lung cancer distribution. (From Mason, T. J., and McKay, W.: Atlas of cancer mortality for U.S counties 1959, Washington, D.C., 1969, U.S. Department of Health, Education and Welfare, p. 76.)

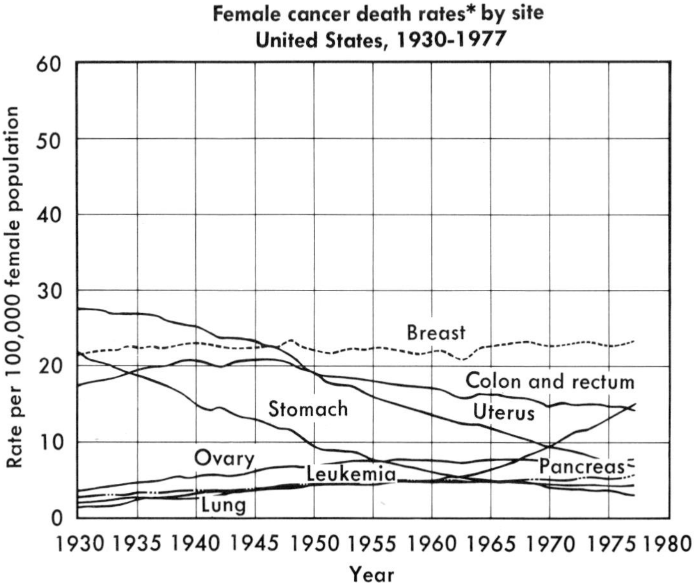

Fig. 9-3. Time trends in female cancer incidence. Note risk of lung cancer. *Rates for the female population standardized for age in the 1940 U.S. population sources of data; National Vital Statistics Division and Bureau of the Census, United States. (From American Cancer Society: Cancer facts and figures, New York, 1980, American Cancer Society, Inc.)

there have been recent reports of increasing incidence in cancer of the uterine corpus during the last decade.[48,50] During the same period, an increase in the sales of menopausal estrogens has been noted.

Rates and ratios. Epidemiologists are interested not only in observing the natural course of diseases such as cancer and studying its etiology, but they are also interested in quantifying the extent to which cancer affects certain populations. Some of the most commonly used approaches to quantification are summarized below and include: prevalence rate, incidence rate, period prevalence, mortality rate, and age-specific mortality rate:

$$\text{Prevalence rates} = \frac{\text{No. of persons with a disease}}{\text{Total No. in group}}$$

$$\text{Period prevalence rate} = \frac{\text{No. of persons with a disease during a period of time}}{\text{Total No. in group}}$$

$$\text{Incidence rate} = \frac{\text{No. of persons developing a disease per unit of time}}{\text{Total No. at risk}}$$

$$\text{Mortality rate} = \frac{\text{No. of persons dying due to a particular cause per unit of time}}{\text{Total No. in group}}$$

$$\text{Age-specific mortality rate} = \frac{\text{No. of persons dying in a particular age group per unit of time}}{\text{Total No. in that age group}}$$

These rates are proportions; that is, they are calculated by determining the number in the total population who have the disease or who die from it compared to the total number of people in the population or those at risk for the disease.

Prevalence rates summarize the proportion of a population affected by the disease at any point in time. This would include the total number of cases, whether they were newly diagnosed or whether they had been diagnosed several years earlier. If one were to consider the prevalence of breast cancer in the female population of the United States for 1980, then one must consider in the numerator the women who were diagnosed in 1975 and are still surviving as well as the women who are diagnosed in 1980. The denominator would include these same women as well as all other women at risk of breast cancer. A variation of this rate is termed period prevalence and describes the number of persons with a disease during a period of time, for example, from 1975 to 1977, per the total number of persons in the group.

Incidence rates describe the occurrence of *new* cases of disease over a specified period of time. Incidence rates imply the rate of development of a disease over time. When calculating incidence rates, epidemiologists consider that persons who have already developed diseases of lifelong duration cannot be counted as new cases more than once. Therefore, the denominator for incidence rates includes only the population at risk of developing the disease rather than the total population. In the case of cancer, we find that the estimated incidence for 1980 is about 785,000 new cases, whereas the prevalence of cancer is estimated to be about 3 million cases. Thus the incidence rate would be calculated as follows:

Cancer incidence rate =

785,000/(total population of US−3,000,000)

In addition to estimating the number of cases of disease compared to the total population, epidemiologists are concerned with rates that reflect the outcomes of disease. *Mortality rates* are commonly used to reflect the number of deaths from certain cancers as compared to the total population. For example, the death rate per 100,000 population for cancer in 1977 was 178.7. Rates may refer to special subgroups of the population as well as to the total population. The age-specific mortality rate refers to the number of persons dying in a particular age group compared to the total number of persons in that same group per unit time. For example, the age-specific mortality rate for breast cancer for women 35 to 54 years of age for 1977 could be calculated by counting all women who died from breast cancer in that age group (8,348) and dividing it by the total number of women who were 35 to 54 years of age in 1977.

Rates allow for comparison of groups and phenomena over time. For example, one might compare the rate of lung cancer among smokers to the rate of lung cancer in nonsmokers. One might also compare the incidence rate of lung cancer for a population during one period of time to the same rate for another period.

Rates can also be compared by determining the ratio of one rate to another. For example, the age-adjusted death rates for lung cancer among women from 1950 to 1952 were 3.9 per 100,000, and from 1975 to 1977 they were 14.0 per 100,000. The rates could be compared as follows:

14.0 for 1975 to 1977
3.9 for 1950 to 1952
$14.0 - 3.9 = 10.1$

This indicates that the death rate for lung cancer has increased by approximately 10.1 per 100,000, and this represents about a 260% increase. In conjunction with the

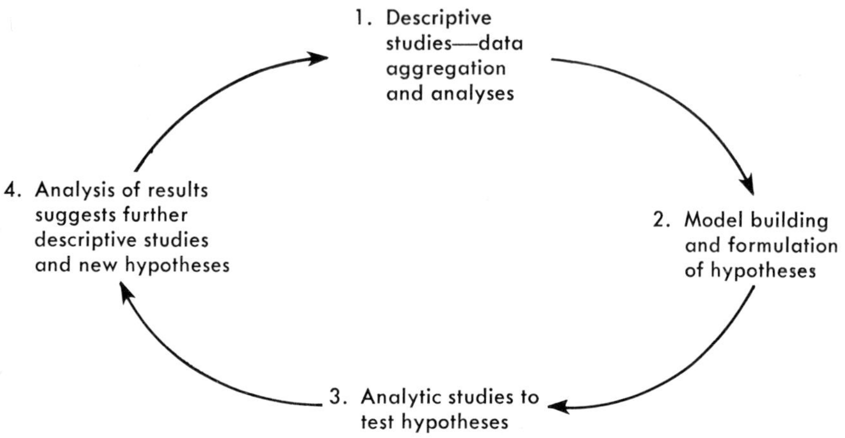

Fig. 9-4. Epidemiologic study cycle. (From Mausner, J., and Bohn, A.: Epidemiology: an introductory text, Philadelphia, 1974, W. B. Saunders Co.)

studies discussed later in this chapter, further application of the use of rates and ratios will be evident.

The cyclic nature of epidemiologic investigations

Although descriptive studies are vitally important in cancer epidemiology, they are the first step in a cycle of investigation. As illustrated in Fig. 9-4, the descriptive study frequently gives rise to hypotheses about the relationship between certain characteristics and health conditions; in some cases a causal model might be suggested.[35] Such thinking provides the basis for further studies that are designed to test hypotheses. These studies are commonly referred to as "analytic studies." Although analytic studies can generate support (or lack of it) for a hypothesis, they do not represent a final point in the search for new knowledge. Usually the analysis of results from these studies suggests further descriptive studies or generates new hypotheses.

CAUSATION AND ASSOCIATION

Epidemiology as a discipline is concerned with a search for causes, with the ultimate goals being prevention of disease and death and promotion of health. To these ends epidemiologists explore hypotheses linking suspected causes to suspected effects, usually disease.

Criteria for causal associations

A hypothesis of causation asserts that X is a factor that determines Y. In other words, whenever X occurs, Y will follow. It is recognized, however, that conditions often obtain where a single factor is a partial or contributory cause. Furthermore, in epidemiologic studies events are usually viewed in a probabilistic rather than deterministic way. Our current frameworks for causation of cancer recognize that a web of causation exists in which multiple variables are involved. Where it was once believed that one could find a single cause that was both necessary and sufficient to produce disease, it is now recognized that most health problems are determined by multiple factors.

There are generally accepted criteria for causal associations: *covariation, causal direction,* and *nonspuriousness.* Covariation means that the dependent variable varies with the independent variable or that a change in X results in a change in Y. A dose-response relationship implies that for a range of X there is a gradient in the degree of Y. Causal direction implies that the cause must precede the effect in time: X → Y (the antecedent-consequent relationship). Nonspuriousness means that we must observe that there are no other variables that cause changes in the dependent variable and are associated with the independent variable.

There are two basic approaches to testing causal hypotheses in epidemiology: observational and experimental. In the *observational* study, the investigator can only perceive and report the natural variation of two variables, whereas in an *experiment* the investigator can manipulate the causal variable under controlled conditions. The observational study will undoubtedly continue to provide a major contribution to the understanding of disease etiology, although experimentation can establish a causal relationship between a factor and a disease more conclusively than observation. Sometimes groups may be similar in every characteristic except an exposure to a specific factor. In this instance, the conditions for making a causal inference are so favorable that a "natural experiment" may be said to occur. An example of a natural (but tragic) experiment was that afforded by the bombing of Japan during World War II. Observation of people who had been exposed to varying amounts of radiation led to the discovery of an increased risk of certain cancers, such as leukemia.

Because of the need to rely on observational methods in epidemiologic studies, additional considerations in establishing a causal relationship are appropriate. Once the noncausal explanations for the association have been excluded, the following additional criteria can be used to explore the likelihood of a causal association:

1. *Strength of the association.* The stronger the association, the less likely it is that it might be produced by unknown confounding factors.
2. *Consistency of the association.* The relationship is repeatedly observed by different investigators, in different samples, and in different places and times by different research designs.
3. *Coherence.* The relationship does not contradict current knowledge about the phenomenon. The finding is coherent with the body of knowledge.
4. *Experimental confirmation.* Confirming an association in an experiment is a powerful way of establishing a causal relationship.[24]

When considering the relationship between two variables, it is important to recognize that they may be:

1. Independent—not statistically associated
2. Statistically associated
   a. Noncausally associated
   b. Causally associated
      (1) Indirectly causal
      (2) Directly causal

Independence between two variables, for example, a characteristic and a type of cancer, can be established by means of statistical tests of significance. If the two variables are statistically associated, that is, associated not simply because of chance, the investigator must then proceed to determine whether the relationship is a noncausal or a causal one.

Noncausal associations

Artifact. Two variables can be statistically but noncausally related simply because of artifact. Such an association would be spurious. It is well known that in a certain proportion of statistical tests, an association will be declared statistically significant when in fact it is not (type I error). In this instance the association may simply be a result of random fluctuation or *chance*.

A second source of artifact is *bias,* that is,

the false labeling of either the characteristic or condition under study. Bias can occur as a result of lack of reliability or validity in measurement, selective recall of the person being studied, or the reverse bias of the investigator. Selective recall may occur when the person either exaggerates part of a history or fails to recall some characteristic such as exposure. For example, the wife of a man who died of lung cancer will probably remember her husband's smoking habits more clearly than the wife of a man who died of a cause not commonly linked to smoking. Sometimes characteristics or conditions are falsely labeled in a study. For example, statistics may indicate that a disease rate has changed when in reality all that has changed is the ability to diagnose it. Sometimes investigators have strong preconceived notions about the relationship between a characteristic and condition. This may result in their being more attentive to these characteristics in persons who have the condition. Sometimes reverse bias occurs when the investigator makes a conscious effort to avoid bias; this leads to underdetection; for example, the person with a mild version of the disease is not labeled as a "case." Bias can be prevented by measuring concordance between observers or diagnosticians whenever possible and establishing the validity, sensitivity, and specificity of measuring instruments.

Another source of artifact is *selection bias*. This occurs when, by some fault in the research design or sampling, it has become easier for people in whom there is an association between the characteristic and disease to be selected into the study or excluded from it. The former results in an inflation of the strength of the association and the latter leads to an underestimation of the association.

Secondary association occurs when the association between two factors is produced by a third factor, termed a *confounding* factor. *Confounding* factors are associated both with the characteristic and the condition. A classic example of a secondary association is that between having a "yellow finger" and lung cancer. Yet it is clearly reasonable to question the causal nature of this relationship. Cigarette smoking, however, is found to be associated both with yellow fingers (nicotine stains) and lung cancer. In this instance, when one controls for the effects of the confounding variable, smoking, the association between yellow finger and lung cancer disappears, thus indicating this was a *secondary association*. Fortunately, confounding factors can be controlled both in the study design and in analytic approaches.

Causal associations

Causal associations may be classified as indirect or direct. An association is said to be *indirect* when the characteristic and condition are related only because they both are encompassed by the actual cause. In other words, if X is causally related to Y and Y is causally related to Z, there will be a causal relationship between X and Z, but the association is indirect. An example of an indirect association is that between the season of the year and Burkitt's lymphoma (BL). The season does not *cause* BL but contributes to the breeding of mosquitos that carry malaria, a factor that seemingly alters the susceptibility of the host to BL.

The *direct* causal association occurs when the characteristic can be associated with the condition with some specificity. Usually, however, the distinction between indirect and direct causal associations is a relative one, and assertion of a direct relationship depends on our current level of knowledge.

A final type of causal relationship is known as *configurational association*. This means that one factor is capable of producing a condition only in the presence of another factor. For example, we know that co-carcinogens are involved in the development of certain cancers; certain malignancies are caused by more than one co-carcinogen, and one of these may be capable of producing cancer only in the presence of the other.

ANALYTIC APPROACHES TO THE ETIOLOGY OF CANCER

Analytic approaches to the study of cancer have been primarily directed toward elucidating etiologic agents or models. Data sources for these studies include not only persons who have disease and their disease-free counterparts but also clinical records and studies in laboratories. Generally, the studies take one of two forms: prospective or retrospective (or some variation of these).

Prospective studies

Prospective studies are a very important form of epidemiologic investigation for testing hypotheses about disease causation. The study population for a prospective study consists of people who initially do not have the disease to be studied. From the reference population, people who are free of the disease are selected. They are subsequently classified according to presence or absence of the characteristic(s) thought to be related

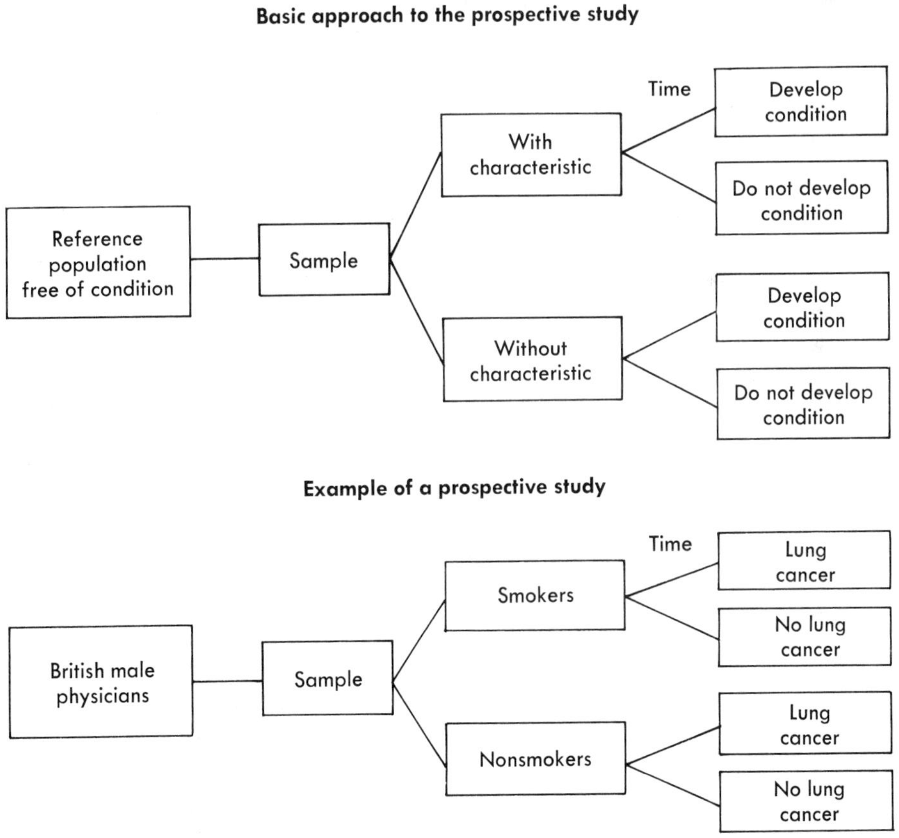

Fig. 9-5. Prospective study.

to the disease. The sample (usually termed a cohort) is then studied prospectively for a specified period of time (often for several years) to determine what proportion of the comparison groups under study develop the disease. Fig. 9-5 includes an example of a prospective study of the relationship between smoking and lung cancer by Doll and Hill.[11,12] These investigators initially identified a sample of British physicians free of lung cancer. Next, the sample was classified with respect to smoking habits. The smoking classification was based on an estimate of the number of cigarettes smoked daily: nonsmokers—0, light smokers—1 to 14 daily, moderate smokers—15 to 24 daily, and heavy smokers—25 or more daily. The sample was then followed for a period of 10 years, and the lung cancer deaths were ascertained. The annual death rate per 1,000 for the sample according to their smoking habits was as follows:

None	0.07
1 to 14	0.57
15 to 24	1.39
25+	2.27

Simple inspection of these results suggests that there was a positive association between the level of smoking and the development of lung cancer. With this in mind, let us consider the process of conducting a prospective study in more detail.

Selecting the cohort. The initial cohort can be selected for a number of reasons: (1) they may have been exposed to the particular factor under study; (2) they may belong to a group where follow-up is facilitated; or (3) they may be as appropriate as any other cohort for this study.

The study by Doll and Hill described earlier used a cohort of physicians listed in the Medical Register of the United Kingdom; because the physicians were legally required to maintain their registration, they were easy to trace. Furthermore, it is likely that they would have better than average access to diagnostic services that would enhance ascertainment of cases. Other cohorts frequently studied might include special occupational groups exposed to disease-producing agents, such as asbestos workers, persons enrolled in prepaid medical plans who will get most of their care through a single source, people taking out life insurance policies, obstetric populations (for neonatal or prenatal experiences), and volunteer groups of subjects, such as persons who volunteer for screening or who are identified by other volunteers. Other cohorts might be selected on the basis of their presence in a single geographic location to either facilitate continued study of the cohort over time or to facilitate quantification of exposure, such as with air pollution studies.[31]

Exposure. Once the cohort has been identified, the investigator must collect data that allow classification of the subjects as exposed or not exposed. As we have seen earlier, it is frequently possible to define several different levels of exposure, for example, the use of four smoking categories. This procedure provides the investigator with an opportunity to assess the effects of a gradient of exposure, sometimes referred to as "dose-response" effect. In other words, the investigator can ascertain whether the incidence of disease increases with the grade of exposure.

Data regarding exposure can be obtained from records, from individual members of the cohort, through testing or examining members of the cohort, or from assessing the environment in which they live. Doll and Hill[12] used mailed questionnaires to ascertain smoking habits from their cohort.

One of the difficult aspects of obtaining data from individual members of a cohort is that there is frequently no response. When a certain proportion does not provide data regarding exposure, it is possible that the loss of the respondents is biased with respect to either exposure, disease outcome, or both. The effects of bias in exposure or bias in disease or outcome differ from the effects of bias in *both* exposure and disease. When persons with high exposure levels fail to respond, the impression of the distribution of the exposure factor in the population will be inaccurate, but the association between the exposure and the disease will probably be accurate. When the nonresponse is biased with respect to disease, for example, the most ill do not respond, the disease rates for the cohort will be underestimated, but the ratio of disease rates among the exposed to the nonexposed will probably be similar to that in the population as a whole. When persons who do not respond to the study are biased with respect to both the exposure factor and the disease, the true relationship between the factor and the disease will be biased. It is often difficult to ascertain which type of bias is operative. Some approaches include more intense efforts to obtain data about exposure from nonrespondents, for example, by sending out a second questionnaire. Comparing the nonrespondents to the respondents on other variables, monitoring outcomes in the nonrespondents, and assessing the disease rates in the cohort over time (normally the effects of selection bias would be most apparent early in the study) may also help.[31]

Another concern in assessing exposure is that people may be exposed to different experiences over time. For example, a heavy smoker may quit smoking or a nonsmoker may start smoking. Thus, it is important to verify the exposure categories periodically during the study.

Comparisons. Comparison groups in the prospective study are entered into the study at its inception. For example, in Doll and Hill's study,[12] the nonsmokers and smokers were entered into the study at the same time. Often, however, other comparison groups are needed. In the case of a study of a special population selected for its exposure experience, for example, rubber workers, an appropriate nonexposed comparison group must be found. Often the experience of the general population at the time the cohort is being followed provides an appropriate comparison. Sometimes comparison cohorts or multiple groups are selected.

Follow-up. The appearance of disease or death is usually the outcome to be ascertained. Procedures may include examination of members of the cohort or the surveillance of other data sources such as death certificates. Doll and Hill[12] used death certificate data in ascertaining lung cancer mortality. There are many difficulties associated with the use of these procedures to assess outcome, not the least of which is migration of members of the cohort, misclassification of disease on death certificates, or changes in diagnostic procedures. When cohort members are examined, there is also the possibility of bias in diagnosis when the examiner is aware of the individual's exposure status. This can be limited by use of objective measures and by keeping information regarding the exposure status from the examiner.

Analysis: rates. The primary focus of analysis of data from prospective studies is the derivation of rates of an outcome (disease or mortality) for the cohorts studied. The rates are then usually compared across exposure groups.

Because of variability in the number of years during which each person in the cohort is observed, a commonly used denominator for calculating rates is person-years. Person-years considers the number of persons observed and the duration of each observation. For example, let us consider the distribution on the following page.

Years of observation	No. of persons
5	30
10	20
15	10

The person-years numerator for this study would be computed as follows:

$$(5 \times 30) + (10 \times 20) + (15 \times 10) = \mathit{500} \text{ person-years}$$

This denominator allows for the variation in entrance dates into the study (for example, often persons in the cohort are enrolled over several years) as well as for loss of certain individuals from the cohort.

The age distribution of the cohort also changes over time. For this reason, separate calculations of rates are usually made for persons in certain age groups.

When persons are lost to follow-up, a situation analogous to failure to obtain exposure information occurs. Losses that are biased with respect to both exposure and outcome will affect the relative rates of disease or death for exposure categories. When losses are large, there may be considerable distortion of estimates of risk. Often investigators compute several estimates based on different sets of assumptions regarding possible biases. For example, the investigator might assume that persons lost to follow-up were lost immediately after entry into the cohort. The investigator then may use only the number of persons examined on each occasion (beginning and end of the study) to compute rates. Another possibility is to make varying assumptions regarding the number of years persons lost to follow-up were actually observed. This may be a useful technique when multiple measures are made of the outcome at varying intervals during the study. Yet another approach might be to calculate a range of rates possible in each exposure category. In this instance, the investigator might first assume that none of the persons lost developed the outcome and, second, that all of them developed the outcome. The usefulness of the latter option, however, is limited inasmuch as the frequency of the outcome measured is often smaller than the proportion lost to follow-up.[31]

Analysis: risk estimates. In addition to calculating rates of disease or death, epidemiologists are concerned about the association between exposure to certain factors and the risk of a particular outcome. Two commonly used measures are the relative risk and the attributable risk. The relative risk (RR) is the ratio of the incidence rate in those exposed to the risk factor (or characteristic) to the incidence rate in the population not exposed. Let us take an example of the relative risk of death of lung cancer for heavy smokers (as compared to nonsmokers). Data from the Doll and Hill study[12] show that the annual lung cancer death rate per 1,000 for heavy smokers and nonsmokers was as follows: nonsmokers = 0.07, heavy smokers = 2.27. Taking the ratio RR (relative risk) $= \frac{I_e}{I_o}$, where I_e is the incidence in the exposed (0.07) and I_o is the incidence in the nonexposed (2.27), we find that: RR $= \frac{2.27}{0.07} = 32$. The relative risk of lung cancer mortality for heavy smokers is 32. Attributable risk (AR_e) is another measure of association between risk factors and outcome. AR_e is the rate of the disease in exposed persons that can be attributed to the exposure: $AR_e = I_e - I_o$. Using the rates from Doll and Hill's study,[12] it can be seen that the incidence for moderate smokers is 1.39. The AR_e for moderate smokers is:

$$AR_e = 1.39 - 0.07 = 1.26$$

In addition, the attributable risk percent ($AR_e\%$) can be computed, where $AR_e\% =$

$\frac{I_e - I_o}{I_e}$. The $AR_e\%$, also referred to as the etiologic fraction among the exposed, is the proportion of disease in the exposed population that is attributable to the risk factor. For moderate smoking exposure, the $AR_e\%$ is $\frac{1.39 - 0.07}{1.39} = 0.949$ or 94.9%.

The population attributable risk (AR_p) is the rate of the disease in the entire population that can be attributed to the risk factor. In the case of Doll and Hill's study,[12] the total incidence of lung cancer mortality in the population was 0.65.

$$AR_p = I_t - I_o$$

OR

$$0.65 - 0.07 = 0.58$$

The population attributable risk percent ($AR_p\%$), sometimes referred to as the etiologic fraction in the population, is the proportion of the disease rate in the total population that is attributable to exposure to the risk factor:

$$AR_p\% = \frac{I_t - I_o}{I_t}$$

In the above case:

$$AR_p\% = \frac{0.65 - 0.07}{0.65} = 89.2\%$$

The comparison of rates can also be achieved for a number of risk factors. Often it is found that two risk factors act synergistically. That is, the joint effect of the two risk factors results in a rate that exceeds the sum of the risks of those exposed to either risk factor individually. Recently, synergistic effects have been observed in workers exposed both to asbestos and to smoking.

Interpretation. Results of a cohort study are interpreted in relation to two primary questions: (1) Are there alternative explanations for the association (or lack of association) between risk factors and outcome? (2) Is the association likely to be a causal relationship? To answer the first question, the investigator must meticulously review all previous steps in the study. The second question can be answered by considering the criteria for causal relationships discussed earlier in this chapter.

Advantages. The fact that the cohort is drawn from a reference population enables the investigator to generalize from the sample to the reference population with some degree of certainty. In addition, it is clear that the characteristic precedes the development of the condition, one of the necessary conditions for a causal relationship. The investigator can directly quantify the risk of developing a condition in the presence of a risk factor. The likelihood of bias in reporting the relationship between the characteristic and the condition is reduced, since the characteristic is described before the outcome is measured. Selective survival, the survival of only special groups until the study is initiated, is not a problem here as it is for retrospective studies.

Disadvantages. Prospective studies are very costly in time, personnel, and follow-up. They are not feasible when the condition being studied is rare. Attrition of persons in the cohort constitutes a considerable problem in interpretation of results. Likewise, there may be attrition among investigators. Finally, other changes may occur over time in the environment, individuals, or treatment of the condition, and these may affect the outcomes.

Historic or reconstructed cohort study

A variation of the prospective cohort study is the historic cohort study. Here the cohort is reconstructed from records of their exposure, and they are then subsequently followed to see who develops the condition. In this case the investigator has a reference

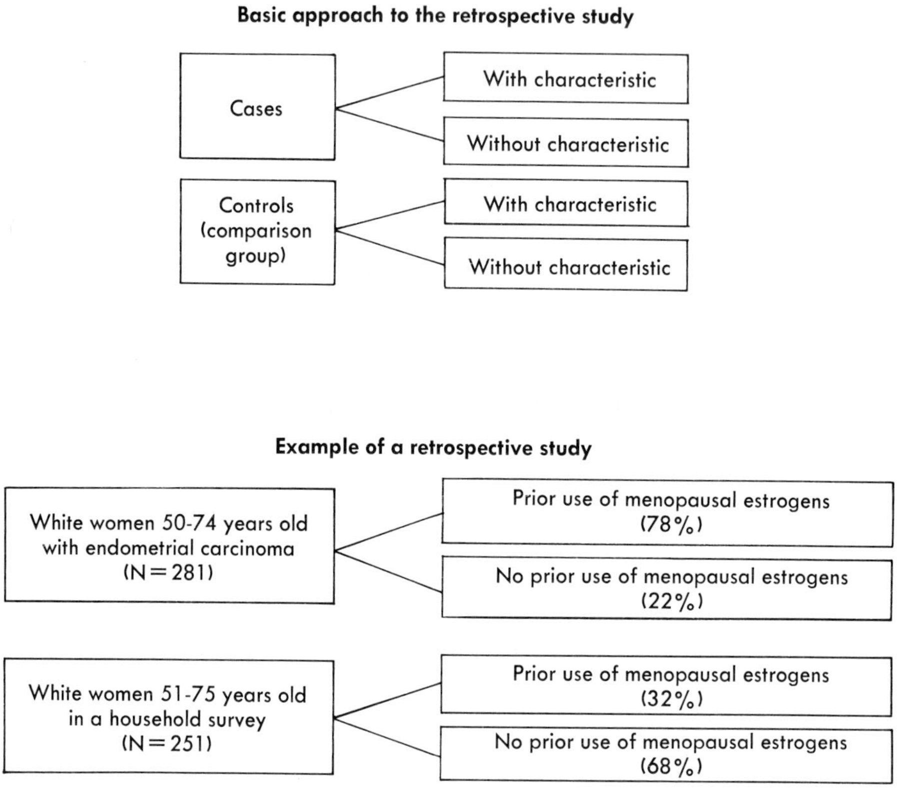

Fig. 9-6. Retrospective study.

population and proceeds from that point in time with the study.

Retrospective studies

Retrospective studies involve comparisons between groups of individuals who have the disease (cases) and groups who do not have the disease. The cases and comparison groups (commonly referred to as controls or referent group) are then compared with respect to current or past characteristics that the investigator believes have relevance to the particular disease being studied.*

Fig. 9-6 illustrates the approach used in a recent study of endometrial cancer and estrogen use.[51] The approach used in this study involved the identification of women with a new diagnosis of endometrial cancer from January 1975 to April 1976 through the assistance of the Cancer Surveillance System, a population-based tumor registry for the western Washington state area. These women were interviewed in their homes approximately 1 year after diagnosis and were asked about their prior estrogen use as well as other reproductive history. The comparison group was drawn from the randomly selected respondents to a household survey who were similar in age and race to the cases. In this previous study comparable

*This approach is also commonly referred to as a case-control study. It is apparent, however, that the "controls" in this case are not equivalent to the controls in an experimental study.

data had been obtained regarding estrogen use in the comparison groups. The investigators then compared the relative proportion of estrogen users and nonusers among the cases and controls.

Selection of cases. In selecting the cases for a case-control study, the criteria for the definition of the disease, the source of cases, and the inclusion of incident or prevalent cases are extremely important considerations. Valid and reliable definitions of the disease are essential. Often the investigator must decide whether or not to include "borderline" cases or how to cope with differences in pathologists' use of diagnostic categories. Weiss and colleagues[51] decided to include women with diagnosis of in situ lesions in the group of cases because of the likelihood that these lesions would develop into unequivocal cancer if untreated (and because their inclusion did not alter the magnitude of the estrogen-cancer association).

Cases may be obtained from persons being treated for the disease at a certain facility or from persons with the disease from a more general population. Weiss and associates[51] were able to identify all the female residents of King County who had a new diagnosis of endometrial cancer through a population-based tumor registry. This procedure was preferable to studying women only from one clinic because it eliminated the biases associated with the use of a certain source of medical care and also allowed computation of rates of the disease in the population.

Inclusion of incident or prevalent cases is also an important consideration. Weiss and associates[51] chose only relatively "new" cases. Such an approach may make it easier to interpret findings. For example, the inclusion of patients with advanced stages of malignant disease might make it difficult to obtain data that clearly pertained to antecedents of the disease rather than consequences of its treatment or advancement.

Selection of controls. Decisions about the source of controls are also important in the conduct of case-control studies. Controls may be obtained from the general population, hospitalized clients, or relatives or associates of the cases. In general, if the cases represent all the affected persons in a defined population, then controls should be selected from that same population. Some of the concerns in the selection of controls relate to whether information on the study factors can be obtained from the control group in a manner similar to that by which it was obtained from the case group, whether to match the controls with the cases to control for a certain confounding factor, whether the controls are similar to the cases in general, and practical and financial considerations. Weiss and associates[51] studied controls from the same county as the cases.

Sampling. Once the source of controls is identified, the investigator must decide whether to study the entire population or sample from the population. Because of the difficulty encountered in enumerating everyone to draw a random sample from a large population, paired sampling is often used. This means that for each case one or more controls is selected. This may be accomplished, for example, by asking the cases to identify someone in the same neighborhood of the same age.

Information about exposure. Sources of data on exposure include the individual being studied or a relative and records such as hospital charts, birth certificates, and employment records. If the data on exposure differ systematically in completeness or accuracy between cases and controls, the association between exposure and disease will be spurious. The validity of exposure data is extremely important; where possible, information about exposure recorded *prior* to discovery of the disease is desirable to reduce bias in reporting. Further efforts to ensure validity include the use of similar procedures for cases and controls. Finally, the sensitivity and specificity of classification schemes should be established in advance of the study (these will be discussed in greater detail later in this chapter). When misclassification with respect to study variables occurs, and occurs to a different extent in cases and controls, then a problem of lack of comparability exists. In some cases, misclassification can lead the investigator to conclude that no difference exists when, in fact, it *does* exist.

Table 9-2. Number of women with endometrial cancer and controls reporting previous menopausal estrogen use*

Menopausal estrogen use	Cases	Controls		Totals
Yes	219 (a)	80 (b)	=	299
No	62 (c)	171 (d)	=	233
TOTALS	281	251	=	532

*Data are interpolated from Weiss, N., Szekely, D., English, D., and Schweid, A.: J.A.M.A. **242**(3):261, 1979. Copyright 1979, American Medical Association. Excludes women who interrupted use of estrogen for >1 year. Frequencies may not be exact owing to rounding error in computations.

Table 9-3. Distribution of women with endometrial cancer and controls according to average daily dosage of menopausal estrogen*

Average dosage of conjugated estrogens or equivalent amount of other estrogens in mg/day	Women (%)	
	Endometrial cancer cases (N = 309)	Controls (N = 272)
Never used	20	63
<0.5	5	7
0.5–1.2	32	12
>1.25	44	18

*Data are from Weiss, N., Szekely, D., English, D., and Schweid, A.: J.A.M.A. **242**(3):261, 1979. Copyright 1979, American Medical Association. Women who only had injections or unknown preparations were excluded from the original calculations.

Analysis. The analysis of a case-control study consists of a comparison between cases and controls of the frequency of the characteristic believed to be related to the condition.

It can be seen in Fig. 9-6 that the proportion of menopausal estrogen users was much greater among the cases than among the controls. The number of women with endometrial cancer and the number of women in the comparison groups who used menopausal estrogen are given in the fourfold table (Table 9-2). Another approach to analysis in retrospective studies involves comparison of the intensity and duration of exposure for the cases and controls (Table 9-3). Such a display offers the advantage of observing dose-response relationships and estimation of risk for a variety of levels of exposure.

In addition to assessing the significance of observed differences between cases and controls, investigators can also estimate the risk of developing the disease associated with the exposure and determine to what extent differences in the two groups might be attributable to a confounding variable.

Because Weiss and associates[51] studied cases referable to a population and because the controls were also representative of the same population, it was possible to estimate rates of the disease in exposed and nonexposed women and also to derive relative and attributable risks from these estimates.[31] Procedures similar to those described for calculating relative risk for prospective studies would be appropriate.

Many retrospective studies, however, cannot be related to a defined population, for example, cases from a single hospital compared with neighbors. Because the populations at risk are then unknown, one cannot estimate rates in the exposed and nonexposed. Using the data in Table 9-2 as an example, an estimate of the relative risk of the disease given exposure to the characteristic can be made for retrospective studies in the following manner: (1) The rate in exposed persons is calculated. In Table 9-2, the rate in the exposed persons is $\frac{a}{a+b}$ or $\frac{219}{299}$ = *0.732*. (2) The rate in the nonexposed persons is also calculated. In Table 9-2, the rate in the nonexposed persons is $\frac{c}{c+d}$ or $\frac{62}{233}$ = *0.266*. (3) The rate in the exposed persons is then divided by the rate in the nonexposed persons: $\frac{a}{a+b} \div \frac{c}{c+d}$ to give *2.75*. The result is an estimate of the relative risk of developing endometrial cancer given exposure to menopausal estrogens. (A more correct name, the relative odds, is usually given this estimate inasmuch as it is the ratio of affected to unaffected individuals in one group relative to the same ratio for the other group.)

The relative risk of developing the disease can also be calculated for each level of exposure. Referring to the data in Table 9-3, it was determined that the relative risk of developing endometrial cancer for the group using <0.5 mg of menopausal estrogens would be 2.5; for women who used 0.6 to 1.2 mg of estrogens, 8.8; and for women using >1.25 mg/day, 7.6.[51] Thus, one can note that women exposed to >0.5 mg of menopausal estrogens had about a threefold increase in the risk of developing endometrial cancer when compared to women using <0.5 mg of menopausal estrogens.

In this study, the investigators noted that age was related both to having endometrial cancer and to estrogen use. It was therefore necessary to take age into account in analyses to prevent any distortion of the estrogen-cancer association.*

*It was noted earlier that a confounding variable is a third variable that is associated both with the disease and the characteristic being studied, and lack of control of the confounding variable may introduce spurious differences between cases and controls.

Adjustment can be made for confounding variables in the study design or in analysis. One way of controlling for the effects of age in such a study would be to match each case with one or more controls of the same or similar age. While this is a useful technique, it is cumbersome and often an appropriate match cannot be found for the cases, or the data for many controls must be ignored. Another approach to controlling for confounding is stratification analysis. This involves examining the relationships between the exposure and disease for each of several strata. In the case of the preceding study, the investigators stratified the cases and controls according to the following age groups: 50 to 54, 55 to 64, and 65 to 74 years of age. In the analysis of relative risk, the investigators then standardized for age. (For further information about stratification analysis, see Mausner and Bahn.[35] For further information about matching, see MacMahon and Pugh.[31])

Advantages. There are several advantages associated with retrospective studies. They are short-term and relatively cheap when compared to cohort studies. The retrospective study is feasible particularly when the disease occurs only rarely. The problem of attrition often associated with cohort studies is less marked in the retrospective study, although people may refuse to participate in the study. As earlier illustrated, these studies can support the estimation of a dose-response relationship and are particularly powerful when the cases and controls were both obtained from a referent population. When a number of retrospective studies conducted by different investigators on different populations confirm one another, confidence can be attached to the conclusions. For example, as Table 9-4 shows, there are now several new studies that suggest an association between menopausal estrogens and endometrial cancer.

Disadvantages. There are, however,

Table 9-4. Association between exogenous estrogen and endometrial cancer

Study	Population	Results
Smith et al.[44]	Clients (N = 317) with adenocarcinoma of the endometrium were compared with 317 clients who had other gynecologic neoplasms (matched for age at diagnosis and year of diagnosis).	Risk of endometrial cancer was 4.5 times greater among women exposed to estrogen therapy than in women not exposed to estrogen.
Ziel and Finkle[54]	Clients (N = 94) with endometrial cancer from the Kaiser Permanente Medical Center in Los Angeles were each compared with two controls selected from the health plan (matched for date of birth and zip code).	Risk of endometrial cancer was estimated to be 7.6 times greater among women exposed to estrogen than among women not exposed. The relative risk increased with the duration of exposure was: 5.6 for 1 to 4.9 years and 13.9 for 7 or more years.
Mack et al.[30]	All (N = 63) residents of an affluent retirement community who had endometrial cancer were compared with women from the same community without endometrial cancer (matched for age and marital status).	Risk of developing endometrial cancer for women taking estrogens was eight times greater than the risk for women not taking estrogens. Risk was greater at higher doses of estrogen.
Antunes et al.[2]	Women (N = 451) with endometrial cancer were compared with women clients (N = 888) without endometrial cancer and from services other than gynecology or psychiatry (matched by hospital, age, race, and date of admission).	Risk of developing endometrial cancer for women taking estrogens was six times greater than for women not taking estrogens. Risk associated with cyclic use was as great as that for continuous use.

Table 9-5. Rates and risk estimates associated with specific study approaches

	Cohort study	Case-control study	Cross-sectional study
Rates	Incidence	Proportion of the cases with the characteristic, unless cases are from an identifiable reference population; then incidence can be estimated directly	Prevalence
Risk estimate	Relative and attributable risk	Relative odds; when cases and controls are from an identifiable reference population, then relative risk is appropriate	Relative and attributable risk

some major disadvantages associated with retrospective studies. First, the reference population for the cases and controls is often unknown, whereas the sample drawn for a cohort study is based on a reference population. Therefore, generalization to a reference is usually not possible. Because there is often not much information about the population from which those with the disease come, it is difficult to give *precise* estimates of risk, although such estimates as the relative odds are commonly used. Because of the retrospective nature of the study, it is often not possible to know whether the exposure characteristic is antecedent to the disease or consequent to it.

Often the investigator must be concerned with bias, which may take the form of selective recall, selection, false labeling, or reverse bias (see earlier discussion). A final problem associated with retrospective studies is selective survival. When this type of study is initiated, only persons who have survived the disease are available for the investigation. Survival may be associated with a variable such as income, which in turn influences access to treatment and survival. Thus, it is easy to see how the representation of certain groups, for example the wealthy, might be artificially inflated. This in turn might give the impression that the wealthy are at greater risk of developing the disease when in fact it is only that the wealthy who have the disease survive.

Interpretation. MacMahon and Pugh[31] suggest two important questions to consider in interpreting findings from a case-control study: (1) "Do the findings reflect the true situation with respect to the presence or absence of association between the disease and the study factor?" (2) "If an association *is* observed, is it a causal one?" In considering the first question, the investigator must refer again to all previous steps of the study, attempting to find alternative explanations for the observed association. In addition, the investigator is concerned with the findings as a whole. In considering the differences between cases and controls, one or only a few sharp differences are more compelling than many differences. The second question can be considered in relation to the earlier discussion on causality.

Cross-sectional studies

Another approach used in epidemiologic investigations is the cross-sectional study. A reference population is identified and for a sample of that population both the characteristic and condition are ascertained simultaneously. Because these studies begin with a reference population, rates such as prevalence can be computed as well as risk estimates (Table 9-5). These studies enable the investigator to generalize to the reference population. Although bias and attrition can present problems, they can be minimized with careful designs. These are short-term, relatively inexpensive studies in comparison to prospective studies. The cross-sectional study does, however, have some disadvantages: it is sometimes impossible to disentangle antecedent-consequent relationships, and selective survival or migration may occur.

Analytic approaches to studying the effectiveness of interventions

Frequently, prevention or treatment programs are conducted with enthusiasm but without careful assessment of their effectiveness and possible undesirable outcomes. Often assumptions about the advisability of a certain therapy dictate the clinical approach rather than the results of careful clinical trials.

A recently reported clinical trial for the treatment of operable breast cancer attempted to assess the relative effects of simple mastectomy with radical postoperative radiotherapy and standard radical mastectomy.[21] Women 35 to 69 years of age with operable breast cancer (international stages I and II and a proportion of stage III cases) were randomly allocated to either of two groups: (1) standard radical mastectomy using a version of the Halstead technique and (2) simple mastectomy plus radical radiotherapy. Prophylactic bilateral oophorectomy was performed on all women between 35 and 60 years of age. Women under 40 years of age who refused oophorectomy were excluded from the study, as were women from 41 to 59 years of age who refused oophorectomy and ovarian radiation. A total of 498 women participated in the study from 1964 to 1971; 242 of these had simple mastectomy and radiotherapy (SM + R), with 256 having a radical mastectomy (RM). A total of 394 clients was available for 5 years of follow-up (191 SM + R; 203 RM). Results indicated similar survival and disease-free survival for the two treatment groups. The survival curves for premenopausal, menopausal, and early and late postmenopausal women were also compared, with the postmenopausal women having a substantially worse prognosis. The size of the primary tumor was negatively associated with survival. In addition, women with tumor deposits in the axillary nodes had a poorer prognosis.

The intervention trial. In an intervention, the investigator manipulates the treatment, which becomes the independent variable, and measures the effect, which becomes the dependent variable. The basic strategy involves an application of the experimental method with some special modifications necessary in view of the concern for the human population being studied.

Study groups. In some studies, it is possible to enroll a study group that receives the treatment and a control group(s) not given the treatment but perhaps a placebo. In other instances, it would be considered unethical to withhold any treatment at all, such as in a study of breast cancer treatment.

The reference population for the study is the group to which the investigator can ideally generalize results of the study. In the preceding example, the reference population would be women between 35 to 69 years of age with operable breast cancer. The experimental population is the actual population being studied, in our example, the women treated at 16 surgical units in hospitals in the southeast region of Scotland. Ideally, the experimental population is as similar as possible to the reference population. Convenience and accessibility, incidence of the disease to be prevented (in prophylactic trials), and size of the population needed to detect statistically significant differences are all important considerations in selecting the experimental group. Because humans have the right to refuse involvement in an experiment, the final complement of the experimental population is not under the control of the investigator. Careful assessment of systematic differences between volunteers and refusals should be made when possible. Usually allocation to the experimental or control group is done *after* the person consents to participate. In an attempt to attain equivalence or similarity of the experimental and control groups, the investigator can randomly allocate participants to one or more treatment or control groups. It is best that a system of randomization is developed in advance of the study to limit the noncomparability between the groups. An example of the selection of participants for an intervention study is shown in Fig. 9-7.

The double-blind trial. The double-blind trial includes two safeguards to prevent bias in the ascertainment of the outcome as a result of knowledge of the group to which the participant was assigned: blind assignment is made of the participants to the study groups,

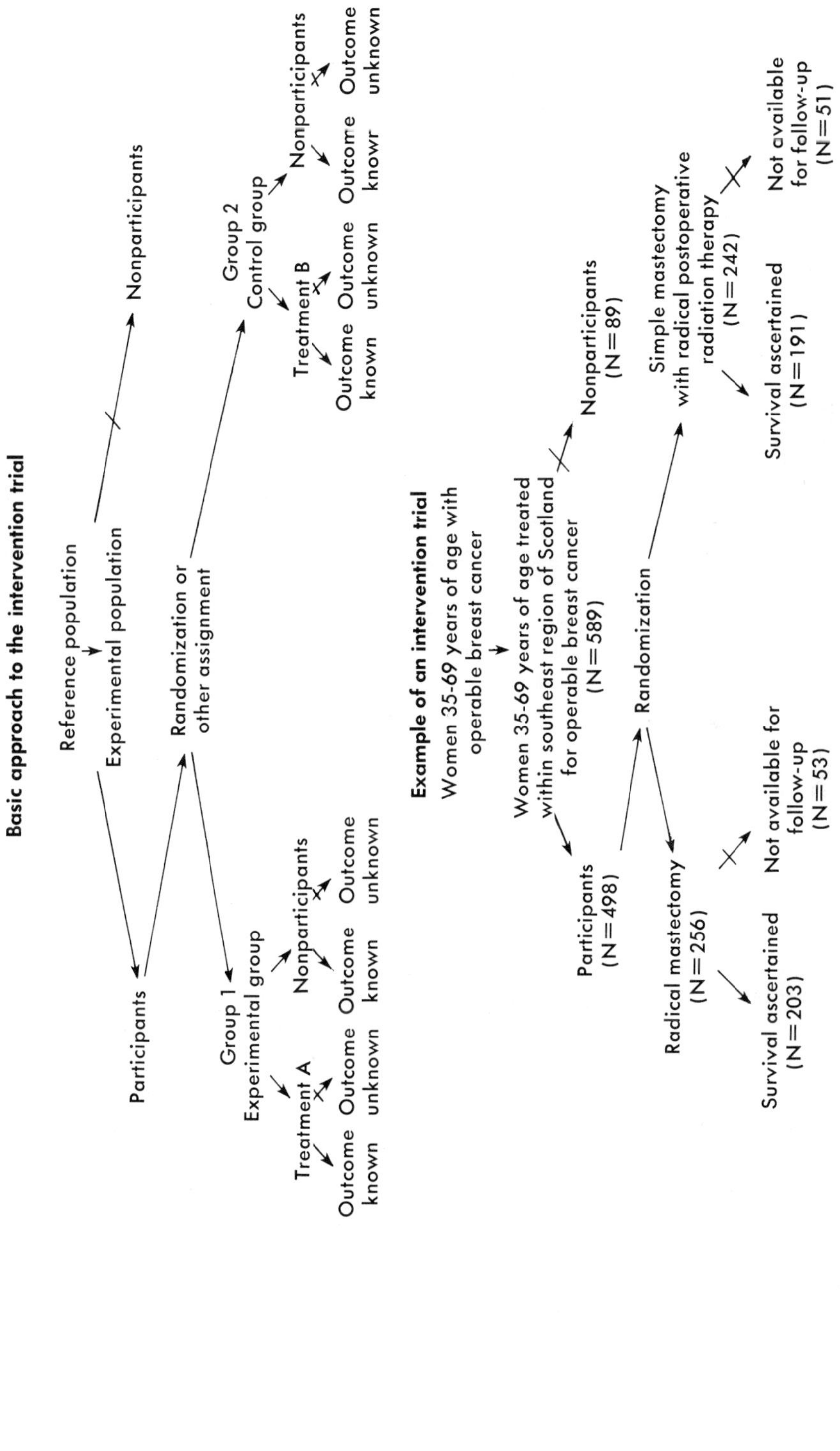

Fig. 9-7. Intervention trial. Hatched lines indicate points of attrition from study.

and a blind assessment of outcome is achieved. First, neither the study personnel nor the participants know to which group they were assigned. While this is feasible in studies of medications, it is clearly impossible in the study of operable breast cancer, where both the staff and clients are obviously aware of the treatment. The second component involves blind ascertainment of outcome. This might be achieved by keeping knowledge of the treatment group from a pathologist or interviewer measuring disease, survival, or other outcomes and from the statistician or epidemiologist analyzing the data.

Protocols

To ensure that each participant in the experimental and control groups receives the same treatment, study protocols are usually developed that describe in detail the types of procedures to be used in both groups. This is particularly important when several investigators from different areas participate in a collaborative trial. In our example, a single protocol was used for surgery and radiation therapy by physicians in 16 different hospitals.

Ascertaining outcomes. Ascertaining outcome in cases where the outcome does not occur for several years, as in the preceding example where 5-year survival rates were measured, presents the same problems that were discussed in conjunction with prospective studies, for example, migration and selective survival. Measures are usually taken to ensure as complete a follow-up as possible, and blind assessment is desirable. A very important concern is the type of outcome measure most appropriate to the study. In the example of the clinical trial for operative breast cancer, the outcome measure was survival at 5 years. Other measures that could have been used are survival at 10 years, morbidity resulting from the two surgeries, and quality of life after treatment. In this case, however, the investigators were concerned with establishing whether or not radical mastectomy had a more positive effect on survival than the method they were currently employing.

Sequential designs are sometimes employed in intervention studies. This means that data are continuously analyzed during the trial, and as soon as statistically significant differences appear, the trial is stopped. For example, if the investigators in the clinical trial for operative breast cancer would have discovered that a much greater proportion of women in the control group were developing recurrence or metastasis than those in the experimental group, they could have stopped the trial and use of the control treatment. It is possible to maintain double-blind procedures and incorporate sequential designs by having investigators not involved in the clinical work analyze the data submitted to them.

Analysis. The analysis of an intervention trial is similar to that for a cohort study. Special attention, however, must be given to those who did not participate in the control group and study group and any systematic differences between those who participated and those who did not. This can be attained by attempting to measure outcome for at least a sample of the nonparticipants. Although some of the women in the southeast region of Scotland chose not to participate in the study and some may have dropped out before follow-up or moved away from the area, ideally their survival could be ascertained and these data included in some analyses of the trial.

ETIOLOGY OF CANCER

Many distinct diseases, all collectively called cancer, can occur in almost all tissues of the body. Although the precise etiology of these diseases is not currently known, it is recognized that all cancers have as a common characteristic a lack of growth control manifested as a lost ability to respond to metabolic signals that control the rate of multiplication. Thus, they continue to grow and divide, eventually invading neighboring tissues (metastasize) and preventing the performance of normal physiologic functions. When this happens, the likelihood of survival diminishes significantly.

The extent to which an individual is at risk from cancer and its debilitating effects is now known to be related to a variety of etiologic factors as determined from epidemiologic studies. These include diet, lifestyle, and iatrogenic causes as well as exposure to chemicals in the environment.

Environmental chemicals. Foremost among the leading candidates in the etiology of cancer today is the host of occupational and other environmental chemicals that humans encounter in the course of everyday living. According to the United States Environmental Protection Agency (EPA) estimates, over 70,000 chemicals are manufactured or processed commercially in as many as 115,000 establishments around the country. The EPA also estimates that about 1,000 new chemical compounds are introduced each year. At least 50 to 60 chemicals are now known to increase the risk of cancer in humans.

Cancer as an environmental chemical disease is not new and, in fact, was discovered over 200 years ago when Percival Pott, a British physician, associated a rare form of neoplasm, scrotum cancer, with the fact that his clients were chimney sweeps and exposed to coal tar in soot. Since that time, clients have been diagnosed with cancer after occupational exposure to numerous chemicals in a variety of industrial situations.[49] Today there is little doubt that many cancers, previously regarded as spontaneous, are caused or promoted by environmental chemicals.[13]

The mechanisms by which chemicals induce neoplastic changes in tissue cells have been the subject of intensive study in recent years. Before these mechanisms can be discussed, it is appropriate to review the highlights of what is known about the general characteristics of the carcinogenic process. Two properties in particular stand out. The first is the obvious multistep nature of the process. The exact number of steps in the development of any malignant neoplasm is not known, although many may occur depending on the organ involved. The second feature is the apparent brevity of the *initiation phase,* in contrast to the subsequent *promotion* or evolution phase, which constitutes most of the time for cancer induction. The initiation phase may last only a matter of minutes, hours, or maybe a few days, whereas the prolonged period of cancer development following initiation may last months or even years.

Research into the mechanisms by which chemicals induce cancer in living tissues has concentrated primarily on the initiation phase, and some insight is now beginning to develop concerning this process. It is now clear, for example, that most chemical carcinogens that initiate cancer are not carcinogenic per se but must first be metabolized in the body to chemically reactive derivatives called ultimate carcinogens, which appear to be the actual carcinogenic agents.[37,38] The process of metabolic activation can occur in various organs and tissues. However, the organ receiving principal attention in this regard is the liver and in particular a group of enzymes, the "mixed function oxidase system," located in a portion of the endoplasmic reticulum. This carcinogen-activating enzyme system has yet to be clearly analyzed for individual chemicals, and many different overlapping activities appear to be involved. However, the activated derivatives (which in the vast majority of cases are positively charged electrophilic molecules) produced through this system can interact with many different components in their target cells to effect carcinogenic change. This especially occurs through interaction with DNA, RNA, or proteins that are involved in the regulation of cellular growth and function. Which of the many possible chemical interactions or physiochemical effects of the ultimate carcinogen is sufficient for initiation is not yet known. However, when DNA becomes the target of an ultimate carcinogen, serious modifications in the cellular information storage and retrieval processes may occur. For example, alterations to DNA by a carcinogenic agent may cause faulty information transfer during DNA replication, which could lead to a breakdown in the processes that normally control cell growth and differentiation. In some cases, tissues possess the ability to repair lesions made to DNA during carcinogenic insult, such that brief or low-level exposure to such substances during a period when the target cells are not actively replicating may not necessarily produce carcinogenic change. However, if the target cells are actively replicating their DNA during exposure to an ultimate carcinogen, an immediate and permanent effect on the information content of the cell may be produced regardless of the presence or absence of DNA repair processes. This situation prevails, for example, in rapidly proliferating tissues such as skin, bone marrow, and intestine, in which brief exposure to an active carcinogen may be sufficient to initiate carcinogenesis.

The nature of the cellular events that follow initiation are still poorly understood. However, a relatively prolonged period may occur between the time of application and removal of a carcinogenic agent and the time of appearance of identifiable neoplastic cells. This has been shown clearly in the case of skin where a potent carcinogen need only be applied once for a period of minutes or hours in order to initiate the molecular events leading to neoplasia. The promotion period can be modified and shortened by the use of many compounds, called promotors or co-carcinogens, the majority of which are themselves not carcinogenic or are only weakly so. In the case of skin, several phenols and fractions of croton oil (for example, phorbol esters) are promoting agents. Presumably, with many carcinogens, the promoting agents are endogenous in origin, such as hormones.[17] Considerable emphasis is now being placed on the epidemiologic research of cancer with regard to identification of substances in food, water, or in the working environment that serve to promote the induction of cancer by known carcinogens in humans. An extensive review of this subject by Falk[14] provides numerous examples of the co-carcinogenic effects of chemicals in the etiology of human cancer.

Life-style. Many life-style factors, including diet, socioeconomic status, place of residence, and even daily stress levels, are now recognized as playing an etiologic role in human cancer. Probably the best documented example of this phenomenom is the dramatic increase in the incidence of lung cancer in both men and women in relationship to cigarette smoking habits.[1] As of 1930 in the United States, lung cancer in males had a very low incidence of the order of 3 cases per 100,000 population. Now it is over 60 per 100,000. An even more dramatic, although only recently substantiated, increase in the incidence of lung cancer has been seen in women.[1] The main cause of this important increase has been traced to cigarette smoking. Epidemiologic studies have shown that the more people smoke, the higher their risk of lung cancer, and that this risk diminishes significantly when smoking is stopped.[10] Cigarette smoking is also known to interact with other chemicals to enhance the risk of different forms of cancer. Thus, there is now clear evidence[26] that smoking and alcohol interact to enhance the production of oral and esophageal cancers. Smokers who are occupationally exposed to asbestos fibers are at a much greater risk of lung cancer than are nonsmokers.[42] Cigarette smoking also increases the risk of cancers associated with ionizing radiation.[10] In fact, it is rapidly becoming clear, as the Surgeon General's Report points out, that cigarette smoking is the single most important, preventable environmental factor contributing to illness, death, and disability in the United States.

Another major life-style determinant of cancer is diet. Although eating habits have evolved over thousands of years so as to avoid items that are immediately toxic, the potential danger associated with dietary omission or excess of certain nutrients or with repeated exposure to harmful supplements or food additives has only recently been recognized. If, for example, a dietary factor is weakly carcinogenic, it may take decades for the effect to be noticed. Much information regarding the contribution of dietary factors in the etiology of cancer has come from recent epidemiologic studies of large groups or migrant populations.[20] From these studies it has been observed that diet might be related to cancer by several mechanisms. Among the more important of these are (1) the distribution of individual nutrients or food components, for example, protein, carbohydrate, and fiber in the diet and (2) the presence of carcinogenic substances that are associated with the production, preservation, or manufacture of goods and beverages.

The proportion and distribution of nutrients in the diet has been shown to be particularly important in the etiology of gastrointestinal cancers.[20] Diets high in abrasive irritant foods such as pickled vegetables, salted fish, and abrasive food grains, for example, have been correlated with an increased incidence of stomach cancer,[6,18] whereas high fat, low residue diets predispose to a high risk of cancer of the colon and rectum.[29] The contribution of the high fat diet to an increased risk of colon cancer is thought to result from metabolism of the cholesterol in the high fat foods to primary bile acids, which in turn undergo bacterial conversion to co-carcinogenic secondary bile acids in the gut.[49] Recent epidemiologic studies have indicated that a decreased risk of colon cancer is associated with frequent ingestion of high fiber vegetables such as broccoli, brussels sprouts, and cabbage, regardless of the fat content of the diet.[18] Whether this is because high fiber foods increase the bulk and hence the mobility of the intestinal contents, thus enhancing the elimination of co-carcinogenic bile acids and other substances, remains to be determined.

In addition to risks posed by the distribution of natural dietary components, the presence of chemical substances deliberately added to the diet may increase the risks of certain types of cancer. Nitrosamines, for example, are a group of carcinogenic substances that can be formed when dietary nitrites, used commonly as meat and fish preservatives, combine with dietary amines in the acid medium of the stomach.[7] Nitrosamines have been implicated in the genesis of both esophageal and gastric cancer.[6] Another group of dietary supplements that have been suspected as being carcinogenic are the artificial sweeteners, saccharin and cyclamate. Both substances have been implicated in the etiology of bladder cancer.[29] The annual consumption of cyclamates in the United States, principally in low calorie beverages, reached into the millions of pounds until the federal ban on their use was imposed in 1969. Saccharin is still in use, but investigations into its possible carcinogenicity continue.

Finally, there is some evidence that our food might contain some substances that could actually reduce the neoplastic response to ingested carcinogens such as those discussed here.[29] These include antioxidants such as BHA (butylated hydroxy anisol) and BHT (butylated hydroxy toluene), and certain trace metals such as selenium[22] and zinc.[9] Further epidemiologic studies will be required to ascertain the contribution of these substances to the association between diet and cancer in human populations.

Iatrogenic cancer. A number of cancers are now recognized as being iatrogenic in nature, that is, as being caused by medical procedures in which clients were exposed to carcinogenic drugs or radiation. Among the best known examples of these are cancers caused by x-rays and radiation. Bone cancers have been seen in clients treated with radium (Ra-224) used for the treatment of tuberculosis.[45] X-radiation used for treatment of enlarged thymus glands has been implicated in the etiology of increased numbers of thyroid carcinomas that are continuing to develop in persons who received such treatment as children.[23] The incidence of leukemia has been reported to be somewhat increased in children who were irradiated in utero when their mothers were subjected to pelvic x-ray examination during pregnancy.[46] Currently, there is considerable controversy as to whether x-rays used for therapeutic or diagnostic purposes should be eliminated or substantially reduced. If it were discovered, for example, that x-rays currently used therapeutically increased the incidence of breast cancer, exceptional caution would be needed in the continued application of mammographic techniques for early detection of that disease.

Among the most unfortunate iatrogenic tragedies to be recognized in recent years is the occurrence of vaginal cancer among young women whose mothers took the synthetic estrogenic drug diethyl stilbestrol (DES) during pregnancy to prevent miscarriages. It is now estimated that as many as 2,000,000 young women may be at risk of vaginal cancer from this cause.[5] There is also evidence that women who take estrogen to relieve the symptoms of menopause may be at higher risk of developing cancer of the lining of the uterus.[5]

There are undoubtedly other examples of iatrogenic cancers, although the extent to which they occur is not known because of the difficult epidemiologic problems in conducting investigations to assess such events. Clearly, prevention is the most effective means of reducing the future incidence of cancer from iatrogenic as well as other personal and life-style factors.

SPECIAL PROBLEMS IN ASSESSING CAUSAL RELATIONSHIPS

Latency periods and competing risks. As discussed in the previous section, a considerable lag period may occur between the time that a neoplastic process is initiated in a tissue cell and the actual manifestation of cancer. This period of cancer development is referred to as the latency period and may vary from several years to many decades, depending on the nature of the particular chemical and the exposure situation involved. During this period of cancer development, an individual may be subjected to numerous other life-threatening events. Thus, the demonstration of causality in epidemiologic studies dealing with late-occurring diseases such as cancer may be obscured by mortality from competing risks that occur during the latency period.

To illustrate, the latency period for vinyl chloride, a cancer-causing chemical used in the manufacture of plastics, may average from 15 to 20 years. During that time some of the workers who are exposed to this carcinogenic substance may develop cancer. However, many others may die from other causes that ensue before cancer is fully manifested, thus failing to be included in the final tally of cancer cases. In this situation the actual incidence of cases of vinyl chloride–related cancer could be significantly underestimated and so, therefore, could the strength of the causal relationship between vinyl chloride and cancer.

One way to deal with the problem of competing risks during the latency period is to conduct an extremely thorough prospective study in which the death outcome of each worker who entered the study cohort was determined over a 20- or 30-year observation period. This approach has obvious limitations, however, in both time and cost as well as other requirements. Alternatively, a retrospective study could be performed to evaluate causes of death over the past several decades. However, this approach would require that records of the occupational and subsequent retirement history of each worker be available for analysis, which is seldom the case. It is therefore necessary to take alternative approaches to supplement knowledge from epidemiologic studies to determine the probable effects of competing causes of death in human populations. One such approach involves studies using animals whose life spans and, hence, latency periods for tumor development are much shorter than those of humans. Rodents, the species often used for this purpose, have life spans of only 2 or 3 years. This greatly facilitates lifetime evaluation of causes of death during the latency period of a particular cancer-causing chemical. In such investigations, the effects of a specific chemical on particular causes of death can be determined as it would in humans by closely monitoring each animal during lifetime exposure to that chemical to determine specific causes of death. In addition, a certain proportion of the animal population would be sacrificed at regular intervals throughout the duration of the study to determine the incidence of diseases, particularly cancer, that might prevail at that time prior to death from possible competing causes. Meaningful analysis of such survival experiments can then be obtained by determining estimates of the net probability of death owing to each specific cause. Such estimates can then be applied to epidemiologic situations, where estimates of probable competing causes of death during the course of development of late-occurring diseases in human populations are desired.

The applicability of results from animal studies to a determination of risks or causality in humans is, of course, subject to considerable controversy because of the inherent differences in both the individual and population characteristics of the species involved. Some of these problems will be further discussed in the following pages.

Problems in animal-to-human extrapolation

Among the problems of major concern to epidemiologists today is the design of studies that will reliably assess causality between exposure to a suspected carcinogenic agent and the malignant disease that ultimately appears in an exposed human population. This problem has become especially important in recent years because of both the increasing numbers and the rising incidence of neoplastic diseases that are seemingly linked to exposure to a growing number of chemicals in the everyday environment. Although epidemiologic studies represent the most direct approach to assessing causal relationships between exposure and disease in humans, it is not practical to consider that such studies could be performed for the vast numbers of potential etiologic relationships that need to be examined. Hence, an alternative approach to this problem has been employed, utilizing data from experimental animal studies to estimate risks and causal associations in humans. This approach, however, carries other inherent problems that must also be considered. One of the most important of these concerns the appropriateness of extrapolating observations made in animals to humans. Another concerns the issue of high-to-low dose extrapolation.

Interspecies extrapolations. In addition to the obvious anatomic and physiologic differences between animals and humans, numerous other factors may act to determine the responsiveness of different species to cancer-causing agents. Lack of knowledge about these factors has given rise to considerable concern about the appropriateness of using observations about incidence and causality in animals to make statements about those events in humans. For example, animal studies are usually conducted in inbred species, involving populations for which individual differences in responsiveness owing to genetic and social variations are minimal. Human populations, in contrast, are heterogeneous in nature and are characterized by a wide variety of social, behavioral, and biologic features that could greatly affect responsiveness to any environmental agent. In addition, animal studies are performed under well-controlled exposure conditions wherein time and dose exposure regimens are maintained. Human exposure situations, on the other hand, can be highly sporadic, depending on the work and residential patterns of individuals comprising the population as well as weather, accidental exposure situations, and other conditions. Thus, where animal studies are useful for deriving information about the time and dose characteristics of a disease process, the data derived from such studies must be used cautiously in making statements about risks or causality in humans until more can be learned about the major biologic and epidemiologic factors affecting the responsiveness of individual species to chemical agents. In this regard, it would seem to be of increasing importance that an interdisciplinary approach be taken toward defining the nature of factors needed for determining responsiveness to cancer- and other disease-causing chemicals among different species including humans. Although there are still numerous problems associated with current approaches to long-term risk assessment from diseases such as cancer, the thoughtful application of both epidemiologic and experimental methodologies to this objective should go far toward providing a better means of assessing the degree of causality between exposure and disease in human populations.

High-to-low dose extrapolation. A second problem involving the use of animal data to make estimates of risks of diseases in humans is the issue of high-to-low dose extrapolation. This issue refers to the biologic and statistical problem of predicting effects in large human populations exposed to low-dose levels of environmental chemicals from data on small populations, whether animal or human, exposed to high-dose levels of that chemical. Current methods of estimating the risk from chronic exposure to low levels of chemical agents in the environment again rely mainly on experiments with laboratory animals. This is because the long latency periods and the demographic and lifestyle characteristics of human populations would render epidemiologic assessments of risks to the many chemicals involved prohibitively long and expensive.

In animal experiments designed to assess risks in low dose–exposed humans, test subjects are typically exposed to doses of the test chemical low enough to minimize early deaths from acute toxicity but high enough to produce assurance of detecting chronic effects including carcinogenicity. Since the number of animals that can be used in testing any one chemical is limited by space and budgetary constraints, it is usually necessary to expose the animals to dose levels far above the anticipated range of human exposure in order to be reasonably sure of detecting chronic effects. To illustrate, assume that humans and animals are equally sensitive to a particular carcinogenic chemical and that this particular chemical carries a risk of producing cancer in one of every 10,000 humans exposed. This would result in about 22,000 cancers in the population of the United States. The chances of detecting this in a group of 50 or so test animals, tested at ambient human exposure levels, are very low indeed. Therefore, much higher dose levels are required to detect the carcinogenicity of the chemical at statistically significant levels. If it were financially and logistically possible to test the chemical at the lower ambient human exposure levels, samples of 10,000 test animals would be required to yield one cancer, over and above any spontaneous tumors that might appear; perhaps 30,000 or more would be needed for statistical significance. Thus, the rationale for higher dose levels on smaller animal populations appears to be justified as the most current practical approach toward estimating the risks of cancer in humans. The design and use of follow-up epidemiologic studies to confirm the estimates of risks made from animal investigations, however, remains a pressing need in assessing actual causality between exposure and ensuing diseases in human populations.

SCREENING

Screening is an extremely important contribution of epidemiology in detecting disease. It is assumed that by selecting from apparently healthy volunteers those persons who have an elevated risk of suffering from a certain disease that treatment will be easier and more effective. Note that an instrument used for screening a population is not intended to be diagnostic; instead, it is intended only to separate those persons with a high probability of disease from those with a low probability of disease. In turn, the former are subjected to further diagnostic tests and to treatment if appropriate.

Screening tests must meet several criteria. First, they must be valid and reliable. The *validity* of the test refers to whether it is able to separate those with the disease from those without the disease. In epidemiology, the validity of a test is commonly assessed by determining its sensitivity and specificity. Sensitivity refers to the test's capacity to identify correctly those with the disease, whereas specificity refers to its ability to identify correctly those who do not have the disease. Such values are determined by comparing results on the screening tool to those derived from a definitive diagnostic procedure. Usually the sensitivity and specificity can be varied by changing the level at which the test is considered positive.

Although the Pap smear has become institutionalized as a cancer screening tool in women's health, there has never been a formal randomized controlled trial of its efficiency in preventing cervical cancer deaths. As an alternative to an experimental trial, Pap smear histories of women with invasive cervical cancer were compared to age-matched neighborhood controls. The results are given in the bottom half of Fig. 9-8. In this example, the smear could be said to have a sensitivity of 62.5% and a specificity of 87%. When the value of the screening tool's results is continuous, for example the level in units of an enzyme, the sensitivity and specificity can be adjusted by changing the cutoff point for "positives" on the test. In some instances, multiple tests can be used to increase the sensitivity of the screening.

Screening results	Disease by diagnosis: Present	Disease by diagnosis: Absent
Positive	True positive (TP)	False positive (FP)
Negative	False negative (FN)	True negative (TN)

$$\text{Sensitivity} = \frac{TP}{TP + FN} \qquad \text{Specificity} = \frac{TN}{TN + FP}$$

Screening results	Diagnosis: Invasive cervical cancer	Diagnosis: No cervical cancer (controls)*
One or more abnormal smears	30	53
No abnormal smear	18	365
Total	48	418

$$\text{Sensitivity} = \frac{30}{30 + 18} = 62.5\% \qquad \text{Specificity} = \frac{365}{53 + 365} = 87\%$$

Fig. 9-8. Illustration of sensitivity and specificity. *These data are adapted from Clarke, E. A., and Anderson, T. W.: Do screening "Pap" smears help to reduce the frequency of cervical cancer? A case-control study. Presented at the Society for Epidemiologic Research, New Haven, Connecticut, 1978.

Reliability (precision) of a screening test refers to the reproducibility of its results. Variation in the method and observer error can be a source of inconsistent results. Standardizing procedures and training observers improve reliability.

The yield of a screening tool refers to the amount of a previously undiagnosed disease that can be diagnosed and treated as a result of the screening. The yield depends not only on the sensitivity of the test but also on the prevalence of unrecognized disease, the extent of previous screening in the population, and the degree to which people will participate in the screening.

There are varying opinions regarding what criteria should be used to judge whether to implement a screening program. The criteria suggested by Wilson and Junger[52] follow:

1. The condition to be screened should constitute an important health problem.
2. For clients with recognized disease there should be an accepted treatment.
3. Facilities for diagnosis and treatment should be available.
4. The disease should have a recognizable latent or early symptomatic stage.
5. A suitable test or examination should exist.
6. The test should be acceptable to the population to whom it is applied.
7. The natural history of the disease, in-

cluding development from latent to declared disease, should be adequately understood.

8. There should be a policy on whom to treat as clients after they are identified as possible cases.
9. The cost of case finding (including diagnosis and treatment) should be economically balanced in relation to possible expenditure on health care as a whole.
10. Case finding should be a continuing process.

Although screening procedures have become institutionalized without careful adherence to these criteria, it is important to recall that screening, itself, is not completely risk free and in some cases could do harm if misapplied, for example, the radiation exposure from mammography.

CANCER SURVEILLANCE PROGRAMS

The surveillance of cancer incidence and mortality is extremely important not only for assessing the occurrence of cancer of various types but also for evaluating the effectiveness of cancer treatment and preventive action programs. Numerous surveillance registries on the federal, state, and regional levels have developed over the past few decades. Some of the more prominent of these are discussed here.

Probably the most extensive information on cancer occurrence is based on mortality data. Within the United States, the National Center for Health Statistics publishes extensive mortality tables every year. These tables include all causes of death, and trends for specific diseases including cancer can be developed by compiling data from separate annual volumes. The National Cancer Institute has used these data to produce a compilation of United States cancer mortality by county covering the period 1950 to 1969.[32] This volume does not give time trends but does provide mortality data by state, sex, and race, including numbers of cases and rates for over 3,000 counties in the United States. Companion volumes of maps have also been published, making it possible to visually identify areas of high cancer mortality for 35 anatomic sites of cancer. Separate maps are available for both white[33] and nonwhite[34] United States populations. The tapes from which the county cancer mortality data were published can be merged with demographic, industrial, and similar data collected by the Census Bureau to provide correlations and leads to further epidemiologic studies. However, since none of these data identify individuals, any work on a case control basis requires working in study communities to identify the cases of interest.

Although cancer mortality data are useful in assessing deaths from cancer in relation to geographic or potential etiologic factors, the effectiveness of cancer treatment and prevention programs can best be evaluated through continuing surveillance of cancer incidence. The major source of such data in the United States at the state level has been the Connecticut Cancer Registry,[4] which was established in 1935. This surveillance registry reports on incidence by all major sites and has served as a prototype for other state and regional population-based registries that have subsequently developed.

At the national level the National Cancer Institute has conducted three sampling surveys of cancer incidence timed to coincide with a census year to give a satisfactory population base for computing rates. The most recent of these, the Third National Cancer Survey, was conducted between 1969 and 1971 and contains data on nine study areas including Atlanta, Birmingham, Colorado, Dallas–Ft. Worth, Detroit, Iowa, Minneapolis–St. Paul, Pittsburgh, and Oakland–San Francisco. It contains both numbers and cases of age-standardized rates for males, females, whites, and blacks for 46 primary cancer sites.

The most comprehensive area cancer incident reporting system maintained by the National Cancer Institute is the Surveillance, Epidemiology, and End Results (SEER) program.[53] This system covers 10% of the United States population and has as its objective the provision of detailed information on the incidence of and survival from (hence, mortality owing to) essentially all malignant neoplasms in the United States. The SEER program is an outgrowth of two earlier NCI programs, including the End Results program[3] and the NCI surveys. Like the surveys, the SEER program is not a random sampling but includes areas where there is technical ability to carry out the work, as well as an appropriate geographic and social mix. The eleven current participants include metropolitan Atlanta, Detroit, New Orleans, San Francisco–Oakland, Seattle–Puget Sound (13 counties), Connecticut, Hawaii, Iowa, New Mexico, Utah, and Puerto Rico. Information is collected on anatomic site, histologic cell type, extent of disease at the time of diagnosis of cancer, demographic characteristics of the patient, as well as data on how the diagnosis was established, treatment given, and subsequent vital status of the client. All data are provided on a population base so that incidence, survival, and mortality data can each be related to the same defined group of individuals at risk.

There is clearly a need to relate incidence data from systems such as the SEER program to possible causal factors. Although occupational and environmental exposure information is scant, some important data sources do exist. Among these are the Social Security Administration, which maintains a continuous work history sample of workers, and the Census Bureau, which maintains occupation and industrial data that are potentially useful in extending ecologic cancer mortality studies. A number of labor unions have also begun collecting data on the illnesses and causes of mortality among their members. Hopefully, the practice of maintaining concise records of occupational histories of all workers in the United States will become commonplace in the near future, so as to permit both early detection of cancer incidence as well as elimination or at least minimization of many cancer causes.

POLICY IMPLICATIONS FROM EPIDEMIOLOGIC STUDIES

Results from epidemiologic studies have been used to influence, either directly or indirectly, implementation of health policies on a number of issues in recent years.[25] In general, these refer to the establishment of measures to protect industrial workers from exposure to toxic substances, to provide for air quality standards, and to establish policies of preventive health behavior.

On the issue of measures to protect industrial workers, results from epidemiologic studies are playing an increasingly important role in influencing the revision of occupational standards toward providing greater levels of protection from occupational health hazards. The first standards designed to protect workers were established early in this century and were oriented principally toward reducing exposure to trace metals such as lead, mineral dusts, and organic solvents. These standards, known as threshold limit values (TLV), defined the permissible limits of exposure during an 8-hour day or a 40-hour work week. Little human data were available at that time, and TLV's were often established on the basis of experiments from laboratory animals or even by analogy with chemicals of similar properties. The principal problem with TLV's as a measure of exposure limitations to toxic chemicals rested in the fact that they did not consider the issue of cumulative toxicity or the fact that many years of exposure to a toxic substance may be required before manifestations of late-occurring effects, such as cancer, appeared. In addition, early industrial exposure standards did not account for individual sensitivities or the ethnic, geographic, and socioeconomic factors that influence the incidence of diseases in a human population.

Hence, it is likely that many adverse health effects were produced during exposure to occupational chemicals because early exposure standards were inappropriately established. A case in point again is the situation involving workers exposed to the carcinogenic chemical, vinyl chloride. This chemical has been found to cause a rare type of liver tumor, hepatic angiosarcoma, in both animals and humans after sufficient exposure time. Early production standards failed to protect workers from this property of vinyl chloride, essentially because animal studies available at the time provided no clue to the carcinogenic properties of vinyl chloride. Essentially no concern existed, in fact, with regard to the carcinogenic potential of this substance until early in 1974 when a vinyl chloride manufacturer in the southeastern United States reported to the National Institute for Occupational Safety and Health (NIOSH) that seven of its employees had died of angiosarcoma. Perhaps little notice of this occurrence would have been taken even at that time were it not for the extreme rarity of this disease in the United States population (0.0128 cases/100,000 persons per year). The occurrence of this rare event at a very high level in the occupational population suggested an etiologic association between vinyl chloride and angiosarcoma, and numerous epidemiologic studies that were subsequently conducted on vinyl chloride–exposed populations bore this out. These studies also showed that vinyl chloride may be the causal agent of other types of malignant tumors as well as serious noncarcinogenic disorders in people with occupational exposure to it (see *Environmental Health Perspectives,* vol. 21, 1977 and *Annals of the New York Academy of Sciences,* vol. 246, 1975).

As a result of these studies, action was initiated on behalf of NIOSH and the EPA both to reduce occupational exposure levels and to establish a national atmospheric emission standard for vinyl chloride to protect people living in the vicinity of vinyl chloride production plants. The types of considerations that go into the establishment of such standards are based on the capabilities of the best available technology for controlling exposure to that chemical as well as knowledge derived from experimental animal and epidemiologic studies, which are used to predict the extent to which potential health hazards can be minimized under reduced exposure conditions. Clearly, the more knowledge that is gained from epidemiologic studies regarding human sensitivities and susceptibilities to long-range chemical-induced diseases, the more the results of such studies will contribute in a significant way toward formulation of a health policy designed to protect human populations from harmful environmental conditions.

Epidemiology has also made contributions to the health policy in the area of identification of factors influencing preventive health behaviors. One particular example of this is the change in the health policy that has occurred since the identification of the hazards of cigarette smoking. In a little more than a decade, advertisements for cigarettes have been banned from television and radio, smoking is restricted to public places, and active media campaigns have been launched to deter people from smoking.

Thus, although the contributions of epidemiologists to health policy may be not readily apparent because of the time lag between completion of research studies and the implementation of related policy actions, their need is nonetheless unrefuted and of growing importance to the definition of policies in a broad spectrum of health-related areas.

REFERENCES

1. American Cancer Society: Cancer facts and figures, New York, 1980, American Cancer Society, Inc.
2. Antunes, C., et al.: Endometrial cancer and estrogen use: report of a large case-control study, N. Engl. J. Med. **300**:9, 1979.
3. Axtell, L. M., Asire, A. J., and Myers, M. H., editors: Cancer patient survival, Report No. 5, Publication No. 77-992, Bethesda, Md., 1977, U.S. Department of Health, Education and Welfare.
4. Christine, B., Flannery, J. T., and Sullivan, P. D.: Cancer in Connecticut, 1966-68, Connecticut State Department of Health, 1971.
5. Clayson, D. B., and Shubik, P.: The carcinogenic action of drugs, Cancer Detection Prevention **1**(1):43, 1976.
6. Correa, P., et al.: A model for gastric cancer epidemiology, Lancet **2**:58, 1975.
7. Crosby, N. T., Foreman, J. K., Polframan, J. F., and Sawyer, R.: Estimation of steam-volatile N-nitrosamines at the 1 ug/kg level, Nature **238**:342, 1972.
8. de-The, G.: The epidemiology of Burkitts' lymphoma: evidence for a causal association with the Epstein-Barr virus. In Sartwell, P., editor: Epidemiologic reviews, vol. 1, Baltimore, 1979, School of Hygiene and Public Health, Johns Hopkins University.
9. DeWys, W., and Pories, W. J.: Inhibition of a spectrum of animal tumors by dietary zinc deficiency, J. Natl. Cancer Inst. **48**:375, 1972.
10. Doll, R.: An epidemiologic perspective of the biology of cancer, Cancer Res. **38**:3573, 1978.
11. Doll, R., and Hill, A. B.: Lung cancer and other causes of death in relation to smoking. A second report on the mortality of British doctors. Br. Med. J. **2**:1071, 1956.
12. Doll, R., and Hill, A. B.: Mortality in relation to smoking: ten years' observation of British doctors, Br. Med. J. **1**:1339, 1460, 1964.
13. Epstein, S. S.: Environmental determinants of human cancer, Cancer Res. **34**:2425, 1974.
14. Falk, H. L.: Possible mechanisms of combination effects in chemical cocarcinogenesis, Oncology **33**:77, 1976.
15. Fraumeni, J., editor: Persons at high risk of cancer: an approach to cancer etiology and control, New York, 1975, Academic Press, Inc.
16. Friedman, G.: Primer of epidemiology, ed. 2, New York, 1980, McGraw-Hill Book Co.
17. Furth, J.: Influence of host factors on the growth of neoplastic cells, Cancer Res. **23**:21, 1963.
18. Graham, S., and Mettlin, C.: Diet and cancer of the colon, Am. J. Epidemiol. **108**:241, 1978.
19. Graham, S., Schotz, W., and Martino, P.: Alimentary factors in the epidemiology of gastric cancer, Cancer **30**:175, 1972.
20. Haenszel, W.: Cancer mortality among foreign born in the United States, J. Natl. Cancer Inst. **26**:37, 1961.
21. Hamilton, I., Langlands, A. O., and Prescott, R. J.: The treatment of operable cancer of the breast: a clinical trial in the southeast region of Scotland, Br. J. Surg. **61**:758, 1974.
22. Harr, J. R., Exon, J. H., Weswig, P. H., and Whanger, P. D.: Relationship of dietary selenium concentration, chemical cancer induction and tissue concentration in rats, Clin. Toxicol. **6**:487, 1973.
23. Hempelmann, L. H., et al.: Neoplasms in persons treated with x-rays in infancy: fourth survey in 20 years, J. Natl. Cancer Inst. **55**:176, 1975.
24. Hill, A. B.: The environment and disease: association or causation? Proc. Roy. Soc. Med. **58**:295, 1965.
25. Holland, W. W., and Wainwright, A. H.: Epidemiology and health policy. In Sartwell, P., editor: Epidemiologic reviews, vol. 1, Baltimore, 1979, School of Hygiene and Public Health, Johns Hopkins University.
26. International Agency for Cancer Research: Annual report, Lyon, France, 1975.
27. Kelsey, J.: A review of the epidemiology of human breast cancer. In Sartwell, P., editor: Epidemiologic reviews, vol. 1, Baltimore, 1979, School of Hygiene and Public Health, Johns Hopkins University.
28. Lilienfeld, A., Pederson, E., and Dowd, J. E.: Cancer epidemiology: methods of study, Baltimore, 1967, The Johns Hopkins Press.
29. Lowenfels, A. B., and Anderson, M. E.: Diet and cancer, Cancer **39**:1809, 1977.

30. Mack, T. M., et al.: Estrogens and endometrial cancer in a retirement community, N. Engl. J. Med. **294:**1262, 1976.
31. MacMahon, B., and Pugh, T.: Epidemiology: principles and methods, Boston, 1970, Little, Brown & Co.
32. Mason, T. J., and McKay, F. N.: Cancer mortality by county: 1950-1969, Publication No. 74-615, Bethesda, Md., 1974, U.S. Department of Health, Education and Welfare.
33. Mason, T. J., et al.: Atlas of cancer mortality for U.S. counties: 1950-1965, Publication No. 75-780, Bethesda, Md., 1975, U.S. Department of Health, Education and Welfare.
34. Mason, T. J., et al.: Atlas of cancer mortality among U.S. non-whites: 1950-1969, Publication No. 76-1204, Bethesda, Md., 1976, U.S. Department of Health, Education and Welfare.
35. Mausner, J., and Bahn, A.: Epidemiology: an introductory text, Philadelphia, 1974, W. B. Saunders Co.
36. Miettenen, O.: Confounding and effect-modification, Am. J. Epidemiol. **100:**350, 1974.
37. Miller, J. A.: Carcinogens by chemicals: an overview, Cancer Res. **30:**559, 1970.
38. Miller, J. A., and Miller, E. C.: Chemical carcinogenesis: mechanisms and approaches to its control, J. Natl. Cancer Inst. **47:**5, 1971.
39. Morris, J. N.: Uses of epidemiology, ed. 3, Edinburgh, 1975, Churchill Livingstone.
40. Omran, A.: Modern concepts of epidemiology. In Omran, A., editor: Community medicine in developing countries, New York, 1974, Springer Publishing Co., p. 3.
41. Schottenfeld, D., editor: Cancer epidemiology and prevention: current concepts, Springfield, Ill., 1975, Charles C Thomas, Publisher.
42. Selikoff, T. J., Hammond, E. C., and Churg, J.: Asbestos exposure, smoking and neoplasia, J.A.M.A. **204:**106, 1968.
43. Shimkin, M.: Some historical landmarks in cancer epidemiology. In Schottenfeld, D., editor: Cancer epidemiology and prevention: current concepts, Springfield, Ill., 1975, Charles C Thomas, Publisher.
44. Smith, D. C., et al.: Association of exogenous estrogen and endometrial cancer, N. Engl. J. Med. **293:**1164, 1975.
45. Spiess, H., and Mays, C. W.: Bone cancers induced by 224 Ra (Th X) in children and adults, Health Phys. **19:**713, 1970.
46. Stewart, A., and Kneale, G. W.: Radiation dose effects in relation to obstetric x-rays and childhood cancers, Lancet **1:**1185, 1970.
47. Susser, M.: Causal thinking in the health sciences, concepts and strategies of epidemiology, New York, 1973, Oxford University Press.
48. Walker, A., and Hershel, J.: Cancer of the corpus uteri, Am. J. Epidemiol. **110**(1):47, 1979.
49. Weisburger, J. H.: Environmental cancer: on the causes of the main human cancers, Tex. Rep. Biol. Med. **37:**1, 1978.
50. Weiss, N., Szekely, D. R., and Austin, D. F.: Increasing incidence of endometrial cancer in the United States, N. Engl. J. Med. **294:**1259, 1976.
51. Weiss, N., Szekely, D., English, D., and Schweid, A.: Endometrial cancer in relation to patterns of menopausal estrogen use, J.A.M.A. **242**(3):261, 1979.
52. Wilson, T., and Jungner, G.: Principles and practice of screening for disease, Public Health Paper No. 34, Geneva, 1968, World Health Organization.
53. Young, J. L., Asire, A. J., and Pollack, E. S., editors: SEER program: cancer incidence and mortality in the United States, Publication No. 78-1837, Bethesda, Md., 1978, U.S. Department of Health, Education and Welfare.
54. Ziel, H. K., and Finkle, W. D.: Increased risk of endometrial carcinoma among users of conjugated estrogens, N. Engl. J. Med. **293:**1167, 1975.

10

Nursing's contribution to case finding and the early detection of cancer

MARILYN FRANK-STROMBORG

Although many advances have recently been made in the treatment of cancer through surgery, radiation, chemotherapy, hormone therapy, and immunotherapy, many authorities believe that the best route for cancer cure today is still early detection before metastases occur.[156,158,211] It is generally acknowledged that in the vast majority of cancers early detection of precancerous and cancerous lesions is beneficial and results in improved survival.[136,218] In the past, nursing's involvement with cancer detection has been minimal. There were a few reports of nurses conducting cancer detection examinations, but these tended to focus on detection of cancer as a secondary activity (such as detection of cervical cancer in a family planning clinic).

Fortunately, several things have occurred in the past few years that have increased nursing's involvement in cancer detection. These are the emphasis on the nurse's role in primary health care settings, growth of the nurse practitioner role, expansion of the nursing role, and inclusion of physical assessment courses in nursing curriculums. These changes have resulted in nurse practitioners giving total physical examinations conducted for the sole purpose of detecting cancer. Client acceptance and satisfaction with nurses doing these examinations in a cancer detection clinic have been documented by Stromborg and Nord.[235] Involvement in cancer detection has not been limited to nurse practitioners. White[253] reports that nurses in rural communities in Texas have been trained in a short period of time to conduct cancer detection physical examinations. Nurses have also been actively involved in performing examinations to detect cancer in mobile detection clinics.[129,141,142] Research has also documented that nurses can perform some of these physical examinations as well as physicians. Copher[47] found that nurses with 6 months additional training can perform pelvic examinations as well and as reliably as fully trained Ob-Gyn residents. Sutnick, Miller, and Yarbo[236] write that the preliminary data from the Preventive Medicine Institute–Strang Clinic also indicate that nurses detect breast lesions with an effectiveness equal to that of physicians.

The scope of the cancer problem that is summarized below mandates that nurses incorporate the principles of cancer detection into their nursing practice regardless of individual clinical settings. In the 70's, there were an estimated 3.5 million cancer deaths, 6.5 million new cancer cases, and more than 10 million people under medical care for cancer.[179] If we truly are to make a commitment to early detection of cancer, then cancer detection must be as much a part of the occupational nurse's role as it is the cancer clinical specialist's role. Case findings should be done by nurses working in day-care centers, public health agencies, acute care settings, physicians' offices, college health centers, schools, factories, and employment health settings.

What does the nurse need to know to be involved in cancer detection? Two basic skills are required for this activity. The nurse must have a thorough knowledge of the known or suspected risk factors for cancer and a basic understanding and competence in physical assessment skills. The bibliography contains a list of textbooks, programmed instruction, and manuals that the nurse wishing to acquire these skills should consult. It is recommended that these assessment techniques be acquired by taking a structured course that offers both theory and supervision of skills.

Through proper utilization of the four cardinal techniques of physical assessment—inspection, palpation, percussion, auscultation—the nurse can detect cancer in the asymptomatic client. Cancer detection can, should, and must take place in any clinical setting and does not require an armamentarium of equipment. The ability to obtain a thorough history, to identify risk factors, and to use physical assessment skills will enable nurses in a multitude of roles to be actively involved in cancer prevention and detection. It is urged that whenever a nurse has professional contact with another person, cancer detection methods be utilized.

To aid nurses in cancer detection, methods of detecting those cancers that commonly occur will be discussed. This discussion will include known and hypothesized risk factors, questions that should be asked when obtaining a history, early signs and symptoms, and diagnostic procedures. In addition, there are controversies surrounding a few of the commonly occurring cancers (such as screening for breast cancer), and these will be detailed.

SKIN CANCER

The risk factors for cancer of the skin have been identified by Shimkin[222] as exogenous, endogenous, and premalignant states or lesions. Exogenous risk factors include ultraviolet radiation from sunlight; ionizing radiation; arsenic; petroleum, including coal tar and creosote preparations; and burn scars. Scars following burns, bites, infections, corrosive damage, and vaccinations have all been implicated in the genesis of skin cancer.[239] Inorganic arsenicals taken internally produce skin cancers that are characteristically multiple, involving unexposed parts of the body and unusual locations.[112] Ionizing radiation refers to x-rays, radium, and atom bomb exposure. Skin cancers from ionizing radiation tend to develop many years after radiation exposure and almost always occur at the edge of the irradiated sites rather than in the center.

Risk factors

Endogenous risk factors include individuals who have fair complexions and individuals with xeroderma pigmentosum or albinism. Xeroderma pigmentosum is a rare, recessively inherited deficiency in one of the enzymes that repairs DNA after ultraviolet injury. Daniels[51] points out that pigmented races have far less skin cancer than people with white skin and that the incidence of skin cancer in white-skinned people is greater in areas of decreasing latitude. Typically, indi-

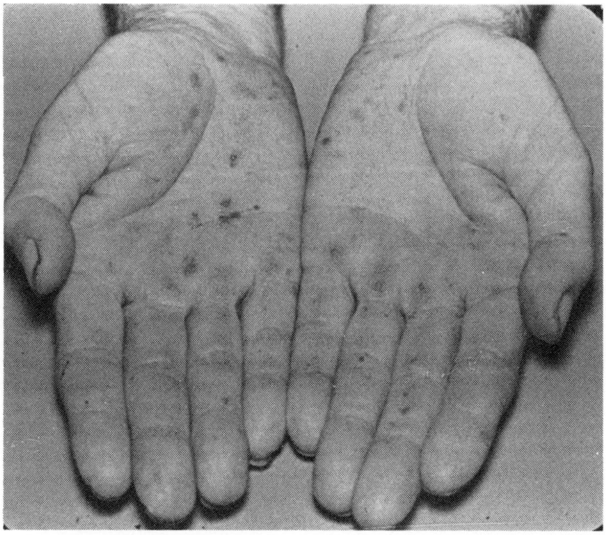

Fig. 10-1. Arsenic keratosis. Arsenic keratosis is caused by exposure to arsenic. This may occur occupationally (metal smelters and agricultural workers using certain herbicides and pesticides). It may also occur in clients who received arsenic medications (such as Fowler's solution or Asiatic pills). Over a period of years, discrete, firm, yellowish keratotic lesions appear on the palms and soles. (From Weinstein, G. D.: Skin cancer: recognition and treatment, New York, 1973, Famous Teachings in Modern Medicine, Medcom, Inc.)

viduals who have a light, ruddy complexion or blonds with thin skin and blue eyes tend more readily than brunettes to have skin cancer.[37]

Premalignant states or lesions are senile keratosis, arsenical keratosis (Fig. 10-1), and leukoplakia (Fig. 10-2). Leukoplakia is a term applied to a thickened patch adherent to the mucous membrane and is premalignant.[54]

Of all the known risk factors, most experts believe that ultraviolet radiation from the sun is the leading cause of skin cancer.[65] Fortunately, the most carcinogenic of the ultraviolet wavelengths can be blocked by sunscreening agents. Light-skinned individuals should be instructed to employ one of the sunscreening agents such as para-aminobenzoic acid (PABA) whenever they go into the sun.[101,256] Client education should also include the advice that sunbathing should *not* be done during the 2-hour period around noon, since two thirds of the day's ultraviolet light comes through during that time.

Nursing interventions

When obtaining the health history, the nurse should inquire if there has been previous exposure to electromagnetic radiation (x-rays, radium), chemical carcinogens (tar and pitch, arsenic), a genetic predisposition (xeroderma pigmentosum), past scarring (thermal burns, corrosive damage), or chronic exposure to solar rays (excessive sunbathing, occupations such as ranchers or sailors). All of these questions will help the nurse identify those persons who are at risk for developing skin cancer. When feasible, client education can assist these high risk individuals in appropriate procedures for re-

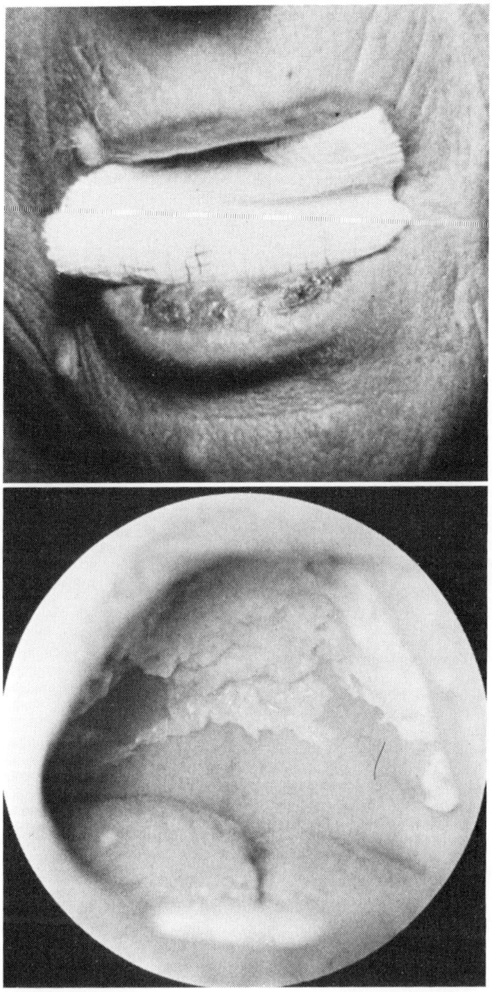

Fig. 10-2. Leukoplakia is a premalignant lesion found in the mouth, genitalia, cervix, and bladder. Clinically, the lesion is a white, flat or slightly elevated plaque, irregular in shape, scaling, ulcerating, or even atrophic. (From Weinstein, G. D.: Skin cancer: recognition and treatment, New York, 1973, Famous Teachings in Modern Medicine, Medcom, Inc.)

ducing exposure to offending agents (such as sun, tar and pitch, arsenic, oils, and paraffins). If exposure has already taken place (that is, medical irradiation, occupational exposure to arsenic), it may be more appropriate to monitor the individual with follow-up visits at established intervals.

Carcinomas of the skin are divided into two main types: basal cell and squamous cell. The incidence, clinical characteristics, and common sites are summarized in Table 10-1. When examining a client, it is important to remember that the vast majority of basal and squamous cell carcinomas of the skin occur on sun-exposed areas.[101] Del Regato and Spjut[60] describe the typical client with car-

Table 10-1. Incidence, clinical characteristics, and common sites of skin cancer*

Skin carcinoma	Incidence	Clinical characteristics	Common sites
Basal cell carcinoma	Most common form of skin cancer; it occurs primarily in clients exposed to intense sunlight, especially fair complected Caucasians with light eyes and hair.	Nodular basal cell carcinoma: elevated lesions with an umbilical, ulcerated center, raised margin, and waxy or "pearly" border; moderately firm. Superficial basal cell carcinoma: plaque, usually with a crusted and erythematous center and a raised, pearly border; often multiple.	Commonly found on the nose, eyelids, cheeks, and trunk; uncommon on palms and soles; metastases are extremely rare.
Squamous cell carcinoma	Less common than basal cell carcinoma, it occurs primarily on areas exposed to actinic radiation.	Appearance varies from an elevated nodular mass to a punched-out ulcerated lesion or a large fungating mass. Unlike basal cell carcinoma, squamous cell tumors are opaque.	Seventy-five percent occur on the head, 15% on hands, and 10% elsewhere. Can metastasize to regional lymph nodes; in more advanced lesions, pulmonary metastasis can occur.

*From Gumport, S., Harris, M., and Kopf, A.: Diagnosis and management of common skin cancers, Publication No. 3373-PE, New York, 1974, American Cancer Society Professional Education Publication.

cinoma of the skin as an elderly man showing signs of chronic exposure to solar rays (farmers, sailors, ranchers, laborers). During examination for possible cutaneous cancers, the nurse must inspect the client's *entire* integument. This is best accomplished in a setting with good lighting (such as a gooseneck lamp) that enables the nurse to project it obliquely across the client's skin surface.

Figs. 10-3 and 10-4 illustrate the typical basal cell carcinoma, while Fig. 10-5 shows a squamous cell carcinoma. There should be a high index of suspicion when inspection and palpation of a client's skin reveal either a firm cutaneous or subcutaneous mass of unusual nature or a persistent ulcer.[95] The definitive diagnosis of carcinomas of the skin is best confirmed by biopsy.

Malignant melanoma. Blonde or red-haired, blue-eyed, pale-skinned, sunlight-intolerant northern European peoples are susceptible to malignant melanoma. Of this group, those who burn but do not tan in sunlight and who freckle excessively have the highest incidence of melanoma development.[31] Yet there is some debate concerning the association between sunlight and the risk of melanoma.[51] Teppo[240] writes that the recognition of sunlight as the only important risk factor of cutaneous melanoma may be

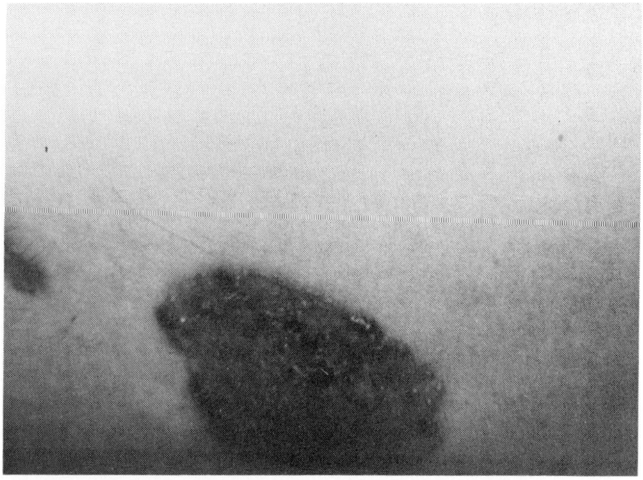

Fig. 10-3. Superficial basal cell carcinoma. Note typical appearance—plaque, usually with crusted and erythematous center. (From the clinical files of Mark J. LeVine, M.D., Fellow in Photobiology, Harvard Medical School, Department of Dermatology, Massachusetts General Hospital, Boston, Mass.)

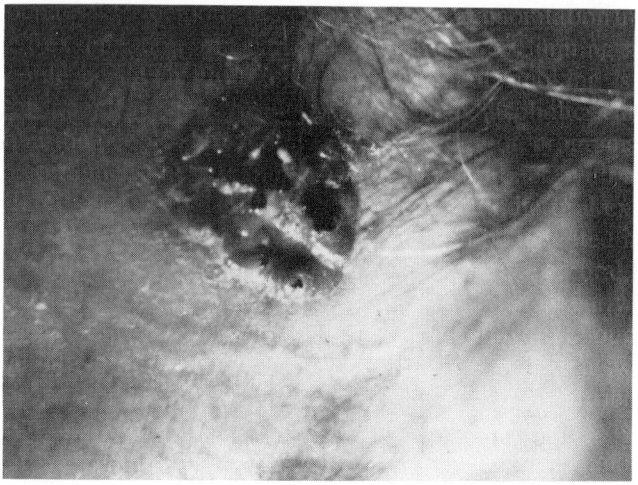

Fig. 10-4. Basal cell carcinoma. Note lesion is elevated with ulcerated center, raised margin, and "pearly" border. (From the clinical files of Mark J. LeVine, M.D., Fellow in Photobiology, Harvard Medical School, Department of Dermatology, Massachusetts General Hospital, Boston, Mass.)

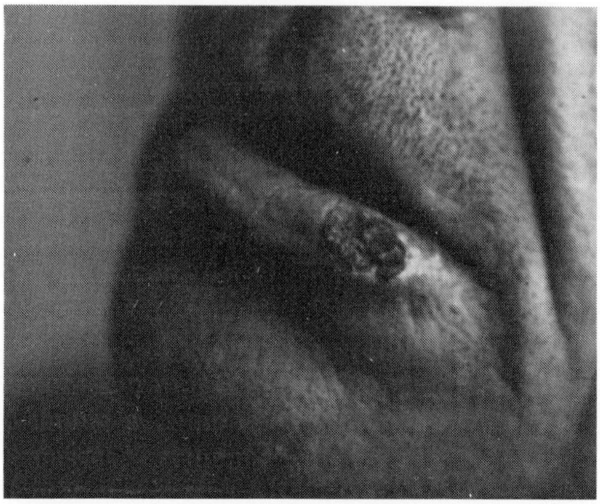

Fig. 10-5. Squamous cell carcinoma. Note this lesion is on the lip (75% of squamous cell carcinomas are on the head). (From the clinical files of Mark J. LeVine, M.D., Fellow in Photobiology, Harvard Medical School, Department of Dermatology, Massachusetts General Hospital, Boston, Mass.)

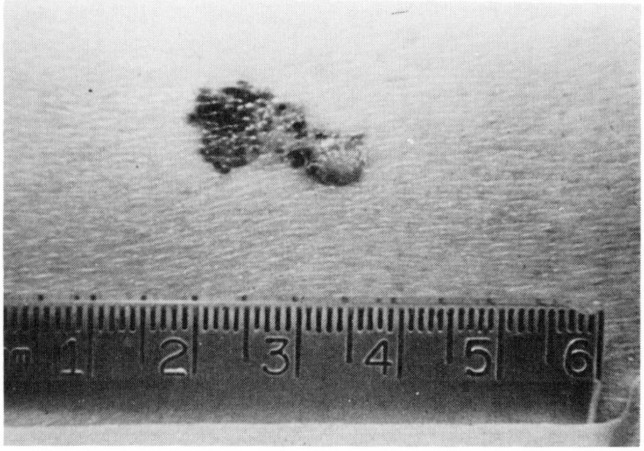

Fig. 10-6. Early melanoma. Note subtle variations in color, outline, and height. Nodule at right side of lesion can be appreciated only by gentle palpation with fingertip. (From Weinstein, G. D.: Skin cancer: recognition and treatment, New York, 1973, Famous Teachings in Modern Medicine, Medcom, Inc.)

an oversimplification of a complex problem. Curious aspects of skin pigmentation protection in melanoma can be found in Africa. Here, melanoma is common but occurs almost exclusively on such nonpigmented areas as the plantar surfaces of the feet, the palms of the hands, and the mucous membranes. American blacks demonstrate a similar melanoma distribution, with sparing of pigmented skin.[31,52]

If individuals are instructed to report any change in a mole, the diagnosis could be

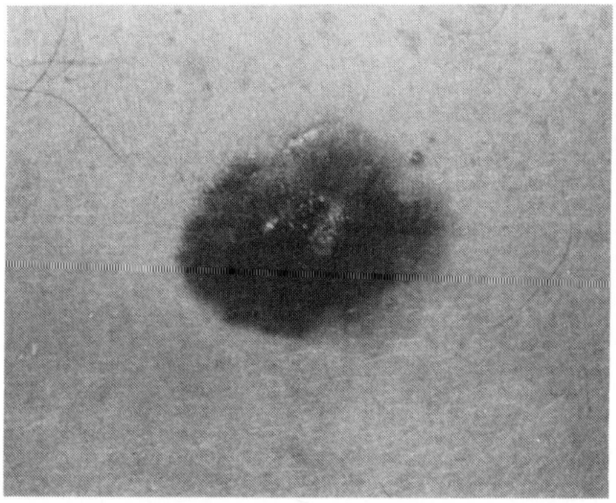

Fig. 10-7. Malignant melanoma showing irregular pattern of coloring, topography, and pigment disbursement into surrounding skin. Colors portending malignancy in a brown or black lesion are shades of red, white, and blue. Of all colors, shades of blue are most ominous. (From Cady, B., Moschella, S., and Legg, M.: Contemporary aspects of malignant melanoma, New York, 1974, Famous Teachings in Modern Medicine, Medcom, Inc.)

made at an early biologic and potentially curable stage. Client education must include instruction that a change in any of the following characteristics merits medical attention:

1. Change in the size of a mole
2. Change in the elevation of a mole
3. Change in the color of a mole
4. Change in the surface characteristics of a mole
5. Change in the surroundings of a mole
6. Change in the sensation of a mole[53]

Client education may also include the suggestion that any nevus that is subjected to *chronic irritation* (that is, from a bra, belt, shoes) be removed.[62]

Many, possibly half, of the melanomas arise in moles or pigmented areas, hence there should be a high index of suspicion in any mole that is changing or enlarging.[117,220] When obtaining a health history, the nurse must inquire whether any of the changes listed above have occurred. A history of change, often extending over a period of weeks or months, in a preexisting mole or the development of a new mole in an adult is of great importance and demands inspection.

The positive signs in order of importance that suggest malignant change include variegated color, irregular border, and irregular surface (Figs. 10-6 and 10-7).[155] Diagnosis is based on the history and clinical appearance of the lesion and is confirmed by microscopic examination after surgical excision.

ORAL CANCER

Risk factors

Several risk factors have been identified as contributory factors in the development of oral cancer. Table 10-2 lists the known or suspected risk factors for cancer of the oral cavity.

When obtaining the health history, it is important to ask about smoking habits and alcohol consumption. Alcoholics, particularly those who smoke heavily, experience a greatly increased risk of cancer of the oral cavity. Rothman points out that "the preponderance of evidence supports the view

Table 10-2. Risk factors for oral cancer[186,204,260]

Risk factors	Site
Chronic ingestion of alcohol	Frequently affects the mouth and tongue
Infectious agents	
Atrophic leutic glossitis	Frequently affects the tongue
Tobacco	
Cigarette smokers	Frequently affects floor of mouth, base of tongue, and buccal mucosa
Pipe smokers	
Cigar smokers	
Chewing tobacco and snuff	
Chewing betel nut and pan	Frequently affects buccal mucosa and base of tongue
Chronic exposure to actinic radiation (sunlight)	Affects lower lip
Chronic irritation from ill-fitting dentures or defective teeth	Generally associated with oral cancer
Plummer-Vinson's disease (a vitamin B–complex and iron deficient condition)	Generally associated with oral cancer
Premalignant lesions	Generally associated with oral cancer
Leukoplakia	
Erythroplakia	

that alcohol does not usually initiate cancer but acts as a cocarcinogen, magnifying the carcinogenic activity of other cancer-inducing agents such as tobacco."[204] Since almost all heavy drinkers are smokers as well, the effect of alcohol cannot be separated from tobacco. In the history, tobacco usage should be measured in pack years by calculating the packs per day times the number of years an individual has smoked.

Since it is sometimes difficult to obtain an accurate history of alcohol consumption, several sources are given in the references that should assist the interested nurse.[18,104,160,197,230] Heinemann and Estes give the following advice about asking alcoholics questions that pertain to their drinking habits:

> Alcoholic patients are notorious for being inaccurate historians, particularly in regard to their drinking. This often relates to their need to deny the reality of alcohol intake. Therefore, questions are posed to elicit *specific* answers. What, when, where, who questions are, as a rule, more productive than how and why questions.[104]

Expressions such as "I'm just a social drinker" and "I don't drink everyday" must be further defined to ascertain if there is alcohol abuse.

Other areas the nurse should include in the history geared to detect oral cancer would be: (1) if the client has noticed any white or red sores in the mouth for over a month, (2) if there are any denture problems or ill-fitting dentures, (3) amount of dental care per year, (4) frequency of oral hygiene, and (5) if the client has an occupation in which there is constant exposure to the sun as with farmers or sailors.[122]

Nursing interventions

Client education first begins with the identification of high-risk clients for oral cancer. Depending on the risk factors identified, the individual could be referred to a physician or a dentist, taught how to inspect and palpate

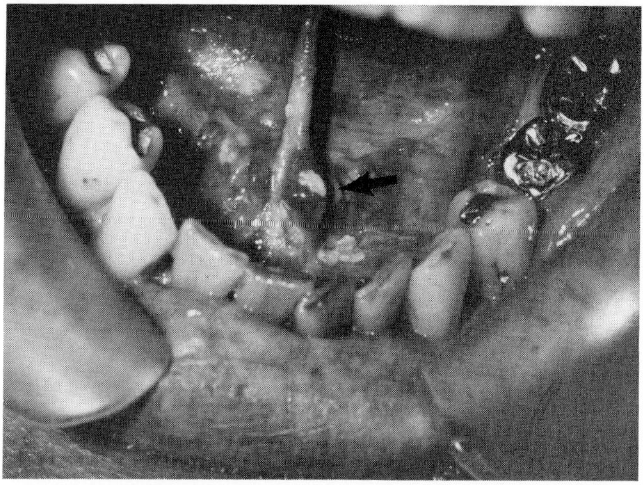

Fig. 10-8. Squamous cell carcinoma of floor of mouth. (From the clinical files of Alan Felsenfeld, D.D.S., Oral and Maxillofacial Surgeon, La Puente, Calif.)

their own oral cavity for the early signs of cancer, or the nurse could conduct the oral examination at predetermined intervals. Grabau and associates[91,92] demonstrated that oral/facial self-examination for early signs of cancers could be taught to a substantial number of people. Their results found that about half the people shown oral self-examinations continued these examinations at regular intervals. Several authors point out that oral self-examination techniques need to be popularized in the same manner that breast self-examination techniques have been.[70,196] Individuals chronically exposed to the sun should be adivsed to wear headgear that will reduce this exposure and to use sunscreening agents on their face and lips.

Since alcoholics who smoke constitute the largest risk group for oral cancers, screening programs should be geared to this population. Several researchers [127] have proved the feasibility of conducting oral screening programs for alcoholics. Any screening programs would have to be conducted in settings where alcoholics could be approached as a group such as reform organizations, Salvation Army facilities for alcoholics, or alcoholic rehabilitation units. While primary prevention by limiting alcohol intake and cessation of smoking is a more desirable goal, many alcoholics cannot be reached by these types of programs. Thus, the more realistic approach with alcoholics is to encourage periodic oral examinations so that cancer can be detected in the early stages.

The majority of oral cancers cause no symptoms in their early stages. An observant client may first notice a white or bright red spot, "sore," or a swelling in his mouth that he frequently attributes to his teeth or dentures, and this leads him to consult a dentist. The most common oral carcinoma is of the lip, particularly the lower lip, with carcinoma of the tongue the second most frequent form of oral cancer. Over 90% of malignant tumors of the oral cavity are squamous cell carcinomas.[59,174] Fig. 10-8 illustrates leukoplakia that appears as a white patch or plaque. Leukoplakia can be keratotic or nonkeratotic. When a white oral lesion is found, the area should be rubbed to see if it can be removed. White lesions that adhere to the surface are classified as keratotic and have a greater probability of malignancy.[130] Erythroplakia, also considered premalignant, is a red plaque or well-defined red patches that have a velvety consistency and often have tiny areas of ulceration.[13] A high index of suspicion should accompany the finding of any oral masses, erythema, whitening, swelling, ulceration, abnormal textures (roughness, induration), limitations of motion (primarily of the tongue), areas of tenderness, or areas that tend to bleed easily.

Physical examination of the mouth includes inspection, digital palpation, and olfaction of the oral cavity. Maneuvers frequently omitted during the oral examination are detailed below.

1. Have the client extend the tongue and move it from side to side. Limitation of normal movement could indicate that a tumor is interfering with muscle action.[23]

2. Palpate the tongue with a gloved hand or finger cot. Palpation may reveal a lesion not visible. Palpation of a hard lesion should be referred for biopsy to establish the diagnosis.[73]

3. Inspect the anterior two thirds of the tongue by grasping the tip of the tongue with a piece of gauze and gently pulling the tongue forward and to each side. Lesions of the base of the tongue are most often overlooked and must be both inspected and palpated. The nurse should be aware that most tongue cancers appear on the lateral surfaces.[3,219]

4. Palpate the lips. In the earliest stages, a cancerous lesion may appear as a small swelling or induration that may be difficult to see but can be palpated. An area of roughness, induration, or granularity is often the best clue to the diagnosis of early carcinoma.

5. Olfaction of breath—an odor of sourness may indicate obstruction and fermentation, while fetid and foul odors may signal necrotic neoplasms indicative of advanced disease.[46] Client education and a dental referral may be necessary if the breath odors indicate advanced dental decay and poor oral hygiene.

6. Palpate the parotid, submandibular, and submental areas.

THYROID CANCER

Thyroid cancer is a relatively rare disease that predominately affects females and the young. It has received national attention because of the data linking irradiation of the head and neck in infancy and childhood to the development of thyroid cancer in adult life.[5,66,110,116]

Risk factors

From 1940 to 1959, it was considered good medical practice to give therapeutic doses of x-radiation and radium applications to the head, neck, or upper thorax to treat various nonmalignant conditions. These nonmalignant conditions included acne, enlargement of the thymus, and hypertrophy of the tonsils. It is now recognized that anyone with a history of such prior irradiation is at significantly increased risk of developing thyroid tumors 5 to 35 or more years after radiation.[75] Other identified risk factors for thyroid cancer are iodine deficiency as well as iodine excess.[19]

A nursing assessment of any client should include a health history to elicit known risk factors for thyroid cancer. If clients give a history of prior irradiation to the head or neck in infancy or childhood for anything other than diagnostic purposes, they should be informed of the findings linking this treatment to thyroid cancer and urged to see their physician. Since it is difficult to locate those people who have such histories, several communities have attempted to reach these individuals through public education programs.[75,146]

Nursing interventions

Nurses are urged to investigate the need for these types of programs in their community and to consider initiating some type of thyroid cancer alert program in their clinical setting (that is, public health agencies, health services in factories and hospitals, ambulatory care clinics, and retirement facilities). Very effective inexpensive educational programs could be conducted using posters, slide-tape presentations, and other types of multimedia programs that would help locate people with histories of childhood irradiation.

In addition to inquiring about childhood irradiation during the history, the nurse should ask if there is a history of persistent hoarseness, difficulty swallowing, or a mass in the neck of increasing size.[66] All these contribute to the suspicion that a thyroid carcinoma may be present.

The usual presentation of the thyroid tumor is as an accidentally discovered lump in the neck noted by the client, a friend, or the examiner. Tumors must reach a size of approximately 0.5 to 1 cm before they can be palpated.[55] The most common of the thyroid tumors is the adenoma, and it can typically be felt as a single lump in an otherwise normal gland. DeGroot[55] points out that the adenoma moves with the gland on deglutition but can be moved within the substance of the gland since it is not directly attached to the trachea.

Inspection and palpation of the thyroid and neck give the most information during physical examination. The normal thyroid is barely visible and usually only in the isthmic region. The examination must include observing the neck while the client swallows water. This maneuver will enable the nurse to identify the isthmus because the thyroid gland is fixed to the trachea and ascends during swallowing.[17,250] The thyroid examination must be thoroughly and skillfully executed to detect tumors. Because thyroid cancer spreads beyond the gland to neighboring lymph nodes, both cervical nodes and salivary glands should also be palpated with great care when examining the thyroid.[77]

Diagnosis of malignancies may be accomplished by radioisotope scans, needle biopsy, and surgical exploration.[55,66] Most malignant lesions are cold on scan, while as many as two thirds of cold lesions may be benign. Most nodules that are "hot" on a scan are not malignant.[63]

BREAST CANCER

Breast cancer is the most common cancer in women and the number one cancer killer in women at any age. In the United States, about 33,000 women die from this disease each year, which is about one woman every 15 minutes.[265] One of every six females develops this disease, and there has been no reduction of the mortality figures over the last 30 years.[192]

Risk factors

Breast cancer appears to be due to a constellation of risk factors rather than to a single one. Following is a list of the risk factors predominantly mentioned in the literature[135,187,208,234]:

- Women over 40 years of age
- Women whose mothers, sisters, or aunts have had breast cancer, especially premenopausal breast cancer
- Women with a history of breast cancer
- Women with a lump, localized pain, or nipple discharge
- Childless women or women with first parity after age 30
- Women with an adverse hormonal milieu,

hypothyroid clients, early menarche (before age 11), or late menopause

Women living in the Western hemisphere or a cold climate, belonging to the upper socioeconomic groups and of the white race

Women with other organ cancers, especially the endometrium

Genetic predisposition, carcinogen exposures, immunodeficiency, and adverse hormonal milieu are the most important of the known risk factors. Some authorities also include the following as risk factors: high dietary fat intake; the triad of obesity, diabetes, and hypertension; chronic psychologic stress; and precancerous mastopathy type of fibrocystic disease.[189,215]

It has been postulated that there are two main types of breast cancer associated with different age peaks and hormonal relationships. The first type occurs in the premenopausal woman with an age peak of 45 to 49, and the second type occurs in the postmenopausal woman with an age peak at 65.[134] Breast cancers develop chiefly in the menopausal and postmenopausal woman, increasing in incidence throughout the woman's life span and reaching the highest incidence peak in clients over 85 years of age. There is about one case of cancer of the male breast for every 100 cases in women. The age distribution is similar, with greater relative frequency among the elderly.

In the 1960's, mammography was introduced and a randomized study was set up in New York by the Health Insurance Plan of Greater New York (HIP) to test the independent value of mammography and physical examination. The data clearly indicated that about one third of the breast cancers were detected by mammography alone, one third by mammography and physical examination, and one third by physical examination alone. There was a mortality decrease in the screened population, but the improvement in mortality was clearly limited to women *over* 50.[192]

In 1973, the National Cancer Institute (NCI) and the American Cancer Society (ACS) set up the Breast Cancer Detection Demonstration Projects (BCDDP) throughout the United States. In these BCDDP, mammography was offered to women over the age of 35. Around 1976, published reports such as Bailar[12] and Breslow and associates[28] indicated that radiation in moderate doses might cause breast cancer if the radiation occurred in young women who were in the childbearing age. With no benefit over physical examinations for those under 50 and a risk estimated at six additional breast cancers per million women screened per rad of exposure per year, the BCDDP centers stopped submitting younger women to this hazard and issued new screening guidelines.

These new guidelines were that mammographic screening would be limited to women over 50 years of age unless the client had a personal or family history of breast cancer, and the informed-consent wording spelled out that there was a small but finite risk of radiation.[190]

There continues to be a great deal of controversy on the issue of mammography. Some authorities[67,209,213,233,234] feel that the present state of the art in mammography would indicate that the risk is minimal as contrasted with the natural incidence of breast cancer. They point out that the radiation dose used in mammography has been substantially decreased by newer techniques and that the tandem technique is necessary for proper yield. The tandem technique consists of clinical examination, mammography, and thermography. A new computer analysis of mammography's risk and benefits suggests that radiologists are reducing radiation doses to such low levels that it *may* be safe to start screening asymptomatic women for breast cancer at 45 or conceivably even at 35.[149] Strax[234] reports that the results of 162,876 examinations at the Guttman Breast Diagnostic Institute in New York City showed that 20% of the cancers were found by mammography alone, 22% by clinical examination alone, and 58% by both. In summary, those who advocate using mammography feel it is a valuable screening technique when used adjunctively with clinical examination (palpation and thermography). They urge that selection of candidates for mammography be based on all risk factors, *not just age*. The nub of the mammography controversy is the lack of statistical proof that mammography reduces mortality among women screened between the ages of 35 and 49, as it did for women over the age of 50 in the HIP study. Controlled clinical trials similar to the HIP study are being carried out in Sweden and may help resolve the breast cancer screening controversy.[149]

Other authorities[10,12,29] argue that under the age of 50, mammography screening is appropriate only for a very small percentage of women known to be at extremely high risk and that average or even moderately increased risks do not overcome the future hazards. They argue against the indiscriminate population-wide screening of women under the age of 50. Bailer writes that "for women below age 35 or those with symptoms of breast cancer at any age, mammography should be the last step before a decision on the need for surgical biopsy, and should be done then if, and only if, the mammographic findings will conclusively determine how or whether biopsy is to be performed."[11] In summary, these critics do not view mammography as a screening tool and urge that it not be used on any woman unless there is good medical reason to do so.

All authorities agree that at the present time, thermography finds its greatest use as an adjunct to mammography and physical examination. It is recommended that thermography not be used as the sole modality in any breast cancer screening program because of the relatively high false positive rate.[137]

While all authorities agree that clinical examination is an essential feature in screening for breast cancers, they have differing opinions on the percentage of cancers that can be detected by this method alone. Overall, most feel that physical examination alone can detect up to 60% of all breast cancers. Hall quotes a much higher percentage and states "approximately 94% of cancerous lesions are potentially palpable and are candidates for early manual detection."[97] Strax[234] limits the value of clinical examination to examination of small glandular breasts, large cancer masses, and premenopausal women.

Nursing interventions

The importance of self-breast examination (SBE) is based on the fact that approximately 95% of breast cancers are accidentally self-discovered. Since some 10% of cancers called interim cancers will become apparent within a year of a negative examination, reliance must be placed on SBE to find these lesions. The majority of American women do not practice monthly SBE. Research has shown that they don't practice SBE because of:

1. Fear and anxiety
2. Lack of specific knowledge about breast self-examination and confidence in how to do it
3. Ignorance of the importance of monthly breast self-examinations as a necessary supplement to physician examinations[120]

Many researchers, including the Gallup Poll,[71] found that personal instruction results in more frequent self-examination (SBE) than do films, pamphlets, or lectures.

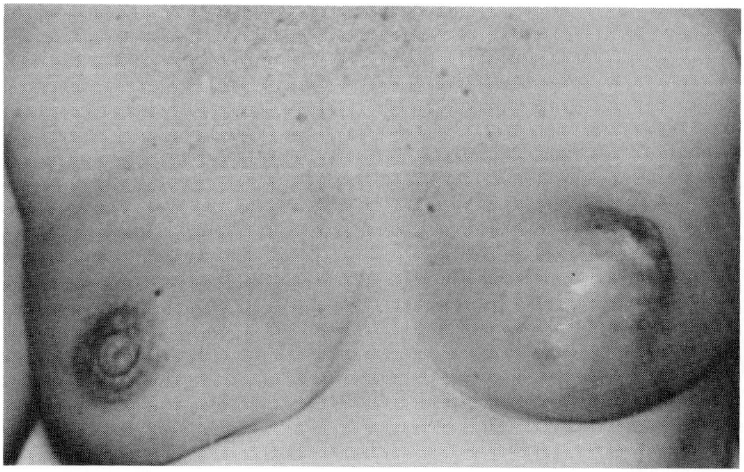

Fig. 10-9. Multiple malignant breast lesions. Note mass on right breast that causes areola and nipple to be eccentrically pointed. Left breast demonstrates inflammatory carcinoma. Note erythema and flattened nipple on left breast. (From Rosemond, G., and Maier, W.: Breast cancer, New York, 1974, Famous Teachings in Modern Medicine, Medcom, Inc.)

Self-instruction includes teaching a woman to do SBE by *using her own hand on her breast under the direct guidance of a professional*. This has been shown to be the single most effective method for ensuring long-term regular SBE. Since women can be taught to detect lesions of 1 cm or less in their own breasts, those who practice regular SBE will detect tumors within a size range that will maximize chances for survival and minimize chances for axillary node involvement.[78,94,97]

Because a high percentage of cancerous lesions are potentially palpable and are candidates for early manual detection, it is important for nurses to include personal instruction in SBE techniques whenever possible.[97] Research documents the effectiveness of personal instruction in self-examination techniques by registered nurses as part of a cancer education program through their place of employment.[90] Primary nursing as well as public health and occupational

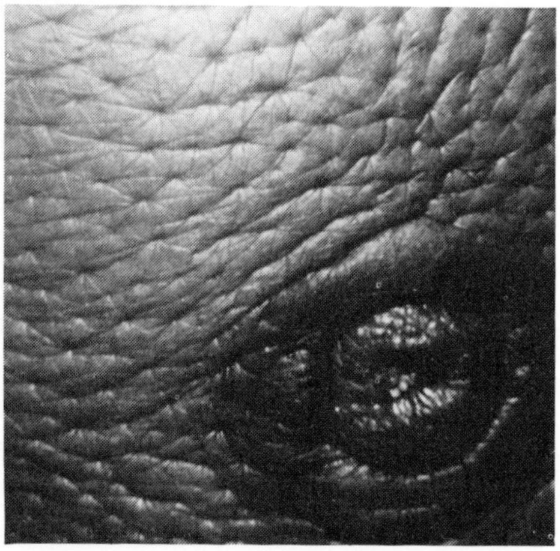

Fig. 10-10. Orange-peel skin (peau d'orange) is another physical sign of underlying malignancy. Skin changes are caused by lymphedema. Edema of skin is indicated when skin is indented deeply with holes that are accentuated orifices of sweat glands. (From Rosemond, G., and Maier, W.: Breast cancer, New York, 1974, Famous Teachings in Modern Medicine, Medcom, Inc.)

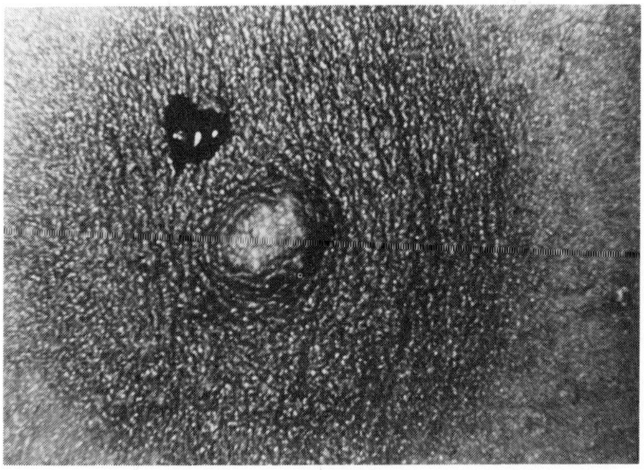

Fig. 10-11. Discharge from breast, demonstrating importance of stripping breasts for discharge during physical examination. This is bloody discharge from areola. (From Rosemond, G., and Maier, W.: Breast cancer, New York, 1974, Famous Teachings in Modern Medicine, Medcom, Inc.)

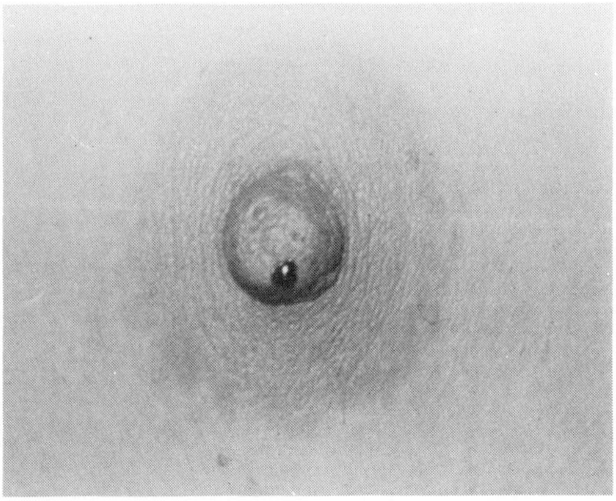

Fig. 10-12. Bloody discharge from single nipple duct. (From Rosemond, G., and Maier, W.: Breast cancer, New York, 1974, Famous Teachings in Modern Medicine, Medcom, Inc.)

health nursing afford the nurse excellent opportunities for SBE client education. To reinforce personal instruction in SBE there could be posters, multimedia such as slide-tape and films, and educational panels portraying the techniques of SBE. But these should reinforce *not* replace personal instruction.

The history should contain questions that will enable the nurse to identify known risk factors for breast cancer. This identification of risk factors is essential for effective client

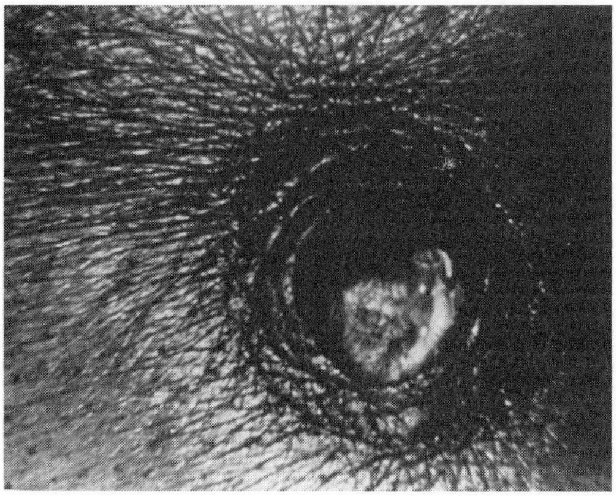

Fig. 10-13. Early Paget's disease. Note tiny vesicle on nipple of client. "Any persistent, unilateral, itchy, vesicular, eczematoid, or ulcerative nipple lesion that is not part of a generalized dermatologic condition should be viewed as Paget's carcinoma of the breast until proved otherwise." (From Rosemond, G., and Maier, W.: Breast cancer, New York, 1974, Famous Teachings in Modern Medicine, Medcom, Inc.)

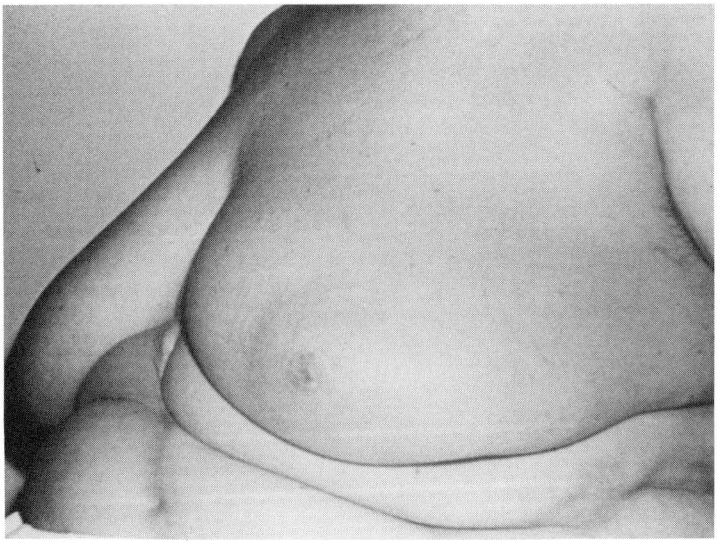

Fig. 10-14. Physical examination of breast with client sitting. No obvious abnormality is observed. (From Rosemond, G., and Maier, W.: Breast cancer, New York, 1974, Famous Teachings in Modern Medicine, Medcom, Inc.)

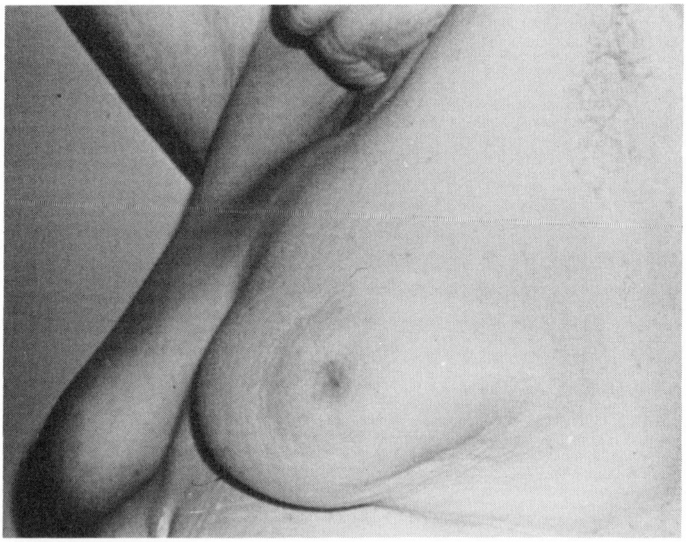

Fig. 10-15. Same client from Fig. 10-14 but demonstrating changes in breast that become obvious with raising of arms. Note skin retraction, which is clearly visible over area of mass. This emphasizes importance of inspecting breasts in all recommended positions. (From Rosemond, G., and Maier, W.: Breast cancer, New York, 1974, Famous Teachings in Modern Medicine, Medcom, Inc.)

education. The chief complaints of clients with breast lesions include lump or mass; pain; nipple symptoms such as discharge, retraction, elevation, and eczema; and skin symptoms such as dimpling, redness, edema, and ulceration. The *most common* presenting complaint of women with breast cancer is a lump or mass in the breast that was detected by the woman through accidental or planned self-examination. Nipple discharge ranks second to a lump as a chief complaint.

Physical examination includes inspection of the breast with the woman lying, sitting with her arms at the side, sitting with her arms elevated, sitting with pectoral contraction, and sitting bending forward. Palpation includes superficial palpation for tissue thickening and palpation for lesions. Palpation for lesions uses a rotary or transverse linear motion of the hands. The breasts are most effectively palpated when the woman is in the supine position, but it is recommended that the following women also be examined in the sitting position: women with present or past complaints of breast masses, women at high risk of breast cancer, and women with pendulous breasts. Cancer usually presents as a solitary, unilateral, solid, hard, irregular, poorly delineated, nonmobile, painless, and nontender lump, most often in the upper outer quadrant of the breast. Figs. 10-9 through 10-15 demonstrate visible examples of breast pathology.

LUNG CANCER

Risk factors

Lung cancer is a common neoplastic disease confronting nurses in both hospital and community settings. There are nearly 91,000 new cases each year in the United States and approximately 80% of these clients are dead

Table 10-3. Risk factors for lung cancer[99,102,103,159,217,222]

Type of exposure	Carcinogenic agent	Individuals affected
Personal	Tobacco and tobacco smoke	People who smoke and people with a family history of lung cancer
Occupational or environmental	Products of coal combustion	Coke oven workers exposed to coke—even gas
	Radon daughters	Uranium workers/miners exposed to radon daughters
	Bis (chloromethyl) ether	Chemical workers
	Asbestos	Asbestos workers in direct mining and manufacturing, construction, insulation, brake lining, shipyards, roofing, installation of asbestos products such as pipes
	Inorganic arsenic	Workers exposed to arsenic compounds—tanners, vintners
	Hexavalent chromate	Chromate manufacturers
	Nickel	Nickel–copper matte refinery workers
	Petroleum	Workers exposed to petroleum mists such as paraffin pressors, lathe workers, and drillers
	Isopropyl oil	Isopropyl alcohol manufacturers
	Iron oxide	Iron ore (hematite workers) and iron foundry workers

in 2 years.[159,180] The incidence of lung cancer has more than doubled for both men and women over the last 25 years. A variety of agents either have been proved to be or are suspected of being respiratory carcinogens in man. Authorities hypothesize that the *most* important environmental carcinogen related to the increased incidence of lung carcinoma is cigarette smoking. The likelihood of developing lung cancer is related to both the amount of smoking and the length of exposure. There are also reports of increased incidence of lung cancers in the occupations shown in Table 10-3. A remarkable synergism between asbestos and cigarette smoking has been found. Asbestos workers who smoke cigarettes have an *eightfold* increased risk of dying of bronchogenic carcinoma as compared with cigarette smokers who do not work with asbestos. They have *92* times the risk of those who neither smoke cigarettes nor are exposed to asbestos.[6,99,216] A similar synergistic relationship has been found between tobacco smoke and exposure to radon daughters in causing bronchogenic carcinoma, especially oat cell carcinoma.[268]

Nursing interventions

When obtaining a health history, it is important to inquire into smoking habits, occupational history, and the general respiratory environment in both the workplace and home. People who are at high risk for lung cancer are those exposed to high levels of respiratory carcinogens in their workplaces, in their general environment, and in their personal environments as affected by such habits as tobacco smoking. The Department of Health and Human Services (formerly DHEW) recommends taking a detailed, lifetime occupational history for nurses who are interviewing an individual who worked in shipyards or believes they were otherwise exposed to asbestos. A detailed, lifetime history must be taken on these people. This is time consuming, but it is important because significant exposures may have been as brief as 1 month and may have occurred many years ago, even during World War II. Because the World War II work force was comprised of many women as well as men, the potential for female client involvement should not be overlooked.[201] If the nurse suspects exposure to other known carcinogenic respiratory agents such as those listed in Table 10-3, the same type of detailed, lifetime occupational history should be obtained.[102,103,161,201]

An occupational history includes dates of employment, average hours worked per week, exposure to potential hazards in the workplace, and personal protective equipment worn on the job. Some examples of potential occupational hazards are as follows:

- Physical—noise, vibration, temperature extremes
- Chemical—mercury, lead, gases, acids, solvents
- Biologic—viruses, fungi, parasites, bacteria
- Psychologic—fatigue, risk of falling or being burned, boredom, rotation of shifts[183]

Since research documents the atmospheric pollutants caused by smoking and the adverse effects of these pollutants on nonsmokers in the same areas, it is important to ascertain if there are individuals in either the client's workplace or home who smoke.[82,181,194,248]

Clients with lung cancer usually report a sign or symptom or show an abnormality on chest x-ray examination. The most frequently reported symptoms are a cough that is productive and often associated with hemoptysis or chest pain. The irritative cough may occur at night accompanied by mucoid expectoration.[59] Other symptoms frequently reported are thoracic pain, respiratory infection, dyspnea, hemoptysis, and loss of weight.[217,266] The four main histologic types of lung cancer—squamous cell or epidermoid, adenocarcinoma, small cell or oat cell, and large cell—have slightly different patterns of spread and clinical courses.[24] In most clients, the first symptoms are local rather than extrapulmonary.[153]

The nurse must have a high index of suspicion in anyone with a history of smoking or occupational exposure to carcinogenic agents who complains of pneumonitis that persists longer than 2 weeks despite antibiotic therapy. Unfortunately, the first symptoms of lung cancer are usually not alarming and may be considered lightly by health professionals. One of the earliest physical findings the nurse may encounter on auscultation of the chest of a client with lung cancer is a unilateral wheeze.

Current prospective studies of asymptomatic persons who have been screened for lung cancer by chest roentgenograms and sputum cytologic examination do not at present show any evidence of a notable reduction in mortality from the disease.[83,154] Boucot and associates[22] at the Medical College of Pennsylvania screened 6,136 asymptomatic men over 45 years of age with chest x-ray examinations every 6 months for 10 years. Cancer was discovered in 121 and they received immediate treatment. Only eight survived 5 years, which was the very same survival rate as when lung cancer is detected in people *with* symptoms.[22] Present recommendations from the National Institutes of Health are that until the value of screening for lung cancer by chest x-ray examination and sputum cytologic examination has been demonstrated, mass screen-

Table 10-4. Resources available to nurses interested in assisting clients in smoking cessation

Smoking cessation groups	"I Quit Clinics" conducted by local American Cancer Societies Smoke Enders—a national commercial organization, 3436 Camino del Rio South, Suite 216, San Diego, California 92108
Other smoking cessation approaches[34,40]	Hypnosis Behavior modification Cold turkey Individual counseling Commercial filters that increasingly decrease the tar/nicotine content Tapering off/gradual withdrawal
Client education material sources	American Heart Association, 7320 Greenville Ave., Dallas, Texas 75231; client education pamphlets such as: "How to Stop Smoking" and "Cigarette Quiz" American Cancer Society—contact local units; numerous, varied client education material; excellent examples are: "The Dangers of Smoking—the Benefits of Quitting" and "If You Want to Give Up Cigarettes." American Lung Association, 1740 Broadway, New York, New York 10019 or local unit; many booklets available such as: "Hey Look—A Smoking Puzzle" and "Women are Kicking the Cigarette Habit." American Health Foundation, 320 East 43rd Street, New York, New York 10017; antismoking material including the pamphlet: "Something New About Smoking . . ." U.S. Department of Health and Human Services, Public Health Service, Center for Disease Control, National Clearinghouse for Smoking and Health, Atlanta, Georgia 30333; client education material including: "Smokers' Self-Testing Kit" and "Facts: Smoking and Health." They have fact sheets that list the "Tar and Nicotine Content of Cigarettes" as determined by the Federal Trade Commission.
Antismoking organizations	Groups Against Smokers' Pollution (G.A.S.P.), P.O. Box 632, College Park, Maryland 20740 A.S.H.—Action on Smoking and Health, 2000 H Street N.W., Washington, D.C. 20006 National Organization of Nonsmokers, 332 South Michigan Ave., Suite 106, Chicago, Illinois 60604 National Interagency Council on Smoking and Health, 419 Park Avenue South, Room 1301, New York, New York 10016 Nonsmokers' Travel Club, 8928 Bradmoor Drive, Bethesda, Maryland 20034
Professional material on smoking	Office on Smoking and Health, Park Building, Suite I-58, 12420 Parklawn Drive, Rockville, Maryland 20857; excellent publications for professionals dealing with all issues of smoking. Examples are: *Health Consequences of Smoking; Bibliography on Smoking and Health; Directory of Ongoing Research in Smoking and Health.* Also antismoking material available for the public World Smoking and Health, American Cancer Society, 777 Third Ave., New York, New York 10017; journal (published 2 to 3 times a year) devoted to all the issues involved in smoking—physical, emotional, economic, and political. Cigarette Cancer Committee, Roswell Park Memorial Institute, 666 Elm Street, Buffalo, New York 14263; "Curriculum on Smoking and Health" for elementary school educators and school nurses; excellent guide for schools instituting antismoking curriculums

ing programs should be limited to well-designed, controlled clinical trials.[212] These clinical trials should have provisions for analysis of results and further diagnostic workup and treatment when indicated.[83]

All authorities agree that the greatest reduction in mortality can be achieved by cessation of cigarette smoking, with additional important benefits from reduction of exposure to other respiratory carcinogens such as those found either occupationally or in the environment.[83,152] One of the nurse's most important roles in helping people to stop smoking is to serve as a role model. Nurses who themselves smoke are a contradiction to all media coverage and scientific research pointing out the physical harm this habit does to the body. Nurses cannot persuade their clients to stop smoking if they themselves have not.[87]

It is the nurse's responsibility to actively and assertively disseminate information on the disease potential of smoking whenever possible. Individuals employed in high-risk occupations should also be informed of the synergistic relationship between smoking and occupations related to asbestos and radiation exposure. Every assistance should be afforded to help those individuals who want to stop smoking. Research documents that fear tactics, nagging, preaching, and threats are not effective in convincing people to stop smoking.[262] Because fear tactics have proved to be ineffective in changing smoking behaviors, there are now serious efforts being made to create a social climate wherein smoking is not an acceptable behavior. This approach reflects the concept of smoking as a social disease.[175] The American Cancer Society's "Smoking Stinks" campaign reflects this new trend.

The most rational approach for nurses to take would be: (1) to conduct educational programs that unemotionally detail the known hazards of smoking, (2) to provide clients with educational material that further explains the health hazards of smoking or high-risk occupations, and (3) to provide specific measures for those people who do desire to stop smoking or decrease occupational risk factors. It is extremely important for the nurse to supply information on the "how to's" of smoking cessation. Many people think seriously about stopping smoking but lack the information to help themselves stop. Table 10-4 shows the groups and approaches that are available for those who desire to stop smoking. Nurses should be familiar with the antismoking resources in their communities so that appropriate referrals may be made.

A three-pronged approach is now being recommended to decrease the number of people who smoke in this country: (1) youth antismoking programs to prevent the acquisition of the smoking habit, (2) smoking-cessation programs to help current smokers quit, and (3) a less harmful cigarette for those who cannot or will not quit smoking.

A nonjudgmental approach should be taken with those individuals who refuse to stop smoking or are unable. If appropriate, they should be urged to smoke cigarettes with tar yields of less than 10 mg, to smoke filtered cigarettes, and to smoke only half of each cigarette. When recommending the above for the individual who prefers to continue smoking, make it clear that switching brands merely *reduces* the hazard at best and may not even do that for smokers who unconsciously increase the number of cigarettes smoked and alter their puffing pattern to get more nicotine and, consequently, more tar and carbon monoxide from each of them.[228]

PROSTATE CANCER

Risk factors

Prostate cancer is second only to lung cancer as the leading site of malignant neoplasm for men.[80] Little, other than sex and age, is known about risk factors predisposing to prostate carcinoma. No infectious etiologic agent has been found after exhaustive research. Incidence is unrelated to socioeconomic class, but race is a risk factor with a very high incidence in blacks. The incidence among blacks is now almost double that in whites.[244] Prostate cancer is also higher in urban areas than rural areas for unknown reasons, although some authors hypothesize that air pollution may account for the difference in rates. Benign prostatic hypertrophy and prostatitis are not thought to have malignant potential.[128] Incidence varies with advancing age.[170] Autopsy data show microscopic lesions in 15% to 20% of men in their 40's and in 60% of men in their 70's. Only one sixth of those studied had clinically apparent disease; a full five sixths of these autopsies revealed prostatic carcinoma as an *incidental* finding unrelated to the cause of death.[128,199]

There are no real symptoms of most cases of early, probably curable, disease. It may be wise in an elderly client with a strong family history of prostatic carcinoma to have rectal examinations twice yearly, although this disease is not known to be genetically transmitted.[84] Most symptoms are related to late complications of stage C or D disease.[169] Inquiries should be made about nonspecific symptoms such as hesitancy, frequency, dysuria, hematuria, weakness of stream, dribbling after voiding, or anuria. One cause of these symptoms is carcinomatous obstruction of the prostatic urethra, but benign prostatic hypertrophy is much more common. Pelvic invasion may lead to vague symptoms of low back pain, sometimes mimicking sciatica, when the seminal vesicles are involved by tumor extension. Bone metastasis may cause bone pain, often in the lumbosacral area, but it may occur anywhere in the skeleton. Of course, far-advanced disease may be associated with the constitutional symptoms of pain, cachexia, weight loss, and anorexia.[258]

Nursing interventions

When obtaining the health history, the nurse should phrase the questions in a manner that will ensure understanding on the part of the client. Shortridge and MacLain suggest:

> . . . rather than asking "Do you have any hesitancy?" ask instead a more specific symptoms-oriented question such as "Do you have to wait for your stream to begin?" or "Does your stream stop while you still have the urge to void?" Such phrasing is more apt to uncover subtle symptoms of obstruction otherwise overlooked.[223]

By far the most important and useful screening for prostatic carcinoma is the digital rectal examination. A stony hard prostate, nodular prostate, or an indurated prostate should be considered to harbor cancer until proved otherwise by invasive diagnostic techniques. Serum acid phosphatase determinations are most helpful in discovering advanced disease, being elevated when spread beyond the prostatic capsule has already occurred.[171] Radioimmunoassay (RIA) is a newly developed, still expensive test that may prove to help detect early disease. Counter-immunoelectrophoresis determinations of prostatic acid phosphatase are currently being studied in a nationwide protocol for a less expensive method of detecting early intracapsular carcinoma.[177,242]

In the detection of early prostate cancer, one of the most important roles the nurse can assume is that of client educator. All male clients over the age of 40 should be informed of the importance and rationale for yearly or biannual rectal examinations. Those individuals with strong family histories of pros-

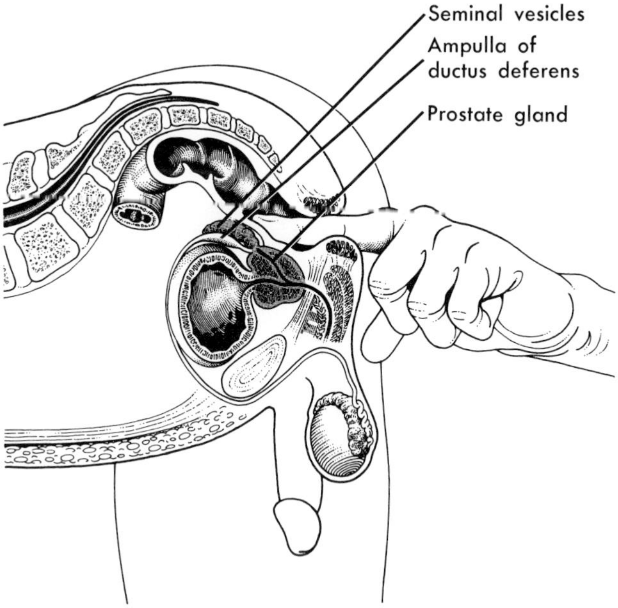

Fig. 10-16. Palpation of prostate. Note that only posterior surface of prostate is palpable through anterior wall of rectum. Normal prostate has symmetric, smooth, firm, rubbery consistency. (Redrawn from Malasanos, L., Barkauskas, V., Moss, M., and Stoltenberg-Allen, K.: Health assessment, St. Louis, 1977, The C. V. Mosby Co., p. 273.)

tate cancer should be urged to request and expect rectal examinations at their annual physical. It is important to stress to these high-risk clients that early detection can result in cure and that rectal examination is the most effective means of detecting early prostate cancer.[88]

No physical examination of the male is complete without including a rectal examination. It is recommended that every male over the age of 40 have a yearly examination, and if there is a positive family history of prostate cancer, they should be examined at more frequent intervals. Nurses conducting physical examinations who omit the rectal assessment because of their embarrassment or discomfort are to be severely criticized. If nurses are unable to rectally examine the male client either because of their discomfort or the client's, it is essential that they request a male physician or nurse practitioner to complete this portion of the examination rather than omitting it. Fig. 10-16 illustrates palpation of the prostate gland.

When examining the prostate gland, the nurse should first palpate the medial sulcus and then proceed to palpate each lateral lobe. While palpating the prostate, note the following: surface, consistency, shape, size, sensitivity, and movability.[148] The earliest palpable change is conventionally considered to be a discrete nodule of firm or stony consistency.[193] Remember that describing the sequence and content of the entire rectal examination prior to beginning will eliminate any surprises and gains the client's cooperation.[223]

COLORECTAL CANCER

Risk factors

The estimated incidence of cancer in the United States shows that colon and rectal cancer has a higher incidence in the total population than any other cancer except skin cancer.[224] Much conjecture is currently being raised about potential risk factors for colorectal carcinoma. Certain disorders and diseases of the colon and rectum are definitely associated with an increased risk of carcinoma. Familial colonic polyposis (autosomal dominant) and Gardner's syndrome (colonic adenomatous polyps with benign tumors such as lipomas, fibromas, and osteomas elsewhere) show malignant degeneration 100% of the time.[81] The presence of villous adenomas is associated with a 40% to 60% malignant degeneration, and some experts feel the very common adenomatous polyp is a premalignant lesion.

There is some controversy as to the premalignant nature of the benign adenomatous polyps; however, it is still recommended that they be removed.[56,198] Ulcerative colitis also places the client at higher risk for colorectal cancer. Factors that further increase the risk for colorectal carcinoma developing in ulcerative colitis clients are: (1) total colonic involvement or pancolitis, (2) family history of colon cancer, and (3) duration of colitis disease greater than 10 years. Clients who have had ulcerative colitis before the age of 15 show a 20% incidence of colon cancer after 20 years of disease.[2] Fraumeni and Mulvihill[81] write that all these known risk factors account for about 6% to 10% of colorectal cancers and argue that judicious screening programs aimed at these high-risk groups could reduce colorectal *mortality* about 6% to 10%.

Much has been written about the type of diet and the incidence of colon carcinoma.[30,139] It is known that highly industrialized countries have a higher incidence of colorectal cancer than the developing nations of the world such as Africa and Asia. Compared to diets in Africa and Asia, the Western world diet is higher in fat, lower in fiber, and colon cultures show higher counts of bacteroides.[50,56] Low fiber content decreases fecal transit time in the bowel and some investigators feel this may allow ingested carcinogens to maintain prolonged contact with the bowel mucosa.[263,264] At the present time there are no good studies to prove or disprove these theories, and the whole subject remains investigational and controversial.

Cancers of the colon and rectum can be conveniently divided into those affecting the right side, or the cecum and ascending colon, and those affecting the left side. By far, the most common location of disease is in the descending colon, rectosigmoid, and rectum, accounting for 75% of all colorectal cancers. The cecum and ascending colon harbor 15%, and the transverse colon contains 10%. Cancers of the right side are most often clinically silent owing to the nature of the typical polypoid lesion, the caliber of the lumen, and the loose consistency of the fecal stream. Left-sided lesions are often circumferential and produce obstruction to the movement of more solid fecal material.[133] Certain clues to the diagnosis should be looked for when interviewing clients:

1. Has there been a *recent change in bowel habits?* Is there a feeling of incomplete evacuation or tenesmus? Has there been any change in the size or caliber of stool? Many victims of this disease complain of alternating constipation and diarrhea, a symptom frequently associated with the common irritable colon syndrome. Even a change in

the frequency of bowel movements or the time of evacuation may be a subtle clue to the diagnosis.[157]

2. *Abdominal pain* is a presenting complaint of 50% to 75% of all clients and is most common with lesions proximal to the sigmoid colon.[56] Symptoms of pain usually relate to partial obstruction and may be intermittent, relieved by passing a stool. An occasional client is acutely ill with peritonitis secondary to perforation or total colonic obstruction.

3. *Anemia and bleeding*[145] are important clues. Does the client have symptoms of fatigue, shortness of breath, weakness, or cardiac symptoms consistent with anemia. Anemia is most common with right-sided lesions and is usually occult in nature. Anemia usually occurs when blood loss exceeds the ability of the marrow to replace lost red cells, so a normal hemoglobin does not rule out blood loss in the gastrointestinal tract. Only 25% of clients with right-sided lesions will notice blood in the stool, but up to 70% of left-sided lesions will cause noticeable blood in the stool at some time. With this knowledge, it is important *not* to attribute blood in the stool simply to hemorrhoids or anal fissures without a complete examination. Many clients notice bleeding only during constipation and it disappears with the use of laxatives. Thus they attribute the bleeding to constipation or to the presence of hemorrhoids.[56] The two most common symptoms of anal cancer are anal bleeding and pain.

4. *Anorexia, weight loss, and malaise* are nonspecific clues to a chronic illness, sometimes carcinoma, and the client should be queried about the presence of these symptoms.

The two most important *screening* tests in asymptomatic clients are examination of the feces for occult blood and the digital rectal examination.[100] When duplicate samples are taken from different parts of the feces each day for three successive days while on a higher fiber, meat-free diet, the guaiac test is highly accurate in detecting occult blood in the stool.[257] A positive test only means there is bleeding in the gastrointestinal tract and that could be anywhere from the mouth to the anus. False positive results should only occur 1% of the time in a well-performed test, and false negative results are very rare. The American Cancer Society currently has an active community screening program utilizing the guaiac test as an inexpensive "do-it-yourself" home test.[190] The *routine* testing of clients, especially those over the age of 40 years, with the guaiac-impregnated or Hemoccult slide test at present provides the *best method* for detecting colorectal carcinoma at an early stage.[76] The Hemoccult slide test has all the qualities of an ideal cancer-screening procedure; it is simple, inexpensive, aesthetically satisfactory, and false negative results are rare. Table 10-5 lists recommended screening procedures for various population groups.

It has long been taught in physical assessment courses that no physical examination is complete without rectal examination. Approximately 50% of all rectal cancers are within reach of the examining finger. The client should be examined in the supine position with the legs drawn up to allow palpation of high rectal lesions. A ridge above the prostate or in the rectovaginal pouch is called a Blumer's shelf and represents metastases to the peritoneal floor. Females should have a thorough pelvic examination to rule out involvement of the uterus, ovaries, and vagina.

Rigid proctosigmoidoscopy is recommended for any client suspected of having cancer, and some experts recommend yearly proctoscopic examinations as part of

Table 10-5. Recommended screening intervals and procedures for colorectal cancer

Population group	Risk factors	Recommendations
Asymptomatic people under 50 years of age[48]		Yearly Hemoccult slide testing; if positive, then sigmoidoscopy and digital rectal examination
Asymptomatic people over 50 years of age[48,163,164]		Stool testing for occult blood supplemented by proctosigmoidoscopy after 50 years of age; proctoscopy every 2 years thereafter
Asymptomatic clients with significant family histories[257]	Positive family histories of colon cancer Relatives of clients with polyposis syndromes or juvenile polyps Positive family histories of multiple carcinomas	Periodic screening beginning at age 20 that includes sigmoidoscopy and Hemoccult slide testing
Individuals with previous colon polyps or previous colon cancers		Hemoccult slide testing and sigmoidoscopy annually; highest risk for a new colon cancer within 5 years of the index cancer
Individuals with underlying premalignant disease of the colon[257]	Ulcerative colitis, granulomatous colitis, genetically acquired polyposis syndromes	Sigmoidoscopy with rectocolonic cytologic lavage every 6 months; colonoscopy with cytologic lavage once a year
Symptomatic clients		X-ray endoscopy

an annual physical examination for all persons over 40 years of age. (Others feel it should be done after the age of 50.)[48] The 25 cm rigid proctoscope should put 60% of colon cancers within reach. Proctosigmoidoscopy is not feasible for large-scale screening because it is expensive, time consuming, and clients are hesitant about having this procedure done. The 55 cm fiberoptic flexible sigmoidoscope and longer colonoscopes can put the entire colon under direct vision. While fiberoptic colonoscopy is the most accurate method for detection of early colonic neoplasms, it is expensive, time consuming, inconvenient, and more hazardous to the client than other modalities. Thus it is reserved for screening certain known high-risk groups such as clients with a history of colon cancer or long-standing ulcerative colitis. Any client undergoing a proctoscopic examination because of irregularities suggesting bowel cancer usually has, in addition, a barium enema x-ray examination of the colon.

Carcinoembryonic antigen (CEA), once hoped to prove itself as a tumor-specific antigen, is not specific for colorectal cancer.[269] A normal level does not rule out colon cancer and elevated levels have been found in cancer of the pancreas plus nonmalignant diseases of the colon, lung, and liver. Since it is so nonspecific, it is not considered a good screening test for colorectal cancer.

Nursing interventions

In colorectal cancer detection, nurses have a variety of roles. Not only are they practitioners, but they are also educators, coordinators, counselors, and researchers. As *educators,* nurses can play an important role in colorectal cancer detection by: (1) informing the public about colon and rectum cancer and (2) encouraging the public's participation in early detection of the disease through the use of a Hemoccult test. Research documents the most effective public education approach to "the cancer nobody talks about" is that public information and educational materials should emphasize the effectiveness of the test and the fact that it can be administered in the privacy of one's home and communicate that the test is convenient and painless and that the results are confidential between the individual and the physician or the screening agent.[33] Nurses working in community organizations, clinics, factories, nursing homes, retirement centers, geriatric day-care centers, and schools are in ideal settings to provide client education and plan and participate in colorectal screening programs. These screening programs could be conducted by community organizations such as the American Cancer Society, local service groups, or community religious groups, with the nurse *coordinating* the efforts.[89,229,255] If the nurse finds that the organizational resources or personnel are limited for community screening programs, efforts should be geared to *first* screen those individuals who are known to be at higher risk for this type of cancer such as people over 40 or people with a positive family history. Colorectal screening programs, using Hemoccult slide tests, do not have to be elaborate to be effective. Richardson[200] documents that a successful colorectal screening program can be achieved without digital rectal examinations, using nonmedical personnel to primarily conduct the program, and with minimal involvement of physicians.

As a counselor, the nurse provides information and support for clients who are at high risk for developing this type of cancer. It is important to emphasize the benefits of periodic examinations, since many high-risk individuals are anxiety ridden about developing colorectal cancer. Providing specific information about available detection procedures, recommended screening techniques, and available community programs for early detection may help alleviate some of their anxiety. Taking the time to listen and answer questions about colorectal cancer may be all that is needed.

In the researcher role, it is extremely important that nurses be knowledgeable about the risk factors for colorectal cancer. Since there is a great deal of speculation about the role of diet in causing this type of cancer, future research reports may establish definitive relationships.[16,221] Nurses should also be knowledgeable enough to be able to evaluate research findings. Those reports that are based on sound, ethical research principles may be judged appropriate for inclusion in client education. Nurses could also plan or participate in a wide range of research projects related to colorectal cancer such as health behaviors, dietary habits, motives that facilitate early detection, and effective educational approaches for changing dietary patterns. Results would certainly benefit existing nursing practice as it relates to the early detection of colorectal cancer.

BLADDER CANCER
Risk factors

Most authorities agree with Whitmore's hypothesis that bladder cancer is "a disease with multiple etiologies, acting either alone or in concert, and including physical, chemical and possibly viral carcinogens, which may vary in etiologic role from place to place or even in the same place at different times."[254] Urban incidence rates for bladder cancer are higher than those in rural areas.[225] This is probably due to industrialization and the presence of many carcinogens. Bladder tumors occur frequently in chemical, rubber, and cable workers and in individuals who are exposed to antioxidants, solvents, or other carcinogens.[32] Caldwell[32] writes that the exposure may be from either skin contact or from the vapor and that the risk is related to degree of exposure to these agents.

In 1895, Rehn first made his observations among aniline dye workers. Rehn felt the men employed in the dyestuffs industry were at increased risk of developing bladder tumors. This fact has now been established, although Rehn's opinion that aniline was the cause has been shown to be incorrect: "Recent studies indicate that aniline itself probably is not carcinogenic, but confirm that intermediate agents used in the manufacture of fuchsin, as well as auramine, undoubtedly are."[32] The following industrial compounds have been identified as bladder carcinogens for humans: beta-naphthylamine, benzidine, chlornaphazine, 4-aminobiphenyl or zenylamine, 4-nitrobiphenyl, and auramine.[44,74,108] The use and manufacture of β-naphthylamine was abandoned in the late 1940's by the British rubber industry, but there is a lengthy latent period, as much as 18 years, before bladder tumors develop.[245]

In summary, those in occupations that involve coal products and aromatic amines have an increased risk of developing bladder cancer. These high-risk occupations include asphalt, coal tar, and pitch workers; gas stokers; still cleaners; dyestuffs users; rubber workers; textile dyers; paint manufacturers; and leather and shoe workers.[43]

Research has shown an association between cigarette smoking and an increased risk of bladder cancer.[39,42] Hammond[98] writes that smoking multiplies the risk of bladder cancer, particularly among men under the age of 65. An association has also been reported between urinary bilharziasis, or schistosomiasis, and bladder cancer. Although the association between bladder cancer and schistosome infection is not conclusively established, "the presence of chronic bacterial cystitis, complicated by urethral strictures, calculi, diverticulae and paralytic stasis has been known to induce epithelial changes in the bladder mucosa, which may progress to invasive cancer."[72] Schistosomiasis is a parasitic disease still prevalent in some parts of the world, such as Africa, Asia, and South America.[239]

A great deal of controversy surrounds the association of bladder cancer and coffee drinking and the use of drinks with artificial sweeteners.[15,19,125,261] There has been no evidence to date to conclusively support or refute the claim that these substances increase the user's risk of developing bladder cancer. Full evaluation of the association between bladder cancer and artificial sweeteners and coffee drinking is still forthcoming. It is important for the nurse to remember that only *one* type of exposure has been so strongly and consistently linked with human bladder cancer as to be generally accepted as a cause of the disease; this cause is exposure to aromatic amines and coal tar products. Although smoking, high sodium saccharin use, and coffee drinking have been linked with bladder cancer, they have not been established as a cause of the disease.

Nursing interventions

When obtaining the health history from a client with urinary complaints, the nurse should elicit a detailed occupational history.[126] Exposure to specific known carcinogenic agents as well as involvement in high-risk occupations and concomitant urinary symptoms should raise the suspicion of bladder cancer. The nurse can use the health assessment and occupational history interview as an opportunity for client teaching. It provides the individual being interviewed with an opportunity to identify his or her own sources of risk. Oleske points out that clients may be unaware of the oncogenic potential associated with certain occupations and personal habits, despite the increased dissemination of cancer prevention information in the mass media.[185] The occupational history includes chronologic history of jobs, exposure to carcinogens, and type of carcinogen transmission such as fumes or contact.[183]

The most common presenting symptom in clients with bladder cancer is gross, painless hematuria. *Any* episode of hematuria requires investigation. Hematuria is characteristically intermittent and often a factor in delay in establishing the diagnosis.[64] Other early symptoms may be an increase in frequency, urgency, and dysuria.[9,254] Pain, loss of weight, and back pain are late symptoms of bladder cancer. Whitmore[254] stresses that there are no *early* physical signs of bladder cancer.

Physical assessment of a client with urinary complaints should include palpation of peripheral lymph nodes, a thorough abdominal examination, a bimanual examination of the female, and a rectal examination. Physical examination may yield evidence of metastatic disease either in peripheral lymph nodes, the liver, or the bones. A pelvic mass may be palpable through the abdominal wall or on bimanual examination of the female. Definitive diagnosis usually rests on cystoscopic examination. Jewett[118] points out that sometimes the final diagnosis will depend on the microscopic examination of a biopsy or on a cytologic smear.

Parkes recommends that any cytodiagnostic screening program for bladder cancer meet the following criteria: "1) Significant exposure to known or strongly suspected carcinogens should be firmly established before any screening program is considered. 2) There should be available clear epidemiological evidence of an enhanced risk of cancer resulting from such exposure. 3) It should be demonstrable that the diagnostic techniques to be applied will have a high degree of efficiency."[188] Thus any bladder screening program should be geared to a population clearly identified as high risk.[44] Parkes describes a bladder cancer screening program in Great Britain that screens workers in British rubber and chemical industries. He recommends screening workers not less frequently than three times a year. This frequency is desirable in view of the possibility that occasional false negative results may be obtained on the basis of a single test.[258] Out of 20,000 high-risk employees, Parkes reports that 200 cases of bladder cancer were detected using cytodiagnostic technique.

The most vital health professional in the recognition of occupational illnesses is the industrial or occupational nurse.

> The industrial nurse is the first to see the worker at the plant, the first to hear about the symptoms and to see the effects of work exposure, the first to make a judgment, an interpretation of these symptoms, and first to record, just what has occurred, and where. It is on the basis of this information provided by the nurse, that the physician on call to a small plant, or the physician in a large plant, makes a further medical interpretation, whether a particular illness is work-related or not.[150]

Therefore, it is essential that industrial nurses, as well as public health nurses and nurses in the community, have an understanding of the chemical carcinogenesis, early warning signs of chemically related bladder cancer, and means of referral and procedural systems for diagnostic and therapeutic measures.[245] Industrial nurses employed in high-risk industries, such as in the rubber industry, paint manufacturers, or textile dyers, have a mandate to investigate the possibilities of bladder cancer screening programs if this is not already available. The cornerstone of any detection program is employee education. The objectives of the employee educational program are as follows: (1) to increase employees' knowledge about the hazards inherent in an industrial setting where there is the possibility of exposure to dangerous chemicals, as in the case of aromatic amines; (2) to dispel myths or superstitions concerning exposure to these chemicals and provide factual information about their toxicity; (3) to increase employee motivation in developing, designing, and participating in medical surveillance and laboratory screening for bladder cancer; and (4) to promote the employees' utilization of safety measures and adherence to necessary precautions that will reduce or minimize occupational exposure to toxic chemicals.

The most convenient, practical approach to early detection of bladder cancer is to have the urine screening programs emanate from the industrial nurse's office. It is toward this goal that occupational nurses must strive.

GASTRIC CANCER

Risk factors

Some clues in the past and family history of clients may raise suspicions as to an increased risk of gastric cancer. This disease is two to four times more prevalent in relatives of affected clients than in control populations. Clients with blood group A seem to have a higher incidence. Clients with atrophic gastric mucosa, with or without pernicious anemia, have a higher risk of developing gastric cancer.[56] It must be emphasized, however, that an atrophic gastric mucosa is common in many elderly people with no evidence of tumor. Clients with a history of partial gastrectomy or gastroenterostomy for peptic ulcer seem to be at increased risk, possibly because of an increased reflux of bile into the antrum. Those individuals with polyps of the stomach certainly have an increased risk, especially if the polyps are over 2 cm in size. Many feel gastric ulcers should be considered potentially malignant until proved benign by endoscopic visualization, biopsy, and complete healing. A certain number of gastric ulcers are in fact ulcerated gastric cancers, sometimes having a benign appearance radiographically.

Certain countries such as Chile and Japan have extremely high incidences of gastric cancer.[167] The incidence in the United States has been decreasing since 1930. In the United States, the incidence is higher in Japanese of the western United States than in other ethnic groups.[163] Several authorities hypothesize that the decreasing incidence of gastric cancer in the United States may be related to the widespread consumption of wheat cereals rich in antioxidants and the extensive use of food antioxidant preservatives such as butylated hydroxytoluene (BHT) and butylated hydroxyanisole (BHA).[19,132]

Lower socioeconomic groups have a higher incidence, with nonwhites having a higher incidence than whites. Persons living on peat soils in the Netherlands and Wales have higher rates of gastric cancer attributed to the high amounts of trace elements in food grown in this type of soil.

Several studies have suggested that the extremely common nitrate food additives that are converted to nitrites may be converted to potentially carcinogenic nitrosamines in the stomach.[108] This is still somewhat controversial, but it has prompted some brisk advertising in the food industry emphasizing foods that contain "no nitrates." Other suspected dietary associations in the etiology of gastric cancer are the consumption of large amounts of smoked foods, particularly fish and mutton; salt in pickled vegetables; and talc-treated rice.[109,144] Interestingly, research documents a negative association between consumption of vitamin C, which is an antioxidant, and stomach cancer. Because of this negative relationship, some experts recommend high-risk individuals increase their daily intake of vitamin C vegetables.[19]

The most common presenting complaint is a vague epigastric discomfort of insidious onset. It may range from a dull and vague postprandial fullness to a severe, steady pain. Anorexia is common when inquiries are made and weight loss occurs in about 50% of clients. About 25% of clients have classic symptoms of ulcers as presenting complaints, as well as complaints of weakness, hematemesis, melena, or change in bowel habit. Dysphagia occurs with tumors in the cardia; nausea and vomiting are quite common with tumors involving the pylorus. Anemia, again, may or may not be symptomatic as an initial symptom. Unfortunately, metastatic complications may cause presenting complaints ranging from malignant ascites and obstructive jaundice to bone pain and shortness of breath from lung metastasis to symptoms secondary to intracranial metastases.

Examination of the asymptomatic client with early gastric carcinoma is almost always unrewarding. Physical examination will reveal a palpable mass in 45% to 50% of clients with advanced gastric carcinoma.[25] About 20% of clients with advanced gastric carcinoma are cachectic and 5% will have palpable peripheral lymph nodes. In any client with symptoms suspicious of gastric carcinoma, the nurse should examine the following areas looking for signs of metastasis: cervical lymph nodes, or Virchow's nodes; peritoneum for ascites or Blumer's shelf; and liver and ovaries for Krukenberg tumors.[132]

A unique quality of spread in gastric cancer is via peritoneal implantation, so that rectal constrictions or shelfs may occur in men and Krukenberg tumors in the ovaries in women. Metastatic involvement of ovaries by stomach cancer occurs with a known frequency and is exceeded only by breast cancer.[206] Abdominal tenderness is only present in 20% of clients with advanced gastric cancer. The ultimate diagnosis rests with a combination of radiologic studies, endoscopy, biopsy, and exfoliative cytologic examination.[41,210]

Nursing interventions

The nurse's role in early detection of stomach cancer is limited to: (1) identification of high-risk populations such as clients with atrophic gastritis, pernicious anemia, achlorhydria, hypochlorhydria, or gastric polyps; (2) client education about the known risk factors for cancer of the stomach and available screening procedures; and (3) referral to physicians or hospitals offering modern techniques of detection such as fiberoptic gastroscopy, diagnostic radiology, and gastric cytodiagnosis. Rubin summarizes the goal of early detection of gastric cancer by stating:

> . . . modern techniques of diagnosis applied to the known high-risk population with genetic, enzymatic, and histochemical defects, to the premalignant states associated with benign conditions, and to those patients whose benign lesions are concealing a malignant neoplasm will enable early discovery of cancer.[205]

Although there continues to be a great deal of speculation about the role of diet in the etiology of stomach cancer related to food additives, contaminants, smoked foods, and salty preserved foods, evidence of the carcinogenicity of a particular food item in man remains to be demonstrated. Thus the nurse is encouraged to continue to review the literature for future research findings that will establish a conclusive relationship. These results could then be incorporated into dietary counseling for high-risk individuals. Until there is conclusive evidence, many of these issues remain speculative.

TESTICULAR CANCER

Although testicular cancer only represents about 1% of all cancers in males, it has been spotlighted as a cancer that can be detected early by self-palpation. Several researchers have noted that testicular cancer is rarely found in blacks and Asians, and that there is an increasing risk with increasing occupational level.[162,173] The peak incidence for testicular cancer is between the ages of 20 and 40 years.

Risk factors

The principal indicator of risk of testicular cancer is undescended testis, or cryptorchidism, or previously atrophic testes. Approximately 1 in 80 inguinal and 1 in 20 abdominal testes will become malignant.[58] Some feel that if orchiopexy is performed before the age of 6, the risk of malignancy may return to normal; otherwise, it continues to be elevated after surgery.[58,168] Henderson points out that "orchiopexy does not necessarily protect against the increased risk of cancer of the involved testis; the contralateral scrotal testis also is at increased risk."[105] A number of factors may be responsible for the increased incidence of testicular tumors in the cryptorchid—gonadal dysgenesis, elevated temperature, interference with blood supply, endocrine disturbances, or perhaps the atrophy itself, which is usually present.[93,165]

The tumor most frequently found in undescended testicles is the seminoma or carcinoma of the spermatic epithelium. This is also the most common type of tumor in testicular cancer and is of relatively low malignancy. Mostofi[166] writes that seminomas comprise from 35% to 71% of testicular tumors.

Hernias and other genitourinary tract anomalies are also highly associated with testicular cancer in children and adults. Other factors that *may* play a role in the development of testicular tumors are trauma; history of orchitis, particularly mumphs; genetic factors; and endocrine abnormalities.[79] One report documented that the 331 male offspring of DES-exposed mothers in that study had a statistically significant higher incidence of testicular abnormalities.[20] Whether or not this will mean a greater risk for testicular cancer in the male offspring of DES-exposed mothers remains to be seen.

The two most frequent early symptoms of testicular cancer are a sensation of discomfort due to the weight of the tumor and painless swelling. These symptoms may be intermittent, which often accounts for the delay in consulting the physician.[121] Clients with choriocarcinoma usually exhibit endocrine disturbances such as gynecomastia and pigmentation of the nipple.[184] The overall presence of endocrine disturbances in all testicular tumors is about 5% and may range from feminization to virilization. Virilization may be observed in children with interstitial cell tumors.[21] Other symptoms, which are numerous, depend on the metastatic spread of the testicular tumor.

Nursing interventions

When obtaining the health history, the nurse should inquire about hernias, cryptorchidism, testicular atrophy, and genitourinary tract anomalies. Other significant questions to include in the health history are: "Is there a scrotal 'heaviness' or heaviness felt in the lower abdomen and groin as well?" "When was the lump first discovered?" "Is there any breast swelling and nipple tenderness?" "Are there signs of early puberty in a child?" "Have you noticed changes in your genital organs or interest in sex?" "Has there been recent trauma?" Although there is no direct proof that trauma causes testicular cancer, many clients with scrotal masses typically link the swelling or lump to a recent trauma.

Physical examination of the testes is best accomplished with the client standing and the nurse seated in front of him. To assess testicular size, shape, consistency, tenderness, and weight, it is recommended that the nurse palpate the scrotal contents with both hands. This will help the nurse differentiate

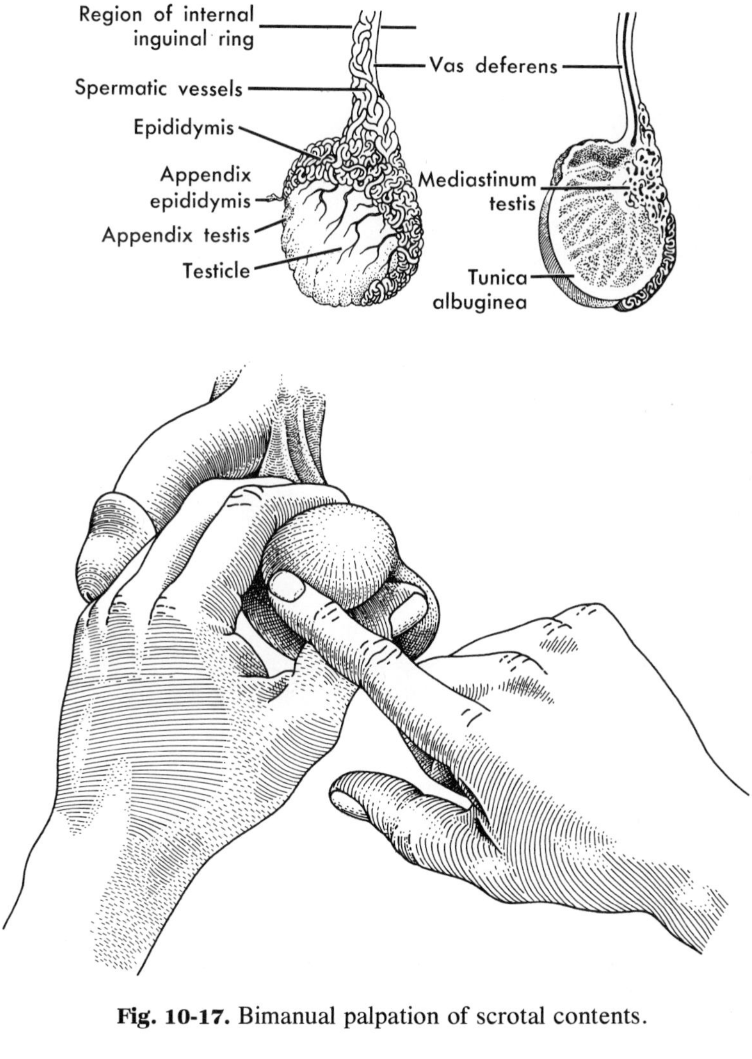

Fig. 10-17. Bimanual palpation of scrotal contents.

the testicles themselves from the other scrotal structures—epididymis, vas deferens, and spermatic cord. Palpating bimanually also improves the chances of detecting any weight differential between the testicles, an important clue to malignancy.[184] Fig. 10-17 demonstrates the procedure for bimanual palpation of the scrotum. The normal testicle has a somewhat rubbery, spongy consistency and the surface should be smooth and free of lumps. The most common sites for tumors are on the testicular anterior and lateral surfaces.[172] Testicular tumors frequently appear as hard painless masses not involving the scrotal wall or spermatic cord. A testicle harboring a tumor is apt to feel heavy. Transillumination is advisable for any testicular swelling and is helpful in distinguishing cystic from solid masses. Transillumination can be accomplished by aiming a small flashlight behind or on the side of the scrotum in a darkened room. Areas that should be checked to ascertain if there has been metastases are palpation of the supraclavicular node areas and palpation of the abdomen for retroperitoneal lymph node metastases. Chest x-ray films, intravenous pyelogram, urinary chorionic gonadotropins, and lymphangiography are used to establish the diagnosis and stage of the disease.[246]

The major obstacle to early detection of testicular cancer is the delay that commonly occurs between initial detection of the lesion in the testis to the time of treatment. Approximately *6 months* will elapse before treatment is either sought by the client or begun by the physician. Borski[21] writes that the following factors contribute to client delays: since the lump is painless, the male (1) assumes it is innocent, (2) hopes that the "tumor" will go away because other men who have had swelling of the scrotum said that theirs went away, (3) feels that the enlarging testis will make him a "better man," (4) feels that the tumor is punishment for past sexual sins, and (5) fears that it is cancer. Conklin and associates[45] studied a group of male college students and found that the majority had never heard about testicular cancer and none knew how to examine their testicles correctly. Yet, 58% of these men had had a health-related course in the past 2 years.

For nursing, this means that a greater emphasis must be placed on testicular cancer in health education. Pediatric hospital nurses, pediatric nurse practitioners, and school nurses must instruct the parents of high-risk males, those who have or had undescended testis, how to correctly palpate the scrotum and what physical findings are significant. These same children should be instructed in testicular self-examination (TSE) as they mature. TSE techniques should be included in health education classes just as self-breast examinations are now routinely included in these classes. For those nurses involved in either consumer health education or professional education, there are several teaching materials available, such as films and pamphlets. The film "Self-Examination of the Testes" can be borrowed free or purchased for $150 from Eaton Laboratories. Memorial Sloan–Kettering Cancer Center[243] has a pamphlet titled "TSE—Testicular Self-Examination," and the American Cancer Society has two pamphlets on this subject, "Facts about Testicular Cancer" and "Testicular Cancer."

The following types of nurses are in ideal clinical settings for teaching TSE and providing education that will dispel the myths that contribute to delay once a testicular lump is found: military nurses, occupational health nurses, office nurses, staff nurses, and school nurses. Teaching TSE should be incorporated into routine physical examinations by the examining health professional. A nursing assessment of any male under the age of 40 should include a health history to elicit any subjective symptomatology and established risk factors for testicular cancer. A man who complains of vague scrotal symptoms should be referred for a careful genital examination, and those men identified as high risk for testicular cancer should be instructed in TSE.

In summary, the best defense against testicular cancer is a well-educated male population that practices TSE and understands the importance of seeking medical attention when a "lump" is discovered. Much progress has been made in the last 10 years in discussing and promoting self-breast examination among women. The time has come for nurses to address the issue of testicular cancer in the same forthright open manner that breast cancer has been discussed so that males will incorporate this health practice into their lives.

GYNECOLOGIC CANCER

Risk factors

The risk factors for cancer of the female reproductive organs vary with the organ affected. The following outline lists the risk factors for each type of gynecologic cancer:

Cervix[105,147,176,195]
- Sexual relations at an early age
- Multiple sexual partners
- Chronic infestation with *Trichomonas vaginalis*
- Low socioeconomic status
- Syphilis
- Herpes genitalis (?)[123]
- Sexual partner is uncircumcised (?)

Vagina
- Exposure in utero to DES

Endometrium[1,143]
- Women over the age of 40
- Triad of obesity, diabetes, hypertension
- Infertility history
- Irregular menses and failure of ovulation
- Adenomatous hyperplasia
- Women receiving conjugated estrogens for menopausal symptoms[4,114,119,131]
- Family history of endometrial cancer
- Stein-Leventhal syndrome and Turner's syndrome (?)

Ovarian[124]
- Upper socioeconomic status
- Reduced fertility or infertility
- History of breast cancer
- Family history of cancer, particularly of the breast, ovary, or colon

When obtaining the health history, the nurse must include questions that will elicit an accurate menstrual, obstetric, gynecologic, and sexual history. The majority of women at risk for cancer of the reproductive organs can only be identified once a thorough and complete gynecologic history has been obtained. Since researchers feel that early coitus or multiple sexual partners is the *key* risk factor for cervical cancer, it is important that the nurse include questions about these two areas.[113] Other areas that should be investigated are past vaginal infections, history of venereal disease, contraception history, past infections with herpes simplex, history of estrogen therapy, frequency of gynecologic examinations and Pap test results, OB history or infertility history, past gynecologic procedures such as cervical cautery and colposcopy, menstrual history, and illnesses such as diabetes, hypertension, and cancer.

As with risk factors, the presenting signs and symptoms of cancer of the female reproductive organs depend on the site affected. Table 10-6 lists the signs, symptoms, physical findings, and recommended diagnostic procedures commonly utilized to arrive at a diagnosis.

Nursing interventions

In addition to assessing risk factors during the health assessment, the nurse should ask specific questions designed to detect the early symptoms of gynecologic cancer. Examples of questions to ask that would aid in

Table 10-6. Presenting early symptoms, physical findings, and diagnostic procedures for cancer of the female reproductive organs

Area involved	*Early* symptoms	Physical findings	Diagnostic procedures
Vagina[106,107,202,241]	Abnormal bleeding or discharge—may seek medical attention because of history of prenatal DES exposure; DES-associated cancer usually occurs in clients 14 years or older	Vividly red focal areas on vagina; indurated, firm, cystic areas in vagina or cervix	1. Complete gynecologic examination 2. Cytology from vagina and cervix 3. Iodine stain (initial visit); investigate areas that appear red or fail to stain 4. Colposcopy
Cervix[231,252]	Dyplasias and carcinoma in situ are not likely to cause symptoms; may have abnormal vaginal discharge or some irregular bleeding or elongation of menstrual period; may have postcoital bleeding or bleeding after douching	May see erosion of cervix	1. Cytology from squamocolumnar junction and endocervical canal 2. Colposcopy when Pap smear is abnormal or stain cervix with Schiller's solution—abnormal epithelium remains uncolored 3. Punch biopsy

Endometrium[27,35,49,96,231]	Seventy-five percent of clients with endometrial cancer are postmenopausal. Postmenopausal vaginal bleeding and spotting; malodorous watery discharge; may be premenopausal history of menstrual irregularities—amenorrhea to hypermenorrhea	Enlarged boggy uterus is indication of advanced disease	1. Cytology using intrauterine endocervical and vaginal pool aspirations 2. Jet wash of endometrium 3. Endometrial biopsy or curettage 4. Pelvic examination under anesthesia
Ovary[14,226]	Peak incidence is between 40 to 65 years of age. Vague abdominal discomfort, dyspepsia, and other mild digestive disturbances; change in abdominal girth	Mass in the ovary (must be 15 cm to be palpated) that is bilateral, relatively immobile, and irregular in shape; suspect any palpable ovary in a postmenopausal woman and any adnexal thickening in a postmenopausal or nulliparous woman Tumors, which are described as a "handful of knuckles," may be felt in the cul-de-sac	1. Pap smear positive in 40% of cases 2. Cul-de-sac taps positive in 90% of cases 3. Laparoscopy

identifying women who may need an examination or referral are:

- Do you have any change in vaginal bleeding or spotting between menstrual periods?
- Do you have any change in your menstrual period (amount or length)?
- Do you have bleeding or spotting although you have stopped having periods (or although you have gone through the "change")?
- Do you have a persistent pain or fullness in the lower part of your abdomen?
- Has it been more than 3 years since you had your last Pap test?
- Was your mother ever treated with hormones during a pregnancy?
- Do you have an odorous vaginal discharge?
- Do you bleed after intercourse or douching?

Including these questions in the health assessment of women will also enable the nurse to do some health teaching. Many women falsely believe that the following are true: postmenopausal bleeding is normal; Pap smears are not necessary until a woman is married; regular pelvic examinations are not necessary after menopause; odorous vaginal discharges are normal; and an early symptom of gynecologic cancer is pain. The necessity of continuing regular pelvic examinations after menopause should be stressed to *all* women along with the fact that any postmenopausal bleeding warrants investigation. It is also important to educate young women in terms of the necessity of Pap smears once they become sexually active, regardless of age. "It is imperative that young women establish good health habits during their reproductive years if they are to perpetuate those habits through their postmenopausal years."[115]

The nurse must recognize that cultural and religious beliefs influence health practices and that folk beliefs are very prevalent about menstruation, menopause, pregnancy, and other topics related to female reproduction. Nurses must make a conscious effort to acquaint themselves with the folk beliefs and health practices of different cultural groups, particularly those with whom they come in contact. By asking open-ended questions during the health assessment that encourage the client to express her health beliefs, the nurse may be able to identify myths and misconceptions that relate to the female reproductive organs. One method of encouraging sharing of culturally determined health beliefs is to open the discussion with the statement, "Many people believe that . . . ." Since many people are reticent to share their health beliefs with health professionals because they are afraid they will be laughed at, it is essential that the nurse avoid making value judgments. By openly identifying and acknowledging that a health belief is held by many people, the nurse facilitates the admission that the clients believe these statements to be true also. Once misconceptions are identified, the nurse has a professional and moral obligation to alter false opinions that will prevent early detection of gynecologic cancer and facilitate corrective education. However, as with any effective teaching, it should take place when the learner is receptive.

A prerequisite to any pelvic examination is a thorough gynecologic history as previously discussed. Since women are frequently anxious about pelvic examinations, it helps to briefly explain what will be done and stress the importance of relaxing during the procedure. Teaching the client a relaxation technique such as breathing deeply and slowly through her mouth will shorten the examination and allow the examiner to successfully complete it. Expensive equipment is not necessary for a thorough pelvic examination. The few necessary items are disposable gloves; stirrup extensions on a regular examination table; specula, one standard and one narrow-bladed for children and elderly women; a good source of light; a cytology kit; and a drape sheet. To assure that the pelvic examination is complete, the following are recommended:

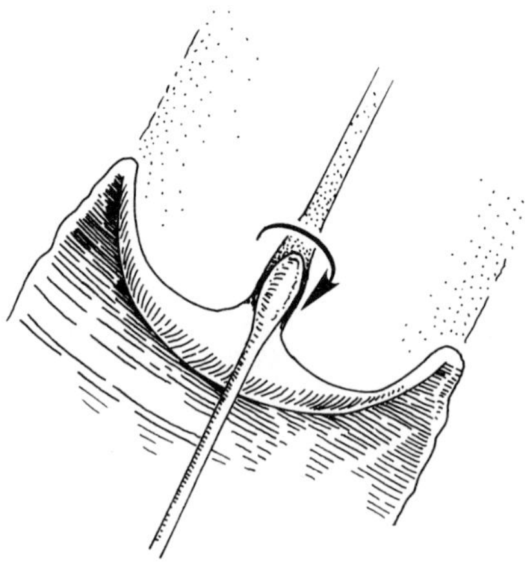

Fig. 10-18. Endocervical smear. (From Fogel, C. I., and Woods, N. F.: Health care of women: a nursing perspective, St. Louis, 1980, The C. V. Mosby Co.)

1. The abdomen must be thoroughly and slowly palpated to detect any masses, areas of tenderness, or inguinal adenopathy.

2. The vulva should be inspected and palpated for signs of cancer of the vulva—excoriation of skin owing to pruritis, ulcers, lumps, leukoplakia, bleeding, and vulvar dystrophies such as atrophy of labia and narrowing of introitus.[68]

3. The vagina should be inspected and palpated for cancer—masses, vaginal bands, texture changes, ulcers, erosions, leukoplakia, pink blush, induration, telangiectasis, or erythematosus. Some authors recommend doing the bimanual palpation before the speculum is introduced into the vagina; others recommend inspecting the vagina and cervix before the bimanual examination.[17,57] Vaginal jelly cannot be used prior to obtaining Pap smear specimens, which may account for the tendency to do the specimen examination *before* doing the bimanual examination. Regardless of individual technique, the examiner may elect to do a Schiller's test on any suspicious area of the vagina or cervix. The mucosa is painted

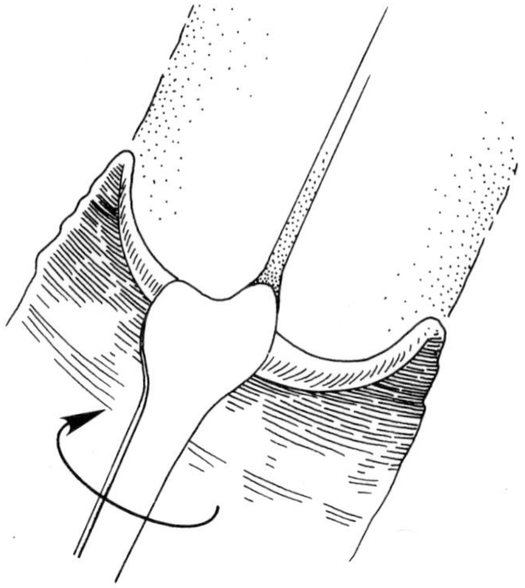

Fig. 10-19. Cervical smear. (From Fogel, C. I., and Woods, N. F.: Health care of women: a nursing perspective, St. Louis, 1980, The C. V. Mosby Co.)

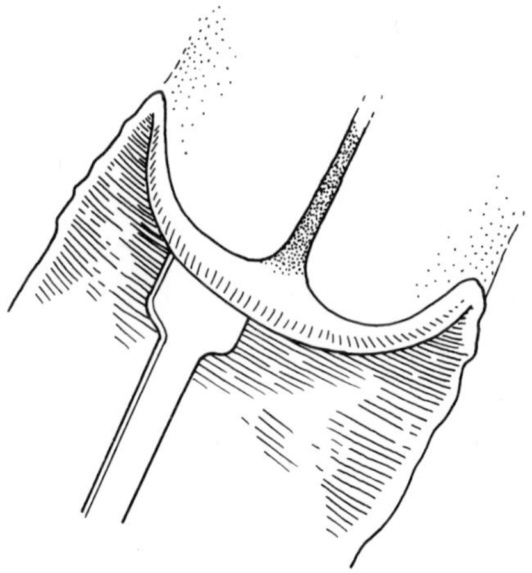

Fig. 10-20. Vaginal pool smear.

with an iodine solution such as Gram's, and the normal mucosa becomes brown while areas of abnormal epithelium remain uncolored. This test is merely an adjunctive aid to colposcopy or used when colposcopy is not available. It indicates a glycogen-free area and delineates biopsy sites.[68]

4. The cervix should be inspected and palpated with a cytologic (Pap) smear being taken. It is generally recommended that *three* samples be taken for the Pap smear: an endocervical smear taken with a cotton applicator, a cervical smear, and a vaginal pool smear taken with an Ayre spatula demonstrated in Figs. 10-18 to 10-20. False negative results between 10% and 20% have been reported in the literature for exfoliative gynecologic cytology.[111] These false negative results may be due to three sources: the trapping effect of the cotton swabs and wooden spatulas, the adequacy of cell collection by the examiner, and the screening by the cytotechnologists.[207] Errors made by cytotechnologists may be minimized in the future by new experimental technology that uses computer systems to screen cervical cells for abnormalities.[8] The effectiveness of automated cytology remains to be proved in future research studies. Del Regato and Spjut[57] recommend *two* bimanual examinations when palpating the cervix, one with the right hand in the vagina and the left hand above the symphysis pubis, and the other with the hands in a reverse position as shown

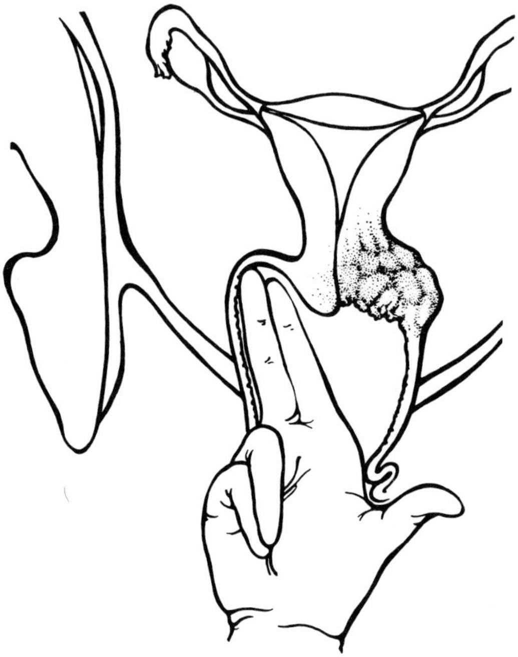

Fig. 10-21. Vaginal palpation with two fingers of right hand allows deep exploration of cervix and right fornix. (From del Regato, J., and Spjut, H.: Cancer of the female genital organs. In del Regato, J., and Spjut, H., editors: Ackerman and del Regato's cancer: diagnosis, treatment, and prognosis, ed. 5, St. Louis, 1977, The C. V. Mosby Co.)

in Figs. 10-21 to 10-24. The rationale is that the same hand cannot reach equally deep into *both* fornices. The nurse inspects and palpates the cervix for position, shape, consistency, regularity, mobility, and tenderness. Since cancer of the cervix is usually symptom free until the lesion is advanced, the diagnosis is frequently determined by the cytology report.

5. A bimanual examination of the uterus and adnexa should be done. The examiner should note the size, shape, mobility, position, tenderness, and consistency of the uterus. Uterine tenderness, immobility, or enlargement merits further investigation by the examiner. Palpation of ovaries in prepubertal girls or postmenopausal women also merits investigation because: (1) the normal ovary and tube are usually not palpable,[54] (2) ovaries in these two groups of women are smaller than the usual ovarian size of 4 cm in their largest dimension, and (3) 3 to 5 years after menopause the ovaries have usually atrophied and are no longer palpable.

6. Rectovaginal palpation as well as rectal palpation should be done. It is extremely important that the anterior rectal wall in the region of the peritoneal rectovaginal pouch, or cul-de-sac of Douglas, be palpated.

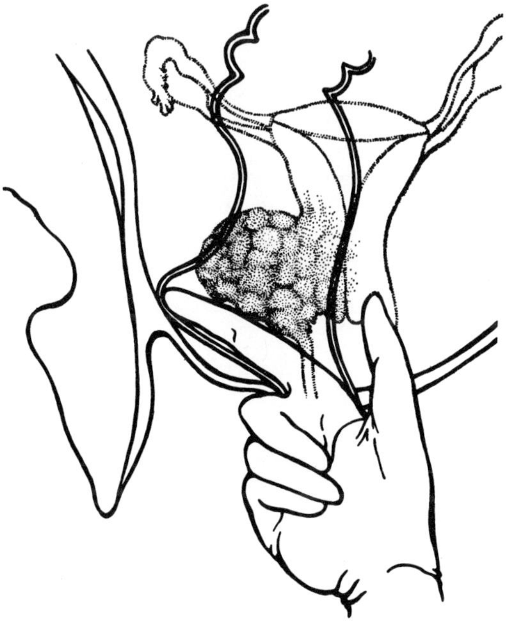

Fig. 10-22. Rectal palpation with right index finger allows complete exploration of right parametrium. When finger can be introduced between tumor mass and pelvic wall, parametrium is probably not totally invaded. (From del Regato, J., and Spjut, H.: Cancer of the female genital organs. In del Regato, J., and Spjut, H., editors: Ackerman and del Regato's cancer: diagnosis, treatment, and prognosis, ed. 5, St. Louis, 1977, The C. V. Mosby Co.)

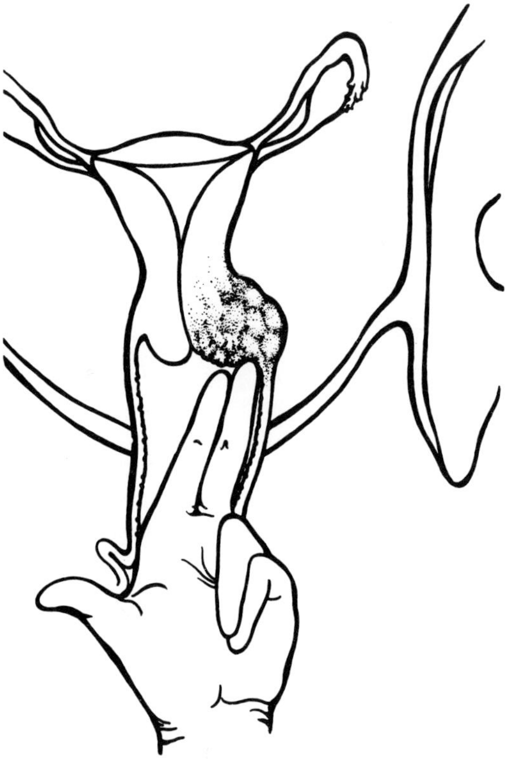

Fig. 10-23. Vaginal examination with left hand allows exploration of left side. Lack of elasticity suggests parametrial extension, but its limits cannot be definitely established by vaginal examination. (From del Regato, J., and Spjut, H.: Cancer of the female genital organs. In del Regato, J., and Spjut, H., editors: Ackerman and del Regato's cancer: diagnosis, treatment, and prognosis, ed. 5, St. Louis, 1977, The C. V. Mosby Co.)

Thickening of this area occurs from spread of cervical carcinoma,[55] while spread from ovarian cancer may be felt as a shelf, nodule, or handful-of-knuckles on rectal palpation.

There is presently debate concerning the necessity of the "yearly Pap smear." The Walton Report from Canada[247] recommends that women who have two initial cytologic studies without notable atypia and normalcy in all subsequent cytologic findings be screened at 3-year intervals until age 35 and thereafter at 5-year intervals until age 60. Women at continuing risk should be screened annually. The American Cancer Society has recently suggested that Pap smears every 3 years are sufficient under similar circumstances. In the United Kingdom it is recommended that below the age of 25, a woman have just two Pap smears taken within a 12-month period, the second to catch a possible false negative. After that, a smear should be taken every 5 years up to age 35, and every 3 years thereafter.[7,191] These recommendations are in contrast with the current standards of the American College of Obstetricians and Gynecologists. They recommend annual examinations to begin with the onset of sexual activity or at

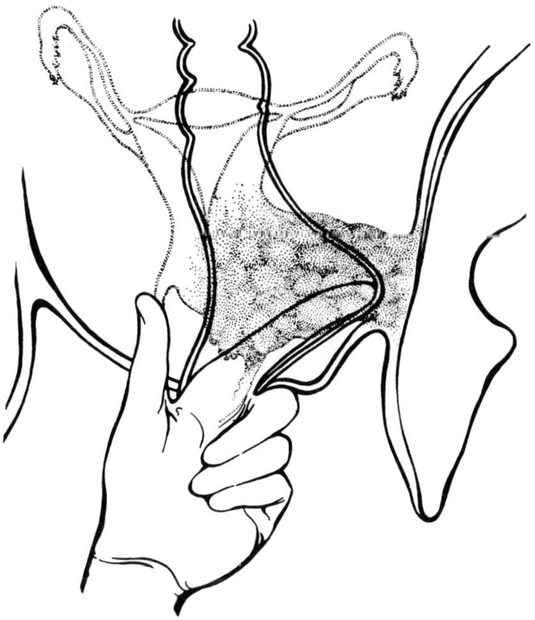

Fig. 10-24. Rectal palpation with left index finger allows complete exploration of left parametrium. When tumor mass is continuous with pelvic wall and there is no "notch" between tumor and pelvic wall, clinical assumption is that tumor has already invaded pelvic wall. (From del Regato, J., and Spjut, H.: Cancer of the female genital organs. In del Regato, J., and Spjut, H., editors: Ackerman and del Regato's cancer: diagnosis, treatment, and prognosis, ed. 5, St. Louis, 1977, The C. V. Mosby Co.)

the latest by age 18. The debate on Pap smear frequency stems from the controversial issue questioning whether the cervical cytology screening programs reduce mortality.

Mortality from cancer of the uterus, including the cervix, has been declining since the 1930's, well before screening with cytology.[27] Some experts credit the decline mainly to better gynecologic care and the growth of hysterectomies. Also mentioned as contributing to the drop in uterine cancer morbidity and mortality are improved socioeconomic factors, better hygiene and education, and changes in contraceptive practices. Researchers Gardner and Lyon[86] conclude that on the basis of all available evidence, a causal association between cytologic screening and the declining mortality and incidence of cervical cancer cannot be established. Contrary to this view, other researchers attribute the decline in the incidence of invasive carcinoma of the cervix to the increased screening for cancer of the uterus and cervix by means of the Pap smear technique both in the United States and in other countries.[36,85,111,140] They point out that the value of the Pap smear is that it can disclose the minutest focus of carcinoma in situ, dysplasia, and overt cancer of the cervix. Breslow[27] states that the absence of a randomized field trial of the value of the Pap test has delayed its widespread use and fuels doubts as to whether the Pap test is effective in reducing mortality from cervical cancer among populations where it was applied. Regardless of position on this issue, all authorities agree that the clients who need this service the *most* use it the *least*. American black women, who suffer cervical cancer at twice the rate of whites, are least likely to have periodic Pap smears or utilize mass screening programs.

Reaching those women who are at high risk for gynecologic cancer is one of the most challenging roles for nurses.

> . . . there is a need to encourage more older women, particularly among high-risk groups, to undergo cervical cytology and pelvic examination, and to insure that females now being screened in their childbearing years continue to undergo this examination in postmenopausal life.[27]

Gaining client acceptance and increasing the availability of screening are areas that will require major effort on the part of nurses if the entire population at *greatest risk* is to be reached. Since cytologic screening is closely tied to obstetric care and contraceptive services, a higher proportion of women are screened among the groups who require such attention than among those who do not. This is effective for screening for cervical and vaginal cancer in the reproductive years but does not reach those women at risk for ovarian and endometrial malignancies (postmenopausal women). Nurses working in retirement centers, extended care facilities, physicians' offices, factories, public health agencies, and ambulatory care settings are urged to provide health education programs that stress the need for gynecologic examinations after menopause as well as during the reproductive years.[178] This education should also include the early signs and symptoms of ovarian, cervical, and endometrial cancer. Female clients being followed routinely for chronic problems (such as hypertension, diabetes, heart condition, or chronic lung disease) should be asked when they had their last pelvic examination. Many times health professionals get complacent when they see clients on a fairly regular basis and forget to address the "whole person." When appropriate, nurses should discuss the myths about menopause with women who are in their late 30's and early 40's. Many times these myths contribute to delay in the early detection of gynecologic cancer.[259]

Nurses are urged to acquire physical assessment skills that will enable them to perform pelvic examinations. Research clearly documents: (1) that nurses performing pelvic examinations are effective in detecting gynecologic malignances, (2) that client acceptance and satisfaction is very high with nurse-conducted pelvic examinations, and (3) that pelvic examinations done by nurses are cost-effective.[235,237] Nurses trained to conduct gynecologic examinations would be in ideal positions to reach those women who are at highest risk for developing the different types of gynecologic cancer but least likely to utilize conventional screening programs or have routine health examinations, such as older women in residential settings or older poor women in the community. Nurses actively involved in conducting pelvic examinations would also increase the availability of screening programs and thus reach more women.

Nurses working in schools, women's studies centers, college health services, adolescent health services, summer camps, and pediatric nurse practitioners should include in all health education the necessity of having Pap smears once a woman becomes sexually active or over 18 years of age. This type of information could accompany discussions of human sexuality and family planning. It is expected that nurses working in family planning, prenatal, and venereal disease clinics include or institute health education programs that detail gynecologic cancer risk factors, early signs and symptoms, and suggested health practices women can take that will lead to early detection.

LEUKEMIA

Risk factors

The risk factors for leukemia are listed in the following outline:[168,182,227,232,231]

A. Chemical radiation
  1. Benzene
  2. Ionizing radiation
    a. X-ray exposure
    b. Exposure to atomic bomb blast
B. Occupational
  1. Poultry farmers
  2. Benzene, explosives and rubber cement workers, distillers, dye users, painters
  3. Radiologists
  4. Radium chemists
  5. Radium miners
  6. Radium dial painters
C. Genetic
  1. Down's syndrome
  2. Bloom's syndrome
  3. Fanconi's anemia
  4. Klinefelter's syndrome
  5. Marked increase in frequency of leukemia in identical twin of a leukemia client
D. Sexual
  1. Males more than females in both (white and black) races
E. Drugs and/or medical treatments
  1. Melphalan
  2. Cyclophosphamide
  3. Chloramphenicol (?)
  4. X-ray treatments for spondylitis
  5. Women exposed to radiation for the induction of artificial menopause

These factors include environmental interactions, genetic factors, viral factors, immunologic factors, and interacting factors.[138] Several microepidemics of leukemia have been reported that might suggest an infectious etiology. However, epidemiologic studies in situations that might reflect an infectious mode of spread have failed to support this suspicion. There is also no conclusive evidence that viruses cause leukemia in humans, although there is clear proof that viruses can cause leukemia in many animal species including primates.

The clinical presentation of leukemia varies with the type of leukemia: acute myelogenous leukemia, chronic myelogenous leukemia, acute lymphocytic leukemia, and chronic lymphocytic leukemia. Because there is a wide range of signs, symptoms, physical findings, and age groups affected for each type of leukemia, they are summarized in Table 10-7.

It is important for the nurse to note the age range for the various types of leukemias and frequent presenting signs and symptoms. School nurses and nurses in preschool and recreational settings should remember that cancer has become the *leading* cause of death from disease in children over 1 year of age, and leukemia is the most common type of cancer to affect children. Whenever there is an index of suspicion of leukemia, either because of the client's age, symptoms, or known risk factors, the following should be done by the nurse during physical assessment. The nurse should: (1) thoroughly examine the cervical and peripheral lymph nodes; (2) palpate and percuss the liver and spleen; (3) thoroughly inspect the skin for systemic signs of leukemia such as pallor, purpura, petechiae, chloroma; (4) inspect the mouth for enlarged tonsils, hyperplasia of the gums, and red friable gingivae; (5) palpate the sternum, bones, and joints for tenderness and pain. Chloroma is a localized tumor mass that has a greenish appearance and may occur in the skin, orbit, or other tissues in granulocytic forms of leukemia.[38]

Nursing interventions

The nursing implications are varied when discussing detection and prevention of leukemia. Probably the most important role the nurse can assume is to help decrease unnecessary exposure to x-rays. There is overall

Table 10-7. Signs, symptoms, and physical findings in leukemia[26,61,69,238]

Type	Age range	Dominant signs and symptoms	Physical findings
Acute myelogenous leukemia (AML)	Nearly equal frequency in all decades	Prodromal of 1 to 6 months—fatigue, dyspnea, palpations, malaise, fever	Pallor, petechiae, purpura, splenomegaly
Chronic myelogenous leukemia (CML)	Uncommon before age 20; increases each succeeding decade	Malaise, easy fatigability, heat intolerance, easy bruising	Splenic enlargement in 90% of cases; tenderness of sternum
Acute lymphocytic leukemia (ALL)	Peak incidence in children in the first decade, especially 2 to 4 years of age; ALL is most common form of childhood cancer	Onset often sudden but may have prodromal period of weakness, malaise, anorexia, fever, tachycardia; frequently present are pain in bone, petechiae, and hemorrhages; may first occur with bleeding after minor procedures such as dental extraction	Enlargement of tonsils, enlargement of spleen and liver; lymph nodes generally enlarged; pallor, petechiae, purpura
Chronic lymphocytic leukemia (CLL)	Rare under 35 years of age; increases in frequency with succeeding decades	Malaise, easy fatigability, weight loss, excessive sweating	Enlarged lymph nodes; enlarged spleen and liver

agreement among various studies of the effects of radiation that children are more sensitive than adults to ionizing radiation. "For children, there are about three cases of leukemia induced per million person-year-rads over a 20 to 25 year follow-up, whereas for adults the corresponding figure appears to be 1 to 1.5."[116,267] It is important for nurses working with children to remember this fact. All efforts should be made by pediatric nursing staff to minimize the x-ray exposure to children undergoing diagnostic x-rays. Care should be taken to make sure that the child is correctly positioned for all x-ray films so that retakes are avoided. It is also important to shield all tissues outside the field to be examined, especially the gonads. The Food and Drug Administration's Bureau of Radiological Health and The American College of Radiology have issued guidelines for the use of gonad shielding. The impetus for the recommendations stem from the belief that x-rays have the ability to produce genetic mutations and chromosomal aberrations. The guidelines include the following: Gonad shielding should be used when the gonads lie within or close to (about 5 cm) the primary x-ray beam. This includes examinations involving the pelvis, hip, and upper part of the femur; examinations of the abdomen or lumbar or lumbosacral spine; intravenous pyelograms; and abdominal scout films for barium enema studies and upper gastrointestinal series. As a basis for judgment, gonad shielding of male clients should be considered for all examinations in which the pubic symphysis will be visualized.[151] In fact, all staff dealing with any aspects of radiation should be properly shielded and cognizant of the long-term effects of radiation. The use of diagnostic x-ray examinations has become so routine that many health professionals have become careless in their techniques and have forgotten that the carcinogenic effects of ionizing radiation are great.

As the client's advocate, it may be necessary for the nurse to: (1) insist on proper shielding of clients and staff, (2) insist that staff who are responsible for holding children during x-ray examinations be rotated so the same staff are not continuously exposed, (3) question if the portable x-ray machine is absolutely necessary or if the client can be moved to the x-ray department to ensure usable films, and (4) make sure that the client is properly positioned so that retakes are not necessary. Along with these actions that may help decrease exposure to ionizing radiation, nurses should strive to educate the public to the fact that x-ray examinations are not necessary for establishing every diagnosis.

Unfortunately, the number of diagnostic x-ray examinations has been increasing rapidly. According to surveys performed by the U.S. Department of Health and Human Services (formerly DHEW), the number of persons receiving medical radiographic examinations rose from 66 million in 1964 to 76.4 million in 1970, and the number receiving dental films rose from 46 million to 59.2 million.[214] Many factors have contributed to this increase such as malpractice suits, which have led to defensive medicine, and client expectations that x-ray examinations must be made to confirm and/or establish a diagnosis. Nurses must involve themselves in increasing consumer awareness of the benefits and *risks* of x-ray examinations. This type of educational approach might help decrease the large number of unnecessary x-ray examinations performed every year by encouraging the public to ask health professionals: "Is this x-ray examination really necessary?"

School nurses and public health nurses working with individuals with Down's syndrome must be aware of the relationship between this genetic condition and increased risk for leukemia. Individuals with Down's syndrome in institutions, sheltered villages, and other types of residential programs should be closely followed by nurses working in these settings for the early signs and symptoms of leukemia so that proper referrals can be made if leukemia is suspected.

CONCLUSION

This chapter has described the risk factors and detection procedures for 12 types or groups of cancer. These cancers were chosen because they represent sites of high incidence or opportunities for cancer prevention and early detection.

Nurses can influence the areas of prevention and early detection by obtaining skills in physical examination and diagnosis as well as utilizing their teaching and counseling skills more fully. A great deal of confusion, controversy, and anxiety exists within American society as to ways that individuals can influence the likelihood that they will develop cancer. Nurses can do a great deal to make these individuals better informed, both in terms of known risks and the earlier utilization of services to detect cancer. Increased involvement in these areas by nurses would help to lower cancer morbidity and mortality as well as enhance professional functioning.

REFERENCES

1. ACOG Technical Bulletin: Gynecologic cancer (No. 24), Chicago, 1973, The American College of Obstetricians and Gynecologists.
2. Ahren, C., Hulten, L., and Kewenter, J.: Precancerous changes in ulcerative colitis and its association with carcinoma of the colon. In Maltoni, C., editor: Cancer detection and prevention, vol. 2, New York, 1974, American Elsevier Publishing Co.
3. American Cancer Society Professional Education Publication: The challenge of oral cancer, Publication No. 3719-PE, New York, 1975, American Cancer Society Professional Education Publication.
4. Antunes, C., et al.: Endometrial cancer and estrogen use: report of a large case-control study, N. Engl. J. Med. **300:**9, 1979.
5. Archer, V.: Occupational exposure to radiation as a cancer hazard, Cancer **39:**1802, 1977.
6. Asbestos exposure, Publication No. 78-1622, Washington, D.C., 1978, U.S. Department of Health, Education and Welfare, National Cancer Institute.
7. Atypical Pap smear in a young woman: red flag or not? Med. World News **19:**16, 1978.
8. Automated scanner for cervical smears shows high accuracy, Med. World News **19:**20, 1978.
9. Bagshaw, M., et al.: Rx of bladder cancer: complex and controversial, CA **23:**81, 1973.
10. Bailar, J.: Mammography: a contrary view, Ann. Intern. Med. **84:**77, 1976.
11. Bailar, J.: Screening for early breast cancer: pros and cons, Cancer **39:**2793, 1977.
12. Bailar, J.: Screening for early breast cancer: pros and cons, Cancer **39:**2783, 1977.
13. Baker, H.: Diagnosis of oral cancer. Part one, CA **22:**30, 1972.
14. Barber, H., Graber, E., and Kwon, T.: Ovarian cancer, Publication No. 3357-PE, New York, 1976, American Cancer Society Professional Education Publication.
15. Barkin, M., et al.: Three cases of human bladder cancer following high dose cyclamate ingestion, J. Urol. **118:**258, 1977.
16. Bass, L.: More fiber—less constipation, Am. J. Nurs. **77:**254, 1977.
17. Bates, B.: A guide to physical examination, Philadelphia, 1974, J. B. Lippincott Co.
18. Bates, R.: The hidden alcoholic: a history that reveals the early clues, Diagnosis, p. 22, 1979.
19. Berg, J.: Diet. In Fraumeini, J., editor: Persons at high risk of cancer: an approach to cancer etiology and control, New York, 1975, Academic Press, Inc.
20. Bibbo, M., et al.: Follow-up study of male and female offspring of DES-exposed mothers, J. Obstet. Gynecol. **49:**1, 1977.
21. Borski, A.: Diagnosis, staging and natural history of testicular tumors. Proceedings of the National Conference on Urologic Cancer, Publication No. 3080-PE, New York, 1973, American Cancer Society.
22. Boucot, K., and Weiss, W.: Is curable lung cancer detected by semiannual screening? J.A.M.A. **224:**1361, 1973.
23. Bowen-Davies, A.: Methods of examination of the mouth and pharynx. In Ballantyne, J., and Groves, J., editors: Scott-Brown's diseases of the ear, nose and throat, ed. 3, vol. 4, Philadelphia, 1971, J. B. Lippincott Co.
24. Boyer, M.: Treating invasive lung cancer, Am. J. Nurs. **77:**1916, 1977.

25. Brandborg, L.: Polyps, tumors, and cancer of the stomach. In Sleisenger, M., and Fordtran, J., editors: Gastrointestinal disease, ed. 2, Philadelphia, 1978, W. B. Saunders Co.
26. Braverman, I.: Skin signs of systemic disease, Philadelphia, 1970, W. B. Saunders Co.
27. Breslow, L.: Review and future perspectives of cancer screening programs. In Nieburgs, H., editor: Prevention and detection of cancer. Part II—Detection. Vol. 1—High risk markers, New York, 1978, Marcel Dekker, Inc.
28. Breslow, L., et al.: Report on NCI ad hoc working group on the gross and net benefits of mammography in mass screening for the detection of breast cancer, Publication No. 77-1400, Washington, D.C., 1977, U.S. Department of Health, Education and Welfare, National Institutes of Health.
29. Bross, I., and Blumenson, L.: Screening random asymptomatic women under 50 by annual mammographies: Does it make sense? Surg. Oncol. **9:**437, 1976.
30. Burkitt, D. P., Walker, A., and Painter, N.: Dietary fiber and disease, J.A.M.A. **229:**1068, 1974.
31. Cady, B., Moschella, S., and Legg. M.: Contemporary aspects of malignant melanoma, Famous Teachings in Modern Medicine, New York, 1974, Medcom, Inc.
32. Caldwell, W.: Cancer of the urinary bladder, St. Louis, 1970, Warren Green, Inc.
33. Callahan, L.: Colo-rectal cancer: clinical trial/community outreach. Proceedings of the Fourth National Cancer Communications Conference, Publication No. 78-1463, Washington, D.C., 1977, U.S. Department of Health, Education and Welfare, Public Health Service, National Institutes of Health.
34. Christen, A., and Cooper, K.: Strategic withdrawal from cigarette smoking, CA **29:**96, 1979.
35. Christopherson, W.: Changing trends in morbidity and mortality in endometrial carcinoma. In Gray, L., editor: Endometrial carcinoma and its treatment, Springfield, Ill, 1977, Charles C Thomas, Publisher.
36. Christopherson, W., et al.: Cervical cancer control, Cancer **38:**1357, 1976.
37. Cipollaro, A.: Cancer of the skin, Am. J. Nurs. **66:**2231, 1966.
38. Clarkson, B.: The acute leukemias. In Thorn, G., et al., editors: Harrison's principles of internal medicine, ed. 8, New York, 1977, McGraw-Hill Book Co.
39. Clemmesen, J.: Environmental and occupational factors in urinary bladder cancer. In Maltoni, C., editor: Cancer detection and prevention, vol. 2, New York, 1974, American Elsevier Publishing Co.
40. Cohen, S.: Hypnosis and smoking, J.A.M.A. **208:**335, 1969.
41. Colcher, H.: Diagnostic fiberoptic gastroscopy. In Rubin, P., editor: Cancer of the gastrointestinal tract. Part one (esophagus, stomach, small intestine), Publication No. 3007.08-PE, New York, 1974, American Cancer Society Professional Education Publication.
42. Cole, P.: Lower urinary tract. In Schottenfeld, D., editor: Cancer epidemiology and prevention: current concepts, Springfield, Ill., 1975, Charles C Thomas, Publisher.
43. Cole, P.: Cancer and occupation: status and needs of epidemiologic research, Cancer **39:**1788, 1977.
44. Cole, P., and Goldman, M.: Occupation. In Fraumeni, J., editor: Persons at high risk of cancer: an approach to cancer etiology and control, New York, 1975, Academic Press, Inc.
45. Conklin, M., et al.: Should health teaching include self-examination of the testes? Am. J. Nurs. **78:**2073, 1978.
46. Conley, J.: How to examine the oro-naso-laryngo-pharynx for cancer. In Rubin, P., editor: Current concepts in cancer: cancer of the head and neck, New York, 1971, American Cancer Society, Inc.
47. Copher, D. E.: Clinical specialist gynecology as a component of the optimal health care system, Clin. Res. **19:**499, 1971.
48. Corman, M., Coller, J., and Veidenheimer, M.: Proctosigmoidoscopy—age criteria for examination in the asymptomatic patient, CA **25:**286, 1975.
49. Creasman, W., and Weed, J.: Screening techniques in endometrial cancer, Cancer **38:**436, 1976.
50. Cutler, S., and Young, J.: Demographic patterns of cancer incidence in the United States. In Fraumeni, J., editor: Persons at high risk of cancer: an approach to cancer etiology and control, New York, 1975, Academic Press, Inc.
51. Daniels, F.: Sunlight. In Schottenfeld, D., editor: Cancer epidemiology and prevention: current concepts, Springfield, Ill., 1975, Charles C Thomas, Publisher.
52. Davis, N.: Pigmented skin tumors, CA **23:**160, 1973.
53. Davis, N., et al.: Primary cutaneous melanoma: a report from the Queensland melanoma project, CA **26:**80, 1976.

54. DeGowin, E., and DeGowin, R.: Bedside diagnostic examination, ed. 2, New York, 1970, Macmillan, Inc.
55. DeGroot, L.: Thyroid carcinoma, Med. Clin. North Am. **59**:1233, 1975.
56. del Regato, J., and Spjut, H.: Cancer of the digestive tract. In del Regato, J., and Spjut, H., editors: Ackerman and del Regato's cancer: diagnosis, treatment, and prognosis, ed. 5, St. Louis, 1977, The C. V. Mosby Co.
57. del Regato, J., and Spjut, H.: Cancer of the female genital organs. In del Regato, J., and Spjut, H., editors: Ackerman and del Regato's cancer: diagnosis, treatment, and prognosis, ed. 5, St. Louis, 1977, The C. V. Mosby Co.
58. del Regato, J., and Spjut, H.: Cancer of the male genital organs. In del Regato, J., and Spjut, H., editors: Ackerman and del Regato's cancer: diagnosis, treatment, and prognosis, ed. 5, St. Louis, 1977, The C. V. Mosby Co.
59. del Regato, J., and Spjut, H.: Cancer of the respiratory system and upper digestive tract. In del Regato, J., and Spjut, H., editors: Ackerman and del Regato's cancer: diagnosis, treatment, and prognosis, ed. 5, St. Louis, 1977, The C. V. Mosby Co.
60. del Regato, J., and Spjut, H.: Cancer of the skin. In del Regato, J., and Spjut, H., editors: Ackerman and del Regato's cancer: diagnosis, treatment, and prognosis, ed. 5, St. Louis, 1977, The C. V. Mosby Co.
61. del Regato, J., and Spjut, H.: Leukemia. In del Regato, J., and Spjut, H., editors: Ackerman and del Regato's cancer: diagnosis, treatment, and prognosis, ed. 5, St. Louis, 1977, The C. V. Mosby Co.
62. del Regato, J., and Spjut, H.: Malignant melanomas. In del Regato, J., and Spjut, H., editors: Ackerman and del Regato's cancer: diagnosis, treatment, and prognosis, ed. 5, St. Louis, 1977, The C. V. Mosby Co.
63. del Regato, J., and Spjut, H.: Tumors of the thyroid and parathyroid glands. In del Regato, J., and Spjut, H., editors: Ackerman and del Regato's cancer: diagnosis, treatment, and prognosis, ed. 5, St. Louis, 1977, The C. V. Mosby Co.
64. del Regato, J., and Spjut, H.: Urinary bladder. In del Regato, J., and Spjut, H., editors: Ackerman and del Regato's cancer: diagnosis, treatment, and prognosis, ed. 5, St. Louis, 1977, The C. V. Mosby Co.
65. DeVore, R.: Sunbathing and skin cancer, Publication No. 77-7021, Washington, D.C., 1977, U.S. Department of Health, Education and Welfare, Food and Drug Adminstration.
66. Division of Cancer Control and Rehabilitation, National Cancer Institute: Information for physicians: irradiation-related thyroid cancer, Publication No. 77-1120, Washington, D.C., 1977, U.S. Department of Health, Education and Welfare, Public Health Service, National Institutes of Health.
67. Dodd, G. R.: Present status of thermography, ultrasound, and mammography in breast cancer detection, Cancer **39**:2796, 1977.
68. Dolan, T.: Cancer of the female genital tract. In Rubin, P., editor: Clinical oncology for medical students and physicians, ed. 5, New York, 1978, American Cancer Society, Inc.
69. Durant, J., and Aomura, G.: Leukemia. In Nealon, T., editor: Management of the patient with cancer, ed. 2, Philadelphia, 1976, W. B. Saunders Co.
70. Early detection of oral cancer may save your life, Buffalo, N.Y., Department of Oral Medicine, State University of New York at Buffalo.
71. Editorial: Public awareness of cancer detection tests: results of a recent Gallup poll, CA **27**:255, 1977.
72. Elsebai, I.: Parasites in the etiology of cancer: bilharziasis and bladder cancer, CA **27**:100, 1977.
73. Engelman, M., and Schackner, S.: Oral cancer examination procedure, New York, 1966, American Cancer Society Professional Education Publication.
74. Fact sheet: Substances known to produce cancer in man, Bethesda, Md., 1974, U.S. Department of Health, Education and Welfare, National Cancer Institute.
75. Favus, M.: Thyroid cancer detection. Proceedings of the Fourth National Cancer Communications Conference, Publication No. 78-1463, Washington, D.C., 1977, U.S. Department of Health, Education and Welfare, Public Health Service, National Institutes of Health.
76. Fazio, V.: Early diagnosis of anorectal and colon carcinoma, Hosp. Med. **15**:66, 1979.
77. Feind, C.: The thyroid. In Nealon, T., editor: Management of the patient with cancer, Philadelphia, 1976, W. B. Saunders Co.
78. Foster, R., et al.: Breast self-examination practices and breast cancer stage, N. Engl. J. Med. **299**:265, 1978.
79. Frank, I.: Urologic and male genital cancers. In Rubin, P., editor: Clinical oncology for medical students and physicians, ed. 5, New York, 1978, American Cancer Society, Inc.

80. Franks, L. M.: Etiology, epidemiology, and pathology of prostatic cancer. Proceedings of the National Conference on Urologic Cancer, New York, 1973, American Cancer Society, Inc.
81. Fraumeni, J., and Mulvihill, J.: Who is at risk of colorectal cancer? In Schottenfeld, D., editor: Cancer epidemiology and prevention: current concepts, Springfield, Ill., 1975, Charles C Thomas, Publisher.
82. Frishman, W.: Involuntary smoking: cardiovascular effects of smoke on nonsmokers, Cardiovasc. Med., March, p. 289, 1979.
83. From the NIH: Treating diabetic retinopathy: guidelines for lung cancer screening, J.A.M.A. **241:**1581, 1979.
84. Furlow, W., et al.: Prostatic cancer: weighing the options, Patient Care **12:**120, 1978.
85. Gambassini, L.: Cytological mass screening of cancer of the uterine cervix in the province of Florence. In Maltoni, C., editor: Cancer detection and prevention, vol. 2, New York, 1974, American Elsevier Publishing Co.
86. Gardner, W. W., and Lyon, J. L.: Efficacy of cervical cytologic screening in the control of cervical cancer, Prev. Med. **6:**487, 1977.
87. Garfinkel, L.: Cigarette smoking among physicians and other health professionals, 1959-1972, CA **26:**373, 1976.
88. Gilbertsen, V.: Cancer of the prostate gland: results of early diagnosis and therapy undertaken for cure of the disease, J.A.M.A. **215:**81, 1971.
89. Gilbertsen, V.: Colo-rectal cancer: clinical trial/community outreach. Proceedings of the Fourth National Cancer Communications Conference, Publication No. 78-1463, Washington, D.C., 1977, U.S. Department of Health, Education and Welfare, Public Health Service, National Institutes of Health.
90. Gowen, G., et al.: Is teaching breast self-examination for cancer effective? Ill. Med. J. **102:**179, 1952.
91. Grabau, J., et al.: A public education program in self-examination for orofacial cancer, J. Am. Dent. Assoc. **96:**480, 1978.
92. Grabau, J., et al.: Oral/facial self-examination for early detection of cancer. In Nieburgs, H., editor: Prevention and detection of cancer. Part I—Prevention, New York, 1978, Marcel Dekker, Inc.
93. Grabstald, H.: Germinal tumors of the testes. CA **25:**82, 1975.
94. Greenwald, P., et al.: Effect of breast self-examination and routine physical examinations on breast cancer mortality, N. Engl. J. Med. **299:**271, 1978.
95. Gumport, S., Harris, M., and Kopf, A.: Diagnosis and management of common skin cancers, Publication No. 3373-PE, New York, 1974, American Cancer Society Professional Education Publication.
96. Gusberg, S. B.: An approach to the control of carcinoma of the endometrium, CA **23:**99, 1973.
97. Hall, D., et al.: Progress in manual breast examination, Cancer **40:**364, 1977.
98. Hammond, E.: Tobacco. In Fraumeni, J., editor: Persons at high risk of cancer: an approach to cancer etiology and control, New York, 1975, Academic Press, Inc.
99. Harris, C.: Respiratory carcinogenesis. In Straus, M., editor: Lung cancer: clinical diagnosis and treatment, New York, 1977, Grune & Stratton Inc.
100. Hastings, J.: Mass screening for colorectal cancer, Am. J. Surg. **127:**228, 1974.
101. Haynes, H.: The front line on skin cancers, Emergency Med. **10:**131, 1978.
102. Health hazards of chromate pigments and paints: hexavalent chromium, Washington, D.C., 1979, U.S. Department of Labor, Occupational Safety and Health Administration Publications Office.
103. Health hazards of inorganic arsenic, Washington, D.C., 1979, U.S. Department of Labor, Occupational Safety and Health Administration Publications Office.
104. Heinemann, E., and Estes, N.: Assessing alcoholic patients, Am. J. Nurs. **76:**786, 1976.
105. Henderson, B., Gerkins, V., and Pike, M.: Sexual factors and pregnancy. In Fraumeni, J., editor: Persons at high risk of cancer: an approach to cancer etiology and control, New York, 1975, Academic Press, Inc., p. 277.
106. Herbst, A., and Cole, P.: Epidemiologic and clinical aspects of clear cell adenocarcinoma in young women. In Herbst, A., editor: Intrauterine exposure to diethylstilbestrol in the human, Chicago, 1978, The American College of Obstetricans and Gynecologists.
107. Herbst, A., Scully, R., and Robboy, S.: Effects of maternal DES ingestion on the female genital tract, Hosp. Prac. **10:**51, 1975.
108. Higginson, J.: Cancer etiology and prevention. In Fraumeni, J., editor: Persons at high risk of cancer: an approach to cancer etiology and control, New York, 1975, Academic Press, Inc.
109. Higginson, J., Terracini, B., and Agthe, C.: Nutrition and cancer: dietary deficiency and modifications. In Schottenfeld, D., editor: Cancer epidemiology and prevention: current concepts,

Springfield, Ill., 1975, Charles C Thomas, Publisher.

110. Hill, C.: Thyroid cancer—iatrogenic and otherwise, CA **26:**160, 1976.
111. Homesley, H.: Evaluation of the abnormal Pap smear, Am. Fam. Physician **16:**190, 1977.
112. Hoover, R., and Fraumeni, J.: Drugs. In Fraumeni, J., editor: Persons at high risk of cancer: an approach to cancer etiology and control, New York, 1975, Academic Press, Inc.
113. Horton, J., and Caputo, T.: Gynecologic cancer. In Horton, J., and Hill, G., editors: Clinical oncology, Philadelphia, 1977, W. B. Saunders Co.
114. Horwitz, R., and Feinstein, A.: Intravaginal estrogen creams and endometrial cancer, J.A.M.A. **241:**1266, 1979.
115. Hubbard, S.: Ovarian carcinoma: an overview of current concepts in diagnosis and management, Cancer Nurs. **1:**116, 1978.
116. Jablon, S.: Radiation. In Fraumeni, J., editor: Persons at high risk of cancer: an approach to cancer etiology and control, New York, 1975, Academic Press, Inc.
117. Jepsen, L.: Malignant melanoma: rare cancer, unique problems, Nursing '77 **7:**38, 1977.
118. Jewett, H.: Cancer of the bladder: diagnosis and staging. Proceedings of the National Conference on Urologic Cancer, Publication No. 3080-PE, New York, 1973, American Cancer Society Professional Education Publication.
119. Jick, H., et al.: Replacement estrogens and endometrial cancer, N. Engl. J. Med. **300:**218, 1979.
120. Keller, K.: Self-examination for breast cancer: an analysis of women's attitudes and actions toward this medical necessity, Today's Clinician, May, p. 49, 1978.
121. Kennedy, B. J.: New concepts in testicular cancer. In Sutnick, A., and Engstrom, P., editors: Oncologic medicine: clinical topics and practical management, Baltimore, 1976, University Park Press.
122. Keough, G., and Niebel, H.: Oral cancer detection: a nursing responsibility, Am. J. Nurs. **73:**684, 1973.
123. Kessler, I.: Venereal factors in human cervical cancer: evidence from marital clusters, Cancer **39:**1912, 1977.
124. Kessler, I, and Aurelian, L.: Uterine cervix. In Schottenfeld, D., editor: Cancer epidemiology and prevention: current concepts, Springfield, Ill., 1975, Charles C Thomas, Publisher.
125. Kessler, I., and Clark, P.: Saccharin, cyclamate, and human bladder cancer: no evidence of an association, J.A.M.A. **240:**349, 1978.
126. Key, M.: Occupational diseases: a guide to their recognition, Publication No. 77-181, Washington, D.C., 1977, U.S. Department of Health, Education and Welfare.
127. Kissin, B., et al.: Head and neck cancer in alcoholics: the relationship to drinking, smoking and dietary patterns, J.A.M.A. **224:**1174, 1973.
128. Klein, L.: Prostatic carcinoma, N. Engl. J. Med. **300:**824, 1979.
129. Kraft, C., et al.: Where R.N.s run a mobile cancer detection unit, RN **37:**27, 1974.
130. Krull, E., Fellman, A., and Fabian, L.: White lesions of the mouth, Clin. Symp. **25:**2, 1973.
131. Landau, R.: What you should know about estrogens, or the perils of Pauline, J.A.M.A. **241:**47, 1979.
132. Lawrence, W.: Carcinoma of the stomach, CA **23:**286, 1973.
133. Leffall, L., and Stearns, M.: Early diagnosis of colorectal cancer, Publication No. 3311-PE, New York, 1974, American Cancer Society Professional Education Publication.
134. Leis, H.: Risk factors in breast cancer, Assoc. Operating Room Nurses' J. **22:**723, 1975.
135. Leis, H.: The diagnosis of breast cancer, CA **27:**209, 1977.
136. Letton, A. H., Wilson, J., and Mason, E.: The value of breast screening in women less than fifty years of age, Cancer **40:**1, 1977.
137. Libshitz, H.: Thermography of the breast: current status and future expectations, J.A.M.A. **238:**1953, 1977.
138. Lichtman, M., and Klemperer, M.: The leukemias. In Rubin, P., editor: Clinical oncology for medical students and physicians, ed. 5, New York, 1978, American Cancer Society.
139. Lowenfels, A., and Anderson, M.: Diet and cancer, Cancer **39:**1809, 1977.
140. Luthra, U.: Cancer of uterine cervix—preventable disease: a study of Indian women. In Maltoni, C., editor: Cancer detection and prevention, vol. 2, New York, 1974, American Elsevier Publishing Co.
141. Lynch, H., Lynch, J., and Kraft, C.: A new approach to cancer screening and education, Geriatrics **28:**152, 1973.
142. Lynch, H., et al.: Multiphasic mobile cancer screening: a positive approach to early cancer detection and control, Cancer **30:**774, 1972.
143. Lynch, J., et al.: Mobile cancer screening: epidemiologic and cancer control model. In Nieburgs, H., editor: Prevention and detection of cancer. Part II—Detection. Vol. 1—High risk markers, New York, 1978, Marcel Dekker, Inc.

144. Macdonald, E.: Epidemiological aspects. In Rubin, P., editor: Cancer of the gastrointestinal tract. Part one (esophagus, stomach, small intestine), Publication No. 3007.08-PE, New York, 1974, American Cancer Society Professional Education Publication.
145. Macdonald, J.: Diagnosis and treatment of colorectal cancer, Med. Times. **106:**105, 1978.
146. McGrath, D.: North Carolina thyroid alert program. Proceedings of the Fourth National Cancer Communications Conference, Publication No. 78-1463, Washington, D.C., 1977, U.S. Department of Health, Education and Welfare, Public Health Service, National Institutes of Health.
147. Maisin, H., et al.: Relative rates of breast and cervix cancers in mass screening: evaluation of high-risk groups. In Maltoni, C., editor: Cancer detection and prevention, vol. 2, New York, 1974, American Elsevier Publishing Co.
148. Malasanos, L., et al.: Assessment of the male genitalia and assessment of the inguinal area for hernias. In Malasanos, L., Barkauskas, V., Moss, M., and Stoltenberg-Allen, K., editors: Health assessment, St. Louis, 1977, The C. V. Mosby Co.
149. Mammography screening: safe at 35? Med. World News **20:**9, 1979.
150. Mancuso, T.: Prevention and control of occupational exposures: an overview. In Nieburgs, H., editor: Prevention and detection of cancer. Part I—Prevention, New York, 1978, Marcel Dekker, Inc., p. 1857.
151. Manny, E., Brown, R., and Shaver, J.: Gonad shielding in diagnostic radiology: recommendation of the FDA and ACR, Postgrad. Med. **65:**208, 1979.
152. Maor, D., et al.: Carcinoma of the lung and cigarette smoking, J.A.M.A. **239:**2766, 1978.
153. Martini, N.: Lung cancer—an overview, Cancer Nurs. **1:**31, 1978.
154. Melamed, M., et al.: Preliminary report of the lung cancer detection program in New York, Cancer **39:**369, 1977.
155. Mihm, M. C., et al.: Early detection of primary cutaneous malignant melanoma: a color atlas, N. Engl. J. Med. **289:**989, 1973.
156. Miller, D.: A new look at cancer detection, Public Health **87:**67, 1973.
157. Miller, S.: The detection of asymptomatic colorectal cancer, Am. Fam. Physician **18:**89, 1978.
158. Milner, L.: An early cancer detection questionnaire for public education distribution, Ill. Med. J. **153:**24, 1979.
159. Minna, J.: What you can do for your patients with lung cancer, Med. Times **106:**68, 1978.
160. Mitchell, C.: Assessment of alcohol abuse, Nurs. Outlook **24:**511, 1976.
161. More than a paycheck: an introduction to occupational cancer, Washington, D.C., 1978, U.S. Department of Labor, Occupational Safety and Health Administration Publication Office.
162. Morrison, A.: Some social and medical characteristics of army men with testicular cancer, Am. J. Epidemiol. **104:**511, 1976.
163. Morton, J.: Alimentary tract cancer. In Rubin, P., editor: Clinical oncology for medical students and physicians, ed. 5, New York, 1978, American Cancer Society, Inc.
164. Morton, P.: Proctosigmoidoscopy in asymptomatic men: a 24-month study, CA **28:**211, 1978.
165. Mostofi, F. K.: Testicular tumors: epidemiologic, etiologic, and pathologic features. Proceedings of the National Conference on Urologic Cancer, Publication No. 3080-PE, New York, 1973, American Cancer Society, Inc.
166. Mostofi, F. K.: Epidemiology and pathology of tumors of human testis. In Grundmann, E., and Vahlensieck, W., editors: Tumors of the male genital system, New York, 1977, Springer-Verlag New York, Inc.
167. Muir, C.: International variation in high-risk populations. In Fraumeni, J., editor: Persons at high risk of cancer: an approach to cancer etiology and control, New York, 1975, Academic Press, Inc.
168. Mulvihill, J.: Congenital and genetic diseases. In Fraumeni, J., editor: Persons at high risk of cancer: an approach to cancer etiology and control, New York, 1975, Academic Press, Inc.
169. Murphy, G.: Prostate cancer, Publication No. 3371-PE, New York, 1974, American Cancer Society Professional Education Publication.
170. Murphy, G.: Prostate cancer: progress and change, CA **28:**104, 1978.
171. Murphy, G., Karr, J., and Chu, T.: Prostatic acid phosphatase: where are we? CA **28:**258, 1978.
172. Murray, B., and Wilcox, L.: Testicular self-examination, Am. J. Nurs. **78:**2075, 1978.
173. Mustacchi, P., and Millmore, D.: Racial and occupational variations in cancer of the testis: San Francisco 1956-1965, J. Natl. Cancer Inst. **56:**717, 1976.
174. Myers, E.: The oral cavity and oropharynx. In Nealon, T., editor: Management of the patient with cancer, ed. 2, Philadelphia, 1976, W. B. Saunders Co.
175. Neeman, R., and Neeman, M.: Complexities of smoking education, J. Sch. Health **45:**17, 1975.
176. Nelson, J., and Nikrui, N.: The cervix. In Nealon,

T., editor: Management of the patient with cancer, ed. 2, Philadelphia, 1976, W. B. Saunders Co.

177. New test for prostate cancer advised as routine, Med. World News **19:**13, 1978.
178. Nikolaus, D.: Cancer screening in the physician's office. In Nieburgs, H., editor: Prevention and detection of cancer. Part II—Detection. Vol. 1—High risk markers, New York, 1978, Marcel Dekker, Inc.
179. 1978 Cancer facts and figures, Publication No. 5008-LE, New York, 1977, American Cancer Society, Inc., p. 3.
180. 1980 Cancer facts and figures, Publication No. 5008-LE, New York, 1979, American Cancer Society, Inc.
181. Nonsmoker's rights. A public health issue, J.A.M.A. **239:**2125, 1978.
182. Nowell, P.: Cytogenetics. In Becker, F., editor: Cancer. Etiology: chemical and physical carcinogenesis, New York, 1975, Plenum Publishing Corp.
183. Occupational history, the Mount Sinai School of Medicine of the City University of New York, Environmental Sciences Laboratory.
184. Office urology: when your patient fears testicular cancer, Patient Care **9:**102, 1975.
185. Oleske, D.: Cancer prevention and nursing practice, Occup. Health Nurs. **23:**13, 1976.
186. Osterkamp, R., and Whitten, J. B.: The etiology and pathogenesis of oral cancer, CA **23:**28, 1973.
187. Papaioannou, A. N.: The etiology of human breast cancer, New York, 1974, Springer-Verlag New York, Inc.
188. Parkes, H.: Mass or selective screening for bladder cancer. In Maltoni, C., editor: Cancer detection and prevention, vol. 2, New York, 1974, American Elsevier Publishing Co., p. 188.
189. Patchefsky, A., et al.: The pathology of breast cancer detected by mass population screening, Cancer **40:**1659, 1977.
190. Pomerance, W.: The cancer-screening dilemma, Postgrad. Med. **64:**42, 1978.
191. Pound of prevention, ounce of cure? Med. World News **19:**46, 1978.
192. Presant, C., Van Amburg, A., and Avioli, L.: Breast cancer, Arch. Intern. Med. **139:**452, 1979.
193. Prout, G.: Diagnosis and staging of prostatic carcinoma. Proceedings of the National Conference on Urologic Cancer, New York, 1973, American Cancer Society, Inc.
194. Public exposure to air pollution from tobacco smoke, Washington, D.C., 1972, U.S. Department of Health, Education and Welfare, Public Health Service, Health Sciences and Mental Health Administration.
195. Rapp, F., and Reed, C.: The viral etiology of cancer, Cancer **40:**419, 1977.
196. Rebstock, K.: Communications in head and neck cancer. Proceedings of the Fourth National Cancer Communications Conference, Publication No. 78-1463, Washington, D.C., 1977, U.S. Department of Health, Education and Welfare, Public Health Service, National Institutes of Health.
197. Reed, S.: Assessing the patient with an alcohol problem, Nurs. Clin. North Am. **11:**483, 1976.
198. Rhoads, J., and Mackie, J.: The colon. In Nealon, T., editor: Management of the patient with cancer, ed. 2, Philadelphia, 1976, W. B. Saunders Co.
199. Rich, A.: On the frequency of occurrence of occult carcinoma of the prostate, CA **29:**115, 1979.
200. Richardson, J.: Colorectal cancer: a mass screening and education program, Geriatrics **32:**123, 1977.
201. Richmond, J.: Physician advisory—health effects of asbestos, Washington, D.C., 1978, U.S. Department of Health, Education and Welfare, Surgeon General of the Public Health Service.
202. Risk of cancer, dysplasia for DES daughters found "very low," J.A.M.A. **241:**1555, 1979.
203. Rosemond, G., and Maier, W.: Breast cancer, New York, 1974, Medcom, Inc., p. 13.
204. Rothman, K.: Alcohol. In Fraumeni, J., editor: Persons at high risk of cancer: an approach to cancer etiology and control, New York, 1975, Academic Press, Inc.
205. Rubin, P.: Comment: early detection. In Rubin, P., editor: Cancer of the gastrointestinal tract. Part one (esophagus, stomach, small intestine), Publication No. 3007.08-PE, New York, 1974, American Cancer Society Professional Education Publication, p. 39.
206. Rubin, P.: Gastric cancer diagnosis. In Rubin, P., editor: Clinical oncology for medical students and physicians, ed. 5, New York, 1978, American Cancer Society, Inc., p. 28.
207. Rubio, C. A.: The false negative smear. II. The trapping effect of collecting instruments, Obstet. Gynecol. **49:**576, 1977.
208. Savlov, E.: Breast cancer. In Rubin, P., editor: Clinical oncology for medical students and physicians, ed. 5, New York, 1978, American Cancer Society, Inc.
209. Sayler, C., et al.: Mammographic screening: value in diagnosis of early breast cancer, J.A.M.A. **238:**872, 1977.
210. Schade, R.: Cytology in early diagnosis. In Rubin, P., editor: Cancer of the gastrointestinal tract. Part one (esophagus, stomach, small intestine), Publication No. 3007.08-PE, New York, 1974,

American Cancer Society Professional Education Publication.

211. Schottenfeld, D.: Patient risk factors and the detection of early cancer. In Kruse, L., Reese, J., and Hart, L., editors: Cancer: pathophysiology, etiology and management, St. Louis, 1979, The C. V. Mosby Co.
212. Schumann, G., and Colon, V.: Sputum cytology, Am. Fam. Physician **19:**81, 1979.
213. Schwartz, G., et al.: Mass screening for breast disease: results, problems and expectations, Obstet. Gynecol. **48:**137, 1976.
214. Seaman, W.: Editorial: Radiation risks: progress and problems, Hosp. Prac. **14:**11, 1979.
215. Seidman, H.: Screening for breast cancer in younger women: life expectancy gains and losses: an analysis according to risk indicator groups, CA **27:**66, 1977.
216. Selikoff, I., and Hammond, E.: Asbestos-associated disease in United States shipyards, CA **28:**87, 1978.
217. Seydel, H., Chait, A., and Gmelich, J.: Cancer of the lung, New York, 1975, John Wiley & Sons, Inc., p. 12.
218. Shapiro, S.: Screening for early detection of cancer and heart disease, Bull. N. Y. Acad. Med. **51:**82, 1975.
219. Shedd, D.: Clinical characteristics of early oral cancer. In Rubin, P., editor: Current concepts in cancer: cancer of the head and neck, New York, 1971, American Cancer Society, Inc.
220. Shelley, W.: Consultations in dermatology, Philadelphia, 1972, W. B. Saunders Co.
221. Shils, M.: Nutrition and cancer: dietary deficiency and modifications. In Schottenfeld, D., editor: Cancer epidemiology and prevention: current concepts, Springfield, Ill., 1975, Charles C Thomas, Publisher.
222. Shimkin, M.: Overview: preventive oncology. In Fraumeni, J., editor: Persons at high risk of cancer: an approach to cancer etiology and control, New York, 1975, Academic Press, Inc.
223. Shortridge, L., and McLain, B.: Primary care and prostate cancer, Nurse Pract. **4:**25, 1979.
224. Silverberg, E.: Cancer of the colon and rectum: statistical data, Publication No. 3019, New York, 1973, American Cancer Society Professional Education Publication.
225. Silverberg, E.: Urologic cancer: statistical epidemiological information, Publication No. 3020-PE, New York, 1973, American Cancer Society Professional Education Publication.
226. Silverberg, E.: Gynecologic cancer: statistical and epidemiological information, New York, 1975, American Cancer Society Professional Education Publication.
227. Smith, P. G.: Leukemia and other cancers following radiation treatment of pelvic disease, Cancer **39:**1901, 1977.
228. Smoking: for most, a sentence to nicotine addiction, Med. World News **20:**61, 1979.
229. Soetebier, W.: Colo-rectal cancer: clinical trial/community outreach. Proceedings of the Fourth National Cancer Communications Conference, Publication No. 78-1463, Washington, D.C., 1977, U.S. Department of Health, Education and Welfare, Public Health Service, National Institutes of Health.
230. Spalt, L.: Screening for alcoholism, Ill. Med. J. **152:**348, 1978.
231. Stanhope, C. R., and Hofmeister, F.: Axioms on the detection, diagnosis, and treatment of uterine cancer, Hosp. Med. **14:**91, 1978.
232. Storer, J.: Radiation carcinogenesis. In Becker, F., editor: Cancer. Etiology: chemical and physical carcinogenesis, New York, 1977, Plenum Publishing Corp.
233. Strax, P.: Screening for breast cancer, Clin. Obstet. Gynecol. **20:**781, 1977.
234. Strax, P.: Mammography—is it right for your patients? Mod. Med. **46:**44, 1978.
235. Stromborg, M., and Nord, S. B.: A cancer detection clinic: patient motivation and satisfaction, Nurse Pract. **4:**10, 1979.
236. Sutnick, A., Miller, D., and Yarbo, J.: A new approach to cancer detection. In Maltoni, C., editor: Cancer detection and prevention, vol. 2, New York, 1974, American Elsevier Publishing Co.
237. Sutnick, A., et al.: Population cancer screening, Cancer **38:**1367, 1976.
238. Tartaglia, A.: Leukemia in adults. In Horton, J., and Hill, G., editors: Clinical oncology, Philadelphia, 1977, W. B. Saunders Co.
239. Templeton, A. C.: Acquired diseases. In Fraumeni, J., editor: Persons at high risk of cancer: an approach to cancer etiology and control, New York, 1975, Academic Press, Inc.
240. Teppo, L., Pakkanen, M., and Hakulinen, T.: Sunlight as a risk factor of malignant melanoma of the skin, Cancer **41:**2018, 1978.
241. Townsend, D.: Techniques of examination and screening of the DES-exposed female. In Herbst, A., editor: Intrauterine exposure to diethylstilbestrol in the human, Chicago, 1978, The American College of Obstetricians and Gynecologists.
242. Trial compares enzyme tests for prostate Ca . . . , Med. World News **19:**73, 1978.
243. TSE: testicular self-examination, Memorial

Sloan-Kettering Cancer Center, New York, New York, 1979.
244. Tulinius, H.: Epidemiology of prostate carcinoma. In Grundmann, E., and Vahlensieck, W., editors: Recent results in cancer research: tumors of the male genital system, New York, 1977, Springer-Verlag New York, Inc.
245. Wakefield, J.: Education of the public. In Fraumeni, J., editor: Persons at high risk of cancer: an approach to cancer etiology and control, New York, 1975, Academic Press, Inc.
246. Wallace, S., and Jing, B.: Lymphangiography: diagnosis of nodal metastases from testicular malignancies. In Rubin, P., editor: Cancer of the urogenital tract. Part two (prostate and testes), Publication No. 3007.06-PE, New York, 1970, American Cancer Society Professional Education Publication.
247. The Walton Report: cervical cancer screening programs, Can. Med. Assoc. J. **114:**1, 1976.
248. Weber, A., Jermini, C., and Grandjean, E.: Irritating effects on man of air pollution due to cigarette smoke, Am. J. Public Health **66:**672, 1976.
249. Weinstein, G.: Skin cancer: recognition and treatment. Famous Teachings in Modern Medicine, New York, 1973, Medcom, Inc.
250. Werner, S.: Physical examination. In Werner, S., editor: The thyroid, ed. 2, New York, 1971, Harper & Row, Publishers.
251. What causes cancer on the farm? Med. World News **20:**31, 1979.
252. Whelan, E.: What is your cancer risk? Med. Times **105:**96, 1977.
253. White, L., et al.: Screening of cancer by nurses, Cancer Nurs. **1:**15, 1978.
254. Whitmore, W.: Bladder cancer, Publication No. 3405-PE, New York, 1978, American Cancer Society Professional Education Publication, p. 3.
255. Williams, S.: Colo-rectal cancer: clinical trial/community outreach. Proceedings of the Fourth National Cancer Communications Conference, Publication No. 78-1463, Washington, D.C., 1977, U.S. Department of Health, Education and Welfare, Public Health Service, National Institutes of Health.
256. Willis, I.: Sunlight, aging, and skin cancer, Geriatrics **33:**33, 1978.
257. Winawer, S., and Sherlock, P.: Approach to screening and diagnosis in colorectal cancer, Semin. Oncol. **3:**387, 1976.
258. Woodruff, M., Zornow, D., and Olson, H.: Cancer of the urologic and male reproductive system. In Horton, J., and Hill, G., editors: Clinical oncology, Philadelphia, 1977, W. B. Saunders Co.
259. Woods, N.: Human sexuality in health and illness, ed. 2, St. Louis, 1979, The C. V. Mosby Co.
260. Wynder, E.: Etiological aspects of squamous cancers of the head and neck. In Rubin, P., editor: Current concepts in cancer: cancer of the head and neck, New York, 1971, American Cancer Society, Inc.
261. Wynder, E., and Goldsmith, R.: The epidemiology of bladder cancer, Cancer **40:**1246, 1977.
262. Wynder, E., and Hoffmann, D.: Tobacco and health: a societal challenge, N. Engl. J. Med. **300:**894, 1979.
263. Wynder, E., and Reddy, B.: Metabolic epidemiology of colorectal cancer. Proceedings of the American Cancer Society's Second National Conference on Cancer of the Colon and Rectum, Publication No. 3032-PE, New York, 1974, American Cancer Society, Inc.
264. Wynder, E., and Reddy, B.: The etiology of cancer of the large bowel. In Maltoni, C., editor: Cancer detection and prevention, vol. 2, New York, 1974, American Elsevier Publishing Co.
265. Wynder, E. L., MacCornack, F. A., and Stellman, S. D.: The epidemiology of breast cancer in 785 United States Caucasian women, Cancer **41:**2341, 1978.
266. Ultmann, J., and Stein, R.: Treating lung cancer: a progress report, Curr. Prescribing, Sept., p. 89, 1977.
267. Upton, A.: Physical carcinogenesis: radiation—history and sources. In Becker, F., editor: Cancer. Etiology: chemical and physical carcinogenesis, New York, 1977, Plenum Publishing Corp.
268. Uranium miners' lung cancer risk rivals smokers', Med. World News **19:**32, 1978.
269. Zamcheck, N.: CEA in cancer of the colon. In Maltoni, C., editor: Cancer detection and prevention, vol. 2, New York, 1974, American Elsevier Publishing Co.

ADDITIONAL READING

The following books and articles are recommended for nurses interested in additional information on cancer screening and physical assessment.

American Journal of Nursing Programmed Instruction: History taking, examination of the eyes, head and neck, ear, abdomen, cardiovascular system, respiratory, neurological, and genital examination of the male and female, New York, American Journal of Nursing.

Bates, B.: A guide to physical examination, Philadelphia, 1974, J. B. Lippincott Co.

Braverman, I.: Skin signs of systemic disease, Philadelphia, 1970, W. B. Saunders Co.

Brown, M., et al.: Student manual of physical examination, Philadelphia, 1977, J. B. Lippincott Co.
DeGowin, E. L., and DeGowin, R. L.: Bedside diagnostic examination, ed. 3, New York, 1976, Macmillan Inc.
Fraumeni, J., editor: Persons at high risk of cancer: an approach to cancer etiology and control, New York, 1975, Academic Press, Inc.
G. I. Series: Physical examination of the abdomen, Richmond, Virginia, 1972, A. H. Robins Co.
Mahoney, E., Verdisco, L., and Shortridge, L.: How to collect and record a health history, Philadelphia, 1976, J. B. Lippincott Co.
Malasanos, L., Barkauskas, V., Moss, M., and Stoltenberg-Allen, K.: Health assessment, St. Louis, 1977, The C. V. Mosby Co.
Prior, J., and Silberstein, J.: Physical diagnosis, ed. 4, St. Louis, 1973, The C. V. Mosby Co.
Sana, J., and Judge, R., editors: Physical appraisal methods in nursing practice, Boston, 1975, Little, Brown & Co.
Sauve, M. J., and Pecherer, A.: Concepts and skills in physical assessment, Philadelphia, 1977, W. B. Saunders Co.
Schottenfeld, D.: Cancer epidemiology and prevention: current concepts, Springfield, Ill., 1975, Charles C Thomas, Publisher.
Stromborg, M., and Stromborg, P.: Primary care assessment and management skills for nurses: a self-assessment, Philadelphia, 1979, J. B. Lippincott Co.
Van Allen, M.: Pictorial manual of neurologic tests, Chicago, 1975, Year Book Medical Publishers, Inc.
White, L., et al.: Cancer screening and detection manual for nurses, New York, 1979, McGraw-Hill Book Co.

IV

MULTIMODALITY CANCER TREATMENT AND ITS IMPLICATIONS ON NURSING CARE

11

Multimodality cancer treatment—a challenge for nursing

LISA BEGG MARINO

The fact that a book such as *Cancer Nursing* has been written demonstrates the advances that have taken place in cancer treatment. The advances, which led to increased client survival, came about slowly at first. Surgery led the way with refinements in the various procedures based on the presumed natural history of cancer. Next, radiation therapy advanced through improvement in equipment as well as understanding of more precise techniques in planning and delivering radiation treatments. Then, a plateau occurred until the wider application of chemotherapy took place. This additional form of therapy led to greater improvements in client survival because of its ability to control disseminated disease. All three of these treatment forms, or modalities, were present by the 1950's, but it was not until the 1960's and 1970's that significant improvements in client survival were obtained. These more recent advances are not generally represented in the overall statistics cited in Chapter 2 because much of the work took place in small research projects. It has been only recently that widespread application of these findings has occurred. For this reason, the major cancer sites affected by the successes registered through the application of multimodality cancer treatment will be discussed. The term "multimodality" cancer treatment is defined as treatment given in combinations.

The combinations can be any or all of the following: surgery, radiation therapy, chemotherapy, and tumor immunotherapy. Detailed definitions of each of these forms of therapy along with the scientific rationale for each are presented in the following chapters. Therapy employing these modalities is responsible for saving many clients' lives.

RECENT ADVANCES IN CANCER TREATMENT

Substantial increases in client survival have occurred in a number of cancers during the last two decades. A summary of these advances, described below, was given in March and June of 1979 in response to congressional inquiries about the impact of the National Cancer Program and the extent of cancer in the aged.[2]

Breast cancer

Breast cancer affects 7% of all American women. Advances in treating this cancer have occurred based on information obtained through laboratory research on preclinical tumor models, hormonal receptors, pilot studies in advanced cancers, and clinical research on the surgical procedures and adjuvant therapy of breast cancer.

The discovery of hormonal receptors in breast cancer tissue, particularly estrogen-binding proteins, during the late 1960's has helped to identify clients who have tumors that are hormonally dependent. This discovery now permits the clinician to more accurately identify clients who will benefit from hormonal manipulation. The manipulation can be either ablative procedures such as oophorectomy or additive therapy with hormones. For those clients who do not have hormone receptors, research is underway to evaluate the efficacy of administering chemotherapy instead of hormonal therapy.

Research on more limited surgical procedures is underway to determine if these procedures will give comparable results in survival while minimizing the morbidity frequently associated with the more traditional mastectomy procedures. One of these research studies, the National Surgical Adjuvant Breast Project, is demonstrating comparable survival in clients treated with total mastectomy with or without radiation therapy as compared with the group that underwent radical mastectomy. This same group, along with a separate project based in Milan, Italy, has demonstrated added benefit to adjuvant chemotherapy following mastectomy. These results are still preliminary, but differences have been documented in premenopausal women with more than three axillary lymph nodes invaded by cancer. The premenopausal group constitutes one third of the total new cases of breast cancer.

In the area of advanced breast cancer treatment, improved therapies are available so that significant control for a period of years can be achieved.

Osteogenic sarcoma

Osteogenic sarcoma, striking predominantly young people, carried an 80% mortality rate postamputation until recently. Within the mid to late 1970's, vast improvement in client survival has been achieved. Now, 60% of clients achieve disease-free survival for 5 years. For those clients who suffer a recurrence, surgery has been very successful in removing solitary metastatic disease sites. The natural history of this tumor follows a hematogenous metastatic pattern to the lungs with clients generally dying from problems associated with this pulmonary metastases rather than the primary site. Postsurgical chemotherapy has been the principal reason for the increased survival, with additional surgery to remove solitary lung metastasis increasing survival to nearly 70% in some research studies.

Nonseminomatous testicular cancer

Nonseminomatous testicular cancer is another cancer whose target is frequently the young. Until the 1960's, this form of cancer was overwhelmingly fatal. Treatment successes came first in the advanced stages with a high rate of short-term regressions. Unfortunately, many clients still died as long-term remissions did not occur. During the 1970's, however, complete remissions were obtained in 80% of the clients, with 50% achieving total cure. These dramatic increases resulted from treatment with multiple chemotherapeutic drugs and the discovery of tumor markers, which allowed the monitoring of residual tumor tissue levels during therapy. Research is now underway to test the adjuvant use of chemotherapy to increase client survival still further.

Small cell and epidermoid carcinoma of the lung

Of the 108,000 lung cancers expected in 1979, 20,000 of them were small cell carcinomas; epidermoid carcinomas constitute another 20,000 cases. Prior to 1972, no effective therapy was available for small cell carcinoma, which had a median survival of only 2 months. Now, chemotherapy and, in selected cases, radiation therapy have achieved a median survival of 1 year; some clients have remained alive for over 2 years.

Epidermoid carcinoma survival statistics have been improved in those clients who have a surgically resectable cancer. Following surgery, intrapleural bacillus Calmette-Guérin is placed in the tumor bed and has led to a preliminary increase in survival.

Acute leukemia in adults

Unlike acute leukemia in childhood, the adult form was a rapidly fatal disease until the 1970's. Most clients died within a matter of weeks or months. The turnabout came after the discovery of two chemotherapeutic agents, daunorubicin and cytosine arabinoside, that individually achieved complete remissions in 40% and 20% of clients, respectively. Research employing both drugs in combination has led to the first long-term survival gains, with 12% of clients surviving for more than 4 years.

Soft tissue sarcoma

Soft tissue sarcomas, affecting mainly children and young adults, have been previously managed by radical surgery. Recurrence rates were high in spite of this approach. The addition of chemotherapy increased response rates to more than 50% and in some cases has replaced the radical surgery with equivalent results. This means that less radical surgery can be undertaken if chemotherapy and radiation therapy are given. This research represents one of the better models for demonstrating increased survival while minimizing morbidity.

Non-Hodgkin's lymphoma

Substantial progress has been obtained in both adult and pediatric forms of non-Hodgkin's lymphoma.

With adults, the early stages of disease have benefited from radiation therapy followed by combination chemotherapy. The more advanced stages have long benefited from combination chemotherapy.

Pediatric non-Hodgkin's lymphomas are different from the adult types, primarily because of the higher incidence of abdominal disease and subsequent transition to refractive acute leukemia. Now, treatment consists of surgical resection and radiation therapy, with a 70% to 80% cure rate in children with limited disease. One of the more difficult disease subsets, mediastinal lymphoma, had been virtually 100% fatal but in a research study employing combination therapy is now demonstrating an 88% 3-year survival rate.

Hodgkin's disease, another form of lymphoma, has been very successfully treated with multimodalities and will be discussed separately later in this chapter.

Ovarian cancer

Although ovarian cancer is the fourth commonest form of gynecologic cancer, it is the leading cause of death within this group of cancers. Research underway to test combination versus single-agent chemotherapy is demonstrating an added benefit from the additional agents. Since success has been achieved in the advanced stages, work is underway to test adjuvant therapy with chemotherapy and radiation therapy in the earlier stages of ovarian cancer.

Colorectal cancers

Along with the lung cancer, colorectal cancers represent the most common sites of cancer in the United States. These large numbers, in excess of 100,000 new cases each year, make it even more tragic that the mainstay of treatment, surgical resection, cures only 40% of the clients. Research utilizing combination versus single-agent chemotherapy in clients with advanced disease is establishing the added benefit from the combination of agents. Now, studies involving adjuvant therapy are underway to see if high-risk groups can benefit from earlier use of chemotherapy, immunotherapy, and, in the case of rectal cancer, postoperative radiotherapy. It is still too early to confirm the long-term benefits of these treatments, but there is at least preliminary data to indicate progress is being made in saving more lives.

Gastric cancer

Gastric cancer, until recently, has been a difficult disease to treat effectively. Now, it appears that modest gains are being made in both early stages and advanced stages of this disease through the use of combination chemotherapy. Median survival of clients with advanced disease has doubled from 6 months to more than 1 year.

Bladder cancer

Before the early 1970's, the 5-year survival rate in clients with bladder cancer was less than 30%. This low rate occurred despite the use of surgical resection and radiation therapy. Fortunately, treatments have been refined and chemotherapy has been added with a doubling in survival rate. Work is continuing to increase the survival rate still further along with initiating adjuvant therapy research.

Malignant melanoma

Malignant melanoma is one of the more fatal tumors known and has been difficult to treat because of problems in accurately staging the extent of disease and determining groups of high-risk clients who would benefit from additional treatment given early. Improvements are coming slowly, with preliminary studies showing that adjuvant chemotherapy and immunotherapy improve survival somewhat. Work is continuing in this area.

Brain tumors

Multimodality treatment utilizing surgical resection, radiation therapy, and chemotherapy is demonstrating improvements in client survival in brain tumors. A major multi-institutional research project is focusing exclusively on these cancers and is the major reason information is being obtained. Newer studies employing the use of drugs that enhance the effects of radiation therapy are now underway.

Head and neck cancers

The multiple cancer sites that are commonly referred to as "head and neck" cancer have been difficult to treat because of the extensive surgical resections that are necessary and the propensity of these tumors to metastasize locally. Refinements in surgical resection, along with the use of radiation therapy, are controlling local disease more effectively. The addition of chemotherapy to the two other forms of treatment is being tested in clients after surgery and after recurrence has been confirmed. Since there are numerous drugs that have been shown to be effective against these cancers, it is hoped that earlier utilization of chemotherapy will prove beneficial.

Childhood cancers

Childhood cancers are one of the most promising areas in cancer treatment. Cancer, a major disease entity and a leading cause of death in children under the age of 15, has been more successfully treated in the last 20 years. Acute childhood leukemia underwent a complete reversal during the 1960's, with many children now surviving 10 to 15 years after diagnosis. Solid tumors, particularly Wilm's tumor, have also shown large increases in survival within the last 20 years. At present, more than 90% of the children diagnosed with Wilm's tumor can be cured through the use of surgery, radiation therapy, and chemotherapy. In selected cases, radiotherapy can be omitted, with surgery and chemotherapy maintaining similar rates of survival. Another solid tumor that has benefited from multimodality treatment is rhabdomyosarcoma. This cancer, treated with surgery, radiation therapy, and chemotherapy, is now 60% to 70% curable.

REASONS FOR IMPROVED CLIENT SURVIVAL

There are two principal reasons that more clients are surviving for longer periods: more accurate diagnostic and staging procedures and the treatment successes achieved through multimodality cancer treatment.

Improvements in the diagnosis and staging of cancer

Along with the changing treatment strategy, refinements or advances in diagnostic and staging procedures have contributed to increased client survival in three important categories: more precise diagnosis and staging allows treatment to be given only to tumor-bearing areas with avoidance of normal tissue; accurate determination of the extent of the disease provides for better timing and feasibility of the various treatment modalities; and periodic diagnostic reassessment enables the clinician to detect recurrence of disease earlier or to monitor treatment response or nonresponse.

History taking. A careful history has always been an important part of the client workup, but its importance in cancer has increased because of the recognition of the interrelatedness of family, social, marital, occupational history, and personal habits with the incidence of cancer. Along with the importance of this information to the client's own cancer, information from many clients might lead to the recognition of important clues to the etiology of cancers. Nutritional history is one example of how information might give clues to the etiology of the gastrointestinal cancers or breast cancers. Occupational history is very important in identifying common agents that may be carcinogenic.

Physical examination. The physical examination is important in ruling out benign conditions such as hemorrhoids following a complaint of rectal bleeding. Since most cancers initially present with a mass, it is important for the examiner (physician or nurse) to carefully evaluate the client. Physical examination performed during treatment aids the clinician in determining response to treatment.

Radiologic studies. Increasingly, diagnostic radiology is playing a more important role in cancer diagnosis, staging, and the monitoring of treatment response. The following is a list of the common studies performed to determine the presence and extent of the cancer:

- Plain chest radiographs
- Abdominal radiographs
- Barium examination of the gastrointestinal tract
- Lymphography
- Angiography
- Venography
- Intravenous pyelogram
- Mammography
- Xerography
- Radionuclide imaging or scanning
- Computed tomography
- Echography

These studies also provide information on response to or complications from treatment. This last function is becoming increasingly important as treatments become more toxic. For example, radiation pneumonitis and esophagitis must be promptly identified so that supportive measures can be instituted.

Laboratory studies. Laboratory values are used to identify a cancer, indicate information as to its extent, and aid in monitoring antitumor effects and toxicities. These tests fall into two broad categories: hematologic and serum chemistries. Additionally, a careful evaluation of these tests aids the clinician in determining if a client can undergo a certain form of treatment as well as continue to receive these treatments. Good examples are the hematologic perimeters that are evaluated prior to each chemotherapy cycle or the serum calcium level prior to initiation of hormonal therapy.

Clinical staging. Pretreatment planning must include pathologic or cytologic verification of the presence of cancer and its histologic classification to enable the clinician to make the best possible choice of treatment. Secondly, the extent of the disease is vitally important in determining which modality or modalities of treatment are most efficacious. Thirdly, staging categories should be compatible with larger series to enable comparison of treatment responses. To encourage this trend, most cancer facilities employ the TNM system, which was initially developed by the International Union Against Cancer (UICC).[1]

This staging system is employed only for previously untreated cancers and classifies the primary site of cancer and its extent and involvement. Table 11-1 gives the general criteria utilized for most of the cancer sites that have been categorized. Each of the specific sites has some tailoring to accommodate any unique features, or in the cases where clinical staging is impossible such as ovarian cancer, criteria are based on surgical exploration and histopathology. The categories are based on knowledge of the natural history of each cancer with the premise that the less extensive the cancer, the greater the long-term survival will be.

This classification is monitored by the American Joint Committee for Cancer Staging and End Results Reporting. It was initially developed in 1959 so that the American medical community would have a clinical staging system for most of the common cancers. Six organizations serve as its sponsors: American College of Surgeons, American College of Radiology, American College of

Table 11-1. TNM classification system*

T† subclasses	Tx—tumor cannot be adequately assessed
	T0—no evidence of primary tumor
	TIS—carcinoma in situ
	T1, T2, T3, T4—progressive increase in tumor size and involvement
N‡ subclasses	Nx—regional lymph nodes cannot be assessed clinically
	N0—regional lymph nodes demonstrably abnormal
	N1, N2, N3, N4—increasing degrees of demonstrable abnormality of regional lymph nodes
M§ subclasses	Mx—not assessed
	M0—no (known) distant metastasis
	M1—distant metastasis present, specify site(s)
Histopathology	G1—well-differentiated grade
	G2—moderately well-differentiated grade
	G3, G4—poorly to very poorly differentiated grade

*From American Joint Committee for Cancer Staging and End Results Reporting: Manual for staging of cancer, 1977, Chicago, 1977, American Joint Committee.
†T = Primary tumor.
‡N = Regional lymph nodes.
§M = Distant metastasis.

Pathologists, American College of Physicians, American Cancer Society, and the National Cancer Institute. The American College of Surgeons administers this effort.

This standardization attempts to classify cancers for comparison with the similar UICC system so that comparisons across countries as to treatment regimens and results can be made. The criteria are based on classifying the cancer as local, regional, or distant; histopathologic analysis and grading of the tumor are also recorded. Most of the time, the TNM system is employed for the initial diagnosis, but it can also be utilized throughout treatment to determine response or nonresponse.

Table 11-1 defines the general terms that are employed for each of the specific sites. The extent of disease can be determined by a number of means such as clinical or diagnostic studies, surgical staging, pathologic staging, "second-look" or retreatment evaluations, and autopsy reports. The system is adaptable to ongoing evaluation if it is combined with some performance scale, classifying clients according to their physical status. The most commonly employed scale is the Karnofsky scale of 0 to 100, with 0 representing the dead client and 100 representing normal activity with no complaints.

To translate the general classification to a particular cancer site, the definitions relating to that site need to be listed. For example, the TNM classification system applied to cervical cancer would be as follows:

Name	Cervix uteri
Primary site	The cervix is the lower third segment of the uterus. Its shape is roughly cylindric, projecting through the upper anterior vaginal wall, connecting with the vagina through the external os. Cancers may originate on the vaginal surface or in the canal.
Areas of nodal involvement	The cervix is drained by the preureteral, postureteral, and uterosacral routes—the parametrial, hypogastric, external iliac, presacral, common iliac, and para-aortic nodes.
Common sites of metastases	Lungs and skeleton

The TNM classification of cervical cancer can be based on clinical and diagnostic studies, surgical or pathologic staging, and "second-look" or retreatment staging. The following classification is based on agreement with the International Federation of Gynecology and Obstetrics (FIGO). The stages include stage 0, which is carcinoma in situ, and stage I, which denotes that the cancer is still confined to the cervix. Stage II indicates extension beyond the cervix but not to the pelvic wall; stage III means extension to the pelvic wall. Stage IV indicates extension beyond the true pelvis or involvement of the mucosa of the bladder or rectum. Most of the stages have subsets identified by an "A" or a "B" to clarify the extension still further as with stage IV A, indicating spread to adjacent organs, and stage IV B, indicating spread to distant organs.[1]

Role of the pathologist. The pathologist has many important functions to play in present-day cancer treatment. Because of the seriousness of a diagnosis of cancer and the complexity and potential hazards to its treatment, the clinician must know with confidence that a cancer does exist and the particular type represented. Along with confirming the diagnosis, the pathologist is pivotal in determining the extent of disease through surgical procedures. For example, after the surgeon removes a woman's breast because of cancer, the surgical specimen is examined by the pathologist to determine if the lines of resection are free of tumor. If they are not, the surgeon may ask for a radiation therapy consultation to determine if additional treatment with radiation therapy is appropriate. Another example is the importance of the pathologic evaluation of the regional lymph nodes. If the presence of a cancer is confirmed histologically, the stage of the cancer will probably change as in the case of a breast cancer going from stage I to stage II with confirmation of histologically positive lymph nodes. Because the stage has been advanced, the choice of treatment may also change. In fact, the recognition of the importance of regional lymph nodes to the natural history and prognosis of a cancer led to the initiation of adjuvant chemotherapy. Clients whose cancer is present in the regional lymph node area have a lower rate of survival and are at a higher risk for recurrence. With these clients, it is justifiable to test newer concepts. In the early 1960's, adjuvant chemotherapy was a new concept that was designed to eradicate the micrometastases that were thought to be present in the person. Since these agents can cause serious toxicities, it is necessary to document client high-risk classification, and so the pathologist is an important member of the cancer team.

Along with aiding the clinical team to confirm the diagnosis and determine the extent of disease, the pathologist fulfills two more important functions: (1) Evaluating tissue for any prognostically important tumor characteristics is becoming more common today. These characteristics, identified within the primary site, can be such parameters as the presence or absence of necrosis and the degree of vascularity. (2) The pathologist is important within research projects seeking newer information as to therapy options. No longer does the pathologist work in isolation, but within cancer teams the pathologist has numerous opportunities to benefit clients under treatment.

Benefits of combined or multimodality cancer treatment

Cancer treatment employing multiple forms of therapy, specifically surgery, radiation therapy, chemotherapy, or immunotherapy, has improved client survival substantially for many forms of cancers. These gains have not been reflected in the overall cancer statistics because many projects are small in nature and therefore account for only a small number of clients. However, many publications have appeared, and translation of these newer forms of treatment are taking place within the general medical community. Acceptance is not complete, however, with heated discussions and controversies still to be resolved totally. Fortunately, most cancer treatment is based on research so that facts are generally more available as is more complete information than would be the case in private clinical practice. Since these problems will not be resolved in the near future, it is important for the nurse to understand the dynamics of the situation so that information can be shared with clients and their families before decisions are made relative to treatment options.

One of the major reasons for controversy within the medical community as to how best to treat persons with cancer has been the traditional versus the newer approach of multimodality treatment. Traditional types of cancer treatment are defined as primarily surgical and radiotherapeutic approaches. Cancer chemotherapy and tumor immunotherapy became treatment modalities during the 1940's and 1950's and led to a major shift in approach to treatment utilizing multiple modalities. Since this shift in approach has had a major impact on cancer treatment morbidity and mortality, further discussion on this change will follow.

Fig. 11-1 illustrates conceptually the traditional approach to cancer treatment. The principal characteristic of the approach is the *sequential* use of the various treatment modalities. Surgery, the mainstay of cancer treatment, is employed initially as the definitive form of therapy. Surgery was limited to those cancers thought to be localized. Limiting surgery to local disease led to more and more radical forms of surgical procedures as the natural history and biologic activity of the various cancers became known. Until recently, cancer had been thought to be a localized disease phenomenon, metastasizing only late in the course of illness. Now, it is firmly established that most cancers demonstrate numerous *micrometastases* that will go on to produce clinical evidence of metastatic cancer if no further treatment is given or the host is unable to contain these cancer cells. During the earlier era, radiotherapy and chemotherapy were not employed until the cancer recurred, except for a few cases where radiotherapy was the only treatment of choice. In fact, chemotherapy was only employed as the last form of treatment in far-advanced cancers.

The classic example of this sequential approach to cancer treatment is that of breast cancer management. In earlier times, the usual treatment for a woman who had a breast tumor was the Halstead radical mastectomy. This surgery—entailing the complete removal of the breast; the skin; the pectoral muscles, both minor and major; the axillary lymph nodes; and the fat—was based on the premise that removal of all these tissues would control the local spread of cancer. The Halstead mastectomy was successful in this regard, but women still subsequently suffered distant disease and death. The eventual outcome usually took many years, so the surgeon generally felt comfortable in pronouncing the women "cured." This "cure" lasted a year or longer with many women returning with complaints of bone pain. Evaluation identified the primary breast cancer as being responsible, and radiation therapy was the next treatment of choice. Radiation therapy was, and still is, very effective for controlling bone metastases so that the woman would be successfully treated and discharged home again. In-

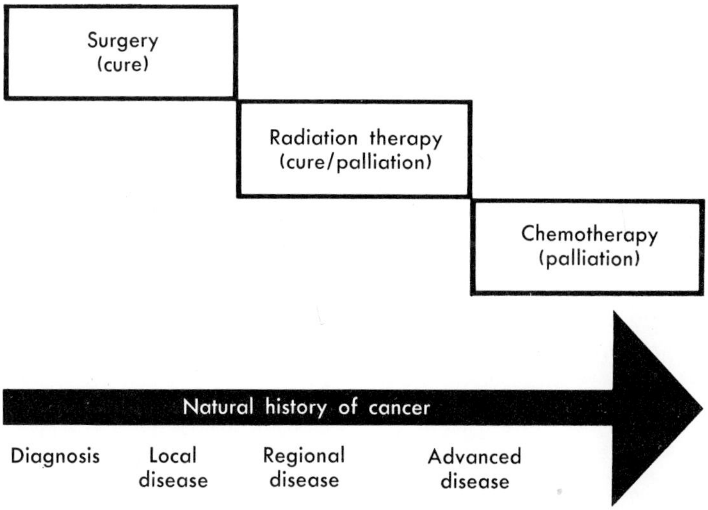

Fig. 11-1. Traditional approach to cancer treatment.

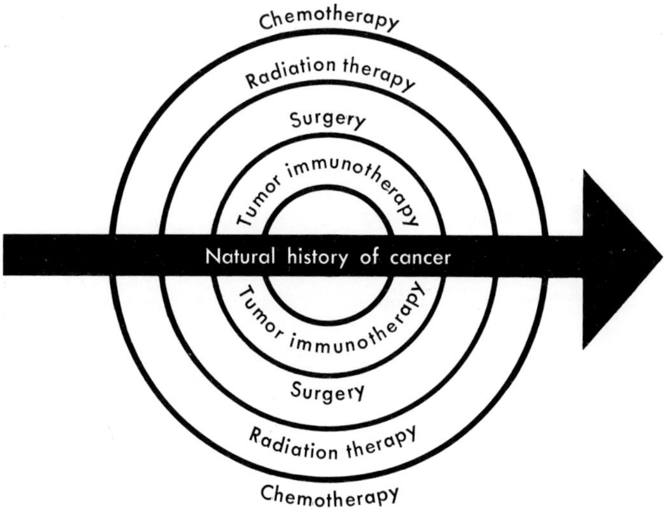

Fig. 11-2. Multimodality cancer treatment.

variably, this client would return after a period of time with more serious disease. Chemotherapy became the last resort for the advanced stage of the disease. Unfortunately, with so much tumor burden, chemotherapy was rarely more successful than brief palliation culminating in the client's death.

This compartmentalization of the modalities of treatment limited the potential benefits greatly. In contrast, multimodality cancer treatment utilizes any or all of the four forms: surgery, radiation therapy, chemotherapy, or immunotherapy. Fig. 11-2 illustrates the conceptual design of this type of treatment strategy. In this strategy, none of the modalities are relegated to a singular role. For example, surgery can be utilized for diagnostic, curative, and palliative purposes. In a reverse from the traditional approach, chemotherapy is employed in the early stages of disease when the tumor burden is much less and the likelihood of eradicating the cancer is improved. In other words, the multimodality approach to cancer therapy more accurately reflects and exploits the natural history of the cancer. If, in the case of osteogenic sarcoma, it is known that this cancer has a propensity to metastasize to the lungs and chemotherapeutic agents are effective, chemotherapy is administered.

As effective as multimodal cancer treatment is, there are two major difficulties with its use. First, instead of having one physician overseeing traditional care, the multimodal approach employs many physicians. These large numbers of health providers make it more difficult for the nurse to coordinate care. However difficult this task may be, it is imperative because of the strong research orientation to multimodal therapy. Second, most of the advances discussed at the beginning of this chapter came about through small or multi-institutional research efforts. Research in cancer is a common occurrence and so it behooves the nurse to understand the rationale for the medical actions and to work to assure that adequate information reaches the client and family. A term that is commonly used to describe these research projects is controlled clinical trials or just clinical trials. These terms generally refer to therapeutic experiments in which clients are randomized to receive a certain treatment. Because these trials have potential risks as well as potential benefits, informed consent has to be obtained to better assure that the client understands that participation is voluntary, and protections are included so that the welfare of the client is assured. The role nurses play in this important area is undergoing substantial change, so the reader is referred to Chapter 5 for a more extensive discussion.

MODELS OF MULTIMODALITY CANCER TREATMENT

Two of the best examples for demonstrating major advances in cancer treatment that have utilized multiple modalities are Wilm's tumor and Hodgkin's disease. Both of these cancers had high mortality rates until innovation led to the use of multiple modalities to control the problems caused by disease progression.

Wilms' tumor

Wilms' tumor, or nephroblastoma, is one of the most common solid tumors of childhood. Evaluation of mortality data for the period 1940 to 1969 demonstrates the improvement in client survival has resulted from treatment advances rather than earlier diagnosis.[5] From a point of surgery employed singularly curing only 11% to 32% of children to the addition of radiotherapy increasing survival to 47%, survival is now estimated to exceed 90% with the utilization of surgery, radiotherapy in selected cases, and chemotherapy.[2] The role of surgery has been expanded from removing the primary tumor to determining the extent of disease by exploring the abdomen for intra-abdominal disease, evaluating the contralateral kidney, biopsying suspicious or enlarged lymph nodes, and placing marker clips to delineate areas needing radiotherapy.[5] Radiation therapy, another mainstay of treatment, has been successfully employed for control of intra-abdominal disease but is now employed successfully for pulmonary metastasis. Chemotherapy has become the third modality and possibly the major reason for the dramatic increase in client survival because of its success in controlling pulmonary metastasis. Three agents, actinomycin D, vincristine, and doxorubicin (Adriamycin), all have shown activity in Wilms' tumor. In fact, because of this activity and improved staging to indicate children with more serious prognosis, radiotherapy can be omitted in selected cases. This omission minimizes morbidity caused by growth retardation. Now, only a subset of children with an unfavorable histology need to receive radiation therapy.

To achieve these high survival rates, the child is under active treatment for 1½ years so that it is important for the nurse to be cognizant of the disruptions in the child's growth and development and to do whatever is possible to minimize these effects. One of the better ways is for the nurse to make a community referral so that resources will be available to the child, the parents, and school officials so that disruptions can be minimized and the child's growth and development promoted.

Hodgkin's disease

Along with Wilms' tumor, the management of Hodgkin's disease serves as a classic example of the successes that are possible with multimodality cancer treatment. Fig. 11-3 chronicles the progress made in treating this form of cancer and illustrates the complementarity of basic and clinical research efforts. Information is contributed by basic scientists, surgical pathologists, diagnostic radiologists, surgeons, radiotherapists, and medical oncologists. Such findings as the natural history of Hodgkin's disease, along

1950's

- Hodgkin's disease was essentially a fatal illness

↓

Basic and clinical research findings that increased client survival

- Disease originates from a single focus
- Disease spreads in orderly fashion from above the diaphragm to entire lymphatic system if untreated
- Histologic subtypes highly prognostic
- Highly accurate pretherapy staging classification system
- Prognostically, lymphocyte predominance and nodular sclerosis subtypes more favorable than either mixed cellularity or lymphocyte depletion subtypes
- Early stages of disease response to radiation therapy
- Combination chemotherapy successful in controlling advanced disease, disease recurrence, and relapse in clients who initially received radiation therapy
- Importance of inducing complete remission early in disease course

↓

1976

- Clients treated by radiation therapy (stages I and II) show long-term (6+ years) control exceeding 90%.[2]
- Clients with previously untreated stages III and IV disease show long-term (10 years) complete remission rate of 72%.[2]

Fig. 11-3. Advances in treatment of Hodgkin's disease.

with the realization of the importance of accurate staging, parallel improvements in supervoltage radiation therapy and chemotherapeutic agents with activity in treating this cancer have had an impact on survival.

Diagnostic evaluation. Careful evaluation of the client to determine the extent of disease is central to a discussion on treatment. Confirmation of the histologic subtype is also important in determining the most appropriate treatment modality to employ. Fig. 11-4 illustrates the major lymph node areas in the body. Evaluation generally is based on physical examination, radiologic examination, exploratory laparotomy, and laboratory studies. Information obtained through these channels is compared with the Ann Arbor staging classification so that treatment regimens are suited to the extent of disease. Chiefly, radiation therapy is employed for stages I and II, with combination chemotherapy being utilized for stage IV, and a combination of chemo- and radiotherapy being tested for stage III Hodgkin's disease.

Treatment of Hodgkin's disease. Treatment for Hodgkin's disease is based on information obtained from the staging procedures.

Various treatment options are available for the different stages of disease, with the past 5 years of research concentrating on refinements of these treatments to increase

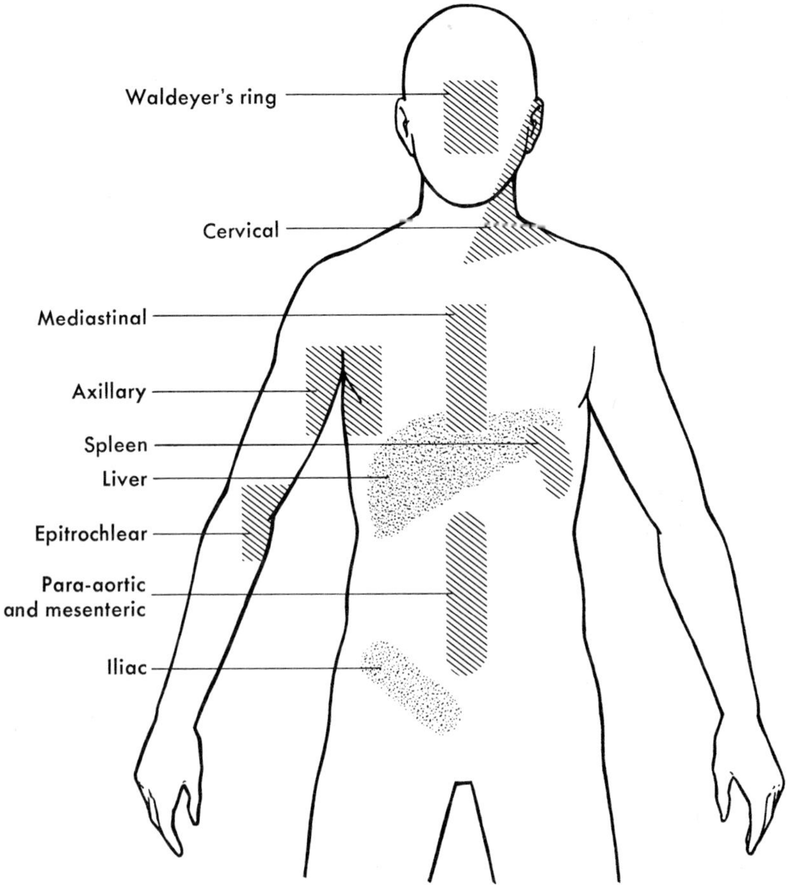

Fig. 11-4. Major areas of lymphadenopathy and organ involvement.

client survival still further. For example, radiotherapy, the mainstay of treating early stage disease, has been varied in the different treatment areas or "fields" to determine whether or not further improvements could be obtained with less extensive radiation treatment.[4] It has also been recognized that meticulous care in designing these fields of treatment is important to sterilize apparent and inapparent disease.[3]

Chemotherapy for the advanced stages of Hodgkin's disease is one of the best examples of tumor response. There are a number of agents that can be used initially or given if recurrence develops following radiotherapy. The principal combinations are MOPP—mechlorethamine (nitrogen mustard), Oncovin (vincristine), procarbazine, and prednisone—and ABVD—Adriamycin (doxorubicin), bleomycin, vinblastine, and Dtic-Dome. With this wealth of agents and the progress that has been made, clinicians are now confident that many more clients can be cured or significant control can be achieved.

Along with these major achievements in client survival, nurses have added opportunities to benefit clients and their families. The entire process of diagnosing, staging, and treating Hodgkin's disease through multimodality methods is complex and difficult. If nurses are willing, they can do a great deal to support the medical team, coordinate care, and provide information, along with carrying out frequent teaching sessions so clients understand what is happening to them and what they can do to better help their cause. A major area needing attention is the reduction of morbidity associated with cancer treatment. As more and more clients live longer with cancer, it becomes more important to minimize the toxicities that are negatively influencing the quality of their lives. Better documentation of what the quality of life is, as well as measures to positively influence that quality, is an appropriate nursing responsibility and interfaces well with nursing's increased research capability.

CONCLUSION

This chapter has presented an update on the advances that have been made in cancer treatment. Most of these improvements in client survival have been achieved in the last 5 to 10 years and therefore are not reflected in the overall cancer statistics.

Treatment employing multiple modalities—surgery, radiation therapy, chemotherapy, and tumor immunotherapy—have been credited with these reversals. Since many of these treatment models originated in small, one-institutional settings, transference to the general medical community has not generally occurred to date. Much controversy continues. For some cancers, heated debate is now taking place as to the virtue and shortcomings of these new models. In some areas, sufficient follow-up time has elapsed to give assurance to these treatments; for others, insufficient time has elapsed to confirm their long-term merits.

The responsibility of nurses in this area is to provide information to the client and family so that they can assess for themselves which options they wish to pursue. Along with information, the nurse has the obligation to work constructively with the medical team to coordinate care and information so that the work is organized and beneficial to the client. Since most multimodality treatments are research oriented, an ethical basis of nursing practice is mandatory. At present, it appears that multimodality treatments have increased benefit to the client, but there is a great need to provide teaching and support during the long, complex period of treatment.

Chapters 12 through 15 discuss in greater detail the individual contributions of surgery, radiotherapy, chemotherapy, and immunotherapy. Content specific to nursing interventions is presented along with interventions for combined therapy models. Chapter 16 discusses an increasingly important concern, namely cancer quackery, detailing what quackery encompasses and how nurses can minimize clients' utilization of the sources. Nursing interventions in legitimate cancer treatment as well as reaction to quack measures will increase as the care becomes even more complex and the issues more blurred. To better aid clients and their families, nurses must become more active in this important area of cancer health care.

REFERENCES

1. American Joint Committee for Cancer Staging and End Results Reporting: Manual for staging of cancer, 1977, Chicago, 1977, American Joint Committee.
2. Hearings before the Select Committee on Aging, Committee Publication No. 96188, House of Representatives, June 19-21, 1979.
3. Lewis, B., and Devita, V. T.: Combination therapy of the lymphomas, Semin. Hematol. **15**(4):431, 1978.
4. Rosenberg, S. A.: Hodgkin's disease and other lymphomas. In Thorn, G. W., et al., editors: Harrison's principles of internal medicine, ed. 8, New York, 1977, McGraw-Hill Book Co.
5. Sutow, W. W., Vietti, T. S., and Fernback, D. J.: Clinical pediatric oncology, St. Louis, 1977, The C. V. Mosby Co.

12

Cancer surgery—its value, client-family needs, and nursing interventions

LISA BEGG MARINO

Surgery has been, and continues to be, the mainstay of cancer treatment. The basic premises for which surgery is performed, however, have changed substantially in the last two decades. What these surgical procedures entail, what they mean to clients and families, and how all this affects cancer nursing practice will be the focus of this chapter.

HISTORY

Surgery for a malignant tumor once consisted of local excision of the tumor. It was not until 1881 that surgery, a subtotal gastrectomy, was performed based on the biology of cancer. Following this surgical technique were the Halstead radical mastectomy in 1890, the Wertheim radical hysterectomy in 1900, and the Miles abdominoperineal resection of the rectum in 1903.[5] All these surgeries were based on the biologic premise that cancer spread by direct contiguity so that an en bloc resection and a lymph node dissection would solve the problem of local control of the tumor and thus be curative. There is no question that all of these procedures did increase direct survival, and in some cases, the client was even cured. However, in the cases where surgery was successful in controlling local disease, many clients went on to suffer distant metastasis attributable to the primary cancer.

From the early 1900's until the early 1970's when multimodality cancer treatment models began to show promise, the advances from cancer surgery came largely from refinements in anesthesia, antibiotic usage, greater availability of recovery rooms and intensive care units, and replacement of blood, electrolytes, and fluids rather than surgery's increased effectiveness in controlling the cancerous spread. In fact, this plateau in client survival continued despite the trend to more and more radical surgery. When the Wertheim radical hysterectomy was not successful for cervical cancer, it was replaced by a procedure called pelvic exenteration. This latter procedure entailed extensive local resection, including the bowel and bladder, which required both an ileal conduit and a colostomy. Needless to say, the adjustments required of the client and family and the resulting morbidity were substantial. This era was also characterized by the philosophy that surgery was not performed unless the cancer could be totally resected. This attitude became a self-fulfilling prophecy in that ". . . a cancer was generally considered incurable if the surgeon found it to be inoperable."[2] If the cancer was not curable, why treat it? Thus the client was doomed. Fortunately, innovation prevailed and multimodality cancer models that proved to be successful were created. Survival rates for many of the cancers increased, and clients and families were able to benefit. Additionally, the areas of cancer treatment in which surgery could contribute were greatly expanded.

CURRENT SURGICAL CONCEPTS

Surgery, within the multimodality cancer therapy model, is only one part of the spectrum of treatment. Now, surgery contributes to the therapeutic management of cancer clients in four major areas: diagnosis and staging, definitive treatment, palliative surgery, and the neurosurgical control of cancer pain. Principles on which the art of surgery is performed are being defined as tumor models become available and the scientific basis for interventions becomes broadened. This knowledge, along with the successes being achieved by the multimodality treatment models, is permitting more limited surgery to be done without sacrifice to client survival.

Surgery as a diagnostic and staging procedure

Surgery's role in the correct ascertainment of a histologic confirmation of the presence of a cancer is crucial to any therapy plan. Reasons such as prognoses varying with the type of cancer present, the seriousness of the condition itself, along with the treatment all combine to make it of paramount importance to accurately document whether or not a cancer exists and if so the histologic type. Along with the major histology, knowledge of the specific subtype is preferred because variations in prognostic significance are now becoming apparent. For example, the two major subtypes within the non-Hodgkin's lymphoma classification are nodular and diffuse. These two patterns in the nodal architecture are the most influential characteristics, followed by whether it is histiocytic or lymphocytic in appearance and poorly or well differentiated. Clients with diffuse histiocytic lymphoma tend to relapse early in their disease course.[4] Knowledge that a person has cancer only answers the preliminary question; further information is needed to accurately plan therapy. Surgeons can obtain this information through three procedures: biopsies, diagnostic laparotomies, or "second-look" operations.

Biopsies. Biopsies can be obtained incisionally, excisionally, or via a needle. Regardless of the technique employed, the cardinal rule is to obtain sufficient tissue for adequate pathologic examination. Incisional biopsies are still being performed, but it is more common that an excisional biopsy be done so that a margin of normal tissue can be examined as well. Problems can occur if the tumor mass is large, in which case only a fragment of tissue would be taken from an incision or a needle. Needle biopsies are becoming more common because of their ease, the reduced need for anesthesia, and the reliability in accurately predicting a cancer. The acceptance of the needle biopsy by surgeons is the principal reason that "two-step" procedures for breast cancer are being done. The advantage of this type of diagnostic surgical procedure is that it allows the client and family time to assimilate the impact of the diagnosis before a decision as to a preferred treatment must be made. The trend toward separate biopsy procedures rather than employing biopsy as a prelude to a major surgical procedure is occurring for many cancers and will probably continue further into the future.

Diagnostic laparotomy. Diagnostic laparotomies are performed when the cancer has a potential for intra-abdominal involvement that cannot be adequately evaluated by radiologic or endoscopic studies. Diagnostic laparotomies are also done prior to radical surgeries such as pneumonectomy for bronchial carcinoma or esophagectomy for esophagal carcinoma so that occult intraperitoneal, lumboaortic, or liver metastases can be ruled out.[6] The most common diagnostic laparotomy performed is a staging laparotomy for Hodgkin's disease. This procedure is quite specialized and is done generally to obtain information for research purposes rather than as a routine procedure. This procedure is employed in those clients whose disease cannot be confirmed by the usual means. Since intra-abdominal involvement would alter the client's stage of disease, documentation as to the presence or absence of disease is important to therapy planning. Numerous biopsies are obtained in addition to a splenectomy and the placement of the radiopaque clips for subsequent radiotherapy. At a minimum, biopsies of the liver, porta hepatis, splenic hilar, mesenteric and iliac lymph nodes, and bone marrow are taken. Additionally, a biopsy of the para-aortic lymph nodes is taken if they prove to be suspicious or positive on preoperative lymphangiogram.[4] Information obtained from this procedure forms the basis for the definitive treatment regimen.

"Second-look" surgical procedures. "Second-look" surgical procedures are considered to be staging mechanisms for those cancers, such as ovarian cancer, that have a propensity to recur locally. For a cancer with this type of natural history, the surgeon will initially perform an oophorectomy, knowing that the residual tumor left behind will be treated by either radiotherapy, chemotherapy, or both. If the client responds to these treatments, the only way to assess whether the response has been complete is for the surgeon to perform a "second-look" procedure. Whether or not any residual disease is still present will determine the need for additional treatment.

Client needs. Many health care providers assume that since biopsies are such minor surgical procedures, the client's needs are also minor. Nothing could be further from the truth. For most clients, the biopsy period is a very stressful period with many unknowns and some "possible knowns" that are completely unattractive. Many people assume that a biopsy is only done to confirm the presence of a cancer. They should, of course, assume the opposite; that is, that the biopsy is being done to rule out a cancer. The ratio of benign versus malignant tumors found through biopsies will vary with the specific organ, but the fact that most biopsies prove to be negative should be shared with the client and family.

Major surgery is performed for a diagnostic laparotomy so that the client becomes a surgical case requiring acute care. Care should be appropriate with the condition of the client, but for many worry over the outcome of the biopsy is present. It is common, particularly with the staging laparotomy done for Hodgkin's disease, that the client has been undergoing tests for a lengthy period. Fatigue in general is quite common as is anxiety.

The same emotions and physical state prevail for the client undergoing a "second-look" procedure. If anything, anxiety is heightened more with this procedure than with biopsies or laparotomies because the procedure is being done to confirm the presence or absence of disease. In all likelihood, the client has had to undergo biopsies earlier in the disease course and may have had to withstand a major surgical procedure and then additional therapy. The client now hopes all this effort was worth it and that the disease has been eradicated.

Implications for nursing interventions. The major areas for intervening with the client and family are: providing support during the stressful periods, providing teaching about the procedures, and providing information on what is being done and why. For example, most biopsies for a breast mass prove to be benign and this information should be shared with the client. The nurse should feel confident that sharing this information is not giving the client a false sense of security but rather puts the procedure in proper perspective. If four out of five breast masses prove to be benign, the client can realistically hope that hers will be benign. If the mass proves to be malignant, then further actions would be required.

Along these same lines, the nurse can help clients deal more effectively with their stress by sharing with them the plan for the diagnostic procedures, why they are being done, and what they can do to help themselves. This approach allows the client and family to participate more fully and gives them a greater degree of control over a stressful situation.

Definitive surgery

The function of surgery has been consistent for some time, but recent investigations have documented the high rate of failure for definitive or "curative" surgery. The basic premise on which cancer surgery had previously been performed, that being control of local disease to cure the client, has now been replaced with the concept of micrometastasis, which requires more systemic treatment. Additionally, the multimodality cancer treatment model requires comprehensive decision making so that the overall plan of treatment is decided prior to any definitive surgery. This plan is consistent with the client's disease state and agreed on by all parties at the onset. Today, it is much more common to see an integrated, long-term treatment regimen than an isolated surgical procedure. Follow-up of the client continues for a lengthy period.

Surgical considerations. As a definitive procedure, surgery is still the most common form of treatment for early cancer. One of the guidelines for determining the feasibility of intervening surgically is that it is technically possible to remove the tumor. "Technically feasible" means that the tumor mass itself can be removed with a margin of normal tissue around it. Surgeons generally refer to the situation as the "lines of resection were free of tumor." Accomplishing this task is important as it indicates the surgeon's perception that all of the tumor was removed and provides sufficient and contrasting tissue for the pathologist to evaluate. Unfortunately, this is not always possible because the surgeon cannot predict what will be found during surgery. For example, the tumor may appear to be operable from clinical and radiologic evaluation, but during surgery it may be determined that the tumor is not completely resectable. This situation can happen with any solid tumor but is more likely to occur with the gastrointestinal and gynecologic cancers. The surgeon would remove as much of the tumor as possible and place the radiopaque clips for radiation therapy planning.

A situation even more common is that of the tumor that is both operable and resectable, but microscopic disease is still found to be present. These "micrometastases" form the scientific basis for adjuvant therapy. This therapy, whether it be radio-, chemo-, or immunotherapeutic, is designed to eradicate the small deposits of tumor before they grow into clinically detectable tumors.

Importance of regional lymph nodes. Another important consideration is the status of the regional lymph nodes. Lymph nodes are important in cancer surgery because metastases from the primary site can occur. Lymphatic spread, along with hematogenous and contiguous spread, is the principal mechanism by which metastasis occurs. The lymphatic system consists of

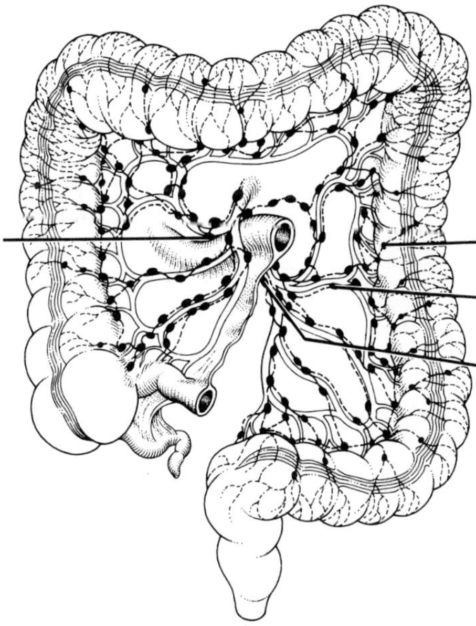

Fig. 12-1. Lymph drainage of large bowel.

lymph vessels, lymph nodes, and lymphoid deposits that are present throughout the length of the alimentary canal. Lymphatic capillaries, present in most body tissue except the epidermis, central nervous system, cornea, and bone marrow, form the lymphatic trunks, which in turn drain into the thoracic and right lymphatic ducts. Both of the ducts empty into the brachiocephalic veins. This system becomes a convenient vehicle for the spread of cancer from the primary tumor to the lymph nodes situated along the lymph vessels and then anywhere in the body.

Fig. 12-1 illustrates the lymphatic drainage of the large bowel and shows the significance that lymph node involvement has on the natural history of colorectal cancer. With this cancer the proximity of the lymph nodes to the intestinal wall is crucial as many of these cancers are found to have invaded the regional lymph nodes at the time of surgery. Invasion of cancer into these nodes allows the cancer to spread to the vessels of the mesentery, mesocolon, and the superior and inferior mesenteric arteries.[3] This common situation, which can be repeated with other solid tumors, partially explains why a major surgical resection can be successfully accomplished only to have the client reappear soon after with a tumor recurrence. In an attempt to reduce these recurrences, many physicians give "high-risk" clients, those who have lymph nodes confirmed to be pathologically positive after a colon resection, some form of adjuvant therapy.

Client needs. Definitive surgical procedures for a diagnosis of cancer are generally difficult for the client because some loss is involved as well as heightened fears of death. Losing a breast or a limb to cancer or suddenly acquiring a colostomy generally requires some major client and family adjustments. Additionally, the client is acutely ill from these major types of surgery so is already in a compromised state. Adjustments, if they are to take place, will take some time. It is very important for the nurse to talk with clients about what the surgery means to them and what they need from the health care providers to cope with this crisis. Likewise, the family will be affected by the surgery and so it is wise to bring them into the discussions as soon as possible. Anxiety on the part of the family is considerable during this period and should be appreciated by the health care group. Hospital routine tends to deaden this sense of apprehension. This is frequently the time when difficulties between family and providers develop.[1]

Implications for nursing interventions. The nurse should concentrate on providing clients with physical comfort measures until they regain some strength. Once clients begin to convalesce, teaching them about care, how to prepare for discharge home, how they can maximize their recovery, along with preparing the client for additional therapy are all important nursing responsibilities. Generally speaking, the more extensive the surgery, the greater will be the adjustments required of the client, so interventions need to be proportional to how the client views the situation. The same premise underlies family interventions; because of the increased numbers and a lessened ability to evaluate the relationships, it may be more reasonable for the nurse to primarily deal with one family member.

Surgery as palliation

Palliative surgery is the major area where the traditional views as to the benefits of surgical intervention have been replaced by more current concepts. It was once thought that surgery should never be undertaken unless there was a good possibility for cure. Anything less than a cure would make the risks too great in relation to the benefits. Today, surgery is routinely employed for palliation when there is no possibility of a cure. Palliative surgery or measures directed at comfort as opposed to cure are routinely done in five situations: removal of a solitary metastasis, cytoreductive surgery, surgical removal of obstructions, ablative surgery, and surgery to place chemotherapeutic equipment. Each of these interventions will be discussed in detail.

Removal of a solitary metastasis. Surgical intervention to remove a solitary metastasis is one of the newer methods of increasing the quality of life for the client. It is most commonly employed for solitary lung metastasis from such cancers as Wilm's tumor and nonseminomatous testicular cancer. The degree of success is increasing as the effectiveness of other multimodalities continues to improve. Most often, chemotherapy is successful in controlling most of the disease, with surgery removing the last major site. Repeated surgeries for recurrent solitary metastasis also increase the client's comfort and thus can be justified.

Cytoreductive surgery. Cytoreductive surgery is another area that has undergone considerable change because previous concepts have been put aside. In earlier years, a surgeon would generally not knowingly operate on a client unless it was possible to remove all of the tumor mass. Now, surgeons routinely perform cytoreductive surgery on primary tumors so that the other treatment modalities, particularly radio- and chemotherapies, will have greater effectiveness on such cancers as ovarian, colon, and the large bulky rectal tumors. In all of these examples, the surgeon knows that cure is not a real possibility, but removal of as much of these primary tumors as possible will make it feasible to give additional treatment because the likelihood of success is much greater.

Surgical removal of obstructions. Surgical removal of obstructions is one of the traditional areas of surgery that has continued and, in some cancers, has been expanded. Most of this type of surgery is done for intestinal obstructions to relieve distressful symptoms in the client, but surgeons routinely remove obstructions involving the kidney and bladder, the bile ducts, and compression of the spinal cord owing to tumor that requires a laminectomy. Surgery is appropriate in these situations because other treatments can be successful in controlling the bulk of the cancer while being inadequate for these select conditions. Therefore, the client's quality of life would be unnecessarily lowered because surgery is effective in minimizing these types of problems.

Ablative surgery. The surgical alteration of the hormonal status of a client with a hormonally dependent cancer is currently a major area of palliative surgery. Removal of the organ is done to reduce the source of the hormone and not because of metastasis to that organ. The most common procedure, oophorectomy, was initially performed by Beatson in 1896.[7] Other surgeries are adrenalectomy, orchiectomy, and hypophysectomy. These operations had been routinely done for recurrent breast cancer for many years. Then, because of the popularity of chemotherapy, they lost some favor. The trend is now back to their utilization because of the ability to predict those clients who will likely benefit from the procedure based on their homone receptors. These are all permanent operations, with adrenalectomy and hypophysectomy considered to be major surgeries because of the need for replacement hormones, especially cortisone.

The boxed material on p. 258 demonstrates a client teaching guide following a hypophysectomy. This guide was developed by concerned nurses with medical input from oncologists so that clients and their families would understand how to provide for their care after their pituitary gland was removed. Once the pituitary gland is removed, the client will need to take over supplying the life-sustaining cortisone; the body is no longer capable of supplying the needed cortisone. The serious and permanent changes in body functioning that result from a hypophysectomy make it necessary for the health care team to carefully evaluate the client's ability to absorb these responsibilities. If the client is determined to be capable of assuming this responsibility, it is still imperative that the entire health care provider team, particularly the nurse, continue to monitor the situation until such a time when the client is confident in self-care and can anticipate dose changes. The guide represented in the boxed material augments the one-to-one teaching that is needed; it can never replace the teaching and monitoring that is necessary. A similar guide for clients who have undergone an adrenalectomy has been used in a similar teaching program. Both of these activities are very important nursing responsibilities and represent valuable contributions to the care of clients undergoing ablative surgery.

Surgery to place chemotherapeutic equipment. Surgery to place chemotherapeutic equipment is more limited but still of value to those select clients whose tumor situations can benefit from a high concentration of drug to an isolated body part or organ. The most common regional chemotherapeutic techniques are perfusion of an entire region, usually an extremity, and intra-arterial infusions, generally to the liver.

Very careful surgical procedures are required as is the careful monitoring of clients throughout and after the procedure.

Neurosurgical management of pain

The control of pain via surgical means continues to be important. Palliation is the appropriate term because, generally speaking, pain can only be reduced on a temporary basis because the cancer itself cannot be eradicated. Despite these limitations, interventions should be made early in the disease course while the client is in a relatively

INSTRUCTIONS FOR THE POSTHYPOPHYSECTOMY CLIENT

Since you have had a hypophysectomy, which means your pituitary gland has been removed, you will need to take cortisone and thyroid medications for the rest of your life.

Cortisone acetate

The regular times you will need to take your cortisone will be the following: the first thing in the morning, in the mid-afternoon, and then around 7 to 9 PM at night. The times for you to take your afternoon and evening doses may vary according to your activities and schedule. For example, if you work from 3 to 11 PM, your busy time will be later than for someone who works from 8 to 5 PM. You will need to tell us when you are the busiest, and we will help you design the best times to take your cortisone. The main thing to remember is that you can never take too much cortisone, but you can take too little!

You are now taking replacement doses of cortisone to keep your body functioning normally. Before your hypophysectomy, your body normally would adjust and react to stressful situations by producing more cortisone. Now, you must think for your body as to when you will need extra doses. Such situations might be the following:

1. When you have the flu, a cold, an infection, or are going to have an operation
2. Happy stresses such as a wedding or a party, going on vacation, or a long shopping trip
3. Sad stresses such as a death in the family or being in situations that upset you

If you think you forgot to take your medication and cannot remember, take another dose! If you are not sure, take more cortisone, not less.

If you develop any of the following symptoms—unusual weakness, excessive fatigue, or nausea—take an extra dose of cortisone. If these symptoms disappear, continue on your regular schedule. Notify your physician if any of the following occur:

1. Unusual weakness or excessive fatigue not relieved by an extra dose of cortisone
2. Diarrhea
3. If you are unable to take your cortisone orally for any reason

Remember, you must always take your cortisone!

Carry some cortisone with you at all times.

Thyroid

Be sure to take your thyroid medication every day. Do not become alarmed if you think you forgot to take a dose. Thyroid is stored in the body for approximately 2 weeks. Missing one dose will not affect you the same day!

Antibiotics

You will be given antibiotic medications for approximately 1 month after surgery. This is just a prevention against the possibility of an infection.

healthy state. The most common procedures are nerve blocks and cordotomies. Chapter 18 discusses these procedures and the nursing care specific to each.

Client needs. The area of palliative surgery creates many needs on the part of the client and family. Most of the needs evolve around the client's weakened state, particularly when surgery is undertaken to relieve obstructions and pain. Most clients needing these types of surgery have advanced cancer that has produced a number of symptoms. Significant relief of symptoms can be obtained by these measures so that encouragement can be given to the client and family.

In the case of surgery to reduce bulky tumors, to remove solitary tumors, to ablate the source of hormones, or to place chemotherapy equipment, clients are generally in the less advanced stages so that physical needs are less but psychologic needs are greater. Identification of the recurrence that is necessitating these procedures is still quite fresh in their minds and the fears of death have only recently been uncovered. Ablative surgery, which causes permanent changes, can disrupt clients' lives a great deal and should be dealt with constructively by the health care provider.

Implications for nursing interventions. Nursing interventions that promote comfort are the key to caring for these clients. Most of these surgical procedures are major and come at a time of lessened physical or psychologic resiliency. The nurse needs to find out what the client's perception of this intervention is so that correct and complete information can be reinforced. A degree of optimism is appropriate as is the assurance that care will be monitored during the course of the illness. Many of these procedures are successful in controlling disease for a lengthy period of time so this information should be reinforced to the client.

Ablative procedures, particularly adrenalectomy and hypophysectomy, require the client to take over a major physiologic role, that being the administration of replacement cortisone. The nurse must carefully evaluate the clients' and families' undertaking of their altered state and work closely with the medical team to assure the clients' complete understanding of what they must do to maintain their physiologic equilibrium.

CONCLUSION

The role of surgery within cancer treatment has undergone substantial revision and expansion within recent years. This modality remains the principal method of treating early cancers and has now expanded to include diagnostic and staging procedures as well as palliation and pain control. Because these procedures encompass the entire spectrum of health care, client-family needs and the nursing interventions that are appropriate will vary. However, reinforcing the underlying concepts of disease control, client-family teaching, and supportive interventions remain the principal nursing responsibilities.

REFERENCES

1. Baudry, F., and Wiener, A.: The family of the surgical patient, Surgery **63**(3):416, 1968.
2. Devita, V. T., Jr.: The evolution of therapeutic research in cancer, N. Engl. J. Med. **298:**907, 1978.
3. Ellis, H.: Anatomical aspects. In Raven, R. W., editor: Principles of surgical oncology, New York, 1977, Plenum Publishing Corp.
4. Lewis, B. J., and Devita, V. T., Jr.: Combination therapy of the lymphomas, Semin. Hematol. **15**(4): 431, 1978.
5. Raven, R. W.: Oncology—a general survey. In Raven, R. W., editor: Principles of surgical oncology, New York, 1977, Plenum Publishing Corp.
6. Veronesi, U.: Surgery in diagnosis. In Holland, J. F., and Frei, E., editors: Cancer medicine, Philadelphia, 1973, Lea & Febiger.
7. Veronesi, U.: Noncurative surgery. In Holland, J. F., and Frei, E., editors: Cancer medicine, Philadelphia, 1973, Lea & Febiger.

13

Nursing management of the radiation therapy client

CAROLYN ST. JOHN ELLIOTT BATTLES

Radiation oncology, or the treatment of cancer clients by radiation therapy, is often misunderstood by health care professionals. However, one half of all cancer clients receive radiation therapy some time in the course of their overall treatment, so the nurse caring for cancer clients should be aware of how radiation therapy affects them. With this basic knowledge, the nurse can form a comprehensive care plan to return clients to their optimal level of functioning. The nurse can also support the client and family during this important phase of treatment.

DISCOVERY

Radiation as a form of cancer treatment was initiated over 75 years ago when a German physicist, William K. Roentgen, discovered a special "ray," which today bears his name. Later a Polish scientist named Marie Curie, after an arduous beginning, discovered radium. The magnitude of Roentgen's and Curie's discoveries induced later scientists such as Einstein, Compton, and Fermi to explore the secrets of ionizing radiation. From the beginning, medicine benefited from the exploitation of the atom in diagnosis and treatment of disease.

Unfortunately, in the early era of radiation therapy, it was a rather crude treatment. The measurement of tissue dose, time-dose fractionization, and the concepts of radioresistant and radiosensitive tissues were not known. The outcome was often fatal at worst, with recurrence from underradiation occurring at the other extreme. Other consequences of erroneous treatment did not appear for years as late effects of treatment. Thus, evaluation of this modality in the early stages of cancer was never really possible.

Myths had developed about radiation therapy, mostly based on the fact that the department was generally located deep within the hospital's subbasement and the treatment was delivered by huge machines in a barren room with the client alone, while a technician watched through a small window. The whole process seemed rather removed and dehumanizing. Fortunately, science does improve, and today radiation therapy is precisely calculated to deliver the correct dose to the area treated while sparing the surrounding normal tissues. It is an acknowledged specialty within medicine with board certification to indicate the physician has fulfilled all the training requirements to be called a radiation oncologist. The client and family are included in planning treatment and instructed in preventive measures to lessen the known unavoidable effects of radiation therapy.

AIMS OF RADIATION THERAPY

Today, the aim of the radiation oncologist in the treatment of cancer falls into three separate categories: cure, palliation, or as an adjunct to other treatment modalities. An example of radiation therapy being the treatment of choice, that is, cure, is with stage I or II Hodgkin's disease. Hodgkin's disease is a malignant proliferation of the reticulum cells associated with infiltration of lymphocytes and eosinophilic leukocytes. These cells accumulate in the spleen, liver, and lymph node chains throughout the body. Radiation therapy is delivered to these sites by total nodal irradiation. Radiation therapy can deliver a cancericidal dose directly to the area affected in contrast to chemotherapy which is delivered systemically. Since Hodgkin's disease is a proliferation throughout the *entire* lymphatic system, surgery would be contraindicated as a form of treatment. However, surgery is very useful in "staging" certain clients so that the exact extent of the cancer's spread can be determined prior to therapy planning.

The second aim, palliation with radiation therapy, may not extend the client's life; however, it does reduce such symptoms as bone pain from bony metastases or drainage from chest wall metastases that is sometimes associated with cancer of the breast. Radiation therapy used palliatively may also be employed to relieve local symptoms such as pathologic fractures, areas of ulceration, or bleeding. Often after a few courses, the client experiences relief of symptoms and healing may begin. Therefore, radiation therapy does play a very valuable role in minimizing the symptoms associated with the advanced stages of cancer.

Radiation therapy is used as an adjunctive treatment in cancers requiring irradiation either preoperatively or postoperatively when surgery is the treatment of choice. For example, the surgeon may remove a colon tumor and the pathology report may reveal that the margins of the dissection were not free of disease or that the tumor extended beyond the resected specimen. In this type of case, radiation therapy may be employed to deliver a cancericidal dose to the local tumor area beyond what was resected through surgery.

Radiation therapy is also employed in those cancers where chemotherapy is the primary treatment. Children with acute leukemia may receive intrathecal methotrexate for leukemic cells that are circulating in the cerebrospinal fluid. These children will often receive brain irradiation in conjunction with this chemotherapy as an additional means of eradicating tumor cells within the brain.

EXPLANATION OF IONIZING RADIATION AND ITS EFFECTS

The nursing care of the client receiving radiation therapy is based on solid knowledge of ionizing radiation and its effects on the cells within the body.

Ionizing radiation occurs when x-rays or gamma rays pass through matter, disrupting or damaging the atoms they come in contact with. Three different effects can result: a cellular effect, a chromosomal effect, or a late effect. The cellular effect can be described as x-rays disrupting the chemical bonds necessary in the reproduction of DNA within the cell. Broken atoms or free radicles no longer fit into the DNA pattern and cause cellular death at the time of mitosis. DNA is

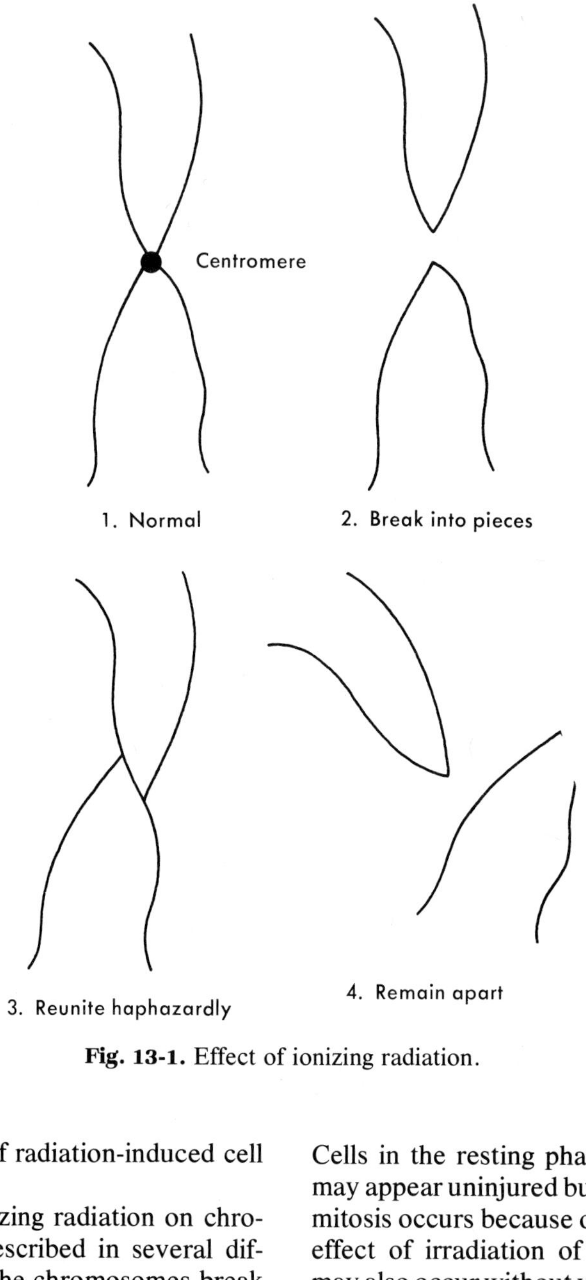

Fig. 13-1. Effect of ionizing radiation.

the primary target of radiation-induced cell death.

The effect of ionizing radiation on chromosomes can be described in several different ways. First, the chromosomes break into pieces, reunite haphazardly or incompletely, or remain apart; or second, they can be injured, resulting in the unequal division of chromosomes at the time of mitosis.[22] Cells in the resting phase of the cell cycle may appear uninjured but will later die when mitosis occurs because of the result of a late effect of irradiation of the cell. Mutation may also occur without visible chromosomal damage, resulting in irreparable changes appearing in later generations.[22] Fig. 13-1 illustrates the chromosomal effect of radiation therapy.

Cancer is basically a disease of the cell, thus the target of radiation therapy is the cell and its components. By precise measurements, radiation therapy can be administered so that beneficial effects to the client can be obtained. Sometimes, the therapeutic effects can totally eradicate the cancer and cure the client as in the early stages (I or II) of Hodgkin's disease. Other times, only palliation can be achieved because the cancer is far advanced. The aim here can only be comfort oriented as in diminishing bone pain. The third aim, radiation therapy used as an adjuvant treatment, is still largely investigational but does show promise for clients who have been determined to be at high risk for later recurrence of their cancer. Determining if a client can benefit from radiation therapy and to what extent is based on how sensitive the particular cancer is to radiation therapy.

RADIORESPONSIVENESS OF VARIOUS FORMS OF CANCERS

Factors determining responsiveness

The sensitivity of a cancer to radiation therapy is called radioresponse; it is determined by three factors: the mitotic potential of the cells, the extracellular environment, and the total dose delivered.

Mitotic potential. The mitotic potential can also be described as the *rate* of mitosis. Cells that divide frequently with a high degree of cell differentiation generally exhibit a greater degree of radioresponse. An example of this is the leukemic cell arising from the hematopoietic system. The hematopoietic system is one of the first systems affected by radiation therapy. This effect is demonstrated by a drop in the blood counts and is dependent on the total amount of bone marrow being irradiated. The bone marrow is the blood-forming organ. The bone marrow produces and differentiates the red cell series, white cell series (except lymphocytes), platelets, and the plasma cells. The bone marrow has a high mitotic potential demonstrated by the fact that it replaces red cells every 120 days and produces white cells in large numbers when they are needed to fight infection.

Extracellular environment. The second factor in evaluating a measurable response is the extracellular environment. This component includes the vascularization and the oxygen available to the tumor itself. Oxygen is a necessary ingredient to the subsequent damage of the DNA. The function of oxygen within the DNA is to combine with the free radicles, thus preventing the reformation with their disrupted electrons and repair of the radicles within the target area. The vascular bed maintains the oxygen supply and the nutritional requirements of the tumor. This is why large tumors generally have a necrotic center. These malignant tumors are not very efficient and therefore do not have the orderly vascular supply most normal, healthy cells have. The peripheral cells of the tumor are destroyed first by the radiation therapy, allowing for the revascularization and reoxygenation of the center so that the radiation therapy can begin to offset the inner cells as seen in Fig. 13-2. The greater the vascularization and oxygenation of the tumor, generally the higher the rate of radioresponse.

Amount of radiation therapy administered. The total dose delivered to the tumor is the last factor in measuring radioresponsiveness. The dose is expressed in rads, which is defined as the radiation absorbed dose. A lethal tumor dose is a dose that achieves 95% tumor control.[22] The dose administered is extremely important because if the tumor has received an inadequate dosage, it can be altered from a potentially radiocurable lesion into a radioincurable one. This unfortunate consequence can occur for several reasons. First, if the tumor is composed of different types of radiosensitive cells, a large number are destroyed by the irradiation. However, the surviving cells produce a more *resistant* cell type. This effect is possibly the result of radiation-induced mutation, which was explained earlier in this chapter. Second, other changes can be observed in the vascular bed such as fibrosis, which can reduce vascularization and oxygenation to the tumor. To have an adequate tumor response, the dose must be a lethal tumor dose administered in the first course of treatment.

Malignant tumors may be classified ac-

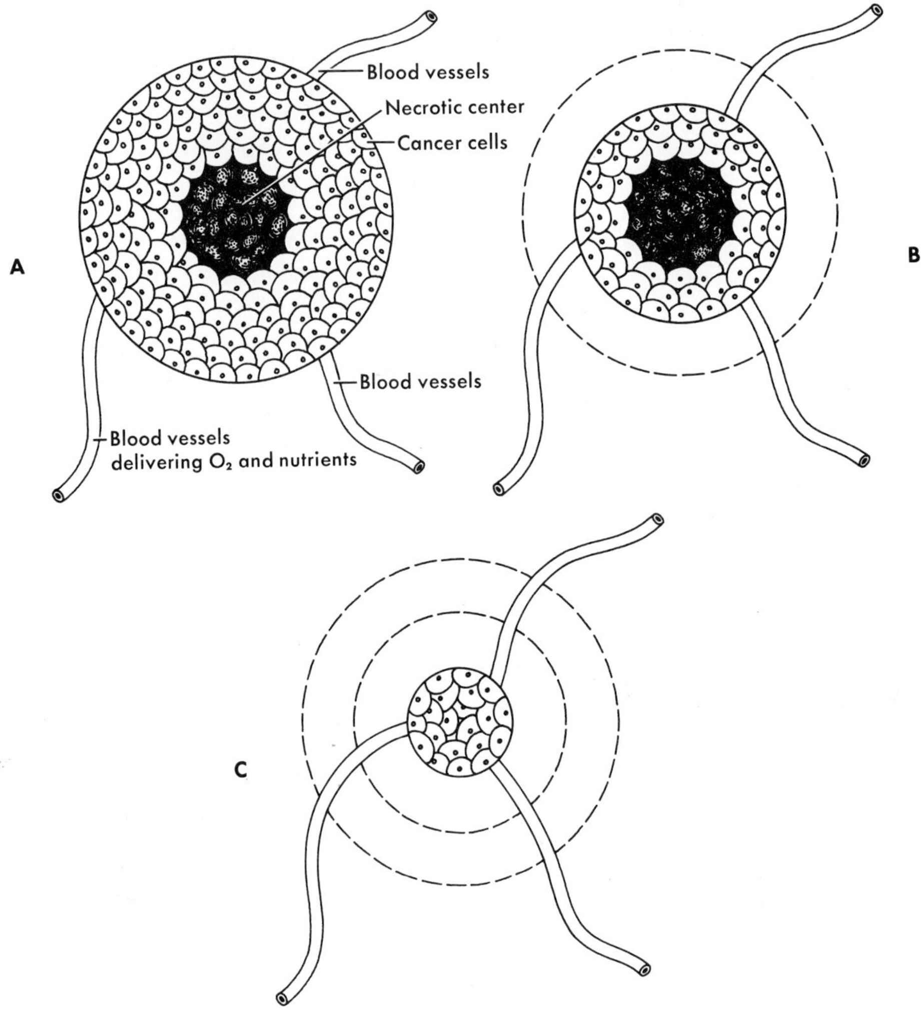

Fig. 13-2. Reoxygenation of necrotic center of tumor. **A,** Malignant tumor in tumor bed. **B,** During radiation therapy, death of the peripheral cell occurs, which allows reoxygenation of the necrotic center. **C,** Near the completion of therapy, the tumor has markedly shrunk because of reoxygenation of the center cells.

cording to their relative radiosensitivity or radioresistance. The differentiation between the two helps in predicting a client's response to radiation therapy.

A malignant tumor eradicated by radiation doses that are well tolerated by the surrounding normal tissue may be classified as radiosensitive.[1,11,22] A good clue to determining radiosensitivity is that a malignant tumor is as radiosensitive as the tissue from which it originates. For example, the tolerance dose or injurious dose of normal bone marrow is approximately 350 to 450 rads.[22] Therefore, malignant tumors arising from the cells within the bone marrow will be radiosensitive at about the same level of rads.

A radioresistant malignant tumor requires large doses to produce some effect, resulting in large amounts of normal tissue damage in and around the tumor[22] and to the vascular bed. This can be demonstrated by the fact that the tolerance dose or injurious dose of the cell within the bone is between 6,000 and 7,000 rads.[22] This is a much higher dose than was necessary for cells originating from the bone marrow. Generally speaking, the higher the dose needed to eradicate the cancer, the greater the risk of damage to the normal surrounding cells. Making an assessment of risk versus benefit of radiation therapy is one of the most crucial decisions the radiation oncologist will make.

METHODS OF DELIVERING RADIATION THERAPY

Along with a determination of radioresponsiveness and overall risk versus benefit, the radiation oncologist needs to determine how best to deliver the cancericidal dose. The two techniques utilized for delivering a cancericidal dose of radiation are through external machines and internal sources.

External radiation therapy

External radiation therapy can be defined as radiation delivered by an external source such as a machine to the skin surface or below. Machines are categorized by the amount of energy they produce and are divided into the kilovoltage and megavoltage energy ranges identified in Fig. 13-3.

Kilovoltage machines. The term "kilo-

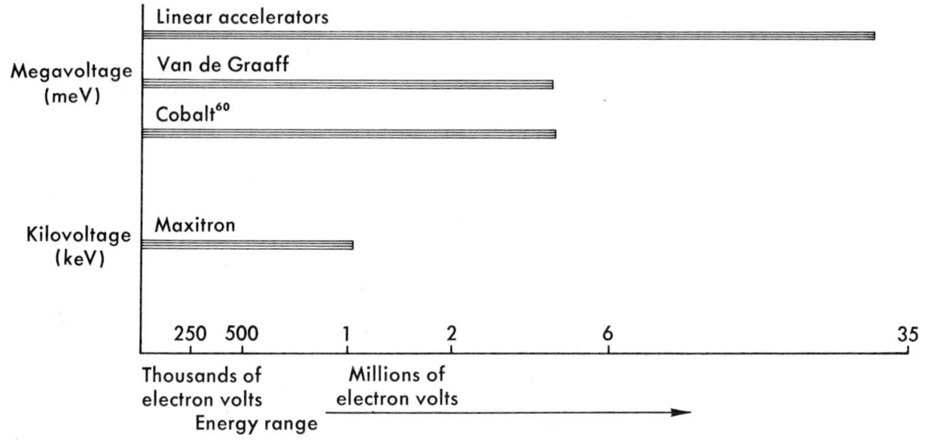

Fig. 13-3. Ranges of radiation therapy equipment.

voltage" refers to thousands of electron volts (keV). The kilovoltage machines were the first machines developed for therapeutic use. Machines in this category produce x-rays that deliver their maximum tumor dose to the skin surface or 1 to 2 cm beneath it.[25] Skin tolerance becomes the limiting factor in the amount of radiation that can be delivered to the malignant lesion. Consequently, these machines are now used only for superficial skin lesions or tumors located near the skin surface such as cancer of the breast and parotid gland. The voltage range of these machines is between 250 to 500 keV. Some examples of this type of machine are the Maxitron and the superficial skin machines shown in Figs. 13-4 and 13-5.

Megavoltage machines. The term "megavoltage" refers to millions of electron volts (meV). Machines in this category have a much wider range of energies. For example, the Van de Graaff generator and the Cobalt[60] machine both deliver about 2 meV. The difference between the two machines is that the Van de Graaff generator produces x-rays, and the Cobalt[60] machine produces gamma rays, which are radiation produced by emissions from the isotope cobalt 60. At the 2 meV energy level, about 50% of the dose is delivered at 10 cm below the skin level.[25] Linear accelerations can produce between 6 and 35 meV. These machines deliver up to 90% of the desired dose at a depth of 10 cm[25] and are shown in Figs. 13-6 through 13-9.

The difference between the machines is determined not only by the amount of energy produced but also by the type of beam produced. Kilovoltage produces soft x-rays of low penetration so that the energy is

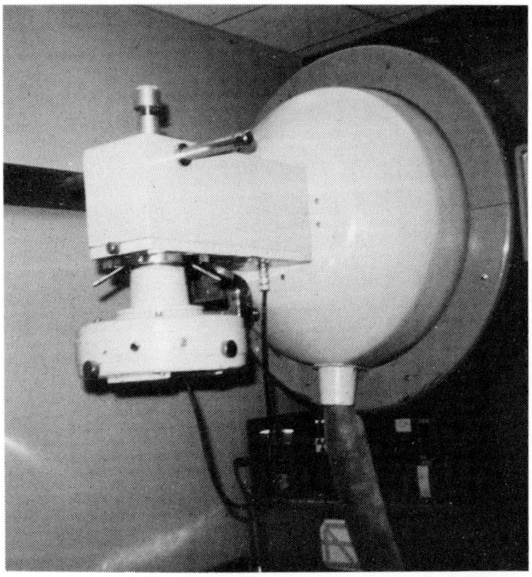

Fig. 13-4. GE 250 Maxitron. (Courtesy of University of Chicago Hospital and Clinics, Chicago, Illinois.)

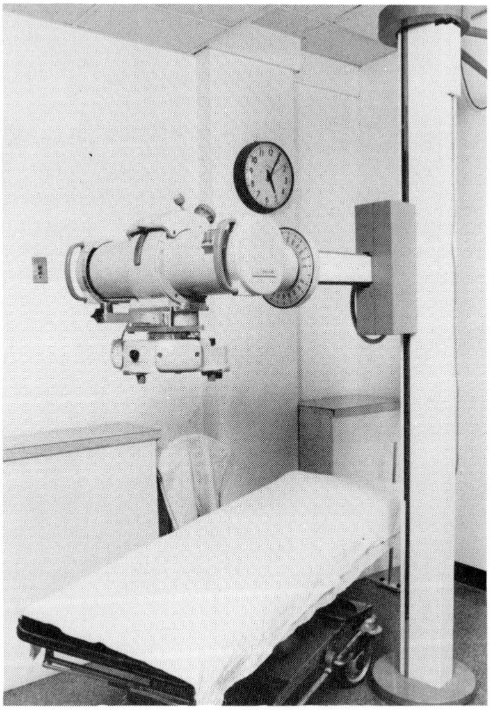

Fig. 13-5. Maximar 250 keV. (Courtesy of M. D. Anderson Hospital and Tumor Institute, Houston, Texas.)

quickly absorbed. Therefore, penetration is not much beyond the superficial tissue.

At the higher energies seen with the meV machines, the edges of the beam are sharper with little side-scatter. Therefore, the maximum dose is not reached until well below the skin level, making skin tolerance less of a limiting factor.

There is also an absorption differentiation between keV and meV machines. In keV machines, there is a large differentiation between the absorption of energy in dense

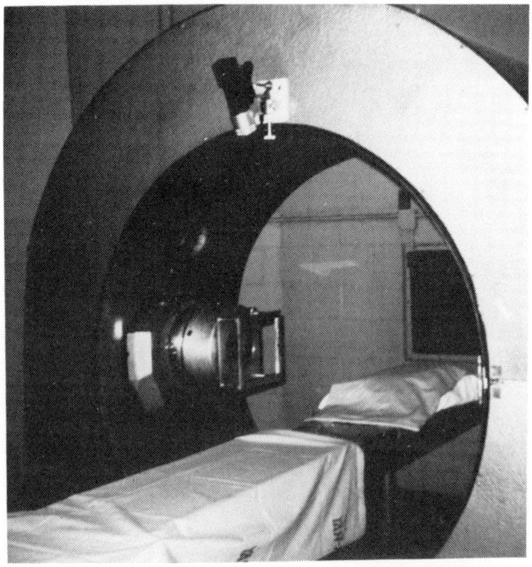

Fig. 13-6. $Cobalt^{60}$ revolver. Source is able to turn 360 degrees. Source in this picture is located in the housing on left. (Courtesy of University of Chicago Hospital and Clinics, Chicago, Illinois.)

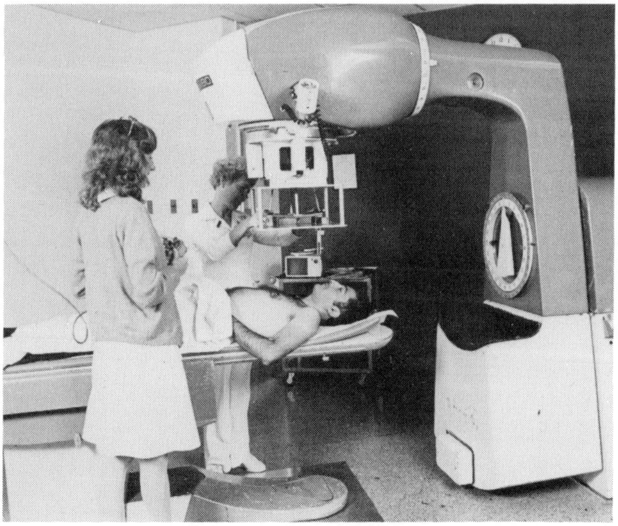

Fig. 13-7. $Cobalt^{60}$. (Courtesy of M. D. Anderson Hospital and Tumor Institute, Houston, Texas.)

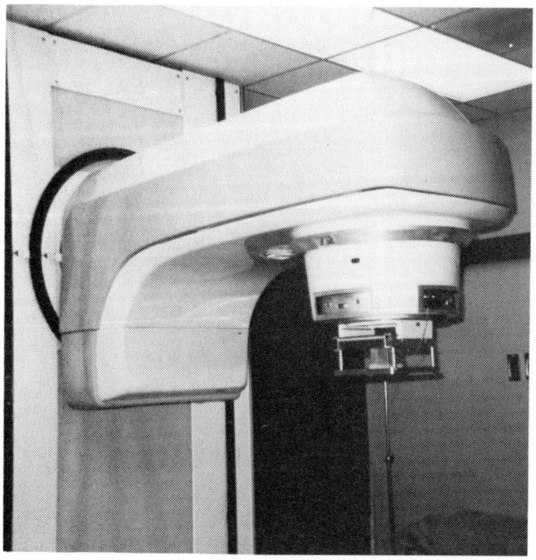

Fig. 13-8. Varian accelerator. (Courtesy of University of Chicago Hospital and Clinics, Chicago, Illinois.)

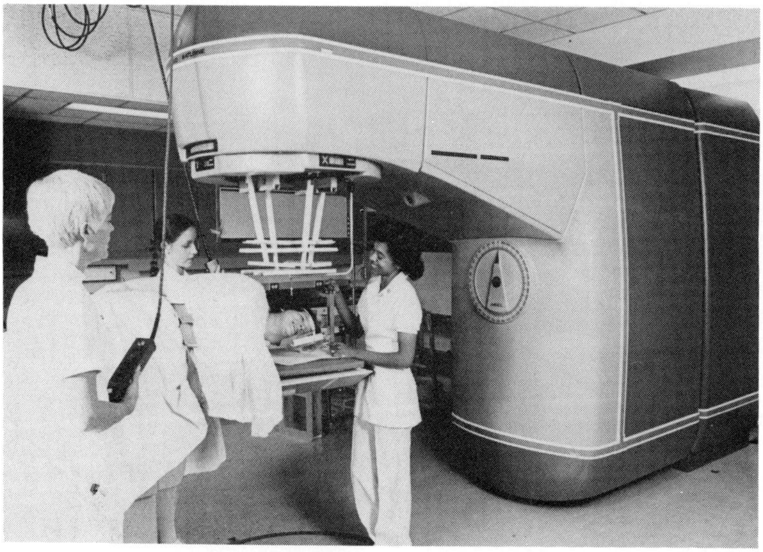

Fig. 13-9. 20 meV linear accelerator. (Courtesy of M. D. Anderson Hospital and Tumor Institute, Houston, Texas.)

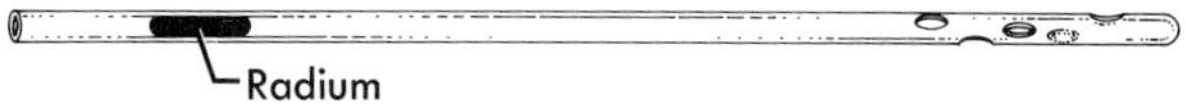

Fig. 13-10. Nasogastric tube with radium implant or radium bougie.

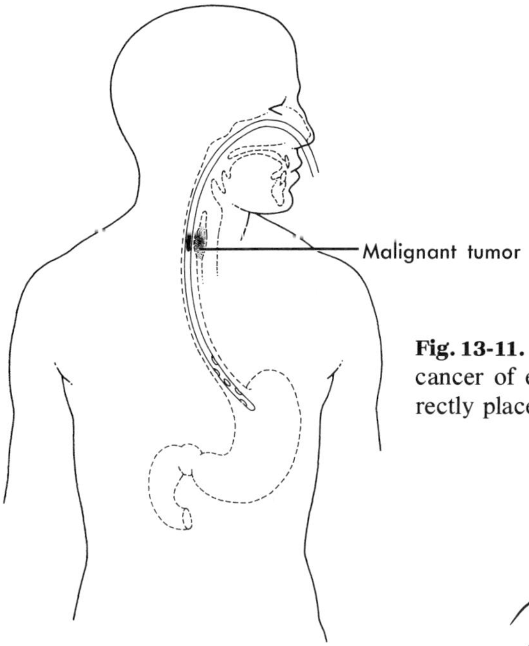

Fig. 13-11. Radium bougie in place for client with cancer of esophagus. Note that radium is correctly placed next to cancer.

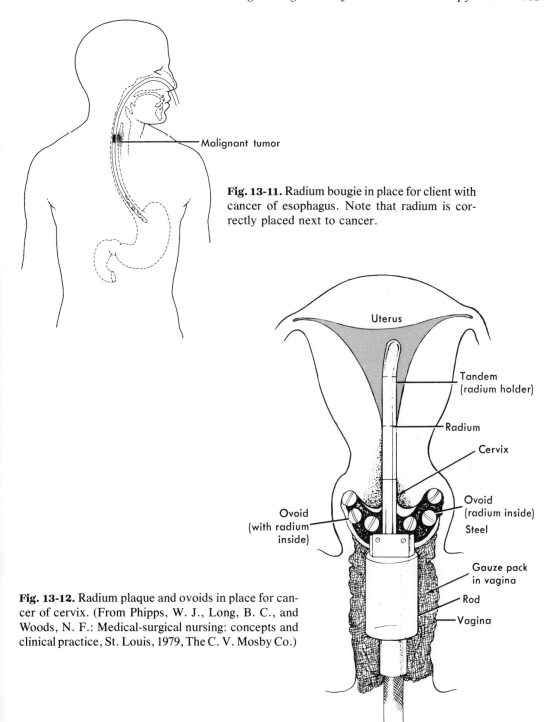

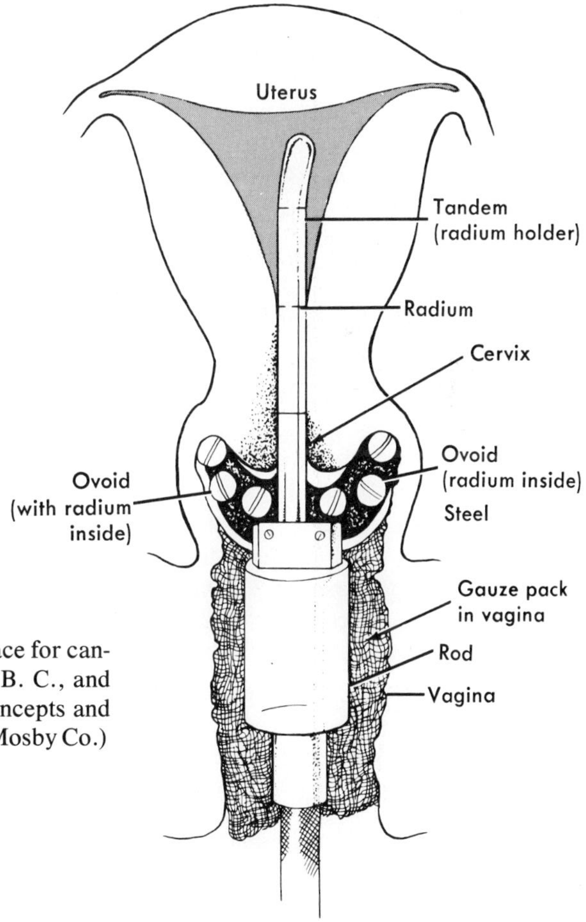

Fig. 13-12. Radium plaque and ovoids in place for cancer of cervix. (From Phipps, W. J., Long, B. C., and Woods, N. F.: Medical-surgical nursing: concepts and clinical practice, St. Louis, 1979, The C. V. Mosby Co.)

and soft tissue. Bones absorb more energy than organs because more energy is required to penetrate them. If an x-ray film is placed under the client, it looks much like a regular x-ray. In meV machines, this absorption differentiation does not exist; the amount of energy absorbed by bone and soft tissue is approximately equal on the x-ray film, with little distinction between bone and tissue. This difference explains the ability of meV machines to deliver a cancericidal dose in the vicinity of bone without causing bone damage.

Internal radiation therapy

The second technique, internal radiation, is the placement of radioactive material intracavitarily or interstitially so as to administer a cancericidal dose to a local area. The material utilized is an isotope such as radium, cesium, ^{32}P, or ^{131}I. These materials can be placed in molds, in bougies for cancer of the esophagus, or in plaques for cancer of the cervix. For example, ^{131}I is swallowed by the client with cancer of the thyroid, whereas ^{32}P is sometimes placed into the peritoneum for cancer of the ovary at the time of surgery.[14] Figs. 13-10 through 13-12 demonstrate these usages.

As was stated previously, specific tissues respond to radiation therapy differently. This difference is termed *tissue tolerance*. Tissue tolerance is an expression of the minimum and maximum dose that would cause injury to the tissue. The higher the dose, the greater the risk of injury to the tissue. Conversely, the lower the dose, the lower the risk to the tissue. However, the lower doses also reduce the tumor response. If treatment of complications is manageable and if treatment by surgery or chemotherapy cannot be utilized should radiation fail, then higher doses may be acceptable[3] in terms of risks to the client. This brings up other factors in determining risk versus benefit from radiation therapy; however, the overriding considerations should remain that cancer is a potentially fatal illness so some risks can be justified in attempting to cure the client. Consequently, if the complications of treatment may severely compromise the client with or without supportive treatments, lower doses become necessary even if tumor control is similarly reduced. Under most circumstances, the worst complication of radiation therapy is the failure to control tumor growth.

EXPLANATION OF THE COMPONENTS OF RADIATION AND ITS EFFECT ON THE TISSUES

There are three specific components that determine the radiation effect on tissues: the dose, the time period to complete the treatments, and the area treated. The determination of the dose by the radiation oncologist is based on: the type of tumor to be treated, such as a seminoma versus a sarcoma; the location of the tumor, such as one located in the pelvis that is surrounded by the radiosensitive normal bone marrow tissue and the gastrointestinal tract versus a tumor in the extremity; and the therapeutic intent of cure versus palliation. Therefore, not only the radiosensitivity of the tumor but also that of the *surrounding normal tissue* may limit the dose.

Tissue tolerance is also a function of dose and the amount of time over which the dose is administered. Six thousand rads given in 6-week intervals will cause fewer complications than 6,000 rads given in only 2 weeks. Generally speaking, the longer time interval allows for normal tissue repair to occur. This is the reason behind the fractionation of therapy such as giving 200 rads/day for 5 days a week for 6 weeks to a total dose of 6,000 rads. Normal tissue maintains reparative mechanisms, while malignant tissue is irreparably damaged following exposure to gamma rays or x-rays. Unfortunately, the administration of large doses over short periods of time disrupts these normal tissue reparative mechanisms as well as affecting malignant tissue. A small amount of this disruption is expected and may be treated symptomatically as the complication occurs. For example, diarrhea is expected to occur during pelvic irradiation.

A large dose of 5,000 rads administered to a large area such as the whole abdomen will also increase the risk of complications. It is for this reason that the radiation oncologist reduces the treatment area to include just the tumor bed itself. In some cases, adjacent structures such as the lymph node chains that drain the area are often included in the treatment area or "port." All treatment plans are individualized so that each client receives treatment only after careful examination and calculation of the extent of the disease to be included in the treatment por-

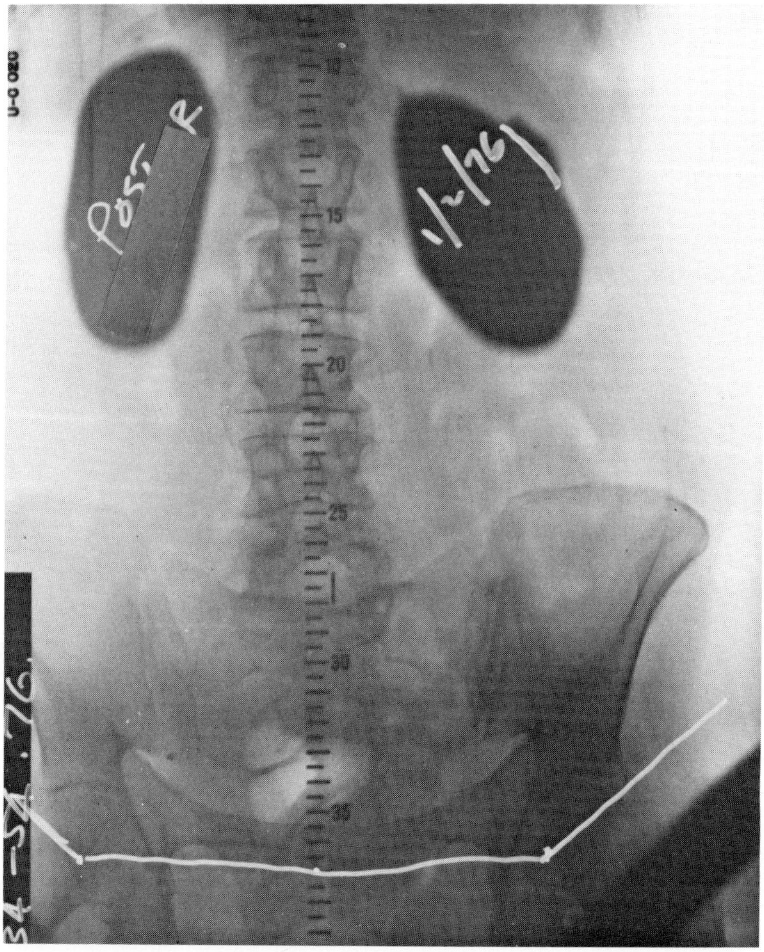

Fig. 13-13. Intravenous pyelogram was used in this case to localize kidneys so tailored shields could be made to their exact size and shape.

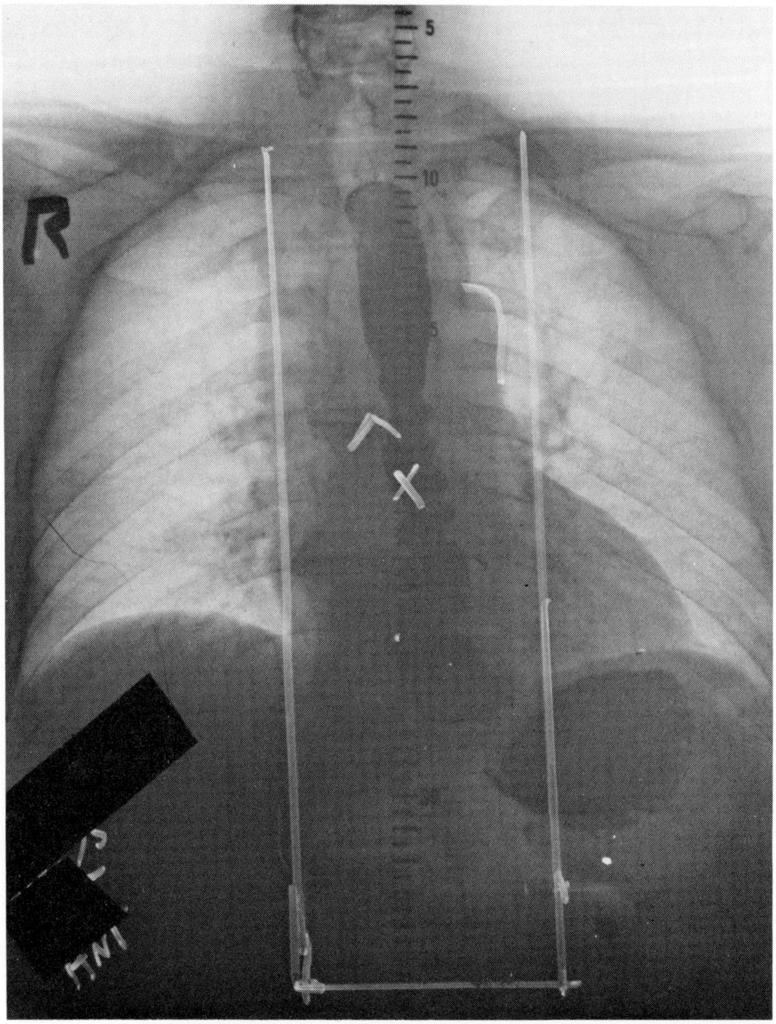

Fig. 13-14. Use of barium swallow for tumor localization. Lesion is located in middle third and appears as ragged edges along esophageal wall.

tal. Often, diagnostic x-ray films as exemplified in Figs. 13-13 and 13-14 are used for tumor localization or for localization of normal tissue such as the kidneys so that they can be shielded during treatment. The surrounding normal tissue is prevented from receiving exposure by an individualized tailored "block."

ACUTE, INTERMEDIATE, AND LATE EFFECTS OF RADIATION THERAPY

Once it has been determined that the client's cancer is amenable to radiation therapy, the radiation therapy team will prepare for the expected consequences of treatment. The major effects of radiation therapy on normal tissue can be divided into three categories. These effects generally occur *only* in the areas actually treated.

Acute effects

The first of the categories is termed acute effects. These effects are related to the dose rate and fractionation rather than the *total* applied dose. These effects always occur during treatment and are usually manageable so that treatment may not be interrupted. Acute effects result from depletion of actively proliferating cells in homeostatic cell-renewal systems such as the hematopoietic system.[3] These effects are treated symptomatically; however, if they become prolonged, therapy may be interrupted. Some examples of acute effects are: nausea, vomiting, low CBC, sore throat, radiation cystitis, diarrhea, mouth ulcers, and dry and moist desquamation of the skin. Nausea, vomiting, and diarrhea are usually controlled by diet and medication. Radiation cystitis may be relieved by forcing fluids and medication. Sore throat and mouth ulcers are relieved somewhat by medication and alterations in the client's diet. Dry and moist desquamations are treated in several different ways as determined by the radiation oncologist.

Intermediate effects

The second category, intermediate effects, includes effects related to fractionation and total applied dose that occur shortly *after* completion of treatment. These effects do *not* cause permanent damage but result from injury to the slower proliferating cell-renewal systems.[3] Examples of intermediate effects are: radiation pneumonitis, radiation-induced pericarditis or myocarditis, radiation-induced electrical paresthesia or Lhermitte's sign, and life-threatening radiation-induced hepatitis and nephritis.[3] Generally, these two life-threatening effects occur only when the entire liver or kidney receives doses above its normal tissue tolerance. The tissue tolerance dose for the kidney is approximately 2,000 to 3,000 rads.[22] Both kidneys are included in a total abdominal port; however, the kidneys are usually shielded or blocked after 2,000 rads to protect them from receiving a dose above their tolerance that would cause nephritis. The same shielding would be done for the liver.

Late effects

The third category of effects is termed late effects. These occurrences are related to the total applied dose given to surrounding normal tissue and occur anywhere from months to years following treatment. Late effects are chronic complications and may not be surgically manageable.[3] Examples of late effects are: tissue necrosis, fistulas, tissue fibrosis, and bone necrosis, especially of the mandible.[3] These late effects can limit the total dose applied to the tumor area, especially in the case of retreatment to an area that has previously received the maximum therapeutic dose.

SUMMARY FOR NURSING ASSESSMENT

The following checklist of important points should be utilized for assessing the radiation therapy client in regard to the treatment received. The important points that were discussed previously include:

1. Cell type and radiosensitivity/radioresistance
   a. Tissue of origin
   b. Mitotic potential of malignant and normal tissue
   c. Extracellular environment of the tumor
   d. Tumor dose applied to the tumor
2. Type of radiation therapy received
   a. External radiation
      (1) Kilovoltage
      (2) Megavoltage
         (a) Van de Graaff generator
         (b) Cobalt 60
         (c) Linear accelerators

b. Internal radiation
   (1) Placement
   (2) Type of isotope
   (3) Time in place
   (4) Total applied dose
3. Radiation effect of specific tissues
   a. Tissue tolerance of normal tissues
      (1) Total dose received
      (2) Fractionation
      (3) Area treated
   b. Major effects (Are they manageable and is the client aware of the complications?)

PLANNING NURSING INTERVENTIONS RELATIVE TO DIET IN THOSE CLIENTS RECEIVING RADIATION THERAPY

After an understanding of how radiation affects the body, the nurse must assess the client to plan interventions and preventive measures specific to the problems associated with the radiation therapy. As previously stated, the side-effects of radiation therapy are the direct result of the damage to the normal tissue surrounding the tumor. The four primary areas of nursing assessment and intervention include the gastrointestinal system, specific effects on head and neck cancer clients, specific effects on clients receiving radiation therapy to the chest area, and specific effects on clients receiving radiation therapy to the abdominal area.

Gastrointestinal system

The first area for nursing intervention is the nutritional status of the client or the effect on the gastrointestinal system. The nutritional status of the client receiving radiation therapy can be easily assessed by determining the client's weight. Weight loss during treatment has been attributed to several causes: inadequate caloric intake, increased caloric need for tissue repair, host-tumor competition for nutrients, and malabsorption with or without clinical symptoms, especially in clients who have received abdominal treatments.[5,12,24,26] Anorexia, diminished appetite, or aversion to food has been reported as the commonest cause of inadequate caloric intake in these clients.[9,21,24,27] Anorexia occurs to some extent in most clients during some period of their radiation therapy. The following techniques may be used in the assessment of the client's weight loss and/or anorexia:

1. Weigh the client at least once a week during treatment.
2. Determine the client's eating habits.
   a. Food likes and dislikes
   b. How often client eats, how many meals and snacks
   c. Quantity of food eaten at each meal
   d. Whether client eats before or after treatment
3. Who prepares the meals, or does the client eat out most often?
4. Have the client make a chart of the actual food consumed for 1 week to determine eating patterns. Use this chart in discussions with the client and significant other(s) to determine if changes have occurred and what alternatives are available for foods the client can no longer eat. Include a discussion of family food preparation to determine alternatives for the client within the family routine.

Some of the nursing interventions for anorexia arise from this basic assessment. For instance, these interventions may include the family in a discussion of how meals can be prepared around the client's favorite foods or foods that are better tolerated. Preparation of the food in an attractive manner should be stressed, such as smaller portions on small plates and attention to color and texture. The client should be encouraged to be in a room other than the kitchen while the food is being prepared since cooking odors may diminish appetite. Meal time should be encouraged as a pleasurable family time, such as a time when the whole family sits down together and discusses the day's activities. A glass of wine or beer, if it is not contraindicated, may be offered prior to the meal to help stimulate the client's appetite. If the client becomes hospitalized, encourage the family members or significant others to bring in favorite foods prepared the way the client likes them. If the nursing unit "orders out," ask the client to join you. Discuss the principles of good nutrition with the client and the person responsible for preparing the meals and structure a diet utilizing favorite foods within a nutritional framework.[24] Sometimes small, frequent meals incorporating high caloric, high protein foods may be more effective in stimulating the client's appetite.

Specific effects on head and neck cancer clients

The following are challenging nutritional problems often experienced by clients receiving radiation treatment to a specific area. Head and neck clients usually experience some degree of difficulty that contributes to their inability to maintain an adequate nutritional intake. Before continuing this discussion, a case study will illustrate the potential problems often encountered by this group of clients.

Mr. J., a 65-year-old male, was diagnosed with squamous cell carcinoma of the tonsil. Mr. J. had a large upper cervical nodal mass that was positive for squamous cell carcinoma at biopsy. Direct and indirect laryngoscopy and bidigital palpation revealed a hard mass in the tonsilar fossa. This mass was also biopsied and was also positive for squamous cell carcinoma of the tonsil. Mr. J. was classified in T_2, N_1, M_0, or stage III disease.

Because of Mr. J.'s previous heart condition, a long history of cigarette smoking, and alcohol abuse, he was not considered a candidate for surgery and was referred to radiation therapy for treatment. The total treatment plan for Mr. J. included 6,000 rads by external radiation to be given in 200 rads/day for 6 weeks. The 200 rads were to be divided into 100 rads to be given anterior and 100 rads to be given posterior per treatment. The treatment area included the primary site and the cervical nodes. Prior to the initiation of therapy, Mr. J. was scheduled to see the dentist for a thorough examination, dental x-ray examination, and possible extraction of damaged teeth. On returning to the radiation therapy area, Mr. J. was further instructed on an oral hygiene regimen to follow, which included brushing his teeth with a soft brush after every meal, followed by a mouth rinse with equal parts of water and peroxide or saline.

A nutritional assessment was also done with Mr. J., including subjective and objective data.

SUBJECTIVE DATA

- Anorexia
- Total lack of concern for a good nutritional intake
- Stated alcohol preference over solid foods

OBJECTIVE DATA

- Underweight
- Dehydrated
- Difficulty in swallowing
- Habit of eating only "fast foods"

Other pertinent data included that Mr. J. lived alone in a boarding house in one room with a small refrigerator and hot plate. However, a friend of Mr. J.'s across the hall would encourage him to share meals together.

The nursing diagnosis based on the data collected was that of a client with poor nutritional intake. The nursing care plan for Mr. J. included the following interventions.

1. Begin health teaching related to the effect of radiation therapy on normal tissues, stressing nutrition's importance for tissue healing. This teaching will be reinforced throughout the treatment period and posttreatment clinic visits.
2. Reinforce oral hygiene regimen to try

and prevent mouth ulcerations that might decrease Mr. J.'s ability to maintain a high nutritional intake.

3. Record body weight weekly.
4. List Mr. J.'s preferred foods and form a diet plan to include as many as possible within a nutritional framework.
5. Talk with Mr. J.'s significant others and determine if Mr. J. ate foods prepared at home or preferred to eat out. Use this information to assist Mr. J. in picking nutritional foods from a menu.
6. Interview Mr. J.'s neighbor to determine his support in changing Mr. J.'s eating patterns.
7. Supplement Mr. J.'s eating patterns with nutritional supplements that can be mixed with milk or water.
8. Discourage Mr. J.'s alcohol intake by explaining the astringent effect of alcohol on the oral mucous membranes and poor caloric intake.
9. Discourage Mr. J.'s cigarette smoking.

Three weeks into Mr. J.'s treatment, he developed mouth ulcerations and increased difficulty in swallowing. Subjective data now also included stated sore throat and mouth. Objective data now also included ulcerations of the oral mucosa that covered the base of the tongue and the anterior and posterior pharynx.[8] Redness and inflammation accompanied the mouth ulcerations.

Other pertinent data given by Mr. J.'s neighbor included that Mr. J. was still maintaining a high alcoholic intake and was only able to take the nutritional supplements and soup as opposed to any solid food.

The nursing diagnosis now included: difficulty in maintaining an adequate nutritional intake owing to difficulty in swallowing.

Mr. J. was rested from treatment for 2 weeks, with instructions to further decrease his alcoholic intake and increase his use of the nutritional supplements and soup to at least 2,000 to 3,000 calories a day. He was also instructed to continue his mouth washes at least 5 to 6 times a day and brush only as tolerated. Mr. J. was seen twice during his break from treatment for assessment of tissue healing, body weight, and reinforcement of his oral hygiene regimen.

On returning to his treatment, Mr. J.'s oral mucosa had healed; however, he had not gained any weight. Mr. J. finished his treatments without further incident by following his oral hygiene regimen and supplementing his nutritional intake.

The interventions for Mr. J. seemed best suited for his life-style. However, the interventions for clients receiving radiation therapy to the head and neck region *are not* limited to the ones employed for Mr. J. As illustrated by the case history, ulcerations of the oral mucosa are a frequent complication. However, these may be controlled, if not *prevented* by good oral hygiene. This is an acute effect caused by the quick response of the oral epithelium to therapy.[11] Some of the recommended management techniques include: determination of the current oral hygiene regimen and reinforcement or instruction of the principles of improved oral hygiene. Clients should be instructed to brush their teeth with a *soft* brush after every meal and before bed.[28] They should also be instructed on mouth irrigations with peroxide, baking soda, or saline at least two to four times a day. Commercial mouthwashes should be avoided because they can produce an astringent effect and further irritate the oral mucosa.[24] Clients should also be encouraged to use dental floss at least twice a day before brushing because this will further remove food particles that might promote cavities and infection.

Clients should also be instructed to avoid hot, spicy foods in the diet. Liquid diets or commercial supplements may be added to the general diet. If the client cannot afford these products, blenderizing nutritious foods prepared for the client may be sufficient.

For clients wearing dentures, it is recommended that they remove them until after the completion of treatment because dentures may become loose fitting during therapy, which will further irritate the oral mucosa. If mouth ulcers continue to cause discomfort, the use of viscous lidocaine (Xylocaine) or other topical anesthetics may be necessary, particularly before meals.

The effect of radiation therapy on the salivary glands occurs early in the treatment. This can become a chronic complication termed xerostomia or dry mouth. These effects occur because irradiation reduces glandular activity, resulting in a decrease in the amount of saliva produced and a reduction in the normal pH of the mouth. The result is thick, scanty mucus ineffective in preventing cavities or lubricating the food for easier swallowing.[8,11] Some recommended interventions the nurse can suggest are:

1. Chewing sugarless gum and sucking sugarless hard candy
2. Drinking water and juices frequently, carrying a vacuum (Thermos) bottle as necessary[24]
3. Moistening food with sauces, gravies, and milk[13]
4. Sipping water between bites of food
5. Prompt diagnosis and treatment of oral candidiasis (Radiation damage to the oral mucosa creates a favorable environment for the growth of *Candida*, producing symptoms of burning and dryness. This condition is seen as creamy patches or streaks that enlarge and coalesce.)

Another effect of radiation therapy to the head and neck area is taste abnormalities. Some clients have reported not only a loss of taste for food but a specific aversion to meat.[7] They often complain the food has no taste or a new, very unpleasant taste and texture. The following are recommended nursing interventions:

1. Suggest alternative foods within the same food group, emphasizing that foods within the same food group will not necessarily taste the same.[7]
2. Have food prepared attractively, utilizing the sense of smell[24] as well as food color and texture.
3. Have the client stay out of the kitchen while food is being prepared so that unpleasant odors do not offset taste.

A late effect of radiation therapy affecting some head and neck cancer clients is tooth loss, occurring 1 to 3 years after completion of treatment.[11] The cause is the effect of radiation on the blood vessels of the jaw, and the result can be observed as crown amputation.[11] The teeth, thus affected, become infected, resulting in bone necrosis. The responsibility of the nurse is to make sure the client is examined by a dentist prior to treatment. The dentist will extract badly decayed teeth and examine the client periodically throughout treatment. The nurse must reinforce the dental regimen, which may include:

1. Prophylactic cleaning of all tooth surfaces and gingival surfaces
2. Utilization of fitted fluoride carriers to surround tooth surfaces
3. Use of topical fluoride for 5 minutes a day after brushing

Specific effects on clients receiving radiation therapy to the chest area

Clients receiving radiation to the chest area, as in extended mantal ports for Hodgkin's disease, experience two acute effects that interfere with their ability to maintain an adequate nutritional intake. The first effect is esophagitis. The esophagus, like the entire digestive tract, is lined with mucous membranes and is affected early in the treat-

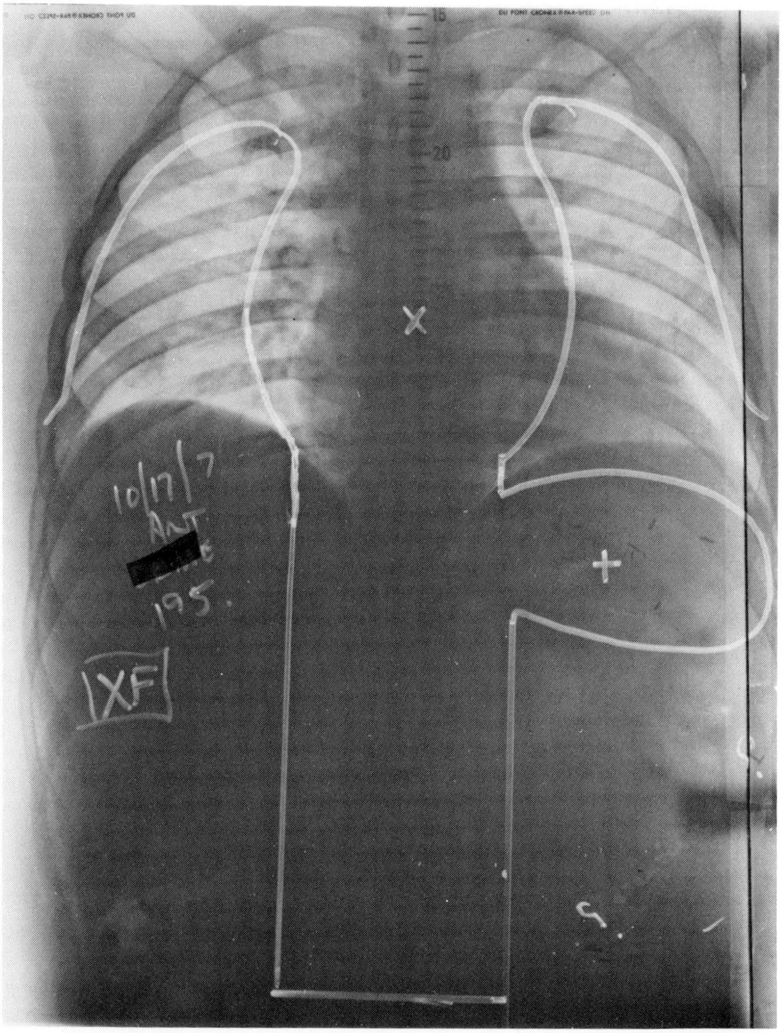

Fig. 13-15. X-ray illustrating extended mantal port. Note area treated includes portion of liver, esophagus, splenic bed, portion of heart, small portion of lung apex, axillary lymph nodes, and larynx up to and including lower jaw. Area shielded is within white marking.

ment.[16] Clients frequently complain of a persistent intensifying sore throat that interferes with the ability to swallow. A decrease in intake occurs in a effort to reduce the discomfort.

The second effect is nausea and vomiting. This effect is the most common cause of decreased nutritional intake; however, the physiologic cause is unknown. The following case study will illustrate some of the nursing interventions employed with clients suffering from these acute effects.

Ms. N., a 26-year-old female, was diagnosed by a staging laparotomy as having stage II nodular sclerosing type Hodgkin's disease. Ms. N. was scheduled to receive 4,000 rads to be delivered to an extended mantal port, 200 rads a day, 100 rads anterior and 100 rads posterior per treatment for 4 weeks.

Because the extended mantal port as seen in Fig. 13-15 extends to the lower jawline, all clients are scheduled to be examined by the dentist and started on a dental regimen. The nutritional assessment of Ms. N. revealed the following data:

SUBJECTIVE DATA

1. Good appetite
2. Vegeterian, including eggs, cheese, and milk
3. Client concerned about weight control
4. Client generally eats only three small meals a day

OBJECTIVE DATA

1. Normal weight for height and bone structure
2. No evidence of anorexia, dehydration, poor eating habits, or difficulty in swallowing

OTHER PERTINENT DATA

1. Ms. N. is currently an elementary education teacher, working part-time while she completes credit toward a master's degree in education.
2. She lives alone, but she often eats her dinner with her family.

The nursing diagnosis of Ms. N. formulated from her nutritional assessment was for a potential decrease in nutritional intake owing to the effect of radiation therapy.

The nursing interventions initiated prior to beginning therapy were:

1. Have Ms. N. chart her meals for caloric intake.
2. Determine Ms. N.'s likes and dislikes.
3. Discuss alternatives with Ms. N. and her significant others to increase protein and calorie sources within Ms. N.'s vegeterian diet preferences.

After 3 weeks of therapy, Ms. N. experienced increased difficulty in swallowing and bouts of nausea that lasted all day. Ms. N. had also lost a total of 10 pounds during therapy. The subjective data changed to: lack of desire for food owing to nausea, ability to eat only one meal a day, and concern about weight loss. The objective data revealed: anorexia, dehydration, 10-pound weight loss, and general fatigue. Ms. N. wishes to continue working and attending school; her therapy was planned so as not to interfere with her schedule.

The following alternatives were discussed with her:

1. Increase caloric intake with increased use of eggs, milk, and cheese.[18,29]
2. Supplement caloric intake with nutritional supplements.
3. Determine when nausea is the worst, that is, pre- or posttreatment and try one small meal before the nausea is worst and one after the nausea subsides.
4. When Ms. N. is nauseous, she should try to eliminate unpleasant sights, sounds, odors, and tastes. Also avoid or limit visual work, motions, and physical activity.
5. Medication may help to relieve symptoms of therapy. Try and determine if medication works best pre- or posttreatment or before eating.
6. Try and maintain a high fluid intake, that is, 1 to 2 L/day. This fluid will help with a sore throat and may be in the form of soup, juices, tea, or nutritional supplements.
7. Encourage periods of activity to be followed by periods of rest to help with the nausea and fatigue.

Ms. N. charted her meals and the periods when nausea was the worst. She found if she ate a small meal prior to therapy and restricted her activity after her treatment, the nausea was not as severe. Also, medication prior to therapy helped alleviate the nausea. She was able to maintain her weight throughout the conclusion of her treatments with nutritional supplements and increased use of eggs and milk in her diet. She found milk often soured in her stomach so use of this as a protein, calcium, and iron source was limited.

Other interventions that can be utilized with a client with esophagitis similar to Ms. N. are:

1. Discourage smoking and try to eliminate alcohol intake.
2. Instruct client to take small bites and chew food well.
3. Avoid hot, spicy foods.
4. Sip water between bites of food.
5. Moisten food with sauces, gravies, or milk.[13]
6. Chew aspirin gum.[24]
7. Blenderize solid food or use liquid diet supplements if condition persists without relief.

Clients on special diets, not only vegetarian diets but also low sodium or low fat diets, can maintain a good nutritional intake that will promote tissue repair with creative nursing interventions. Often, discussions with the client and significant others will determine a diet plan and alternatives necessary for maintaining a good nutritional intake.[19]

Clients with severe nausea or vomiting also need creative nursing interventions. Some of these interventions not previously discussed are:

1. Change the client's eating patterns after determining likes and dislikes.
   a. Several small, nutritious meals a day
   b. Attractively arranged food
   c. Small portions on small plates
   d. Varying meals, that is, eating a large meal before therapy and eating sparingly afterwards or not eating before therapy and eating a large meal afterwards
2. Encourage the client to stay out of the kitchen while meals are prepared; eliminate unpleasant odors that may stimulate nausea or vomiting.
3. Instruct the client to avoid motions, such as rapid or frequent change in position, because quick changes in equilibrium can stimulate vomiting.

Specific effects on clients receiving radiation therapy to the abdominal area

Clients receiving radiation treatment to areas within the abdomen, such as for pelvic malignancies, generally experience nausea, vomiting, and diarrhea. This is because the mucosa is second only to the bone marrow in its radiosensitivity. The small intestine, while rarely the location of the malignant lesion, represents the surrounding normal tissue that reacts quickly to radiation therapy.

Diarrhea is an acute effect that, if unmanageable, may cause the interruption of treatment or malabsorption.[12] The following are recommended nursing interventions:

1. Dietary changes including
   a. High carbohydrate, high protein, low fat, low residue diet
   b. Use of elemental diets that contain no bulk, produce little residue, and may help protect the irritated mucosa
   c. Increasing fluids to offset loss
2. Utilizing anticholinergics and the opium derivatives

PLANNING NURSING INTERVENTIONS RELATIVE TO SKIN CARE IN THOSE CLIENTS RECEIVING RADIATION THERAPY

The second area for development of nursing interventions is in managing acute skin reactions that occur in most clients receiving radiation therapy. These effects are acceptable and manageable complications. They are characterized by a radiodermatitis or radioepitheliitis owing to the loss of the epidermal or epithelial layers.[16] Two types of reactions are observed; dry and wet, with the "dry" reaction usually preceding the "wet" reaction. A dry desquamation is characterized by drying and scaling of the skin, while a wet desquamation is characterized by a weeping of the skin. This reaction is due to the upper layers of the skin having been shed leaving the derma exposed.[16] An *inappropriate* term for this type of reaction is a radiation *"burn."* It is *not* a burn and should not be treated as such. Severe reactions usually require a rest from treatment until healing occurs.

There are several different ways to manage these reactions; the following case study will illustrate several interventions.

Ms. B. was a 56-year-old obese female with epithelial carcinoma of the ovary, stage III, which translates to disease in one or both ovaries spread beyond the pelvis but still confined to the peritoneal cavity.[16] Ms. B. was referred for radiation therapy postoperatively to be completed before starting chemotherapy. The radiation portal for Ms. B. included the entire abdomen for 2,000 rads, which was cut down to a banjo port for another 2,000 rads and was further reduced to a pelvic port for the final 2,000 rads. A banjo port includes the periaortic lymph nodes and the pelvic port as illustrated in Fig. 13-16.

Aside from the expected manageable complications of nausea, vomiting, and diarrhea, Ms. B. experienced a severe skin reaction around her umbilicus. This, too, is an expected complication. Ms. B. first developed a dry reaction, which was due to the friction of her clothes on the area; she then progressed to a wet reaction.

SUBJECTIVE DATA

1. Complaints of pain and burning around umbilicus
2. Complaints of drainage on clothes
3. Inability to wear clothes

OBJECTIVE DATA

1. Weeping from exposed derma layer around umbilicus
2. Redness and inflammation around umbilicus

NURSING DIAGNOSIS

1. Potential source of infection caused by skin reaction to radiation therapy

Ms. B. was rested from treatment to allow for tissue healing. During that period, she was shown how to irrigate the area at least twice a day with warm water or saline made from 1 tablespoon salt added to 1 quart of water, wash the area gently with a mild soap and pat dry, and expose the area to the air as much as possible. The application of a prescribed antibiotic or steroid cream is necessary if these measures are not effective. This was not indicated for Ms. B.

Preventive measures had been taught to Ms. B. prior to initiating radiation therapy. The following preventive measures should be utilized for any client receiving radiation therapy to any area of the body.

1. Instruct the client to discontinue use of colognes and deodorants, substituting baby oil and baby powder.
2. Instruct the client not to scrub the treated area with harsh soap, wash cloth, or brush, or vigorously rub the area with a towel.
3. Instruct the client not to use medications or ointments on exposed or radiated skin unless prescribed by the therapist.
4. Discourage the client from using a hot water bottle or heating pad on the area.
5. Men receiving head and neck irradiation should only shave with an electric razor.
6. Because radiation therapy increases the sensitivity of the skin, the client should discontinue exposing the radiated skin to sunlight for prolonged periods.

Clients receiving extended mantal radiation may develop these reactions in the axilla and the nape of the neck and these clients are instructed in the preceding preventive measures.

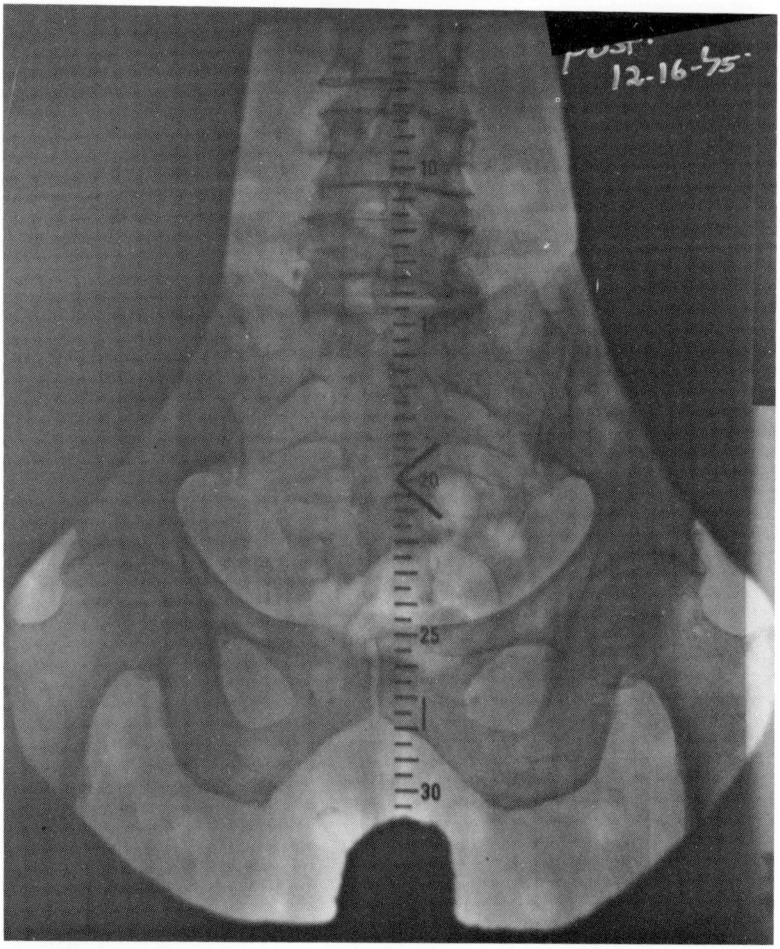

Fig. 13-16. X-ray illustrating "banjo port" for cancer of ovary. Area treated includes periaortic lymph nodes (which stand out as whitish clusters because of dye injected into them), pelvic bone marrow, large intestine, and portion of small intestine.

Clients receiving brain irradiation not only lose their hair but may also develop a dry reaction, especially around the ears, followed by a painful wet reaction. Hair loss occurs on all areas treated but is most distressing on the head. These clients should wash the head with a mild shampoo, pat it dry, and let it be exposed to air as much as possible. The head should not be covered with a wig all the time, but rather a cotton scarf, which is more comfortable and allows the scalp to "breathe."

Late skin reactions are late effects that the client should be aware of because they are chronic complications. These are the result of permanent damage to the blood vessels of the skin and include telangiectasia, delayed wound healing, and necrosis.[2] Pigmentation also occurs because of stimulation of melanoblasts by radiation to produce melanin pigment.[16] The late effect on the dermis consists of fibrosis and is associated with telangiectasia. The client must be careful of the exposed or irradiated areas permanently, utilizing the preventive measures previously described. These effects are the result of total dose and the type of energy utilized. This can be explained simply by the principle of the higher the dose, the greater the risk of complications. After completing a course of treatment, the radiation oncologist may decide that the client needs an additional "boost." This usually occurs after evaluation of the initial treatments and is utilized to further control the primary tumor. All skin reactions result in some permanent or late change, although it may not be significant; also, superficial lesions are more prone to skin reactions than deep tissue lesions.[16] The energy utilized also plays a part in the development of late skin changes. As previously stated, megavoltage has a skin-sparing effect because it delivers its energy *below* the skin surface. Kilovoltage, on the other hand, delivers its maximum dosage *at* the skin level or just below it, and thus produces more skin reactions.

PLANNING NURSING INTERVENTIONS RELATIVE TO MYELOSUPPRESSION IN THOSE CLIENTS RECEIVING RADIATION THERAPY

The third area for planning nursing interventions is in relation to the effect of radiation therapy on the normal bone marrow. The bone marrow is one of the most radiosensitive tissues of the body. Those clients receiving radiation therapy to the abdomen are especially prone to problems because this area includes the pelvis, where over 40% of the bone marrow is located in the adult. These clients must be observed closely for lowered blood counts. Clients who receive radiation to the chest area have approximately 25% of their bone marrow affected and must also be observed for lowered blood counts. The red blood cell, granulocytes, and platelets are all formed in the bone marrow, and the main effect of the irradiation on the bone marrow is a drop in these elements. The following are assessment data that may be collected from these clients:

SUBJECTIVE DATA

1. Complaints of easy fatigability
2. Complaints of shortness of breath
3. Anorexia
4. Cold or flu that seems to "hang on"
5. Easy bruisability

OBJECTIVE DATA

1. Hemoglobin less than 10
2. Hematocrit less than 30 for women, less than 35 for men
3. White blood count less than 6,000

Depending on the severity of the effect on the bone marrow, the client may be rested from treatment. If the blood count does not return to normal or becomes chronically low, the client may require blood transfusions during treatment to prevent lengthening the treatment and decreasing its total effectiveness.

Repopulation of the bone marrow begins 10 to 15 days after irradiation. Erythropoiesis begins also at this time and granulocytopoiesis begins a few days later.[16]

PLANNING NURSING INTERVENTIONS RELATIVE TO PSYCHOSOCIAL ISSUES IN THOSE CLIENTS RECEIVING RADIATION THERAPY

The nurse planning the care for the client receiving radiation therapy must remember the three systems that are first affected by irradiation: the gastrointestinal system, the integumentary system, and the hematopoietic system. However, the diagnosis of cancer evokes several emotional crises. These crises are related to cancer's diagnosis, treatment, and prognosis.[4,6] This section will be limited to emotional support of the client receiving radiation therapy. The primary responsibility of the nurse is to support the client through an individualized, comprehensive plan of care, communicated, documented, and utilized by *all* who are involved with the client's care.[20] This plan should not only include the measures previously described but also measures for the emotional needs of the client and family.[30] The following represent three areas for nursing diagnosis and treatment.

Anxiety caused by radiation therapy can be the result of fear of the unknown or misconceptions surrounding radiation and its use in the treatment of cancer. Fear of the unknown causes thoughts of: Will it hurt? Will I get sick? How long will the treatments last? Will I be disfigured? Nausea has often been attributed to anxiety.[24] Open communication should be established between the health care providers, client, and family. All procedures should be explained, and the client and family encouraged to ask questions when some point is unclear. The inclusion of the family will help them cope with their feelings and support the client.[6,30]

Misconceptions about radiation therapy and its use in cancer treatment are related to fear and anxiety. Often the client has heard about other clients' problems and may be convinced the same problems will occur. The nurse should listen to the client and try to alleviate any fears caused by misconceptions.

The change in body image also affects clients receiving radiation therapy. Most clients receiving treatment will pass through stages much like the grieving process. Some authors identify the stages as shock, denial or defensive retreat, acknowledgment of reality, and finally, adaptation.[17] Nursing interventions are based on the actual stage that the client is in. The nurse should accept the client's behavior without reinforcing it. Only when the client reaches the adaptation stage will a new integrated body image based on the reality of the situation occur. The family or significant others should also be aware that the client is trying to live with a potentially fatal disease. The family must also understand the stages the client is passing through and continue to be accepting and supportive while beginning to accept and work within the restrictions of the situation.

An example of a client passing through the stages prior to adapting to the reality of her situation is Ms. T.

Ms. T. was an 18-year-old female with Hodgkin's disease. She was initially referred to radiation therapy while she was still hospitalized. She was consistently late for her appointment and on arrival at the department demanded instant attention. She would fight constantly with her parents, often resulting in a shouting match between them. The nurses' notes in Ms. T.'s hospital record revealed this type of attention-seeking behavior also occurred on the nursing unit.

Erickson states that adolescence is the period when individuals attempt to form their own identity versus role confusion.[10] Maslow has also determined a hierarchy of needs in the following descending priority: physiologic, safety, belongingness, self-esteem, esteem from others, and self-actualization.[15]

At 18, Ms. T. was just beginning to find out who she was within her world. Diagnosis and treatment of her disease were especially threatening to her safety, self-esteem, and self-actualization needs. The following subjective data were assessed from Ms. T.'s behavior.

SUBJECTIVE DATA

1. Stated disbelief over what was happening to her
2. Stated fear of the disease and the treatment
3. Fear of loss of independence from family
4. Fear of loss of peer acceptance
5. Uncertainty about her future

OBJECTIVE DATA

1. Lack of desire to interact with family, friends, or staff
2. Loss of appetite
3. Desire to maintain control as evidenced by her selecting her own time to meet her appointments
4. Shock as evidenced by her anger over her situation

Other pertinent data revealed Ms. T. to be an active high school senior preparing to enter college in the fall. She was well liked by her peers and was currently treasurer of her class. The nursing diagnosis formulated from this assessment was anger and denial related to her disease and treatment.

The nursing interventions utilized to help Ms. T. adapt to her situation were:

1. Treat Ms. T. as a young adult.
2. Encourage her to be responsible for keeping her appointments and allowing her to determine when it would be most convenient. This would be especially important when she left the hospital and returned to school.
3. Sit down and openly discuss the treatment with Ms. T. and her parents. Encourage them to understand that Ms. T. should continue to go to school and prepare for college.
4. Encourage them to talk together and work out alternatives for helping each other acknowledge the reality of the situation and adapt to the changes.

Ms. T. and her family worked out together the best time for her treatments, so disruption of her daily routine was at a minimum. After being released from the hospital, Ms. T. kept all her appointments at the time she determined. She seemed to adapt to the necessary changes to continue her therapy. She was still fearful of the future but was determined to continue her plans within the limitations of her disease and treatments.

A change in life-style is related to the change in body image. Encouraging the client and family to become involved in the plan of care and discussions about the treatments will allow the client to voice objections and determine alternative measures within the therapeutic plan. Most clients are treated as outpatients and independence should be encouraged. Clients may return to work as long as they do not overextend themselves. The nurse should encourage verbalization about resentment concerning the restrictions during treatment, especially with young children and adolescents. During these discussions, alternatives may be explored and found to be more compatible with the client's life-style.

CONCLUSION

The nursing care of clients receiving radiation therapy should be based on the data collected concerning the type of therapy, area treated, and expected complications. Nursing interventions should be based on this data and preventive measures instituted prior to actually starting treatment. A plan of care carefully developed and openly communicated will maintain consistency in the care of these clients.

REFERENCES

1. Ackerman, L. V., and del Regato, J. A.: Cancer diagnosis, treatment, and prognosis, ed. 4, St. Louis, 1975, The C. V. Mosby Co.
2. Barnes, P. A., and Rees, D. J.: A concise textbook of radiotherapy, Philadelphia, 1972, J. B. Lippincott Co.
3. Bloomer, W. D., and Hellman, S.: Normal tissue responses to radiation therapy, N. Engl. J. Med. **293:**80, 1975.
4. Bohnke, H. D., editor: Guidelines for comprehensive nursing care in cancer, New York, 1973, Springer Publishing Co., Inc.
5. Bounous, G., et al.: Dietary protection during radiation therapy, Strahlentherapie **149:**476, 1975.
6. Crate, M.: Nursing functions in adaptation to chronic illness, Am. J. Nurs. **65:**72, 1965.
7. DeWys, W. D., and Walters, K.: Abnormalities of

taste sensations in cancer patients, Cancer **36:**1888, 1975.
8. Dreizen, S., et al.: Oral complications of cancer radiotherapy, Postgrad. Med. **61:**85, 1977.
9. Elliott, C. S.: Radiation therapy: how you can help, Nursing '76 **6:**34, 1976.
10. Erickson, E. H.: Childhood and society, ed. 2, New York, 1963, W. W. Norton & Co., Inc.
11. Fletcher, G. H.: Textbook of radiotherapy, Philadelphia, 1966, Lea & Febiger.
12. Green, N., Gerald, I., and Smith, W. R.: Measures to minimize small intestine injury in the irradiated pelvis, Cancer **35:**1633, 1975.
13. Hegedus, S., and Phelham, M.: Dietetics in a cancer hospital, Perspect. Pract. **67:**235, 1975.
14. Hilkemeyer, D.: Nursing care in radium therapy, Nurs. Clin. North Am. **2:**83, 1967.
15. Maslow, A.: Motivation and personality, New York, 1954, Harper & Row, Publishers.
16. Moss, W. T., Brand, W. N., and Battifora, H.: Radiation oncology: rationale, technique, results, ed. 5, St. Louis, 1979, The C. V. Mosby Co.
17. Murray, R.: Principles of nursing intervention for the adult patient with body image changes, Nurs. Clin. North Am. **7:**697, 1972.
18. Nutrition and cancer, New York, 1972, American Cancer Society, Inc.
19. Nutrition, New York, 1974, American Cancer Society, Inc.
20. Prosnik, C. R.: Treatment for malignant disease, Part 1. The nurse and patient, Part 2, RN **34:**42, 1971.
21. Rotman, M., Rogow, L., DeLeon, G., and Heskel, N.: Supportive therapy in radiation oncology, Cancer **39:**744, 1977.
22. Rubin, P., editor: Clinical oncology for medical students and physicians, a multidisciplinary approach, ed. 5, Rochester, 1978, American Cancer Society, Inc.
23. Rubin, P., and Casarett, G. W.: Clinical radiation pathology, vol. 1, Philadelphia, 1968, W. B. Saunders Co.
24. Schreier, A., and Lavenia, J.: The nurse's role in nutritional management of radiotherapy patients, Nurs. Clin. North Am. **12:**173, 1977.
25. Schulz, M. D.: Treatment by irradiation. In Cancer—a manual for practitioners, Boston, 1970, Nimrod Press.
26. Sobo, A. O., and Johnston, I. D.: The effect of therapeutic irradiation of the abdomen on intestinal absorption in man, Am. J. Gastroenterol. **60:**616, 1973.
27. Theologides, A.: Nutritional management of the patient with advanced cancer, Postgrad. Med. **61:**97, 1977.
28. Trowbridge, J. E., and Carl, W.: Oral care of the patient having head-neck irradiation, Am. J. Nurs. **75:**2146, 1975.
29. Williams, E. R.: Making vegetarian diets nutritious, Am. J. Nurs. **75:**2168, 1975.
30. Worby, C., and Babineau, R.: The family interview: helping patient and family cope with metastatic disease, Geriatrics **74:**83, 1974.

14

Chemotherapy and the cancer nurse

SUSAN MOLLOY HUBBARD

Cancer has emerged as an important area of clinical specialization for physicians and nurses over the last decade. This development is related to the successful use of chemicals for the treatment of clients with widely disseminated cancers not amenable to treatment with surgery and radiotherapy. Since the initial demonstration that the systemic administration of mechlorethamine or nitrogen mustard could produce dramatic, albeit temporary, regressions of disease in clients with widespread lymphoma, it has been established that drugs alone can cure cancer.[37,50] The advent of effective combination chemotherapy regimens in clients with leukemia and disseminated lymphomas has permitted new approaches to be developed for the management of clients with many of the common neoplasms such as carcinoma of the breast.

However, the impact of cancer chemotherapy is not well appreciated. Despite the fact that the incidence of cancer is increasing, analysis of age-specific trends in cancer mortality in Americans since 1960 indicates that the death rate has *decreased* 20% for individuals under 45 years of age.[6,119] Fig. 14-1 illustrates the trend in cancer mortality between 1954 and 1976 for specific age groups. This improvement can be attributed to the successful treatment of certain cancers with effective chemotherapeutic programs. Death from cancer in persons under 30 years of age has decreased precipitously largely due to the impact of chemotherapy on the lymphomas and childhood neoplasms (Fig. 14-2).[6] Currently, it is expected that half of all children with cancer can be cured utilizing programs that employ cytotoxic drugs, often in combination with surgery or radiotherapy.[36] It should be recognized that chemotherapy can effectively palliate metastatic disease in a growing number of cancers, prolonging survival and improving the quality of life for many clients formerly considered untreatable.

Since nurses have always been intimately involved in the administration and evaluation of all drugs prescribed by physicians, it is consonant that they should play an important role in the development of systemic chemotherapy for cancer. This chapter will discuss the scientific rationale for the use of systemically administered drugs against cancer, currently available chemotherapeutic agents, and newly expanded nursing roles

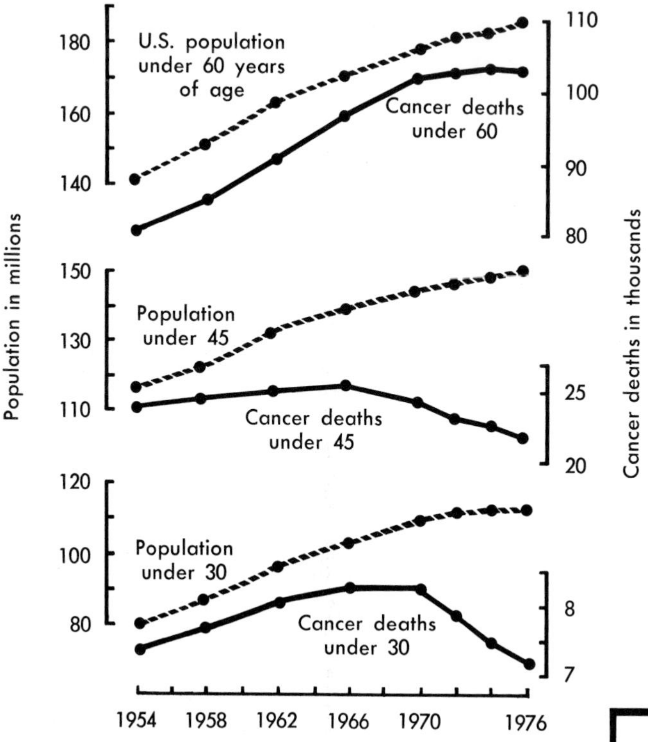

Fig. 14-1. Cancer mortality and United States population trends, 1954-1976. (Source of data: U.S. Public Health Service Statistics.)

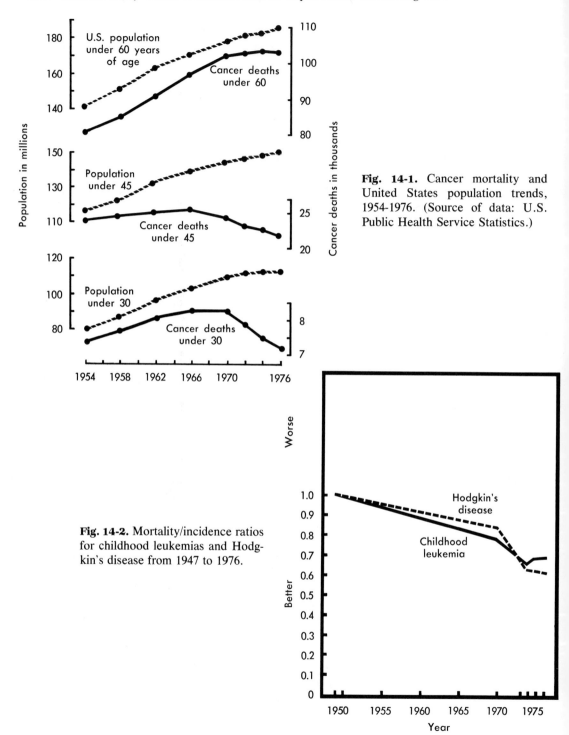

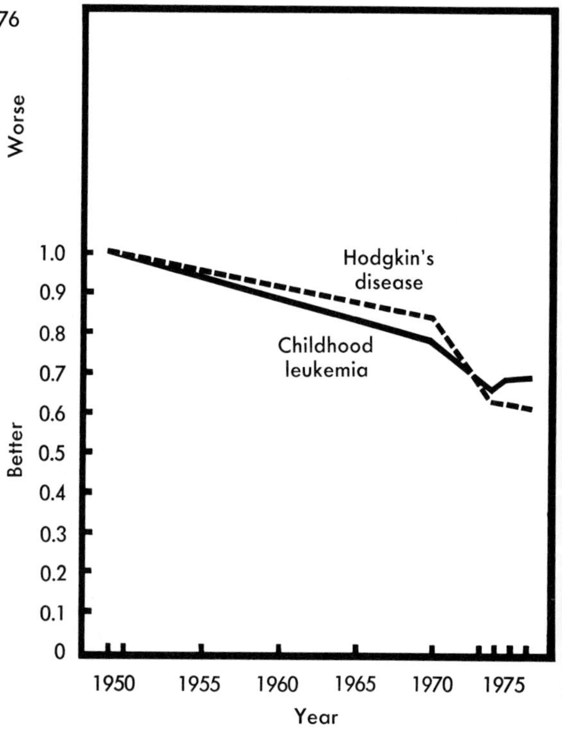

Fig. 14-2. Mortality/incidence ratios for childhood leukemias and Hodgkin's disease from 1947 to 1976.

that have emerged as drug treatment has become a more effective treatment modality.

BIOLOGIC CONSIDERATIONS

Cellular replication

The basic unit of all plant and animal life is the cell. Most cells have the inherent capacity to multiply through mitosis, a complex process of cellular replication. Cellular "growth" is influenced by many factors within the cell's environment. Knowledge concerning the normal behavior and characteristics of cellular growth and proliferation is essential to understand the complex nature of cancer and the rationale on which successful treatment is based. Bacteria and other unicellular organisms multiply until they exhaust the available supply of nutrients or until toxic waste products accumulate in their environment. When the organism is multicellular, complex levels of cellular organization and regulation occur with different cells performing specific vital functions required to sustain life. In multicellular organisms, unrestricted replication of any one of these cells is detrimental to the welfare of the community of cells. Regulation of the capacity to reproduce is necessary. Control of growth is provided by a complex set of biochemical events that can be termed a cellular "brake." This brake inhibits continued multiplication as the array of cells reaches a critical size and "crowding" begins to occur. While this regulatory system is not completely understood, it operates in toto as a feedback mechanism that begins to operate as cells come in contact with other cells, a concept that is known as "contact inhibition."[1] When cells are lost through injury or death, the feedback mechanisms release the brake for a specific period. During this period, cells multiply and regrowth occurs. Wound healing and regeneration of cells in the liver following injury are demonstrations of a normal release of this cellular brake, since the cells cease multiplication appropriately when the damage is repaired.

Neoplasia can be defined as the development of unrestricted cellular proliferation. Neoplasms are characterized by unregulated cellular growth and multiplication that fails to conform to the normal controls governing growth for a particular tissue. These new growths or tumors may be initiated by circumstances occurring in the organism's internal or external environment that abnormally release the cellular brake. In tumors, cells no longer cease replication when they reach a critical mass. Such uncontrolled growth will eventually lead to the death of the organism. Neoplastic growths can be either benign or malignant. Malignant tumors, commonly known as cancers, are the focus of this chapter.

Cell cycle

A brief discussion of the events that pertain to cell reproduction is essential for an understanding of the fundamental principles of tumor growth. The process begins in the nucleus of the cell and the entire period from a single reproduction to a second reproduction is known as the *cell cycle*.[55] Basically, the cell cycle can be divided into two periods, mitosis and interphase.[84] Mitosis, a relatively brief period in the cycle, is the time during which actual cell division takes place and can be divided into four stages as depicted in Fig. 14-3. Interphase encompasses the entire period of cellular growth that occurs between cell divisions. Interphase is a vital period of the cell cycle, because it is during this period that DNA replication occurs. Interphase can be divided into several distinct phases utilizing the G or Gap terminology as shown in Fig. 14-3.[32,55] At the completion of cell division or mitosis, cells enter a phase that is known as Gap 1 or G_1 phase. During this period, DNA syn-

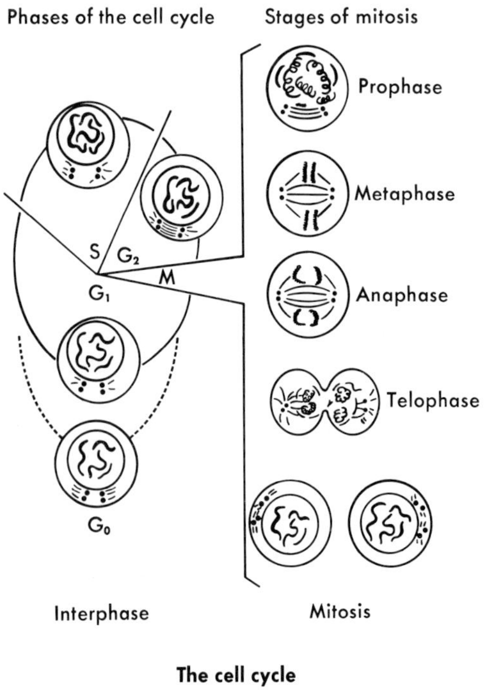

Fig. 14-3. Phases of cell cycle and stages of mitosis.

thesis ceases except for repair of damaged DNA, but RNA and protein synthesis continue actively. Somatic cellular growth (cellular enlargement) mainly occurs in this G_1 period, which is also known as the postmitotic period. At a critical point late in the G_1 period, a nuclear signal initiates a burst in RNA synthesis and the cell becomes committed to undergo mitosis. Following this burst of RNA synthesis, the synthetic period (S phase) of the cell cycle begins. During S phase, the DNA of the cell doubles in preparation for mitosis, resulting in two identical sets of chromosomes that contain all of the cell's genetic material. A complete set of chromosomes will occupy the nuclei of each of the two daughter cells produced during mitosis. RNA and protein synthesis continue actively during the S phase. Following DNA replication, the cell enters a premitotic phase referred to as Gap 2 (G_2) phase. During this phase, DNA synthesis ceases although RNA and protein synthesis continue. Then the cell undergoes mitosis, during which the genetic material is segregated into two daughter cells.

At a cellular level, antineoplastic agents can exert lethal effects by creating adverse conditions that prevent cells from dividing. These mechanisms involve the inactivation of essential enzymes; damage to structural proteins; inhibition of DNA, RNA, or protein synthesis; or direct interactions with DNA. Normal cellular replication is dependent on the orderly synthesis of these substances. Interference with the processes that occur during the normal cell cycle creates conditions that prevent normal cellular replication required for the cell to sustain life.

The cytotoxic effects of chemotherapeutic drugs can differ with regard to the portion of the cell cycle that is affected. Some drugs act primarily on cells that are synthesizing DNA. These drugs interfere with cellular metabolism by inhibiting essential enzymes or competing with normal cellular constituents required for DNA synthesis. Since DNA synthesis occurs during the S phase of the cell cycle, these *antimetabolite* drugs are only effective against cells that are in the S phase when the agent is administered. Cells in other phases of the cell cycle and those that enter the S phase after the drug is bound, metabolized, or excreted will not be damaged. Some antimetabolite agents that have the capacity to interfere with DNA formation also have the capacity to inhibit RNA and protein synthesis, which makes them cytotoxic to cells in other phases of the cell cycle.

Other types of chemotherapeutic drugs exert their lethal effect by *arresting mitosis* during the metaphase stage (Fig. 14-3). These agents inhibit the proper assembly of proteins that form the mitotic spindle apparatus. While the lethal effect of these drugs is expressed during mitosis, the damage may result from exposure of the cells to the drug during earlier phases of the cell cycle. Antimetabolites and mitotic inhibitors are all considered *cycle-specific* agents, since their lethal action is dependent on administration during specific phases of the cell cycle.

A final group of drugs exerts a direct effect on DNA. They prevent separation of the helical structure and thus block successful cell division. The lethal damage produced by these alkylating agents occurs in all phases of the cell cycle. These drugs are lethal to cells in resting phases of the cycle, although damage may not become apparent until the cells enter the S phase. Alkylating agents, however, also covalently bind (in a relatively nonspecific fashion) to most cellular constituents, and multiple mechanisms of lethality are possible for this class of drugs.

Kinetic considerations in relation to cancer treatment

While individual cancer cells often do not divide faster than normal cells, tumor "doubling time" (the time required for a given mass to double its volume) is often shorter for tumor tissue.[87] This can be attributed to a number of related variables. Only a portion of cells in a given cell population that are potentially capable of undergoing mitosis will do so at any given time. A fraction of viable cells, with the capacity to divide, can remain in a "resting" phase for prolonged periods of time. The ratio of dividing cells to resting cells in a mass (the growth fraction) will affect the doubling time in the mass. The growth fraction in a tumor varies at different times and contributes to changes in doubling times and tumor volume. Given a specific cell cycle length, a tumor with a large growth fraction will double faster than a tumor of the same size with a small growth fraction if the loss of cells from each mass remains constant. Loss of cancer cells from the mass through death or metastases is an important factor that affects the rate of tumor growth. A high rate of cell loss can prolong the tumor doubling time even in tumors with high growth fractions.[87]

Cells that are not in cycle but remain viable and capable of undergoing mitosis under proper circumstances are said to be in a quiescent phase known as G_0. The existence of the G_0 "resting" phase is critical to our understanding of tumor growth and chemotherapeutic strategy. These cells, not actively synthesizing DNA, are far less vulnerable to damage from irradiation or drug therapy.[114] Additionally, there is evidence that some cancer cells may be blocked from proceeding from one phase of the cell cycle to another for long periods, thus creating other periods when the cell may be more resistant to therapy.[47] Treatment programs that can "recruit" tumor cells out of these resting states might provide complete eradication of all viable cancer cells in the host.[74] These resting states have an important impact on the scheduling of treatment. They provide a major rationale for combining therapies with different sites and mechanisms of action and for exploring different schedules of administration.[108,115]

The behavior and growth characteristics of normal and neoplastic cells can be compared and contrasted graphically as depicted in Fig. 14-4. The initial slope shown by the rising solid line represents the exponential growth that is characteristic of the early somatic growth in the normal embryo or in rapidly enlarging tumors. When tissues reach their mature adult size, an equilibrium between the rates of cell birth and cell death is maintained by normal tissues. This steady state is represented by the solid horizontal line. In cancer, cells continue to multiply despite overcrowding, violating the feedback mechanism of contact inhibition. However, as the tumor increases in size, the time required for the mass to double also increases. Continued exponential growth, which would be rapidly and predictably lethal, cannot be maintained because of the limited supply of essential nutrients and accumulation of waste products in the surrounding environment.[32] This retardation of the tumor growth rate is depicted by the dotted lines.

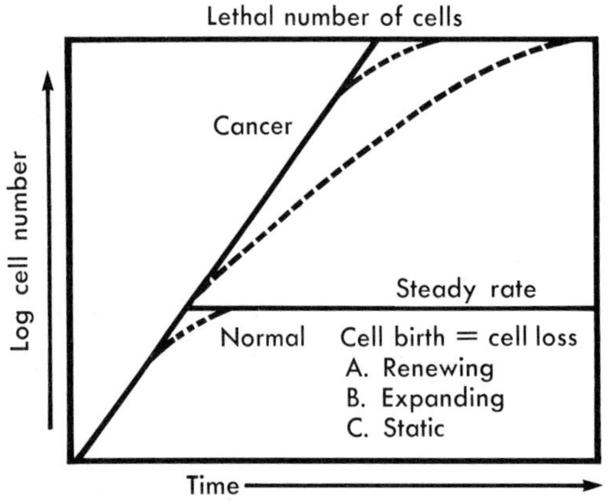

Fig. 14-4. Comparison of normal and neoplastic growth.

Growth characteristics of individual cells in a given tumor mass can be divided into three general categories (Fig. 14-5). Cells in compartment A are actively replicating and most susceptible to injury. Compartment B consists of cells in the G_1 and the G_0 resting phases. Cells in this compartment are relatively insensitive to modalities that interfere with mitosis or the synthesis of essential proteins required for successful cell division. Cells can generally move between compartments A and B, and cells in both compartments are mitotically competent. Compartment C consists of cells that have lost the capacity to divide. Essentially they contribute only mass to the tumor.[109]

The theoretical tumor growth curve depicted in Fig. 14-6 illustrates the number of times a tumor that is growing at a constant rate must double itself from the time of its inception until it reaches a lethal volume in man. The figure correlates the number of tumor cell doublings with the approximate number of cells and the size of the tumor mass. A tumor is generally undetectable with currently available diagnostic techniques until it has doubled 27 times, which is approximately equal to two thirds of its total

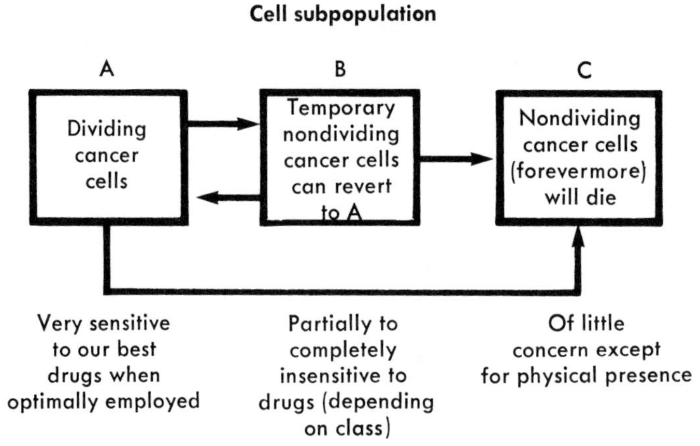

Fig. 14-5. Schematic illustration of cell types in individual tumor.

growth potential. When a tumor can first be visualized radiographically, it has a mass of 0.5 cm^3. The smallest palpable tumor is approximately 1 cm^3 in size and contains more than 1 billion (1×10^9) cancer cells (30 tumor doublings). After 35 tumor doublings, the tumor as an aggregate mass of cells could be 30 cm in diameter. With 5 additional doublings (40 doublings) the tumor mass contains 1 trillion cells (1×10^{12}), sufficient to kill the host.[36]

Based on these figures, cancers are "advanced" by the time they can be diagnosed by currently available techniques. Multiple tumor masses, containing up to 1 billion tumor cells, can exist throughout the body and be undetected by careful physical examination. Therefore, the vast majority of clients with clinically detectable cancer have disease that is biologically in the late stages of its growth. In most cases, these cancers are shedding viable tumor cells that are capable of establishing metastases in other sites throughout the body. Many clients who appear to have early, localized cancers at diagnosis actually have microscopic dissemination that is clinically undetected.

Animal experiments have demonstrated that often a single cancer cell innoculated into the body can multiply, as theoretically shown in Fig. 14-6, to a level that is lethal to the host. This has considerable clinical significance. The therapeutic implication is that a cancer cannot be considered cured until the last cancer cell is destroyed. Treatment that is stopped when disease is no longer clinically evident may leave large numbers of undetected residual tumor cells in the body. The length of time required for a specific therapy to produce a cure is dependent on many biologic factors such as the number of viable tumor cells, the rate of growth, the ratio of dividing tumor cells to

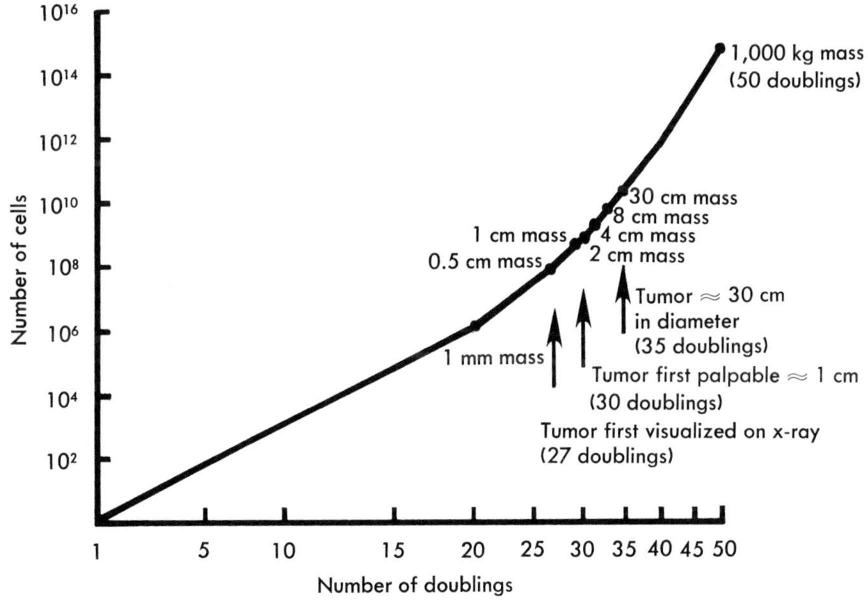

Fig. 14-6. Theoretical tumor growth curve illustrating volume. (Modified from DeVita, V. T., Young, R. C., and Cannellos, G. P.: Cancer **35:**98, 1975. Reprinted with permission.)

resting cells, and the capacity of the host's immune system to eradicate residual tumor when the volume of cancer cells is sufficiently reduced. An understanding of the kinetics of growth in both normal and cancerous tissue has provided a rational basis for successful treatment programs, which often attempt to exploit differences between normal and abnormal growth characteristics.[117]

Rationale for the use of drugs in cancer treatment

The modern era of utilizing cytotoxic drugs in cancer treatment has its roots in the successful development of drugs for the chemotherapy of infectious diseases.[20] The antitumor potential of chemicals was documented as long ago as 1865 when potassium arsenite was shown to produce responses in chronic leukemias and lymphomas.[79] The antistreptococcal activity of sulfonamides was shown to be due to an antimetabolite action, inhibition of folic acid synthesis.[124] This understanding of antimetabolites led to the synthesis of the first folic acid antagonists capable of producing remissions in childhood acute leukemia.[41] There are several analogies between infections and cancer. Both, when truly localized, can be eradicated with localized forms of treatment such as surgery. Disseminated infections and cancer must be treated systemically if all pathogens or malignant cells are to be eradicated. Host defenses play an important role in both the dissemination of infections and cancers and the ability of the body to destroy abnormal organisms and tumor cells. Localized forms of treatment can potentiate the effect of the systemic treatment by decreasing the volume of abnormal organisms or tumor cells that must be eradicated to produce a cure of disease.

Many experiments have indicated that

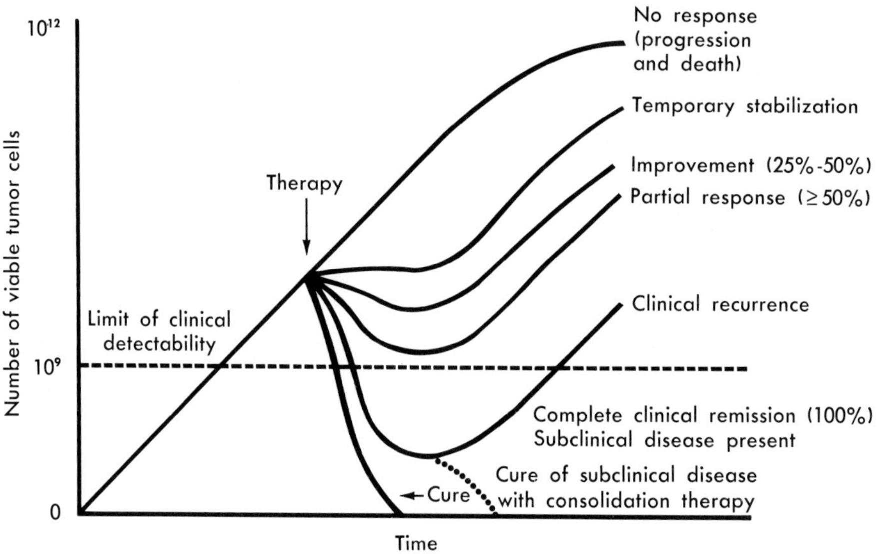

Fig. 14-7. Possible responses to chemotherapy. (From Medical-surgical nursing: a conceptual approach, by D. A. Jones, M. A. Juronec, and C. A. Dunbar. Copyright © 1978 Mc-Graw Hill Book Co. Used with permission of McGraw-Hill Book Co.)

antibiotics kill a constant fraction of susceptible organisms rather than a fixed number.[109,116] This dose-response relationship is known as *first-order kinetics* and is applicable to the destruction of cancer cells by antineoplastic agents. This concept of cell kill by first-order kinetics means that a given dosage of an agent will destroy a fixed percentage of the abnormal cells rather than a specific number of cells. If a specific agent can destroy 50% of the cells, it will decrease 1,000,000 neoplastic cells to 500,000 cells and 100,000 cells to 50,000 cells, and so forth. This means that in clients with clinical evidence of cancer, and hence large numbers of tumor cells, total cell kill generally can be achieved only when repeated doses of the drug are administered. One viable residual tumor cell has the capacity to replicate and to kill the host with recurrent tumor if not eradicated by the treatment program or by the body's immune system.

Drug combinations also kill cells according to first-order kinetics, but an effective combination can destroy an even greater percentage of cancer cells. Repeated administrations of effective combinations therefore would reduce tumor cell volume to a greater degree than would single agents with each course of treatment. Reduction of tumor volume by chemotherapy is illustrated in Fig. 14-7. The rate of clinical regression of disease is dependent on the percentage of tumor that is destroyed, the rate of cell removal, and the rate of regrowth of both sensitive and resistant cancer cells after therapy. It is essential to recall that the volume of cells required for a mass to be clinically detected is approximately 1 billion (1×10^9) cells. Below this level of detectability there are large numbers of cancer cells that represent microscopic or subclinical disease. A major problem in evaluating the effectiveness of a therapeutic modality is the assessment of whether residual disease is present after therapy and the measurement of the volume of residual tumor cells in clients who appear clinically free of disease.

CHEMOTHERAPEUTIC AGENTS IN CLINICAL USE

In the past 30 years, over 60 drugs have been proved effective for use in clients with cancer. Forty (including hormonal agents) are now commercially available. Chemotherapeutic agents can be classified by chemical structure or by biochemical mechanism of action. A commonly utilized classification separates drugs into six broad categories: alkylating agents, antimetabolites, plant alkaloids, antibiotics, steroid hormones, immunologic agents (see Chapter 15 for discussion), and a category of miscellaneous agents that cannot be categorized easily. Fig. 14-8 illustrates the mechanism of action of certain chemotherapeutic agents at the cellular level as they are currently understood. Table 14-1 summarizes currently utilized chemotherapeutic agents by class. Dosage, route, schedule of administration, major toxicities, and nursing implications of treatment are listed briefly. Side-effects that are unique to a specific drug will be briefly described in this section. General toxicities associated with cancer chemotherapy will be discussed in a later section.

Alkylating agents

Alkylating agents comprise a class of chemical compounds that, among other actions, disrupt the structure of DNA. Structurally, alkylating agents contain one or more alkyl groups that bind covalently to cellular macromolecules such as DNA. This can result in coding errors, breaks in the DNA molecule, and cross-linkage between DNA strands, which interferes with mitosis by preventing separation of the strands in the DNA helix. The antitumor activity of alkylating agents is *not* cell cycle specific. Al-

Text continued on p. 306.

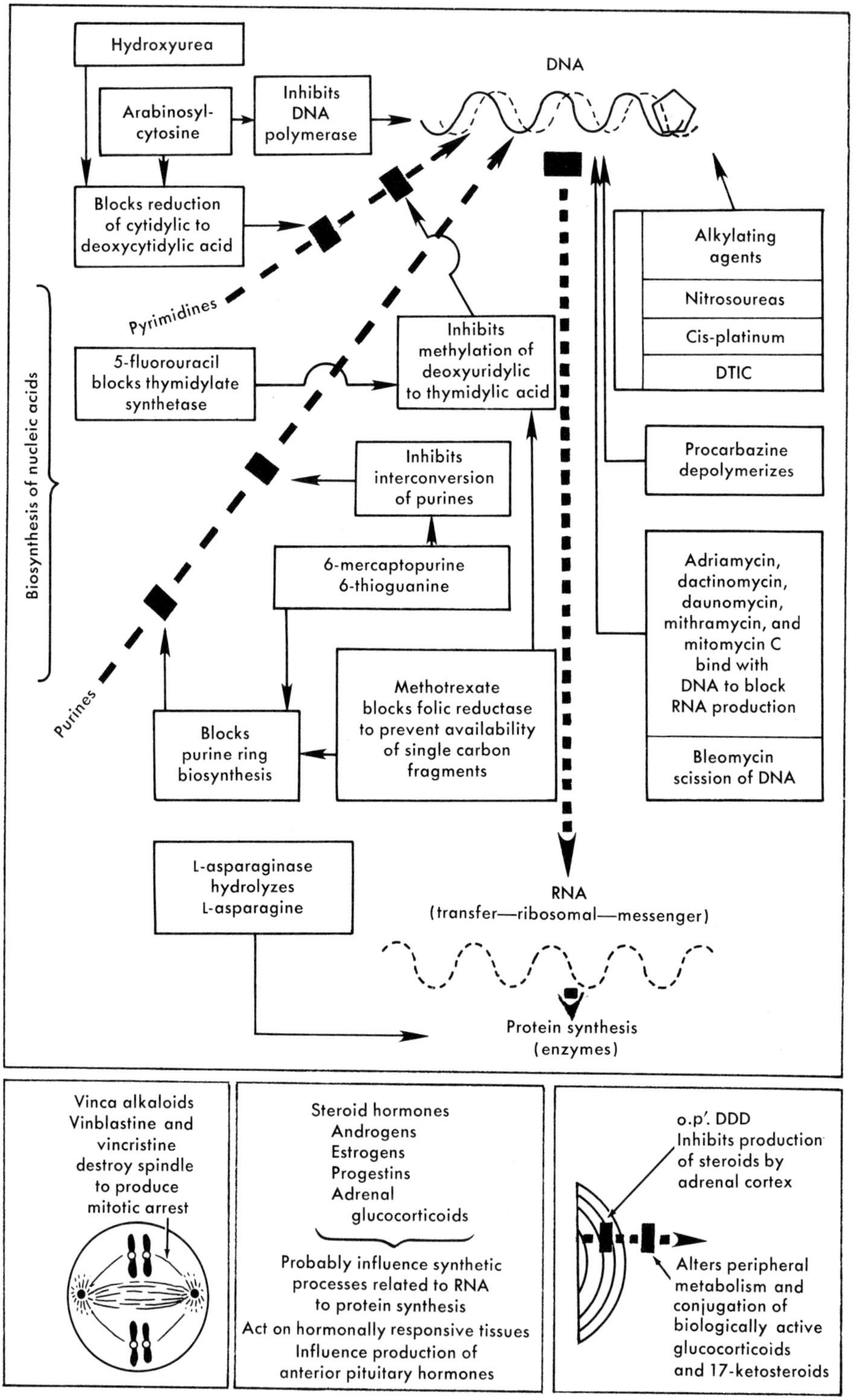

Fig. 14-8. Mechanism of action of chemotherapeutic agents at cellular level. (Reprinted with permission from ACS and Krakoff, I. H.: CA **27**[3]:140, 1977.)

Table 14-1. Chemotherapeutic agents

Currently available chemotherapeutic agents	Dose, route, schedule	Acute toxicity	Bone marrow toxicity (1+ [mild] to 4+ [severe])	Other toxicity	Nursing implications comments
Alkylating agents					
Mechlorethamine (HN_2, nitrogen mustard [Mustargen])	0.4 mg/kg IV q3-4 wk 0.2-0.4 mg/kg (intracavitary)	Severe nausea and vomiting (N/V) in ½-2 hr lasting 2-12 hr Fever, chills, malaise (intracavitary)	4+	Powerful vesicant—avoid extravasation Avoid skin contact Temporary/permanent sterility	Administer in well-established intravenous line to reduce chemical phlebitis; may discolor veins Rapid alkylating action Intracavitary instillation produces intense inflammatory reactions May cause tinnitis and skin rashes
Cyclophosphamide (CYT, Cytoxan, Endoxan)	500-1,500 mg/m² IV q3-4 wk 60-120 mg/m² PO qd continuous	N/V is dose related—occurs 4-12 hr after administration and lasts 8-10 hr Continuous oral use may cause chronic nausea and anorexia	3+	Alopecia in 50% occurs in 3 wk Hemorrhagic cystitis, sterility Hepatotoxicity Hyperpigmentation Ridging of fingernails	Maintain high levels of hydration, 2-3 L/day with large IV doses to induce frequent voiding and prevent cystitis Causes less severe thrombocytopenia At high doses may have an antidiuretic effect with impairment of fluid elimination Client immunosuppressant
L-phenylalanine mustard (L-PAM, Melphalan)	0.2 mg/kg PO qd × 5 d q4-6 wk 0.05-0.1 mg/kg PO continuously	Minimal N/V	3+	Prolonged use may produce persistent thrombocytopenia and mucositis Sterility	Five-day schedule in use for adjuvant therapy in breast cancer Well tolerated by most clients Renal excretion

Continued.

Table 14-1. Chemotherapeutic agents—cont'd

Currently available chemotherapeutic agents	Dose, route, schedule	Acute toxicity	Bone marrow toxicity (1+ [mild] to 4+ [severe])	Other toxicity	Nursing implications comments
Chlorambucil (Leukeran)	0.05-0.2 mg/kg PO qd	Rare N/V seen at high doses	3+	Prolonged use may produce persistent pancytopenia	May be useful in autoimmune hemolytic anemia Well tolerated by clients
Busulfan (Myleran)	0.05-0.2 mg/kg PO qd	Rare N/V	3+	Hyperpigmentation of skin Pulmonary fibrosis (busulfan lung) Gynecomastia, sterility Adrenal insufficiency	Continuous daily administration Renal excretion
Triethylenethiophosphoramide (Thio-Tepa, TSPA, TESPA)	0.2 mg/kg IV qd × 5 q3-4 wk 10-30 mg/m² IV q3 wk	N/V is dose related	3+	Can cause allergic reactions Dermatitis	Can be given intramuscularly and subcutaneously Intracavitary use for control of effusions associated with fever and headache Bladder instillation for superficial bladder tumors
Carmustine (BiCNU)	200 mg/m² IV q4-6 wk	Severe N/V in 4-12 hr lasting 12-24 hr	4+	Delayed myelosuppression in 4-6 wk Pulmonary fibrosis Brown discoloration of skin	Burning sensation, localized pain, and general flushing during IV administration owing to alcohol diluent Crosses blood-brain barrier Cumulative marrow toxicity

[illegible]	[illegible] q4-6 wk	Moderate to severe N/V in 2-6 hr	[illegible]	Delayed myelosuppression	Give on empty stomach; if taken at bedtime, acute effects reduced Cumulative marrow toxicity, crosses blood-brain barrier
Semustine (methyl CCNU)	200 mg/m² PO q4-6 wk	High incidence of moderate to severe N/V in 1-4 hr	4+	Renal failure with prolonged administration reported Delayed myelosuppression More pronounced thrombocytopenia	Give on empty stomach at bedtime
Streptozoticin	500 mg/m² IV qd × 5d q3-4 wk 1,500 mg/m² IV q wk	High incidence of moderate to severe N/V in 1-4 hr Diarrhea	0	Renal tubular acidosis can lead to anuria; monitor renal function, proteinuria, glycosuria Reactive hypoglycemia caused by sudden insulin release Hepatotoxicity	Pain at infusion site Administer over 1 hr with 1-2 L normal saline Test urine for protein and glucose prior to each dose; discontinue dose if grossly positive
Triazenoimidazole carboxamide, dacarbazine (Dtic-Dome)	150-250 mg/m² qd × 5d q4 wk 1,000-1,200 mg/m² q4 wk	Moderate to severe N/V in most patients especially at high doses	3+	Flulike syndrome Metallic taste Mild hepatotoxicity Cumulative myelosuppression	Protect from light; N/V decreases with daily × 5 schedule Burning sensation during infusion Avoid extravasation; may cause thrombophlebitis
Antimetabolites					
Methotrexate (MTX, Amethopterin)	20-80 mg/m² IV, IM or PO q wk	Mild to moderate nausea Occasional vomiting	3+	Mucositis, especially buccal ulcerations Rare diarrhea; some alopecia; fatigue	Maintenance therapy in acute leukemia Renal excretion; monitor renal function with use

Continued.

Table 14-1. Chemotherapeutic agents—cont'd

Currently available chemotherapeutic agents	Dose, route, schedule	Acute toxicity	Bone marrow toxicity (1+ [mild] to 4+ [severe])	Other toxicity	Nursing implications comments
Antimetabolites—cont'd Methotrexate—cont'd				Hepatic fibrosis; pneumonitis; ocular irritation	Avoid aspirin and other compounds that displace MTX from plasma proteins
	15 mg/m² intrathecal q wk	None		Arachnoiditis Neurotoxicity	Administer in Elliot's B solution; use preservative-free MTX Monitor CSF levels; intrathecal dose related to systemic circulation; decrease or omit systemic dose
	2-10 gm/m² q3-4 wk given in 6 hr infusion with calcium leukovorin 15 mg q 3 hr × 8 Starting 2 hr after end of MTX infusion	Mild to moderate N/V	+/− (unusual)	Lethal without rescue Renal failure at high doses to precipitation of drug in renal tubules Alkalinize urine with sodium bicarbonate to prevent crystallization; maintain urine pH 7 Maintain urine output 150 ml/hr	Use preservative-free MTX Monitor serum MTX levels; *do not* discontinue leucovorin rescue until MTX levels are less than 1×10^{-8} molar Monitor creatinine clearance, BUN Monitor urine output and urinary pH closely
6-Mercaptopurine (6-MP)	1-2.5 mg/kg PO qd	Occasional N/V	2+	Stomatitis Hepatotoxicity Drug fever	Hepatic metabolism; renal excretion Reduce dosage in clients with hepatic/renal abnormalities

					Reduce dosage with allopurinol administration to 30% owing to delay in degradation of drug
6-Thioguanine (6-TG)	1-2 mg/kg PO qd	Occasional N/V	2+	Stomatitis Diarrhea	Hepatic metabolism; renal excretion Reduce dose with hepatic/renal dysfunction No dose reduction needed with concomitant allopurinol
5-Fluorouracil	7.5-12 mg/kg IV qd × 5d then qod until toxicity or q wk	Mild to moderate N/V	3+	Chronic N/V after prolonged administration Stomatitis, diarrhea Ataxia, alopecia Photophobia, ocular irritation	Oral administration of intravenous preparation Investigational for oral use—absorption erratic Stomatitis indication to interrupt therapy Intra-arterial infusions 20-25 mg/kg qd × 8-21d
Cytosine arabinoside (ARA-C), Cytosar, Cytarabine)	100 mg/m² q12 hr IV or SC for 7-21d 100 mg/m² continuous infusion × 10d 20-30 mg/m² intrathecal use	Dose-related N/V	4+	Alopecia, fever Diarrhea, stomatitis Hepatotoxicity Neurotoxicity with intrathecal use	Hepatic metabolism—use with care in hepatic dysfunction Intrathecal administration for MTX-resistant CNS disease—use preservative-free diluent Transient immunosuppression
5-Azacytidine	150-300 mg/m² IV × 3-5d	Dose-related N/V Diarrhea in 50%	4+	Rapid infusion may cause hypotension Hepatotoxicity	Very unstable after reconstitution—use within 6 hr Ringer's lactate provides optimal pH and stability

Continued.

Table 14-1. Chemotherapeutic agents—cont'd

Currently available chemotherapeutic agents	Dose, route, schedule	Acute toxicity	Bone marrow toxicity (1+ [mild] to 4+ [severe])	Other toxicity	Nursing implications comments
Antimetabolites—cont'd					
5-Azacytidine—cont'd					Can be given subcutaneously Continuous infusions produce less N/V N/V decreases with each daily dose
Plant alkaloids					
Vincristine (Oncovin, VCR)	0.5-2 mg/m^2 IV q wk	Rare N/V Metallic taste	+/− (unusual)	Paresthesias, loss of DTR's, footdrop Motor weakness, hoarseness, constipation, abdominal pain Jaw pain, alopecia Tissue necrosis	Hepatic metabolism and excretion—dose reductions necessary in hepatic dysfunction Increased toxicity in elderly and immobilized clients and clients with hepatic dysfunction Stable in solution for 14d if refrigerated Prophylactic use of stool softeners and laxatives
Vinblastine (Velban)	6 mg/m^2 IV q wk 0.1-0.4 mg/kg IV q wk	Occasional N/V	3+	Stomatitis, diarrhea Cumulative myelotoxicity Headache Tissue necrosis	Minimal neurotoxicity Stable in solution for 30d if refrigerated Hepatic metabolism—reduce dose if hepatic dysfunction exists
Etoposide (VP-16)	50-60 mg/m^2 IV × 5d	Mild N/V Bronchospasm and hypotension (if infused	3+	Alopecia Anorexia	Antihistamines may relieve bronchospasm Administer over 30-45 min

Dactinomycin, Actinomycin D (Cosmegan)	0.015 mg/kg IV × 5d q3-4 wk	Moderate to severe N/V in 2-5 hr lasting 12-24 hr	3+	Alopecia, stomatitis, diarrhea Erythema and skin rash Prolonged anorexia, glossitis, tissue necrosis	N/V decreases with daily schedule; severe skin reactions in areas of previous irradiation Dosage in micrograms (μg)
Mithramycin (Mithracin)	0.025-1.05 mg/kg IV qod to toxicity 0.025 mg/kg IV for tumor-related hypercalcemia	Moderate N/V in 6 hr lasting 12-24 hr	3+	Fever, stomatitis, facial flush, tissue necrosis Coagulation abnormalities and bleeding Severe thrombocytopenia CNS alterations, neuromuscular hyperexcitability Azotemia, hypocalcemia, hypokalemia	Increased N/V with rapid infusions Increased toxicity in clients with renal and hepatic dysfunctions—interrupt therapy when BUN, SGOT, LDH become abnormal
Mitomycin-C (Mutamycin)	2 mg/m² IV qd × 5d 15 mg/m² IV q6-8 wk	Mild to moderate N/V in 1-2 hr lasting 2-3d	4+	Malaise Renal and hepatic toxicity Tissue necrosis Stomatitis, diarrhea	Myelosuppression is delayed and cumulative and may last 2-3 wk
Doxorubicin hydrochloride (Adriamycin, ADM)	45-75 mg/m² IV q3-4 wk	Moderate N/V in 50% of clients	4+	Cardiotoxicity; irreversible CHF Complete loss of body hair in 3-4 wk Stomatitis, diarrhea Hepatotoxicity Tissue necrosis	Reduce dose with hepatic dysfunction; cardiotoxicity and N/V increased with use with cytoxan Total dose limitation of 550 mg/m² Red discoloration of urine; skin reactions in areas of prior irradiation

Continued.

Table 14-1. Chemotherapeutic agents—cont'd

Currently available chemotherapeutic agents	Dose, route, schedule	Acute toxicity	Bone marrow toxicity (1+ [mild] to 4+ [severe])	Other toxicity	Nursing implications comments
Antitumor antibiotics—cont'd					
Doxorubicin hydrochloride—cont'd					CHF may occur 6 mo after end of therapy
Daunomycin hydrochloride (Daunorubicin, rubidomycin DNR)	30-60 mg/m² IV × 3d	Moderate to severe N/V	4+	Cardiotoxicity Complete alopecia in 3-4 wk Tissue necrosis	Stomatitis and diarrhea uncommon Total dose limitation of 450-500 mg/m² Red discoloration of urine Dose reduction in hepatic dysfunction
Bleomycin (BLEO) (Blenoxane)	5-15 U/m² IV, IM, SC q wk 5 U/m² IV, IM, SC, BLW	Minimal N/V Anaphylactic reactions Bronchospasm Hypertension	1+	Pulmonary fibrosis at doses of 300 U/m² Chills, malaise Hyperpigmentation Stomatitis, alopecia Skin lesions progressing to ulcerations Fever to 103°-105° F	Antihistamines may relieve febrile reactions Local pain with IM/SC use Total dose limitation of 300 U/m² Pulmonary fibrosis can develop early Anaphylaxis precautions and use of test doses
Miscellaneous agents					
L-asparaginase (Elspar)	10-500 IU/kg IV qd × 14-28d	Moderate to severe N/V in 50% Fever, chills Urticaria Anaphylaxis	0	Progressive malaise Hyperglycemia, acute pancreatitis, hepatotoxicity Coagulation abnormalities CNS toxicity, azotemia	Urticaria seen in 30% after repeated exposure Anaphylaxis can occur after repeated exposure Desensitization can be done by using test doses Solution is unstable; discard after use

[illegible] (Matulane)	100-200 mg/m² PO × 14d or continuously	Moderate to severe N/V, which subsides with daily use	3+	Allergic skin rash CNS alternations, somnolence, hyperexcitability Ataxia, confusion Immunosuppression	Crosses blood-brain barrier Avoid all CNS depressants and alcohol Use phenothiazines with care Avoid foods rich in tyramine to prevent hypertensive crisis
Hydroxyurea (Hydrea)	25 mg/kg PO continuous 100 mg/kg IV × 3d	Minimal N/V	3+	Skin rash Alopecia Gastrointestinal ulceration	Rapid reduction in peripheral blast counts in 24-48 hr when given intravenously
Hexamethylmelamine (HXM)	6-12 mg/kg PO qd × 21d continuously	Severe N/V	1+	Peripheral neuropathy Somnolence, depression, hallucinations Diarrhea	Exacerbation of VCR neuropathy N/V may be dose-limiting toxic effect; give in divided doses
O,p'-DDD (mitotane, Lysodren)	2-10 gm/PO qd continuously	Severe N/V	0	Diarrhea Mental depression, lethargy, somnolence Dizziness Skin rash	N/V is often dose limiting
Cisplatin (DDP, Platinol)	60-120 mg/m² IV q3-4 wk 15-20 mg/m² × 5d	Severe N/V	1+	Renal tubular necrosis Ototoxicity Peripheral neuropathy	N/V decreased with prolonged infusions Renal function must be monitored closely Hydration to ensure urinary output 150 ml/hr Anaphylactic reactions after repeated exposure

though replicating cells are more vulnerable, alkylating agents are effective against resting cells as well as those that are dividing or preparing to divide. In addition to exerting a direct effect on the structure of DNA, other molecules in the cell's nucleus can be alkylated by these drugs. Among these are enzymes that participate in the formation of the new DNA strands. The variability in therapeutic activity between alkylating agents depends on which molecules are damaged by alkylating activity.

The nitrogen mustards

Mechlorethamine. Mechlorethamine (nitrogen mustard or HN_2) was the first of the alkylating agents. Studies of soldiers exposed to lethal doses of mustard gases during World War I demonstrated evidence of selective atrophy of lymphoid tissues and profound leukopenia.[73] This observation led to interest in using mustard gas derivatives in clients with advanced lymphomas and leukemia. In the late 1940's, nitrogen mustard was successfully used to induce short remissions in clients with advanced lymphomas.[50] Nitrogen mustard can react to produce two active alkyl radicals. Its action is extremely rapid. Within a few minutes after administration the active drug is no longer detectable and is bound to proteins and other molecules. Its clinical use is limited by very severe nausea, vomiting, and bone marrow depression. It is a powerful vesicant that can cause severe tissue necrosis if extravasated into subcutaneous tissues. It may also cause chemical phlebitis, discoloration, and thrombosis of veins used for injections. Lymphoid tissue is particularly susceptible to the alkylating action of mechlorethamine, and its major therapeutic use is for the treatment of Hodgkin's disease and other lymphomas. Because of its rapid action, nitrogen mustard has been used as a sclerosing agent in the management of malignant pleural effusions. This use is often associated with an intense inflammatory reaction accompanied by high fever.

Cyclophosphamide. Cyclophosphamide (Cytoxan, CYT) is a cyclic mustard, a synthetic derivative of mechlorethamine that was rationally designed in hopes of producing selective activity against cancer cells. Some tumor cells demonstrated elevated levels of phosphatase activity, so scientists synthesized an agent that would remain inert until activated by this class of enzymes.[25] Theoretically, cyclophosphamide would be activated at the tumor site and have little effect on normal tissue. In practice, it was found that most tumors did not have this enzyme and the compound is activated by enzymes in hepatic microsomes that alter the drug at a different site than originally proposed.[96] Despite these disappointments, cyclophosphamide has proved to be a highly effective antineoplastic agent against a broad spectrum of neoplasms that spans from the hematoreticular malignancies to solid tumors.[80] It is more stable in solution than mechlorethamine and can be given orally.

Like other alkylating agents in the mustard class, cyclophosphamide is most active against rapidly replicating cells and causes bone marrow depression, alopecia, and gastrointestinal toxicity. Active metabolites are excreted in urine and these metabolites can produce hemorrhagic lesions in the bladder. Prolonged administration may be associated with hyperplastic changes of bladder epithelium that are associated with chronic cystitis.[93] The urinary concentration of cytotoxic metabolites should be minimized by increasing the urine volume through forced hydration.[95] It is noteworthy to mention that high-dose cyclophosphamide infusions (>50 mg/kg) can be associated with impairment of water excretion, manifested by dilutional hyponatremia, weight gain, and inappropriately concentrated urine in well-hydrated clients.[31] The mechanism for this side-effect is thought to be related to a direct effect of a metabolite on the distal renal tubule. Other unusual effects include skin hyperpigmentation, cardiac and pulmonary damage at high dosages,[91] and a sensation of dizziness during rapid intravenous injection.

Cyclophosphamide is a potent immunosuppressant. It has been used effectively in the management of clients with organ transplants, certain vasculidities, and in disorders associated with altered immune reactivity such as rheumatoid arthritis and Wegener's granulomatosis.[43,48] Since cyclophosphamide can produce sterility and the drug is known to be teratogenic, the benefits and risks of this agent for clients during reproductive years should be carefully considered and discussed openly with clients.[5,40]

Phenylalanine mustard. Phenylalanine mustard (L-PAM) is another synthetic derivative of mechlorethamine. It can be administered orally and its administration is not associated with hemorrhagic cystitis. Nausea, vomiting, and alopecia are also far less pronounced. Bone marrow suppression is the most marked side-effect. L-PAM is useful in the therapy of multiple myeloma and breast, ovarian, and testicular cancers.[80]

Chlorambucil. The slowest acting mustard compound is chlorambucil. It is given orally and has relatively little acute toxicity. Chlorambucil is particularly active against cells of lymphoid origin. It has clinical value primarily in the therapy of chronic lymphocytic leukemia and non-Hodgkin's lymphomas.[80]

Busulfan. Busulfan is a sulfur mustard that is given orally. Its toxic effect is primarily exerted against granulocytic cells of the bone marrow. Its use is limited to treatment of chronic hematologic malignancies. Prolonged use may result in pulmonary fibrosis, which may be fatal, especially if the client is not carefully monitored for this complication.[72] The drug can also produce hyperpigmentation of the skin and, rarely, a syndrome resembling adrenal insufficiency.

Triethylenethiophosphoramide. Triethylenethiophosphoramide (Thio-Tepa) is an alkylating agent that can be used to control malignant effusions. Unlike mechlorethamine it does not cause an intense inflammatory reaction following intracavitary administration. It can also be instilled directly into the bladder in clients with superficial bladder tumors.[121] When it is given systemically, it causes minimal gastrointestinal disturbance.

Nitrosoureas. The nitrosoureas are a family of compounds that have activity similar but not identical to classical alkylating agents. They have both alkylating and carbamylating activity (formation of a covalent bond with free amine groups of certain amino acids) and may also act by inhibiting DNA repair. The nitrosoureas are highly reactive and produce active metabolites that are not as yet fully characterized.[97] Three of these compounds, 1,3-bis (2-cloroethyl)-1-nitrosourea (BCNU, carmustine); 1,(2-cloroethyl)-3-cyclohexyl-1-nitrosourea (CCNU, lomustine); and 1,(2-cloroethyl-3-4-methylcyclohexyl-1-nitrosourea (MeCCNU, semustine) have been evaluated clinically and were found to have activity in a variety of neoplasms.[97] They also have similar toxicities. All are highly lipid soluble, facilitating transport across the blood-brain barrier. This biochemical property has led to clinical trials of these agents in brain tumors and other cancers that develop central nervous system metastases. In general, they have activity in brain tumors, Hodgkin's disease, melanoma, some primary lung cancers, multiple myeloma, and perhaps colon and gastric cancer. An unusual toxic effect seen with the administration of nitrosoureas is a delayed myelosuppression that occurs 3 to 6 weeks after administration.[37] This contrasts with the pattern of myelosuppression seen with most other agents, which occurs 7 to 10 days following administration. Myelosuppression appears to be cumulative. Recent reports implicate nitrosoureas as a cause of renal failure after prolonged use.[120] Pulmonary fibrosis has been reported in clients receiving BCNU therapy. While CCNU and methyl CCNU are available for oral administration, BCNU is only available as a lyophilized powder that must be reconstituted in aqueous alcohol for intravenous administration.

The nitrosoureas were developed as a result of the combined efforts of the Southern Research Institute and the drug development program at the National Cancer Institute to rationally synthesize compounds that are structurally similar to chemicals known to have activity. Continued research has led to clinical trials of two analogues, streptozoticin and chlorozoticin, that have less bone marrow toxicity. Streptozoticin is useful in clients with recurrent Hodgkin's disease refractory to conventional therapy.[111] Streptozoticin is transported across the membranes of islet cells of the pancreas. This property makes it useful for the treatment of islet cell tumors.[18] While streptozoticin has little myelosuppressive toxicity, it has renal toxicity and can cause mild elevations in hepatic enzymes. Chlorozoticin is presently undergoing phase II clinical trials, and final definition of its clinical usefulness and toxicity awaits further study.[2]

Triazenoimidazole carboxamide. Triazenoimidazole carboxamide compounds are also similar to alkylating agents in their activity. They require hepatic microsomal enzymes for activation. The most clinically useful compound is 5-(3,3 dimethyl-1-triazeno)-imidazole-4 carboxamide (dacarbazine [Dtic-Dome]). It is capable of producing responses in malignant melanoma, soft tissue sarcomas, and Hodgkin's disease.[26] Gastrointestinal absorption of dacarbazine is variable and incomplete, so it is generally given intravenously. Toxic effects consist of myelosuppression, nausea and vomiting, and a flulike syndrome accompanied by fever, chills, and malaise.

Antimetabolites

An antimetabolite is a compound that resembles a normal metabolite so closely that it enters a metabolic system but differs from the normal metabolite sufficiently to interfere with normal metabolic pathways. Incorporation of this fraudulent structural analogue either blocks or interferes with normal biosynthesis of DNA and RNA. Since the lethal effects of antimetabolites are exerted primarily during the synthetic phase of the cell cycle (S phase), they are considered *cell cycle specific* in action.

Since antimetabolites exert their cytotoxic effect primarily on cells that are actively synthesizing DNA, they tend to produce toxic side-effects in normal tissues that have a high rate of replication. Rapidly dividing tissues of the body include the cells of the bone marrow, the cells that line the gastrointestinal tract, the skin, and the gametes. The appearance of toxicity in these normal tissues limits the administration of antimetabolites.

Folate antagonists

Methotrexate. Methotrexate (MTX), a folic acid antagonist, was the first clinically effective antimetabolite to be successfully utilized against human tumors. Methotrexate and its related analogues are potent inhibitors of the enzyme dihydrofolate reductase.[65] This enzyme is responsible for converting dihydrofolic acid to tetrahydrofolic acid, which is an essential precursor for thymidine synthesis.[25] Inhibition of thymidylate synthesis interferes with the formation of DNA. Although RNA and protein synthesis are also inhibited, the thymidylate block is considered the most important mode of action. Cytotoxic effects of methotrexate require the presence of free intracellular drug above a specific threshold for each tissue.[23] In addition, the toxic effects on the target tissue are primarily a function of the duration of exposure to concentrations above this threshold and the peak level achieved.[94] Experiments have demonstrated that methotrexate has an affinity for dihydrofolate reductase, which is 10,000 times higher than that of dihydrofolic acid.[25] This means that if a cell contains methotrexate, the enzyme will complex with the methotrexate in preference to dihydrofolic acid. Because methotrexate also inhibits protein and RNA synthesis, which occur in G_1, cells preparing to begin DNA synthesis may be unable to enter the S phase. Inhibition of entry into the S phase, where the cells become vulnerable to the cytotoxic effect of methotrexate, effectively limits the number of cells that will be killed with prolonged methotrexate administration.[16] Major toxic effects of methotrexate are related to its effect on replicating tissues, such as cells of the bone marrow and gastrointestinal mucosa, and also to its excretion by the kidneys, since high concentrations of the drug can lead to crystallization and plugging of renal tubules.

The cytotoxicity of methotrexate can be reversed by *leucovorin* (5-formyl tetrahydrofolate).[49] This compound is readily converted to the reduced folates, which are required for purine and pyrimidine synthesis, thus bypassing the block produced by methotrexate. Reversal of potential methotrexate toxicity by leucovorin provides the pharmacologic rationale for the timing and use of leucorvorin to "rescue" normal cells following "high-dose" infusions of methotrexate.[10] These infusions would otherwise produce lethal toxicity to normal tissues. Pharmacologic data about individual methotrexate levels and excretion patterns are absolutely essential for safe administration of high-dose schedules.

Following intravenous administration of conventional dosages, transport of methotrexate across the blood-brain barrier is poor, so intrathecal administration of methotrexate was proposed to attain high concentrations of drug in the cerebrospinal fluid.[61] Intrathecal methotrexate has become widely employed in the prophylaxis and treatment of leukemic and carcinomatous meningitis. When administered intrathecally, methotrexate can produce arachnoiditis, nausea, and vomiting but only occasionally causes serious neuropathies.[12] However, use of intrathecal methotrexate can produce myelosuppression owing to prolonged leakage of the drug from the spinal fluid into the systemic circulation.[11,62]

The major route of elimination of methotrexate is through the kidney, with approximately 90% of unchanged drug excreted in urine.[25] Any impairment in renal function can produce a marked increase in circulating levels of methotrexate and hence increases in bone marrow and gastrointestinal toxicity. Delayed excretion patterns may produce life-threatening toxicity characterized by profound pancytopenia and extensive ulcerations of the gastrointestinal mucosa. When "high-dose" infusions are employed, methotrexate doses ranging from 50 to 250 mg/kg are administered and renal insufficiency can be produced if the urine is not alkalinized.[118] It is imperative that clients receiving high-dose infusions be given intravenous hydration with sufficient fluid and sodium bicarbonate to maintain a high output of alkaline urine prior to treatment and 36 hours after treatment with methotrexate to prevent irreversible damage to the kidneys.[11] Since methotrexate is bound to plasma proteins, toxic effects can be increased by displacing the drug from plasma albumin by concomitant administration of salicylates, sulfonamides, phenytoin, tetracycline, and chloramphenicol.[77] Other toxic effects seen with methotrexate include dermatitis, hepatic dysfunction, and pulmonary toxicity.

Purine antagonists

6-Mercaptopurine. 6-Mercaptopurine (6-MP) is another antimetabolite that is a structural analogue of hypoxanthine, a purine compound that is an essential component of normal DNA biosynthesis. 6-MP acts by interfering with a number of enzymatic purine synthetic pathways. Its major utility is in the management of acute lymphocytic leukemia.[75] It is well absorbed when given orally and has caused relatively mild gastrointestinal toxicity. 6-Mercaptopurine is metabolized by the liver and excreted in urine and can produce cholestatic jaundice, which is reversible with discontinuation of the drug. The enzyme xanthine oxidase plays an essential role in the degradation of 6-mercaptopurine. This enzyme is inhibited by the administration of allopurinol, a drug used to prevent hyperuricemia caused by rapid tumor breakdown. Since allopurinol administration delays degradation of 6-mercaptopurine, the dosage of 6-mercaptopurine should be reduced to approximately 30% in clients receiving allopurinol to avoid increased toxicity.[102]

6-Thioguanine. 6-Thioguanine (6-TG) is another purine antagonist that has utility in the treatment of acute leukemias, both in children and adults. It inhibits purine biosynthesis and is also fraudulently incorporated into DNA and RNA.[75] It is generally well tolerated and can be given orally. It is partially metabolized by the liver and is excreted in urine and feces. Its metabolism is less affected by allopurinol administration.

Pyrimidine antagonists

5-Fluorouracil. 5-Fluorouracil (5-FU) and two related compounds, 5-fluorodeoxyuridine (5-FUDR) and ftorafur, are fluorinated pyrimidine analogues. They were synthesized because it was found that animal tumors incorporated greater amounts of uracil than normal tissues.[103] It was hypothesized that a compound that was structurally similar to uracil could have cytotoxic effects. 5-Fluorouracil was the first such agent to be synthesized. It is a potent inhibitor of thymidylate synthetase and blocks the formation of thymidylate essential for DNA formation.[24] It is also incorporated into RNA and alters RNA synthesis, which enables it to act in phases of the cell cycle other than the S phase. 5-Fluorouracil must be converted to its active metabolite, 5-fluorodeoxyuridilate, to inhibit thymidylate synthetase. Degradation of the drug occurs in the liver. As a result, the dosage of 5-fluorouracil often must be reduced in clients with severe hepatic dysfunction. The hepatic degradation of 5-fluorouracil has been used to therapeutic advantage. Clients with liver metastases can be treated with hepatic arterial infusions of 5-fluorouracil with little systemic bone marrow or gastrointestinal toxicity owing to the hepatic degradation of the drug.[3]

A variety of different schedules and routes of administration have been studied. 5-Fluorouracil has been given daily as a rapid intravenous injection, or in prolonged intravenous or intra-arterial infusions. The intravenous preparation has been used for oral administration, but recent data suggest that the oral route may have less therapeutic efficacy.[117] Nausea is not a prominent side-effect, but mucositis and diarrhea can be severe and, when they appear, are indications to interrupt therapy. Myelosuppression is the major dose-limiting toxicity. Photosensitivity and skin rashes are not unusual. Neurotoxicity, presenting as ataxia, somnolence, and pyramidal tract signs, has been reported to occur.[24]

Cytosine and deoxycytosine analogues

Cytosine arabinoside. Cytosine arabinoside (Ara-C) is a pyrimidine nucleoside analogue that acts as a competitive inhibitor of DNA polymerase and is also fraudulently incorporated into DNA and RNA.[24,54] Its action is *S phase specific*. Cytosine arabinoside is used primarily in the therapy of acute myelocytic leukemia. It is poorly absorbed orally and when given intravenously has a short plasma half-life because of rapid metabolism by the liver. Various schedules of administration have been used to maximize its cytotoxicity to leukemic cells and thus maximize its therapeutic effect. The most common schedules employ prolonged constant infusions (up to 10 days), subcutaneous injections, or rapid intravenous administration every 12 hours. Hematologic toxicity is dose-limiting. Because of extensive hepatic metabolism, liver dysfunction can occur, and the drug should be used with caution in clients with liver disease. Cytosine arabinoside is a potent immunosuppressive agent. It has significant antitumor activity when given intrathecally and can be useful in the management of clients who have become resistant to intrathecally administered methotrexate. When given intrathecally, it can produce arachnoiditis and neurologic abnormalities.[8]

5-Azacytidine. 5-Azacytidine is an analogue of cytidine that has antileukemic activity and is not cross-resistant with cytosine arabinoside. The drug inhibits DNA, RNA, and protein synthesis by disrupting the transcription of nucleic acid sequences.[24] It also exerts a direct effect on early pyrimidine biosynthesis.[54] It is given intravenously and often produces severe dose-related nausea, vomiting, and diarrhea, occasionally associated with fever. Studies have shown that continuous 24-hour intravenous infusions administered over 5 days can decrease these toxic effects while preserving myelosuppressive and antitumor activity.[81] However, reconstituted solutions of 5-aza cytidine are very unstable and must be administered within 6 hours. This instability necessitates reconstitution in Ringer's lactate solution, administration of the drug in divided doses, and maintenance of temperature below 25° C, to ensure less than 10% decomposition over 6 hours. Its major clinical use is in the therapy of acute and chronic myelocytic leukemia.

Plant alkaloids

Alkaloids are organic compounds that are formed in plants. Many, such as morphine, atropine, and quinine, have effects that have been exploited therapeutically. Two *vinca alkaloids, vincristine* and *vinblastine,* have been isolated from the periwinkle plant (*Vinca rosea* Linn) and are therapeutically useful in cancer treatment. These two alkaloids are remarkably similar in chemical structure but have significant differences in their spectrum of antitumor activity and toxicities. They are not cross-resistant. Both are *cell cycle–specific* agents that block mitosis during the metaphase stage by interfering with the assembly of the mitotic spindle. Cell death results from disruption in the orderly arrangement of chromosomes within the nuclear cytoplasm and also from interference with DNA and RNA synthesis in earlier phases of the cell cycle. Both are poorly and erratically absorbed with oral administration and are potent irritants to skin and subcutaneous tissues, so they must be administered intravenously. Both are rapidly cleared from plasma and excreted by the biliary system. Increased toxicity can occur in clients with abnormal biliary excretion, and hepatic dysfunction may necessitate dose reductions.

Vincristine. Vincristine has a broad spectrum of antitumor activity. It can induce transient complete remissions when used as a single agent in acute lymphocytic leukemia and advanced Hodgkin's disease. Relatively little myelosuppression generally occurs with vincristine administration. This has made it a useful component of combination chemotherapy regimens in a great number of neoplasms. Its principal side-effect is neurotoxicity, which is cumulative and dose limiting. Neurotoxicity is generally manifested as peripheral neuropathies that involve sensory disturbances (numbness and tingling of fingers and toes) and motor disturbances (progressive loss of deep tendon reflexes, footdrop, ataxia, constipation, abdominal pain, or paralytic ileus caused by injury to abdominal nerve plexuses).[123] Alopecia occurs in 20% to 30% of clients. Toxicity is often greater in elderly clients. Since neurotoxicity is cumulative and can become irreversible if treatment is continued in the face of progressive toxicity, clients must be evaluated for the degree of neurologic toxicity prior to each dose of vincristine. The dosage should be reduced if clients develop painful or disabling neuropathies. Prophylactic use of stool softeners and/or laxatives is often effective in reducing constipation and preventing intestinal obstruction, especially in the elderly. Complete reversal of neurotoxicity is gradual and may occur over prolonged periods. Extravasation of both vincristine and vinblastine into subcutaneous tissues during intravenous administration will cause severe tissue necrosis, hence they must be administered with great care. Additional side-effects include a metallic taste, parotid pain, vocal cord paresis, cranial nerve palsies, inappropriate secretion of antidiuretic hormone, and muscle wasting. Rare but serious complications include visual disturbances, convulsions, and coma.

Vinblastine. Vinblastine has its greatest utility in the treatment of lymphomas and breast and testicular cancers. Neurotoxicity and alopecia are less common than with vincristine, but myelosuppression and gastrointestinal toxicity including stomatitis and diarrhea are common.[45] Paralytic ileus may also occur with vinblastine administration.

Epipodophyllotoxins. Epipodophyllotoxins are semisynthetic agents that also act as mitotic inhibitors. Two drugs in clinical use are VP16-213 and VM26. Both cause myelosuppression, alopecia, varying degrees of nausea and vomiting, and diarrhea. VP16-213 may also cause hypotension and/or bronchospasm during rapid intravenous administration, hence the drug should be infused over 30 to 60 minutes. It must be administered in saline solutions to achieve optimal stability of the compound. Responses have been documented in lymphomas, leukemia, and small cell carcinoma of the lung.[22]

Antitumor antibiotics

Antitumor antibiotics constitute an important class of agents. Antibiotics are compounds produced by organisms to interfere with the growth of other organisms in their environment. Important drugs in this class are actinomycin-D, mithramycin, mitomycin-C, bleomycin, and the anthracycline derivatives daunomycin and doxorubicin (Adriamycin). All were identified as a result of research to identify new antibiotics for infectious diseases. The antibiotics exert their antitumor effect through a number of mechanisms described in reference to the specific agents.

Daunorubicin (daunomycin) and doxorubicin (Adriamycin). Daunorubicin and doxorubicin are two of the most important new chemotherapeutic agents that have been introduced into clinical trials in the last decade. They are anthracycline antibiotics and structurally are quite similar. Anthracycline antibiotics interfere with DNA synthesis and DNA-dependent RNA synthesis by *intercalation* (insertion of a compound between the bases in the DNA strands) with DNA, which can lead to uncoiling of the DNA helix.[122] The maximal lethal effects are exerted on cells in the S phase of the cell cycle.[71] Both doxorubicin and daunomycin undergo extensive hepatic metabolism and biliary excretion. Some metabolites are excreted in the urine and may color the urine red following administration. Both drugs cause myelosuppression, gastrointestinal toxicity, and almost complete loss of body hair.

Cardiac toxicity is the most serious side-effect of anthracycline antibiotics.[24] Two clinical patterns of cardiotoxicity have been observed. The first consists of transient electrocardiographic ST-T wave changes, brief periods of supraventricular tachycardia, and atrial and venticular extrasystoles following routine intravenous administration. Acute reversible reductions in ejection fraction have been documented utilizing cineangiography.[17,51] The second cardiotoxicity is a dose-related, cumulative, cardiomyopathy that appears as congestive heart failure. It can occur suddenly and may not always be preceded by electrocardiographic abnormalities. This cardiomyopathy occurs with greater frequency in clients who have received cumulative doses in excess of 550 mg/m^2 and may appear up to 6 months following the cessation of therapy. This drug-related cardiac failure has a high mortality rate. Microscopic studies of cardiac tissues have revealed dose-related necrosis of cardiomyocytes.[27,63] However, it has also been suggested that structural similarities between anthracycline antibiotics and digitalis may result in competition for the same receptor site in the myocardium, thus accounting for the poor response to digitalis that has been seen in this cardiomyopathy.[4] Anthracyclines also disrupt DNA synthesis in the myocardium.[101] Development of cardiac failure is thought to be caused by repeated administration of anthracyclines that produce repeated episodes of acute, reversible cardiac toxicity. A prior history of cardiac irradiation or concomitant administration of cyclophosphamide and other anthracycline antibiotics increases the risk of cardiotoxicity. In addition, these agents are powerful vesicants, producing severe local tissue necrosis if extravasated.

Doxorubicin (Adriamycin) has a broad spectrum of antitumor activity. It appears to be the most effective chemotherapeutic agent for soft tissue sarcomas and bladder and breast carcinomas and has great value in the therapy of lymphomas, leukemia, and carcinoma of the lung and thyroid.[13] Because of its hepatic metabolism, it must be administered with care in clients with impaired liver function. When the total cumulative dose exceeds 550 mg/m^2, the risk of congestive heart failure increases markedly.

Daunorubicin has been reported to have a more limited spectrum of activity, but this may be the result of inadequate evaluation in a wide spectrum of tumors.[80] Its chief use is in the treatment of acute leukemia. The total cumulative dose should be limited to 500 mg/m^2. Nausea and vomiting are more common with daunomycin administration than with doxorubicin.

Bleomycin. Bleomycin is a complex mixture of polypeptide antibiotics that is particularly active in epithelial carcinomas of skin and external genitalia, the lymphomas, and testicular carcinomas.[14] Bleomycin causes fragmentation and scission of DNA strands, and progression of cells through the premitotic resting phase (G_2)

and mitosis is inhibited.[24] The clinical activity of bleomycin may be related to preferential localization of the drug in skin, lung, and certain malignant tumors. It is also an important agent because of its lack of myelotoxicity and immunosuppression. A variety of doses and schedules have been employed and the drug can be given intramuscularly, subcutaneously, or intravenously. Recent studies have employed prolonged intravenous infusions, a schedule known to enhance the activity of other agents active in specific phases of the cell cycle.[106] The primary route of excretion is renal. Toxic effects of bleomycin include febrile reactions accompanied by chills and flulike symptoms. Hypertension, bronchospasm, and/or anaphylaxis occur less frequently. For this reason, several test doses (2 units) are often given at the initiation of bleomycin therapy (particularly in clients with lymphoma who experience this reaction most often). Gastrointestinal toxicity, including stomatitis, can occur, especially with intensive schedules of administration. Alopecia is also seen. The most serious dose-limiting toxic effects are cutaneous and pulmonary toxicities. Both appear to be cumulative and dose-related effects. Skin changes include erythema, hyperpigmentation, hyperkeratosis, and desquamation. Lesions generally begin to appear at cumulative doses of 150 units and are accompanied by pain, pruritis, and hypersensitivity. The hands, feet, fingertips, pressure areas (especially the elbows), and sites that have been irradiated are especially prone to the development of cutaneous toxicity. Progressive worsening of skin toxicity results in the formation of bullae and ulcerations that necessitate interruptions or cessation of therapy. Pulmonary fibrosis is the most serious toxicity and can be fatal in some clients. The clinical syndrome often presents with cough and dyspnea. Physical findings include bibasilar rales. At onset, chest x-ray films may appear normal or demonstrate minimal changes, but as the toxicity develops, bibasilar infiltrates appear and may be progressive. Pulmonary fibrosis develops in 5% to 10% of clients and is fatal in approximately 1% of cases.[14] Pulmonary function studies have not reliably predicted the onset of pulmonary toxicity. Decreases in forced vital capacity and/or diffusion capacity are common even in asymptomatic clients. Pulmonary fibrosis occurs more frequently in elderly clients, those with underlying pulmonary disease or previous pulmonary irradiation, and in those who have received cumulative doses in excess of 400 units. However, pulmonary fibrosis has been reported at a total dose of 50 units. The cumulative total dosage should not exceed 400 units to minimize the risk of irreversible pulmonary toxicity.

Actinomycin-D. Actinomycin-D was the first antibiotic successfully used in cancer treatment. The pharmacology of this drug has been thoroughly studied and its mode of action is well described.[46] It forms hydrogen bonds with single strands of the DNA molecule. It intercalates with DNA, which interferes with DNA-dependent RNA synthesis. It is *not cell cycle specific*.[46] Actinomycin-D is widely used in the therapy of Wilm's tumor, testicular cancer, neuroblastoma, rhabdomyosarcoma and choriocarcinoma.[44] It is a potent myelosuppressive and immunosuppressive agent. Actinomycin-D also causes severe nausea and vomiting, which gradually decrease on successive days when the drug is administered on a daily schedule. Skin reactions may occur, especially in areas that have been irradiated. Alopecia is common. Ulcerations of the gastrointestinal mucosa may be a dose-limiting toxicity. It is a powerful vesicant if extravasated. Since it is excreted primarily by the biliary system, the drug must be administered with caution in clients with preexisting hepatic dysfunction. In contrast to most other chemotherapeutic agents, dosages of actinomycin-D in the *microgram range* are sufficient to achieve therapeutic effects. The dose, therefore, is generally calculated and expressed in *micrograms*.

Mithramycin. Mithramycin is an antibiotic that is clinically useful in embryonal cell carcinoma of the testes.[66] It is thought to inhibit DNA-dependent RNA synthesis by binding to DNA. Mithramycin causes myelosuppression, especially thrombocytopenia, and can depress hepatic synthesis of clotting factors. The clotting abnormalities may result in acute, fatal hemorrhage, a complication that is often preceded by an episode of facial flushing.[67] Gastrointestinal toxicity and renal and hepatic damage can occur, so this agent should be administered with caution to clients with renal or hepatic dysfunction. It is a powerful vesicant and can cause local tissue necrosis if extravasated. Mithramycin affects calcium metabolism and has utility in the management of clients with refractory hypercalcemia of varying etiologies, including non-neoplastic causes.[92]

Mitomycin-C. Mitomycin-C is an antitumor antibiotic that has some antitumor activity in several solid tumors that were completely unresponsive to available chemotherapeutic agents when it was introduced into clinical trials. Its dose-limiting toxicity is severe myelosuppression at doses required for therapeutic effect. It inhibits DNA synthesis by complexing with DNA following intracellular activation.[29] Mitomycin-C has been used less frequently in recent years since more effective therapy has been developed for most settings in which it was formerly used.

Miscellaneous agents

A number of drugs either cannot be easily classified in any of the groups described previously or their mechanisms of action are unknown or poorly understood. While little may be known about their mechanisms of action, acute and chronic toxicity of many of these drugs are well documented and should be understood prior to administration.

L-asparaginase. L-asparaginase is the only enzyme to be used successfully in cancer treatment. It converts L-asparagine, an essential amino acid involved in protein synthesis, to L-aspartic acid, thus depleting the pool of L-asparagine.[21] While normal tissue can independently synthesize this amino acid, many leukemic and some lymphoma cells cannot and require exogenous L-asparagine. Initially, it was postulated that this agent would selectively kill tumor cells by exploiting this biochemical difference between normal and malignant cells. Unfortunately, L-asparaginase also interferes with protein synthesis, causing considerable toxicity to the liver, pancreas, kidneys, and nervous system. In addition, resistance to the drug often develops rapidly. Resistance appears to be caused by increased production of L-asparagine synthetase, an enzyme that converts L-aspartic acid to L-asparagine and thus renews the supply of this amino acid.[21] In spite of rapid development of resistance, L-asparaginase is effective in inducing remissions in acute leukemia and causing relatively little bone marrow toxicity. Its major life-threatening toxicity is anaphylaxis, which occurs in 15% to 30% of clients.[56] Less severe hypersensitivity reactions are common and also develop rapidly. These reactions are often mediated by circulating drug antibodies that can be detected and monitored by serologic techniques. The use of such techniques can reduce the incidence and severity of hypersensitivity reactions, and these techniques are utilized *prior to each dosage*.[21] L-asparaginase is obtained from two microorganisms, *Escherichia coli* and *Erwinia corotovora*. The *Erwinia* preparation can be used in clients who have been sensitized to the *E. coli* preparation.[58] While myelosuppression is rare, hemolytic anemia and coagulation abnormalities are not uncommon. Liver dysfunction, neurologic toxicity, acute hemorrhagic pancreatitis, and hyperglycemia (related to depressed serum insulin levels) also occur.

Procarbazine. Procarbazine is a derivative of methylhydrazine. Hydrazines, a class of drugs that inhibit monoamine oxidase (MAO) enzymes, are useful in the treatment of depression. Procarbazine is an extremely active antitumor agent used in the treatment of lymphoma, especially Hodgkin's disease, and in small cell carcinoma of the lung.[105] Its precise mechanism of action is unclear, but after undergoing oxidation, it may depolymerize or denature DNA, inhibit mitotic activity, and cause chromatin breaks.[24] Procarbazine is absorbed rapidly when given orally and crosses the blood-brain barrier. Rapid drug metabolism occurs in the liver and metabolites are eliminated in urine. Principal toxicities are myelosuppression and central nervous system changes such as somnolence, confusion, cerebellar ataxia, and hyperexcitability. Nausea is common but often subsides with daily administration. Procarbazine potentiates the effects of CNS depressants such as alcohol, barbiturates, and phenothiazines. As expected, it also inhibits monoamine oxidase, an enzyme that converts tyramine to a nonvasoactive metabolite.[19] Sympathomimetic drugs and food rich in tyramine such as beer, ripe and aged cheeses, and chianti should be eliminated from the diet during procarbazine administration to avoid hypertensive reactions. Procarbazine is a potent immunosuppressant and is highly mutagenic in several animal species.[113]

Hydroxyurea. Hydroxyurea interferes with DNA snythesis during S phase. Given in a large single dose, hydroxyurea can markedly reduce the number of peripheral blood myeloblasts within 24 hours in clients with busulfan-resistant chronic myelogenous leukemia.[70] It is absorbed rapidly and excreted in urine. Bone marrow suppression is dose limiting, but marrow recovery occurs soon after cessation of therapy. Other toxic effects are uncommon.

Hexamethylmelamine. Hexamethylmelamine is a synthetic compound that has an unknown mechanism of action. It functions, at least in part, as an antimetabolite interfering with pyrimidine metabolism; its biochemical structure resembles an alkylating agent, and covalent binding of metabolites to tissue proteins appears to occur.[82] It is clinically useful in the treatment of ovarian and lung cancer.[15] Its major dose-limiting toxicities are nausea, vomiting, and diarrhea. It also causes neuropathy that may exacerbate previous vincristine neurotoxicity.[82] Alterations in sensorium are also seen and can be manifested as somnolence, confusion, depression, agitation, or hallucinations.

Ortho para'-DDD. Ortho para'-DDD (o, p'-DDD) is a compound that is related to the insecticide DDT. It is a potent inhibitor of adrenocorticosteroid synthesis and activity.[9] It is used almost exclusively in the treatment of adrenocortical carcinoma. Its toxicity primarily consists of gastrointestinal disturbances, skin rash, and neurotoxicity, such as somnolence, lethargy, and diplopia. Significant myelosuppression is rare.

Cisplatin. Cisplatin (Platinol), which has recently been made commercial, is a derivative of the heavy metal platinum and represents a new class of antitumor agents. Its mechanism of action is thought to be related to cross-linkage of DNA strands. This cross-linking interferes with DNA transcription and repair.[99] Its action is *cell cycle nonspecific*. It is administered intravenously, binds to plasma proteins, and is excreted in urine. It has significant antitumor activity in testicular and ovarian carcinomas and is undergoing extensive evaluation in a variety of "drug-resistant" solid tumors.[100] Its major side-effect is nephrotoxicity, which can be irreversible and fatal if renal tubular necrosis develops. Hydration and forced diuresis with mannitol and/or furosemide can be used prophylactically to prevent renal tubular damage.[100] A urine output of 150 ml/hour should be established and maintained for several hours before and after treatment with cisplatin to reduce renal toxicity. Serum creatinine and urinary creatinine clearance should be determined prior to each dose. Dose reduction for abnormal renal function is mandatory. Cisplatin produces severe nausea and vomiting, which are generally unresponsive to conventional doses of antiemetics. Additionally, it causes mild to moderate myelosuppression. Tinitis and high-frequency hearing loss are dose related and cumulative. Peripheral neuropathy and seizure activity have recently been reported.[100] A less common but serious and life-threatening toxicity is the development of hypersensitivity and anaphylactic reactions occurring within minutes after administration.[100] Clients receiving this agent should be observed carefully in the immediate postadministration period.

ENDOCRINE THERAPY

The growth of cancers derived from organs that are responsive or dependent on hormones may often be affected by alterations in hormonal balance. Endocrine therapy of such cancers has been employed to exploit this dependence. Endocrine therapy includes the administration of exogenous hormones in large, nonphysiologic doses or the ablation of organs responsible for hormone production or activation. Table 14-2 lists these agents. Carcinomas of the breast, prostate, thyroid, and uterine endometrium are known to be responsive to hormonal manipulations. Hormonal therapy also includes the use of corticosteroids. These compounds can inhibit mitosis and are cytotoxic to cells of lymphocytic origin. This makes corticosteroids valuable in the treatment of the leukemias and lymphomas. In general, side-effects of endocrine therapy are identical to adverse effects associated with hormonal imbalance caused by excessive or inadequate synthesis of specific hormones.

Research into the mechanism of hormonal action has revealed that steroid-binding receptor glycoproteins exist in hormonally dependent or responsive tissues.[64] Binding of hormones to these receptor sites can alter the synthesis of RNA and protein in target tissues. Receptors for estrogens, androgens, progesterones, and corticosteroids have been identified in the cytoplasm of cells and probably explain their antitumor activity.[78] Unresponsiveness to hormonal manipulation is now thought to be primarily related to the absence of these steroid-binding receptor proteins in tumor tissue.[85]

Ablative procedures

Ablative therapy has been utilized to produce regressions of metastatic breast and prostatic cancer.[68] Ablative procedures remove the source of circulating hormones that stimulate or support neoplastic growth. *Oophorectomy* is often beneficial in premenopausal women with breast cancer, especially those clients who have developed osseous and soft tissue metastases. Approximately 50% of women who experience tumor regression after castration will respond to adrenalectomy or hypophysectomy when they develop recurrent disease since the adrenal cortex is a limited source of estrogen-like hormones. Clients who do not respond to oophorectomy are unlikely to respond to additional ablative surgical proce-

Table 14-2. Hormonal agents in clinical use

Drug	Dose, route, and schedule	Side-effects	Therapeutic indications
Androgens		Nausea, vomiting, and anorexia at high doses	Breast cancer: premenopausal females and estrogen receptor (ER) positive tumors
Testosterone proprionate (Oreton)	50-100 mg IM tiw	Masculinization and increased libido (hirsutism, baldness, voice change, acne)	Aplastic anemia
Testosterone enanthate (Delatestryl)	600-1,200 mg IM qw	Occasional hypercalcemia	
Testolactone (Teslac)	100 mg PO or IM tiw	Fluid and salt retention, congestive heart failure	
Fluoxymesterone (Halotestin)	10-20 mg PO qd	Stimulation of erythropoiesis	
		Hepatotoxicity and obstructive jaundice	
Dromostanolone propionate (Drolban)	100 mg IM tiw	Less masculinization with calusterone	
Calusterone (Methosarb)	0.3 mg/kg PO qd		
Estrogens		Nausea, vomiting, and anorexia	Breast cancer: postmenopausal females with ER(+) tumors
Diethylstilbestrol (DES, stilbestrol)	1-15 mg PO qd	Feminization; gynecomastia	Metastatic prostatic cancer
		Fluid and salt retention	
Diethylstilbestrol diphosphate (Stilphostrol)	150-1,000 mg PO or IV qd	Decreased libido	
		Hypercalcemia	
Chlorotrianisene (Tace)	12-25 mg PO qd	Uterine bleeding	
Ethinyl estradiol (Estinyl)	0.5-1 mg PO tid	Increased mortality from cardiovascular complications in males	
Conjugated equine estrogen (Premarin)	5 mg PO tid		

Antiestrogens			
Tamoxifen (Nolvadex)	10-40 mg PO qd	Mild nausea Mild leukopenia and thrombocytopenia Vaginal bleeding, pruritus Hot flashes Transient increase in bone pain and flare in skin and soft tissue disease Rare hypercalcemia	Advanced breast cancer in postmenopausal females and ER(−) tumors
Progestins		Mild nausea Minimal fluid retention Skin rash Occasional hypercalcemia Mild LFT abnormalities Thromboembolic phenomena (phlebitis, CVA, pulmonary emboli)	Endometrial carcinoma Ovarian carcinoma
Hydroxyprogesterone caproate (Delalutin)	0.5-1 gm biw		
Medroxyprogesterone acetate (Provera—PO)	20-80 mg PO qd		
(Depo-Provera—IM)	200-600 mg IM biw		
Megesterol acetate (Megace)	40 mg PO qid		
Adrenocortical steroids		Immunosuppression, infection Gastrointestinal disturbance, ulcers, bleeding Hyperglycemia, glycosuria, diabetes Fluid and sodium retention, hypertension, potassium-wasting edema, cushingoid appearance Adrenal atrophy, osteoporosis Emotional lability, euphoria, psychosis Acne, cataracts, muscle wasting (NB: Preparations vary in their mineralocorticoid potency)	Frequently used in drug combinations for leukemia, Hodgkin's disease, multiple myeloma, and non-Hodgkin's lymphomas Also used to reduce edema around tumor masses in CNS metastases and spinal cord compression
Prednisone (Deltasone)	40-60 mg/m^2 PO qd		
Prednisolone (Delta Cortef)	40-60 mg/m^2 IM qd		
Methylprednisolone (Medrol)	10-125 mg/day IV, IM		
Hydrocortisone (Cortef—PO or IM) (Solu-cortef—IV or IM)	100-500 mg/day IV, IM		
Dexamethasone (Decadron)	0.5-16 mg/day PO, IV, IM		

dures. Postmenopausal women whose disease has regressed following the exogenous administration of estrogens may also respond to adrenalectomy or hypophysectomy. The median duration of response to hormonal ablation is 16 to 18 months.[110]

One percent of all breast cancer occurs in men.[88] In those males with breast cancer, surgical castration produces regression of metastatic disease in 67% of clients, and half of these will respond to subsequent ablative procedures.[88] In prostate cancer, both orchiectomy and exogenous estrogen administration produce regression of tumor, often lasting 2 to 3 years in duration.[68]

Aminoglutethimide

Aminoglutethimide, a potent inhibitor of steroid biosynthesis, is a drug that can be used to achieve a medical ablation of adrenal steroid production ("medical adrenalectomy") in clients in whom surgical adrenalectomy is contraindicated.[107] As with clients who have had their adrenal glands removed, exogenous administration of corticosteroids that are not converted into estrogen-like hormones is necessary to prevent the clinical syndrome of adrenal insufficiency. Side-effects seen with aminoglutethimide therapy include skin rash and lethargy; these often subside during treatment.

Estrogen

Estrogen administration will produce antitumor responses in 35% of postmenopausal women with breast cancer and in 50% of males with prostatic cancer.[7] Estrogens are metabolized in the liver and excreted in urine. Side-effects include fluid retention, hypertensive cardiovascular complications, nausea, thromboembolic phenomena, hypercalcemia, and feminization. The incidence and severity of side-effects may vary with individual preparations and doses.

Androgen

Androgen administration can produce responses in 20% of women with breast cancer, especially postmenopausal women with osseous metastases.[69] Androgens also undergo hepatic metabolism and renal excretion. They cause fluid retention, hypercalcemia, and varying degrees of masculinization. Virilizing effects include hirsutism, baldness, increased libido, hoarseness, deepening of the voice, and acne. Because androgens have anabolic effects, increased appetite, weight gain, and a sense of increased well-being may also be noted. Because androgens stimulate erythropoiesis, they are also used in the treatment of aplastic anemia.

Progestins

Progestins are progesterone and its analogues and certain synthetic derivatives. Natural progestins are produced by the corpus luteum and placenta. They can produce responses lasting several years in 30% of women with metastatic endometrial cancer.[38] They are also used to treat clients with metastatic renal cell carcinoma, but a recent review of studies employing these agents suggests that the therapeutic benefit may be minimal or nonexistent.[57] Progesterones generally produce fewer adverse effects than estrogens and androgens.

Antiestrogens

Antiestrogens are nonsteroidal synthetic agents that recently have been discovered to have antitumor activity in metastatic breast cancer. Antiestrogens compete with estrogens for the same receptor sites in target tissues and exert part of their effect by preventing estrogen binding. Antiestrogens can produce regression of disease in approximately 50% of clients whose tumor cells *have estrogen-binding proteins*.[89] Masculinization is uncommon. The most common toxicities are mild myelosuppression, mild nausea, hot flashes, hypercalcemia, vaginal bleeding, pruritis, and discharge. Antitumor responses may be preceded by a transient increase in bone pain or a flare in skin and soft tissue disease in clients who have metastatic disease in these sites. Tamoxifen is the only antiestrogen in clinical use in this country. Recent data suggest that this agent can produce responses in renal cell carcinoma but the data are preliminary.

Corticosteroids

Corticosteroids can be administered to modify the growth of neoplasms. Naturally occurring glucocorticoids are produced in the cortex of the adrenal gland and play a role in the regulation of carbohydrate metabolism. Protein metabolism, hematopoiesis, anti-inflammatory responses, immunosuppression, and production of gastrointestinal secretions are all influenced by glucocorticoids. The lympholytic action of corticosteroids has made them valuable agents in the treatment of lymphatic leukemias, myeloma, and malignant lymphomas. *Prednisone* or *prednisolone,* the synthetic counterparts of the naturally produced glucocorticoids, *hydrocortisone* and *cortisone,* are the agents most commonly used for antitumor therapy. They can be used in combination with other chemotherapeutic agents because of their lack of bone marrow toxicity. However, corticosteroids may cause many adverse effects, including suppression of adrenal function, atrophy of the adrenal gland, hypertension, fluid retention, hyperglycemia, gastric ulcers, osteoporosis, psychosis, emotional instability, cataracts, muscle wasting, acne, increased appetite, cushingoid features, and increased susceptibility to infection.[42] They also have anti-inflammatory properties that are useful in the management of cerebral edema. It must be remembered, however, that this anti-inflammatory property has the disadvantage of masking the principal signs and symptoms of infection.

Thyroid hormones

Thyroid hormones can be utilized to treat certain papillary thyroid carcinomas that are dependent on thyroid stimulating hormone (TSH) secretion for growth.[28] Thyroid hormones act by inhibiting pituitary secretion of TSH.

DRUG DEVELOPMENT AND CLINICAL TRIALS

General concepts and methodology

As it became clear that drugs could be used effectively to treat cancers, it became evident that a national program to identify, develop, and evaluate new compounds for antitumor activity was essential. This led to the establishment of the drug development program by the National Cancer Institute (NCI) and guidelines for clinical studies to evaluate the usefulness of compounds with identifiable antitumor activity. Even in the 1970's curative therapy was not yet available for most clients with metastatic cancer. Involvement of these clients in investigational studies to develop more effective therapy is an essential component of client care. Therapeutic experiments, known as *clinical trials,* are performed at the bedside and have always required the tacit participation of nurses who provide essential supportive care for clients participating in these studies. In recent years, nurses have recognized that tacit participation in clinical research is inadequate in terms of optimal client care, fulfillment of the nurse's professional goals, and the execution of good clinical research.[59] This recognition has philosophic and practical implications for nursing as a profession. Philosophically, it has meant that nurses must abandon passive, dependent roles in research and assume responsibility for full collaboration with physicians in the conduct of clinical trials. Practically, it has meant that nurses must become highly sophisticated, both intellectually and technically, in order to actively participate in the research process. Clinical specialization in medicine and nursing has become the major way that scientific and technologic advances revealed by research are rapidly translated into clinical practice. Clinical specialization in cancer nursing has facilitated the active participation of nurses in this process. The cancer research nurse has emerged as a *clinical specialist* who shares primary responsibility with physicians for physical and emotional care of clients and the ethical conduct of good research.[98] Such nurses often provide continuity of care over long periods. While cures are the primary goal of cancer treatment research, it is important to recognize that participation in research can increase understanding of the disease process, the psychosocial impact of cancer on the individual, and the long-term implications of treatment.[59,60]

A clinical trial is an experiment that is designed to answer a question that has therapeutic implications. A successful trial produces a valid answer that is biologically, ethically, and legally correct. Successful execution of clinical research is dependent on complete and accurate assessment of changes in client status. The nurse can make unique and invaluable contributions to these therapeutic experiments. To illustrate these contributions, the role of the nurse in the development of cancer chemotherapy will be reviewed.

The new drug-screening program

A new drug screen has been established by the NCI to identify compounds with antitumor activity from both natural sources and chemical synthesis. Compounds are chosen on the basis of known activity that influences cell growth because they represent a chemical structure specifically designed and synthesized to affect cell growth or because they are observed to have possible antitumor activity while being administered for other purposes. These chemicals are evaluated for antitumor activity against a panel of human and animal tumors of specific histologic type. In addition to leukemia, this assay includes xenographs of human tumors of breast, lung, and colon that can be grown in athymic, or genetically "nude," mice. If an agent demonstrates significant antitumor activity, it undergoes preclinical toxicologic screening. In these studies, the compound is analyzed for dose and schedule dependency; parameters of drug absorption, metabolism, distribution, and elimination are investigated during this phase of study. In an attempt to predict toxicity that may be encountered in human clinical trials, several species of animals are studied for qualitative and quantitative organ system toxicity using a wide range of drug doses. Maximum tolerated dosages are established in mice, rats, dogs, and monkeys. If a drug continues to exhibit significant antitumor activity in the absence of prohibitive toxicity to vital organ systems, it is considered for clinical evaluation in humans. It is at this stage of development that newly identified compounds are administered to clients with advanced cancer. Only 1 out of every 5,000 compounds seen in the new drug screen eventually enters clinical trial. One out of 50,000 compounds will progress through the three phases of clinical study to commercial availability as a unique addition to the antitumor agents already employed in cancer treatment.

The cost of successfully evaluating a new chemotherapeutic agent is at least several million dollars.[37] Nonetheless, a critical need exists for new agents that have activity in the common solid tumors, such as lung, colon, and pancreatic carcinomas.

Phase I clinical trials

The phase I clinical trial represents the first time a new compound is given to humans. The goal of a phase I study is to establish a maximally tolerated dose in humans, to define drug toxicity, and to arrive at an optimal dose and schedule for further clinical trials. At the initiation of the phase I trial, available preclinical data should support the scientific rationale for study in humans, predict specific toxicities, and provide a guide for the selection and escalation of dosage. The nurse's role in this type of study includes understanding all available pharmacologic and toxicologic data generated in the screening process. Preclinical toxicology in animals may predict the onset and character of side-effects in humans. While animal studies do not consistently or accurately predict specific side-effects, these studies provide guidelines to reduce the risk of unexpected serious toxicity. The initial human dose is one third the minimum toxic dose (MTD) established in the most sensitive animal species in which the drug was evaluated. This dose is chosen to minimize the risk of unpredicted toxicity in early phases of the phase I clinical trial. While the principal investigator's goals include retrieval of sophisticated pharmacologic data, safety must remain a paramount consideration.

The nurse contributes to the optimal comfort and safety of clients by recognizing and interpreting real and potential problems that may occur with the administration of a new compound (see outline below):

Phase I clinical trials

I. Purposes
  A. To establish a maximally tolerated dose in humans
  B. To define toxicity to normal organ systems
  C. To generate data about the clinical pharmacology of the agent
  D. To establish an optimal dose and schedule for further clinical trials
II. Nursing goals
  A. To guarantee optimal client safety and comfort
  B. To facilitate the achievement of the research goals
III. Responsibilities
  A. Knowledge of available preclinical pharmacologic and toxologic data
    1. Scientific rationale for use in man
    2. Mechanism of drug action
    3. Appropriate route(s) of administration
    4. Parameters of drug metabolism
    5. Factors that alter drug metabolism
    6. Acute and chronic side-effects in species evaluated
    7. Dose-limiting toxicity in sensitive species
    8. Cumulative or delayed side-effects
  B. Application of preclinical toxicology to clinical trials in man
    1. Translation of potential adverse reactions in humans to enable recognition of early organ system toxicity
    2. Recognition of potential for unpredicted and unexpected adverse reactions in terms of
      a. Magnitude
      b. Timing (onset, duration, reversal)
  C. Knowledge and understanding of ethical considerations
    1. The nature of the clinical trial (applicable to *all* phases of study)
      a. Therapeutic intent
      b. The ratio of known and/or anticipated side-effects to benefits
      c. Available therapeutic alternatives
    2. The nature of informed consent
    3. Client selection
  D. Clinical expertise
    1. Practice skills—physical and emotional support

2. Clinical observations—complete and accurate

E. Execution of the clinical trial
   1. Assessment of client status
      a. Physical assessment, serial laboratory values
      b. Education of clients to report subjective and objective changes
      c. Discrimination between drug-related effects and disease-related effects
   2. Documentation of changes in the client's medical record
      a. Acute, chronic, delayed, or cumulative effects
      b. Therapeutic effect
   3. Participation in protocol decisions concerning
      a. Dose escalation
      b. Schedule manipulation
      c. Delineation of organ system toxicity
      d. Generation of clinically useful pharmacologic data
      e. Decision to proceed to phase II trials

A nurse involved in any phase I trial must recognize unusual side-effects or signs of unexpected, cumulative, or delayed toxicity. Physicians must rely on the nurse to use knowledge about drugs and the disease to discriminate between toxicity and the complications that may be caused by disease progression. The clinical observations of the nurse are critical in the evaluation of the client's status.

Calculation of dosage

Tables 14-1 and 14-2 show the commonly used dosages of chemotherapeutic agents presented in terms of body weight or body surface area. Body weight dose calculations are expressed as milligrams per kilogram of weight. Body surface dose calculations, the preferred unit of measure, are expressed as milligrams per square meter of body surface area. Dosage calculated in terms of body surface area (BSA) minimizes the variation in total dose between fat and thin persons and provides comparable dosages for adults and children.

In phase I studies, dose is escalated when it can be demonstrated in several clients that no toxicity that might cause severe harm to the client has been seen. A knowledgeable nurse who monitors the serial evaluations of specific organ function can provide valuable information about whether it is safe to proceed to the next dose. In this situation, data analysis is clearly a form of client advocacy. The nurse in phase I trials can note evidence of subtle, early toxicity and cumulative toxicity as it evolves. A nurse's observations can significantly affect the decision to proceed to further clinical trials or to delete the compound from subsequent clinical study on the basis of unacceptable toxicity.

The nurse also plays an important role in ensuring that the conduct of the research is consistent with ethical standards. Clients must be properly informed concerning the nature of any phase I drug trial, since no known therapeutic benefit can be offered to these clients—only the potential hope that the compound may be developed into a more effective chemotherapeutic agent than those presently available. This hope must be balanced carefully against the known and anticipated risks inherent in a new drug trial. Obtaining the informed consent is the physician's legal responsibility, but the ethical responsibility for ensuring and maintaining voluntary and informed consent is shared by all members of the professional team.[59,60] Informed consent is an ongoing process, a learning experience for the client. In phase I clinical trials, the nurse is frequently the focal person to whom clients turn for supplemental information and data about the progress of the study.

Most clients receiving phase I agents have

advanced metastatic cancers and little or no chance of deriving benefit from established treatment modalities. Those clients with extensive prior therapy and progressive disease may tolerate toxic effects poorly and therefore require highly skilled nursing care. To improve survival for all future clients by contributing to the development of new and more effective therapy, clients who participate in a phase I trial are entrusting the members of the research team with a significant portion of their remaining lives. Nurses must always emphasize the value of their contribution, regardless of the outcome of the drug trial.

The phase I trial is complete when (1) effects of the drug are established at specific dosages and schedules, (2) dose-limiting toxicities and reversibility are described, and (3) pharmacologic data on metabolism, tissue distribution, and clearance are obtained. The decision is then made whether to proceed to the phase II trial.

Phase II clinical trials

Phase II clinical trials are designed to demonstrate whether antitumor effects can be shown in clients with a variety of common, or "signal," tumors. Signal cancers are the leukemias, lymphomas, melanoma, colorectal cancer, and cancers of the lung, breast, pancreas, ovary, and brain. In phase II studies, it is important to evaluate the agent in a broad spectrum of cancers and to carefully document clinical responses in each tumor in which the compound has activity. This is crucial because drugs that are minimally active in one type of cancer may be highly active in another tumor. Phase II studies are disease oriented. Evaluation of response in clients with a variety of tumors is performed to determine if significant antitumor activity exists. In phase II trials, a combination of objective and subjective changes is considered in the evaluation of a response. The objective criteria used to describe responses to therapy follow.

Complete remission (CR). Complete remission means complete regression of all evidence of cancer by all criteria (physical, radiologic, biochemical) and a return to normal performance status. All residual symptomatic abnormalities must be related to side-effects of therapy. The duration of complete remission must exceed 1 month (remissions are always expressed in terms of duration).

Partial remission (PR). Partial remission means objective regression of 50% of all measurable tumor accompanied by subjective improvement. The duration of partial remission should be expressed in months. The appearance of any new lesion or increase in the size of residual lesions terminates the partial remission.

Improvement (I). Improvement means there is objective tumor regression of 25% to 50% with subjective improvement. In some studies improvement means that (1) significant subjective improvement has occurred without objective tumor regression or (2) regression of some, but not all, measurable lesions has occurred.

No response (NR). No response means that objective change in the tumor mass is not seen or the response represents less than 25% regression. No significant subjective improvement is seen.

Progression (P). Progression indicates growth of objective disease or appearance of new metastases.

• • •

The nurse utilizes knowledge about the disease process to help interpret the effect a new drug has on tumor growth or regression (see outline below):

Phase II clinical trials

I. Purposes
   A. To identify antitumor activity in a spec-

trum of metastatic human cancers (applicable to single agents and/or new combinations)
   - B. To establish dose and time relationships with observed responses
   - C. To validate phase I data on toxicity to normal tissue
- II. Nursing goals
   - A. To provide clinical expertise
   - B. To facilitate the achievement of the research goals
- III. Responsibilities
   - A. Knowledge about the disease process and its natural history
     1. Responsiveness to other available therapies
     2. Definition of methods to determine response and treatment failure
        - a. Parameters for measurement and quantification of regression of disease by
          - (1) Physical assessment
          - (2) Biochemical parameters
          - (3) Diagnostic techniques
     3. Knowledge concerning the impact of prior drug treatment
     4. Knowledge about the influence of disease-related abnormalities on drug administration and drug effect
   - B. Use of clinical expertise to maximize the impact of tumor regression on the client's life and to minimize adverse effects
     1. Control of environmental factors
     2. Anticipation of adverse effects
     3. Development of effective measures to prevent or minimize toxicity
     4. Education of clients to
        - a. Minimize or avoid adverse effects
        - b. Maximize personal control and participation in therapy
     5. Psychologic support of clients to assist in coping with treatment failure
        - a. Preparing for further therapy
   - C. Documentation of clinical events
     1. Accurate
     2. Comprehensive

Nursing responsibilities include physical assessment of clients, evaluation of subjective changes reported by the client, and evaluation of chemically determined serial laboratory studies. A nurse must understand that disease-related abnormalities can affect drug administration. For example, hepatic metastases, causing impaired hepatic function, may increase the toxicity of a drug that depends on the liver for metabolism or excretion.

In phase II trials, nursing care is important in maximizing the impact of the response on the client's quality of life. As in phase I trials, the nurse must demonstrate autonomy, making decisions to control or manipulate factors in the client's environment to minimize the risk of drug-related toxicity. Meeting the client's physical and emotional needs and teaching him how to anticipate, minimize, or even avoid potential complications are important aspects of nursing responsibility for clinical research trials.

In phase II clinical trials, one frequently must deal with the physical and emotional problems encountered when tumor regrowth occurs following a gratifying but temporary response to the drug. Nurses must anticipate and minimize potential complications so that subsequent treatment with other forms of therapy will not be compromised or delayed. Client education can increase the client's sense of control and also the feeling of participation in the research effort.

Phase III clinical trials

Phase III clinical trials are also disease oriented and are the logical outgrowth of the phase II trials. Drugs that have demonstrated activity in certain cancers are carefully evaluated for the magnitude of tumor regression that they produce in large numbers of clients with that disease. Generally, phase III trials are randomized or comparative trials in a given disease. The responsiveness of a specific disease is studied by comparing an investigational therapy against a standard form of treatment. In phase III studies, the response rate, the speed of response, the magnitude of antitumor regression, and the duration of remission are evaluated. To be of value, a phase III agent must demonstrate activity comparable to conventional agents or provide significant antitumor activity with altered or reduced toxicity (see outline below):

Phase III clinical trials

I. Purposes
   A. To compare a new agent (combination) against a standard form of treatment
   B. To determine the impact of the therapy on survival
   C. To assess the impact of the therapy on the quality of life
II. Nursing goals
   A. To provide clinical expertise (practice skills)
   B. To provide continuity of care
   C. To facilitate achievement of research goals
III. Responsibilities
   A. Assessment of response characteristics in *untreated* clients
      1. Response rate
      2. Speed of response
      3. Percentage of complete regressions
      4. Duration of response
   B. Assessment of adverse effects
      1. Confirmation of acute and chronic toxicity
      2. Delineation of long-term complications of therapy
   C. Provision of supportive nursing care
      1. Continuity of care
      2. Client education
   D. Knowledge about the principles of comparative trials
      1. Ethical guidelines
      2. Protocol design (methods of randomization and data analysis)

Because phase III trials focus on therapeutic efficacy, the trials are designed to compare the investigational treatment against a standard treatment by utilizing a controlled randomized clinical trial. For such studies to be ethical, certain guiding principles must be observed in the design and execution of the study. Nurses collaborating in these trials must be knowledgeable about the design of the trial and capable of explaining the study design and its rationale to clients and colleagues. The investigational drug must have substantial antitumor activity that has been demonstrated in phase II trials to support randomization between the investigational treatment and another more established therapy. The client population and the variables to be studied must be identified and carefully described. Clients entered into these clinical trials are generally *newly diagnosed* and have received no prior therapy with radiation or chemotherapy. To truly assess the impact of each therapy on the natural history of the disease, clients must be divided into treatment groups or "arms" of a trial by random assignment to avoid bias in selection of therapy. Clients must also be stratified with regard to variables that are known to influence prognosis or response to treatment. In addition, the treatment and follow-up period must extend over time periods that are adequate to allow meaningful analysis of therapeutic efficacy by the quality and length of survival. Clinical observations must be recorded in a fashion that is precise, reliable, and minimizes bias. The criteria for treatment failure must be clear, and therapeutic failures or recurrent disease must be identified early so that alternate forms of therapy can be instituted.

An appropriate statistical model for analysis of data should be identified during the formulation of the research study so that an adequate number of clients will be accrued during the study for a meaningful comparison to be performed.

A final phase of the new drug development process is the evaluation of chemotherapeutic agents in treatment programs that are potentially curative. In this type of trial, drugs are often utilized in combination with other active agents or in combination with other effective treatment modalities. These are sophisticated, long-term studies. Nurses play a major role in providing the continuity of care that assists clients to cope with the problems associated with a prolonged period of intensive therapy. They bring experience with the disease to the research trial that complements the knowledge and expertise of the oncologist. Together they can design a comprehensive and realistic plan of care. The nurse, as a client advocate, must thoroughly understand the rationale for the study and be able to explain it to clients. In this way, nurses can ensure that client consent is truly informed and voluntary. Nursing assessment, diagnoses, interventions, and evaluations are critical for trials that often involve complex treatment regimens and have potential for serious and life-threatening complications.

Many of these clinical trials, including studies with phase I and phase II agents, take place in ambulatory care clinics. Increasingly, nurses are actively involved in the administration of chemotherapeutic agents. It is essential that these nurses have a comprehensive understanding of each of the diseases and drugs under investigation, that they have a high level of clinical expertise, and also that they have the ability to recognize and deal with acute changes in the client's condition as they evolve. Ambulatory management affords clients a greater measure of control over their lives and frequently permits the maintenance of a more normal life-style during therapy. However, it necessitates that all clients, their families, and all members of the health care team involved in providing supportive care be knowledgeable about the drugs, their side-effects, and the measures that can be used to prevent or reduce the complications of treatment. Research nurses have assumed major responsibilities in the development of educational programs designed to increase the level of sophistication about antineoplastic agents at all levels.

Combination chemotherapy: rationale for development

Single agents are generally unsuccessful in providing long-term complete remissions in clinically advanced cancer, where the volume of tumor cells is high ($>1 \times 10^{12}$ cells). Potentially curative dosages of a single agent may be so high that life-threatening or fatal toxicity precludes their use. Furthermore, repeated administration of tolerable dosages over prolonged periods of time can result in the development of resistant tumor cell lines. Various mechanisms for drug resistance to chemotherapeutic agents have been proposed, including rapid repair of drug-induced DNA damage (alkylating agents), development of alternate metabolic pathways (antimetabolites), inadequate drug activation (antimetabolites), and increased inactivation of drugs (cytosine arabinoside).

Observation of this development of resistance to single drugs has stimulated the development of treatment programs using drug combinations to circumvent the mechanisms of resistance and to achieve reduction of the tumor cell population to a number that can be destroyed by the host's own defense mechanisms. Effective combinations exploit pharmacologic differences in the sites and mechanisms of action and toxicities of drugs to achieve antitumor activity which can be described as "synergistic." A synergistic therapy is one that produces response rates greater than those expected from the sum of the activities of the drugs used alone. The development of effective drug combinations has dramatically increased the percentage of clients who obtain complete remissions with chemotherapy. The use of these combinations has prolonged the durations of remission in many diseases and is improving overall survival in an increasing number of clients.

An excellent illustration of a drug combination that has become the definitive therapy for a disease is the MOPP combination, which was first studied in advanced Hodgkin's disease. The MOPP combination consists of four drugs, *M*echlorethamine (nitrogen mustard), *O*ncovin (vincristine), *P*rocarbazine, and *P*rednisone. The combination exemplifies basic principles that are employed in the rational design of drug combinations. Firstly, each drug in the MOPP combination has demonstrated antitumor activity in Hodgkin's disease when administered as a single agent. Secondly, the agents in the combination have differing sites and mechanisms of action that inhibit neoplastic growth. (Alkylating agents are often administered in sequence with antimetabolites to take advantage of differences in growth characteristics of cancer cells and the sensitivity of normal host tissues.) The selection of several active agents with differing actions may, in effect, create multiple lesions in the tumor cell that prevent rapid repair of damage, delay regrowth, and prevent or delay the development of resistance.

Differences in the patterns, sites, and timing of toxicity to normal tissues permit the use of full therapeutic dosages of each agent without unacceptable or prohibitive toxicity to the host. Frequently, myelosuppressive agents are combined with drugs that are nontoxic to the bone marrow. Because effective combinations prevent or delay regrowth of the tumor, therapy may be administered in intermittent cycles and still achieve progressive reduction in the volume of malignant cells.

Cyclic administration of drug combinations permits recovery of bone marrow, immunologic function, and repair of other normal tissue to occur during the intervals between one cycle of therapy and another. Finally, both the rate of complete remission and the duration of remission obtainable with effective combination programs is far greater than the data on the single agent activity of each agent would have predicted. With the MOPP regimen it is consistently possible to achieve complete remissions in 80% of previously untreated Hodgkin's disease clients with widely disseminated disease. Of special importance is the fact that 68% of clients attaining a complete remission with this combination are continuously disease free 10 years following the completion of therapy.[33]

Since the most reliable measurement of the magnitude of reduction in tumor volume is the duration of time clients remain clinically free of recurrent disease after all therapy has been stopped, long-term follow-up of clients is crucial in determining the true value of a combination program.

At least three major problems currently exist in our ability to rationally design curative drug combinations for tumors that are known to be responsive to a number of available single agents. There is only a limited understanding of interactions between drugs or of the potentially beneficial or disadvantageous pharmacologic effects such interactions cause, both at the cellular and systemic levels. The activity of many drugs potentially can be enhanced or depressed when combined with other agents (such as 6-MP and allopurinol). To maximize the efficacy of combination chemotherapy, extensive study of the clinical pharmacology of drugs is essential. The second problem is an inability to accurately measure the volume of residual tumor in clients after they achieve a complete clinical remission. The difficulty in documenting the presence or absence of residual disease often complicates decisions concerning how long a therapy

Table 14-3. Advanced cancers currently treatable with chemotherapy

Cancer cures in a significant fraction of clients	Complete remission (%)	Active chemotherapy (active agents)	Current survival
Acute lymphoblastic leukemia of childhood	90	Multiple drug combinations with CNS radiation and intrathecal methotrexate (vincristine, prednisone, methotrexate, 6-mercaptopurine, cytosine arabinoside, 6-thioguanine, doxorubicin, daunomycin, L-asparaginase)	50% of all clients treated with active combinations and CNS radiation are in continous complete remission 10 years later.
Advanced Hodgkin's disease (stages III and IV)	80	Combination chemotherapy such as nitrogen mustard, vincristine, procarbazine, and prednisone (MOPP) and ABVD (nitrogen mustard, cyclophosphamide, procarbazine, vincristine, vinblastine, carmustine, doxorubicin, bleomycin, dacarbazine)	64% of complete responders are in continuous complete remission 10 years later.
Diffuse histiocytic lymphoma	50	Combination chemotherapy such as COPP (cyclophosphamide, nitrogen mustard, vincristine, doxorubicin, prednisone, bleomycin, cytosine arabinoside, high-dose methotrexate)	80% of complete responders are in continuous complete remission 10 years later.
Burkitt's lymphoma	90	Combination chemotherapy (cyclophosphamide, methotrexate, vincristine, cytosine arabinoside, prednisone)	50% of complete responders are in continuous complete remission 10 years later; in early stages 60% are in continous complete remission with cyclophosphamide alone 10 years later.

Choriocarcinoma	90	Combination chemotherapy (methotrexate, cyclophosphamide, 6-mercaptopurine, actinomycin D, vinblastine)	75% cure in metastatic disease, 90% cure in early stages with methotrexate alone, longest survivors over 20 years.
Nonseminomatous testicular carcinoma	75	Combination chemotherapy (methotrexate, actinomycin D, chlorambucil, vinblastine, bleomycin, mithramycin, doxorubicin, cisplatin	70% of complete responders are in continuous complete remission 3 years later.
Ovarian carcinoma	33	Combination chemotherapy (L-phenylalanine mustard, chlorambucil, cyclophosphamide, 5-fluorouracil, triethylenethiophosphoramide, hexamethylmelamine, cisplatin, methotrexate, progestins)	40% of complete responders are in continuous complete remission 10 years later.
Acute myelocytic leukemia	60	Combination chemotherapy CNS prophylaxis (cytosine arabinoside, 6-thioguanine, daunorubicin, cyclophosphamide, 6-mercaptopurine, methotrexate)	20% of complete responders are in continuous complete remission 5 years later.
Skin cancer	70	Topical use of 5-fluorouracil, nitrogen mustard, dinitrochlorobenzene	Excellent control with topical therapy in 70%.
Ewing's sarcoma	*	Radiation plus combination chemotherapy (cyclophosphamide, vincristine, actinomycin D, doxorubicin, carmustine)	66% of complete responders are in continuous complete remission 5 years later.
Wilms' tumor	*	Surgery, radiation, and combination chemotherapy (cyclophosphamide, vincristine, doxorubicin, actinomycin D)	80% of complete responders are in continuous complete remission 5 years later.
Embryonal rhabdomyosarcoma	*	Surgery, radiation, and combination chemotherapy (cyclophosphamide, vincristine, doxorubicin, actinomycin D)	60% of complete responders are in continuous complete remission 5 years later.

*Chemotherapy is not used alone. An integrated multidisciplinary treatment approach is now employed.

must be given in each client to achieve the maximal antitumor response. For this reason there is ongoing research aimed at the detection of circulating "tumor markers," substances produced by tumor cells that can be detected at very low concentrations in the blood when residual tumor is present in the client.[90] The carcinoembryonic antigen (CEA) is such a substance and is often measured in clients with a variety of solid tumors.[53] Finally, data concerning the biochemistry and biology of cancer cell growth are as yet incomplete, and additional fundamental research in this area is needed. Without a more complete understanding of this problem, the rational design of new antitumor drugs with selective toxicity for cancer cells is very difficult.

Despite these problems, there have been impressive improvements in cure rates for a variety of cancers. Table 14-3 lists 12 neoplasms in which combination chemotherapy can *cure* a significant percentage of clients with metastatic disease. Excluding skin cancer, which is often localized and rarely fatal, the statistical impact of these therapies is relatively small, since the neoplasms listed comprise only 10% of cancers and 8% of all cancer deaths.[34] Although these are not the most common cancers, they occur in a relatively youthful population, and the economic and social impact of cure is great. While in some cases (choriocarcinoma and Burkitt's lymphoma) cures have been seen with highly effective single-agent chemotherapy, most often cures are achieved using combinations of drugs. In Hodgkin's disease, acute lymphoblastic leukemia of childhood, and diffuse histiocytic lymphoma, unmaintained remissions following combination chemotherapy extend beyond 10 years.

Following is a list of metastatic cancers that comprise 26% of all malignancies and 26% of cancer deaths.

Metastatic cancers that respond to chemotherapy and have significant prolongations in survival

Carcinoma of the breast
Multiple myeloma
Lymphocytic lymphoma
Prostatic carcinoma
Adrenocortical carcinoma
Malignant insulinoma
Small cell (oat cell) carcinoma of the lung
Sarcoma of soft tissue
Endometrial carcinoma
Malignant carcinoid tumors
Neuroblastoma
Chronic lymphocytic leukemia
Chronic myelocytic leukemia

In clients with these tumors, combination chemotherapy can *prolong* life.[34] Complete remissions are less frequent, however, and only a small fraction of clients remain disease free for prolonged periods of time. Administration of chemotherapy *earlier* in the course of the disease may have a great potential for improving cure rates in these diseases, since available drugs exist that are clearly active in clients with widely metastatic disease.

Combination modality and "adjuvant" therapy

In 1977, approximately 700,000 clients received a diagnosis of some type of cancer, excluding skin cancer. Approximately 500,000 had malignancies that appeared to be localized, and 200,000 had clinically detectable metastases. Forty percent of all clients (280,000) will be free of disease following localized forms of treatment such as surgical resection or radiotherapy. However, following treatment with surgery or radiation, approximately 220,000 clients will develop recurrent disease owing to the presence of undetected microscopic metastases at diagnosis.[35] Considerations of the biology of tumor cell growth and the impact of tumor cell volume on the response to treatment with drugs (first-order kinetics) have provided the basic rationale for use of multiple therapeutic modalities. Combined modality treatment programs utilize surgery, radiation, chemotherapy, and immunotherapy in specific sequences to maximize the curative potential of each. Furthermore, these programs have stimulated the development of "adjuvant" therapy for those clients who are at high risk of developing recurrent cancer following "curative" surgery or radiotherapy. Adjuvant programs involve the use of prophylactic systemic therapy in an attempt to completely eradicate occult residual disease. Since measurable disease cannot be identified in clients given adjuvant therapy, only treatment programs with proved efficacy in advanced cancers of the same type should be employed. Furthermore, the absence of measurable disease necessitates the use of *randomized controlled trials* to document improvement in disease-free survival of treated clients compared to an untreated control group. Since systemic treatment with chemotherapy cannot be administered to clients without significant risk of developing short- or long-term complications, the potential benefits and risks of such programs must be carefully weighed. Use of adjuvant programs that effectively eradicate residual cancer cells has great potential for changing the primary surgical management of many tumors, permitting use of less extensive and less disfiguring surgical techniques.

Complications of therapy

Acute and chronic side-effects occur with the use of most chemotherapeutic agents. Clients who understand the treatment plan and the potential toxicities can actively participate in their own therapy to reduce or prevent complications related to treatment. The ability of clients to become involved in the management of their disease is, to a great degree, dependent on the quality of their interactions with their physicians and nurses. As in all human interactions, the nature and quality of the professional relationships among physicians, nurses, and their clients are related to their personal attitudes. The development of a therapeutic relationship is dependent on the generation of mutual trust. Demonstration of true concern for cancer clients must be accompanied by a demonstration of professional competence and knowledge about the specific neoplasm, available therapies, side-effects associated with treatment, and ultimately, the prognosis for survival. A nursing assessment of the client's interpretation of the meaning of the diagnosis is critical if client perceptions or misconceptions are to be understood. Clients have traditionally found nurses to be more approachable than many physicians, which allows the nurse to explore the client's fears and anxieties through informative discussions. Nurses must remember to talk in terms of probabilities rather than absolutes. It is important to keep future options open and to provide hope while preparing clients for difficult realities that may lie ahead. Through the development of a therapeutic relationship, nurses develop a pathway for effective client education in the area of treatment-related morbidity.

Acute and chronic side-effects of the commonly used chemotherapeutic agents have been listed in Tables 14-1 and 14-2. Several will be highlighted because of the frequency of their occurrence and the discomfort they cause the client. Unique toxicity to organ systems induced by specific drugs has been previously discussed.

Gastrointestinal side-effects

Nausea and vomiting. Nausea and vomiting are the most commonly encountered complications of antineoplastic agents.

Symptoms may appear shortly after administration, be delayed by 8 to 12 hours, and persist for periods up to 24 hours with gradual resolution of symptoms. While they may occur as separate problems, nausea and vomiting frequently appear as a clinical syndrome associated with physiologic changes such as dizziness, pallor, tachycardia, and diaphoresis. The incidence and severity of symptoms are known to be dose related with some, but not all, agents. Induction of symptoms may be related to (1) direct irritation of the gastrointestinal tract (such as ipecac); (2) stimulation of a chemoreceptor trigger zone in the medulla oblongata that is sensitive to certain blood-borne compounds; (3) a central effect on the vomiting zone, a motor and reflex center in the floor of the fourth ventricle that regulates and coordinates the sequence of events during emesis; (4) anticipatory anxiety; or (5) a combination of factors.[86] Symptoms can often be ameliorated with the prophylactic and regular use of phenothiazines and/or sedatives. These agents have a variety of actions including depression of the vomiting center and blocking the effect of drugs on the chemoreceptor trigger zone. Delta-9-tetrahydrocannabinol (THC), the major active ingredient of marijuana, has been employed with some success in clinical settings where conventional antiemetics have failed.[104] Nursing measures should include documenting the onset, intensity, and duration of symptoms and the individual response to intervention. Clients should be encouraged to use antiemetics liberally and advised about the timing, scheduling, and side-effects of antiemetics so that maximum relief can be achieved. Current research in the management of nausea and vomiting includes studies on diversion and relaxation techniques to reduce symptomatology as well as new antiemetic preparations.

Anorexia. Anorexia may occur in conjunction with nausea and vomiting, or it may be related to physiologic changes (such as gastrointestinal obstruction by tumor and loss or distortion of taste) induced by tumor. Anorexia may also stem from emotional disturbances, especially depression and anxiety. Identification of a probable etiology will guide the selection of appropriate therapeutic measures. Intervention may include nutritional counseling, dietary modification, or use of nutritional supplements and intravenous parenteral nutrition to prevent severe nutritional deficiencies.

Diarrhea. Diarrhea may occur as a result of gastrointestinal mucosal irritation secondary to a direct toxic effect of the drug on the bowel. Antidiarrheal agents are often useful. When significant diarrhea occurs, hydration must be increased, especially when drugs that are nephrotoxic or eliminated in urine have been administered.

Constipation. Constipation is generally related to a direct effect on the nerve supply of the bowel causing hypomotility. Prophylactic use of stool softeners and laxatives is warranted with vincristine, the most common etiologic agent.

Cutaneous and mucosal toxicity

Mucositis or stomatitis. Mucositis or stomatitis is a serious and potentially life-threatening complication that is frequently seen with antimetabolites and antitumor antibiotics. Mucositis occurs when renewal of the epithelial cells lining the gastrointestinal tract is inhibited by chemotherapeutic agents. Toxicity is manifested as erythema, pain, and ulceration of the mucosa of some or all of the entire gastrointestinal tract. Ulcerations of the bowel are associated with watery diarrhea and, with more severe toxicity, bleeding. Dose reductions and/or interruptions in therapy are often necessary. Local analgesics, debridement, and topical antibacterial and antifungal therapy can prevent superinfection with opportunistic organisms.

Alopecia. Alopecia is a common complication of chemotherapy that, while not serious, has a profound psychologic impact on clients. Preparation of the client should include arrangements for a wig, empathy, and reassurance that regrowth of hair often occurs during continued treatment.

Rashes. Macular or pustular *rashes,* desquamation, and epidermolysis may occur as a direct effect of the drug on the skin or as an immunologically mediated allergic reaction. Areas of previous irradiation are particularly susceptible to dermatologic toxicity. Dose reductions, interruption, or cessation of therapy may be necessitated by severe toxicity.

Hyperpigmentation and retardation of nail growth. The cytotoxic action of chemotherapeutic agents can cause hyperpigmentation and retardation of nail growth. Clients should be reassured that these side-effects of therapy are not related to disease progression.

Hematologic effects

Myelosuppression. Myelosuppression is the most common dose-limiting toxicity that is associated with chemotherapeutic drugs. Severe leukopenia may result in life-threatening or fatal complications. Bone marrow suppression is manifested as anemia, thrombocytopenia, and leukopenia and can sometimes be managed with blood component therapy.

Anemia. Anemia is a reduction in the number of circulating red cells and the level of hemoglobin. In the absence of concurrent cardiovascular disease, many clients will be asymptomatic if the hemoglobin level remains above 8 gm/dl. When clients develop symptoms such as tachycardia, tachypnea, dizziness, and excessive weakness, packed red blood cell transfusions are utilized to prevent serious cardiovascular complications.

Thrombocytopenia. Thrombocytopenia is a reduction in the number of circulating platelets, which increases the risk of bleeding from all mucous membranes, skin, and into the central nervous system or sites of trauma. Life-threatening hemorrhage can occur in any thrombocytopenic client, but this is uncommon unless peripheral blood platelet counts fall below 20,000 cells/mm^3. Use of prophylactic platelet transfusions in these clients has reduced the incidence of fatal hemorrhage by more than 50%.[125] If available, platelets obtained from histocompatible donors should be used when prolonged periods of thrombocytopenia are anticipated.[125] Administration of certain drugs such as mithramycin and L-asparaginase can produce coagulation abnormalities that further increase the risk of serious bleeding when platelet counts are low. Assessment for evidence of increased bruising, petechiae, or oozing from mucous membranes, and counseling of clients to avoid physical trauma and drugs such as aspirin that compromise platelet function are important nursing interventions.

Leukopenia. Leukopenic clients are particularly susceptible to infectious complications. This increased risk is often due to a combination of granulocytopenia and impaired immunocompetence. As clients become progressively more granulocytopenic, the risk of developing sepsis increases dramatically. The classic signs and symptoms of infection are often absent because of the lack of granulocytes. Early recognition of infection is difficult but essential. Febrile clients who are profoundly granulocytopenic should be hospitalized, cultured promptly, and treated empirically with systemic, broad-spectrum antibiotics until the source of the fever is identified.[76] Fever is due to infection in the vast majority of leukopenic clients. Infection with gram-negative bacilli, fungi, parasites, and other opportunistic organisms is a common cause of death in these clients. Granulocyte transfusions are useful in the supportive care of clients who are expected to be leukopenic for prolonged periods. Hypersensitivity reactions to histoincompatible leukocytes are commonly seen with these transfusions despite attempts to administer histocompatible cells.[83]

Immunosuppression

In addition to having a direct effect on normal hematopoiesis, many commonly used chemotherapeutic agents are potent immunosuppressants. Impairment of the host's immune system increases the risk of infectious complications. Return of normal immune function may take as long as 1 to 2 years following the cessation of all therapy.[52] Current chemotherapeutic programs are designed to provide intensive therapy that alternates with rest periods on a regular schedule to enhance immunologic recovery.

Hyperuricemia can occur following the administration of chemotherapeutic agents when there is rapid lysis of tumor cells. High serum uric acid levels are due to breakdown of nucleoproteins in these cells. Uric acid is excreted by the kidneys. At high concentrations uric acid precipitates in the renal tubules and can cause serious or irreversible kidney failure.[30] Allopurinol prevents the formation of uric acid and should be given prophylactically with hydration prior to the initiation of chemotherapy when rapid cell lysis is thought possible. This is particularly important in clients with acute leukemia and lymphoma where the use of chemotherapy can produce rapid and dramatic reductions in tumor volume. As previously noted, the dose of 6-MP should be decreased when allopurinol is given.

Long-term effects of chemotherapy

Reproductive capacity. Certain chemotherapeutic agents can affect testicular and ovarian function. An important long-term complication of drug therapy is the potential for sterility in treated clients. Sterility may be temporary or permanent. Spermatogenic cells are highly proliferative cells, and this high rate of mitosis predisposes them to damage by cytotoxic drugs. Testicular biopsies in clients following MOPP chemotherapy have demonstrated evidence of seminiferous tubular atrophy with markedly diminished or absent spermatogenesis in most male clients.[112] In females, irregular menses and amenorrhea may also be produced. While spontaneous return of gonadal and reproductive capacity may occur following the cessation of therapy, clients in their reproductive years must be informed that irreversible sterility is a potential complication, both in men and women.[33]

Long-term storage of spermatozoa in special facilities may be considered in young males planning future families. Chemotherapy may cause sublethal chromosomal damage to male or female gametes so the risk of fetal abnormalities following therapy is real. This risk is poorly defined to date. However, several chemotherapeutic agents (such as procarbazine) are highly mutagenic in animals. It is important to remember that while chemotherapy *may* cause infertility, methods of contraception should be discussed with clients, since many agents are teratogenic and pregnancy should be avoided during therapy.

Hepatic, pulmonary, and renal effects. Prolonged administration of chemotherapeutic agents may reversibly or permanently damage the liver, lung, and kidney. The incidence and severity of such effects are not fully appreciated at present. However, the potential for such toxicity must be considered when the decisions about the duration of therapy is made, especially in clients receiving adjuvant therapy for undetectable residual cancer and in clients with metastatic disease who now can be cured with chemotherapy. Both methotrexate and 6-mercaptopurine may cause chronic hepatotoxicity. Toxic effects include hepatic fibrosis, jaundice, and ascites. Prolonged treatment with busulfan, methotrexate, and carmustine have been linked to the development of diffuse interstitial and intra-alveolar pulmonary infiltrates. These infiltrates may gradually resolve when therapy is terminated or may result in progressive deterioration in pulmonary function despite discontinuation of the agent. Treatment with streptozoticin, "high-dose" methotrexate, cisplatin, and recently, semustine is associated with renal toxicity.[120] The incidence of permanent renal damage and renal failure following cessation of therapy with these agents is not yet appreciated.

Carcinogenesis. Studies have demonstrated that alkylating agents, antimetabolites, antitumor antibiotics, and procarbazine can induce chromosomal abnormalities.[113] Use of single agents, or drug combinations with irradiation, also produces cytogenetic aberrations. This strongly suggests that these drugs may have potential carcinogenic activity. Reports of second malignancies in clients who have been treated with chemotherapeutic agents are appearing with increasing frequency. However, it is not established whether this indicates an increasing incidence of second neoplasms, a greater awareness of this potential complication, or an inherent predisposition of cancer clients to develop multiple primary neoplasms. Little data are available concerning the prevalence of second malignancies in cancer clients prior to the use of chemotherapy because without treatment the survival of clients with systemic tumor was short. However, a clear association between an increased prevalence of cancer and immunodeficiency states has been established in animals and clients with congenital immunodeficiency syndromes (that is, Wiskott Aldrich syndrome, ataxia telangiectasia), and in renal transplant recipients who receive immunosuppressive drugs. The pathogenesis of drug-induced second malignancies may be related to the immunosuppressive effect of chemotherapy that permits cells damaged by drugs or radiation to proliferate and become clinically manifest as a second tumor. A growing number of cancer clients are receiving chemotherapeutic agents and are experiencing prolongation in survival and improvement in the quality of life from treatment. Yet the greater and more prolonged use of antitumor agents may place an increasing number of clients at risk for developing drug-induced second neoplasms. As this complication has become recognized, it has become increasingly important to monitor clients in long-term complete remission for the occurrence of second tumors and to inform them of this potential complication. Clients who are receiving adjuvant therapy for suspected occult metastases should also be monitored for second tumors. Comparison of this group of clients to untreated controls should provide important data on the carcinogenic effect of the agents used in such studies.

RESEARCH METHODOLOGY

It is essential for nurses involved in clinical research trials to understand the components of a good research study so that they can interpret data and make sound judgment on the validity of the conclusions that are drawn. Decisions concerning the use of specific methodologies involve clinical expertise, a keen power of observation, and a willingness to test traditional values and concepts. Certain elements of experimental design are basic to all good research. Briefly they include (1) a clear statement of the *problem* or *hypothesis* that is to be studied with a description of how it was formulated and how it relates to a larger conceptual or theoretical framework; (2) a careful review and *synthesis* of current data and *references* from the literature that relate to the problem or hypothesis; (3) evidence of *pretesting* to determine the reliability (reproducibility) and validity of the instrument that will be utilized to measure the phenomena under investigation; (4) utilization of a suitable *study design,* which takes into consideration the manner in which results are to be analyzed, problems associated with sampling, multiple variables, and methods to control variables and observer bias; (5) *analysis* of data utilizing appropriate statistical methods; and (6) careful *interpretation* of results with a statement of conclusions that validly can be drawn from the data.

Analysis of the observations made in a randomized controlled trial involve asking a statistical question about the differences observed between the sample "arms" that have been studied. The researchers must determine whether the differences are due to the therapy under evaluation and whether they are "significant." Statistical tests that are applied to the data give the probability that observed differences can be attributed to chance. This is generally expressed as a *p value,* the difference between the mean (average) values of the variable for each sample. If p is less than 0.05 ($p < 0.05$), the probability that such a difference could occur by chance is relatively rare, less than 5%. Lesser p values imply that a chance difference is even more unlikely. In clinical research, client management decisions are based on the results of clinical trials and the assumption that differences between the study variables were caused by the therapy that was studied. To minimize the risk of drawing unwarranted conclusions about the data, the degree of probability or "level of significance" must be taken into consideration. As a generally accepted convention, most researchers conclude that a p value ≤ 0.05 implies that the populations under study differ with respect to the variable in question if the study is well designed and appropriate statistical tests have been used. It must be remembered that statistical tests are only tools used to compare samples. A poorly designed research study can produce a statistically significant difference between groups but not explain the cause for these differences because of improper selection of subjects or failure to consider important variables.

Development of a full collaborative role for nurses in clinical trials includes active involvement in the collection and analysis of research data. This entails accurate and comprehensive documentation of nursing observations made in all clinical settings where clients receive drug therapy and follow-up care. This is frequently facilitated when the nurse is actively involved in the administration of therapy. Collecting ongoing clinical observations is, in this situation, a form of client advocacy as well as a research function. Maintaining current information enables toxicity to be documented and managed as it evolves and maximizes the safety of the trial for clients. Nurses also review medical records to document and quantitate the biologic effect of investigational agents and the impact on survival and quality of life.

The pivotal role assumed by research nurses in the execution of clinical trials can maximize the nurse's potential to develop the research skills essential for independent nursing research. Clinical experiences gained through collaboration in biomedical research can enable nurses to develop the capacity to define and analyze variables as well as the ability to organize, interpret, and integrate research data. This trend in cancer nursing carries broad implications for the entire nursing profession. Methodology employed in biomedical research can readily be employed to define nursing questions amenable to clinical investigation and to guide independent nursing research studies.

Involvement in collaborative research can enable nurses to conceptualize a research problem by demonstrating how such a project develops from abstract concepts into concrete, well-defined questions. Collaboration in research can assist nurses to organize assumptions in a disciplined manner, to identify useful instruments to measure phenomena, and to learn to use statistical techniques meaningfully. Finally, one learns how to communicate effectively in writing, to explain concepts clearly, and to summarize the results of research for publication. By opening one's ideas to question and disproof, a nurse can learn to take the necessary intellectual risks that are required when initiating an independent research study. The potential for developing creative and innovative research is maximized by learning to look at problems in unconventional ways. Willingness to consider new ways of organizing and providing nursing service is crucial if nursing is to improve the quality of nursing care and practice in the future.

SUMMARY

The cancer nurse has evolved a broad role with a direct impact on nursing in three areas: *practice, education,* and *research.*

In *clinical practice,* nursing specialization in cancer care has generated new nursing expertise and has opened up new avenues of interaction with physicians, auxilliary personnel, and clients. Nursing specialization has demonstrated that expanded nursing roles enable nurses to competently assume a greater portion of the total client care responsibility. In an era when many of the traditional functions of the nurse are either being subsumed or questioned, the importance of "role expansion" should not be underestimated. For example, the cancer nurse has become an important liaison between physicians and clients and their families. The experience required to develop this role has been facilitated by considering the cancer nurse as an integral member of the primary health care team. Close affiliation with the oncologist facilitates integration of a comprehensive nursing care plan into the overall medical treatment of clients.

The impact of the clinical nurse specialist on improving quality of care given to cancer clients has broad implications for *nursing education.* The clinical specialist in cancer has facilitated more rapid dissemination of current information on practice and research to the nursing profession and stimulates improvements in the quality of client care and nursing practice. Additionally, the cancer nurse performs a vital service in educating clients about their disease and proposed management.

Collaboration between nurses and oncologists in *research* has demonstrated that nurses have a significant contribution to make to the operation of clinical trials. Sophistication in research design and methodology is valuable in the development of independent nursing research that can provide new scientific knowledge. Development of such sophistication will facilitate true collaboration with physicians, evolving a full partnership in client care with joint decision making and joint accountability for health care and health maintenance.

REFERENCES

1. Abercrombie, M.: Contact inhibition: the phenomenon and its biological implications, Natl. Cancer Inst. Monogr. **26:**249, 1967.
2. Anderson, T., McMenamin, M., and Schein, P. S.: Chlorozoticin, 2- 3(2-chloroethyl-3-nitrosoureido)-D-glucopyramose an antitumor agent

with modified bone marrow toxicity, Cancer Res. **35:**761, 1976.

3. Ansfield, F. L., et al.: Intrahepatic arterial infusion with 5-fluorouracil, Cancer **28:**1147, 1971.
4. Arena, E., et al.: Influence of pharmacokinetic variations on the pharmacologic properties of adriamycin. In Carter, S. K., DiMarco, A., and Ghione, M., editors: International symposium on adriamycin, Berlin, 1972, Springer Verlag, p. 96.
5. Ashby, R., et al.: Aspects of the teratology of cyclophosphamide, Cancer Treat. Rep. **60:**477, 1976.
6. Axtell, L. M., Asire, A. J., and Myers, M. H., editors: Cancer patient survival, Report Number 5, DHEW Publication No. 77-992, Washington, D.C., 1976, U.S. Department of Health, Education and Welfare.
7. Bailar, J. C., and Byar, D. P.: Estrogen treatment for cancer of the prostate: early results with 3 doses of diethylstilbesterol and placebo, Cancer **26:**257, 1970.
8. Bard, P. R., et al.: Treatment of central nervous system leukemia with intrathecal cytosine arabinoside, Cancer **32:**744, 1973.
9. Bergenstal, D. M., et al.: Chemotherapy of adrenocortical cancer with O, P' DDD, Ann. Intern. Med. **53:**672, 1960.
10. Bertino, J. R.: Rescue techniques in cancer chemotherapy: use of leucovorin and other rescue agents after methotrexate treatment, Semin. Oncol. **4:**203, 1977.
11. Bleyer, W. A.: The clinical pharmacology of methotrexate, Cancer **41:**36, 1978.
12. Bleyer, W. A., Drake, J. C., and Chabner, B. A.: Neurotoxicity and elevated cerebrospinal-fluid methotrexate concentrations in meningeal leukemia, N. Engl. J. Med. **289:**770, 1973.
13. Blum, R. H., and Carter, S. K.: Adriamycin: a new anticancer drug with significant clinical activity, Ann. Intern. Med. **80:**249, 1974.
14. Blum, R. H., Carter, S. K., and Agre, K. A.: Clinical review of bleomycin: a new antineoplastic agent, Cancer **31:**903, 1973.
15. Blum, R. H., Livingston, R. B., and Carter, S. K.: Hexamethylmelamine: a new drug with activity in solid tumors, Eur. J. Cancer **9:**155, 1973.
16. Borsa, J., and Whitmore, G. F.: Cell killing studies on the mode of action of methotrexate on L-cells, Cancer Res. **29:**737, 1969.
17. Bristow, M. R., Mason, M. W., and Billingham, M.: Doxorubicin cardiomyopathy: evaluation by phonocardiography, endomyocardial biopsy, and cardiac catheterization, Ann. Intern. Med. **88:** 168, 1978.
18. Broder, L., and Carter, S.: Pancreatic islet cell carcinoma: result of therapy with streptozoticin in stage II patients, Ann. Intern. Med. **79:**108, 1973.
19. Brunner, K. W., and Young, C. W.: A methylhydrazine derivative in Hodgkin's disease and other malignant neoplasms. Therapeutic and toxic effects in 51 patients, Ann. Intern. Med. **63:**69, 1965.
20. Burchenal, J. H.: From wild fowl to stalking horses: alchemy in chemotherapy (David A. Karnofsky Memorial Lecture), Cancer **35:**1121, 1975.
21. Capizzi, R. L., et al.: L'asparaginase: clinical, biochemical, pharmacological and immunologic studies, Ann. Intern. Med. **74:**893, 1971.
22. Carter, S. K., and Livingston, R. B.: Plant products in cancer chemotherapy, Cancer Treat. Rep. **60:**1141, 1976.
23. Chabner, B. A., and Young, R. C.: Threshold methotrexate concentrations for in vivo inhibition of DNA synthesis in normal and tumorous target tissues, J. Clin. Invest. **52:**1804, 1973.
24. Chabner, B. A., Myers, C. E., and Oliverio, V. T.: Clinical pharmacology of anticancer drugs, Semin. Oncol. **4:**165, 1977.
25. Chabner, B. A., et al.: The clinical pharmacology of antineoplastic agents (Parts I and II), N. Engl. J. Med. **292:**1107, 1159, 1975.
26. Comis, R. L.: DTIC (NSC 45388) in malignant melanoma: a perspective, Cancer Treat. Rep. **60:**165, 1976.
27. Cortes, E. P., Lutman, G., and Wanka, J.: Adriamycin cardiotoxicity: a clinicopathologic correlation, Cancer Chemother. Rep. **6:**215, 1975.
28. Crile, G.: Endocrine dependency of papillary carcinoma of the thyroid, J.A.M.A. **195:**721, 1966.
29. Crooke, S., and Bradner, W.: Mitomycin C, a review, Cancer Treat. Rev. **3:**121, 1976.
30. DeConti, R. C., and Calabresi, P.: Use of allopurinol for prevention and control of hyperuricemia, N. Engl. J. Med. **274:**481, 1966.
31. DeFronzo, R. A., et al.: Water intoxication in man after cyclophosphamide therapy: time course and relation to drug activation, Ann. Intern. Med. **78:**861, 1973.
32. DeVita, V. T.: Cell kinetics and the chemotherapy of cancer, Cancer Chemother. Rep. **2:**23, 1971.
33. DeVita, V. T.: The consequences of the chemotherapy of Hodgkin's disease (David A. Karnofsky Memorial Lecture), Cancer. In press.
34. DeVita, V. T.: Principles of cancer therapy. In Petersdorf, R., editor: Harrison's principles of internal medicine, ed. 9, New York, 1979, McGraw-Hill Book Co., p. 1597.
35. DeVita, V. T., Henney, J. E., and Stonehill, E.:

Cancer mortality: the good news. In Salmon, S., and Jones, S., editors: Adjuvant therapy of cancer, vol. 2, New York, 1979, Grune & Stratton, Inc.

36. DeVita, V. T., Young, R. C., and Canellos, G. P.: Combination versus single agent chemotherapy: a review of the basis for selection of drug treatment in cancer, Cancer **35:**98, 1975.
37. DeVita, V. T., et al.: Clinical trials with 1,3-bis (2-chloroethyl 1 nitrosourea, (NSC 409962), Cancer Res. **31:**332, 1971.
38. DeVita, V. T., et al.: Perspectives in research in gynecologic oncology, Cancer **38:**161, 1976.
39. DeVita, V. T., et al.: The drug development and clinical trials programs of the division of cancer treatment, Cancer Clinical Trials. In press.
40. Fairley, K. F., Barrie, J. V., Johnson, W.: Sterility and testicular atrophy related to cyclophosphamide therapy, Lancet **1:**568, 1972.
41. Farber, S., et al.: Temporary remissions in acute leukemia in children produced by folic acid antagonist, 4 aminopteroylglutamic acid (aminopterin), N. Engl. J. Med. **238:**787, 1948.
42. Fauci, A., Dale, D., and Balow, J. E.: Corticosteroid therapy: mechanisms of action and clinical considerations, Ann. Intern. Med. **84:**304, 1976.
43. Fauci, F. S., Haynes, B. F., and Katz, P.: The spectrum of vasculitis, Ann. Intern. Med. **89:**660, 1978.
44. Frei, E.: The clinical use of actinomycin, Cancer Chemother. Rep. **58:**49, 1974.
45. Frei, E., Franzino, S., and Shnider, B.: Clinical studies of vinblastine, Cancer Chemother. Rep. **12:**125, 1961.
46. Friedman, P. A., and Cerami, A.: Actinomycin. In Holland, J. F., and Frei, E., III, editors: Cancer medicine, Philadelphia, 1973, Lea & Febiger, p. 835.
47. Frindel, E., and Tubiana, M.: Radiobiology and the cell cycle. In Baserga, R., editor: The cell cycle and cancer, New York, 1971, Marcell Dekker, Inc., p. 391.
48. Gershwin, M. E., Goetzl, E. J., Steinberg, A. D.: Cyclophosphamide: use in practice, Ann. Intern. Med. **80:**531, 1974.
49. Goldin, A., et al.: Effect of delayed administration of citrovorum factor on the antileukemic effectiveness of aminopterin in mice, Cancer Res. **14:**43, 1954.
50. Goodman, L., et al.: Use of methyl-bis (B-chloroethyl) amine hydrochloride for Hodgkin's disease, lymphosarcoma, leukemia, and allied and miscellaneous disorders, J.A.M.A. **132:**126, 1946.
51. Gottdiener, J. S.: Noninvasive assessment of cardiac dysfunction in the cancer patient, Cancer Treat. Rep. **62:**949, 1978.
52. Green, A. A., and Borella, L.: Immunologic rebound after cessation of long term chemotherapy in acute leukemia, Blood **42:**99, 1973.
53. Hansen, H. J., et al.: Carcinoembryonic antigen (CEA) assay, J. Hum. Pathol. **5:**139, 1974.
54. Heidelberger, C.: Pyrimidine and pyrimidine nucleoside antimetabolites. In Holland, J. F., and Frei, E., III, editors: Cancer medicine, Philadelphia, 1973, Lea & Febiger, p. 768.
55. Howard, A., and Pelc, S. R.: Synthesis of deoxyribonucleic acid in normal and irradiated cells and its relation to chromosome breakage, Heredity **6**(Suppl):261, 1953.
56. Hrushesky, W.: Analysis of the clinical studies of L'asparaginase *E. coli* 2, CTEP NCI Monograph, 1978.
57. Hrushesky, W., and Murphy, G.: Current status of the therapy of advanced renal carcinoma, J. Surg. Onc. **9:**277, 1977.
58. Hrushesky, W., et al.: The other asparaginase, Med. Pediatr. Oncol. **2:**441, 1976.
59. Hubbard, S. M.: The practice of cancer nursing. Proceedings of The Second National Conference on Cancer Nursing, New York, 1977, American Cancer Society, Inc., p. 23.
60. Hubbard, S. P., and DeVita, V. T.: Medical oncology, drug development, and the chemotherapy nurse, Am. J. Med. **76:**450, 1976.
61. Hyman, C. B., et al.: Central nervous system involvement by leukemia in children. II: Therapy with intrathecal methotrexate, Blood **25:**13, 1965.
62. Jacobs, S. A., et al.: Altered plasma pharmacokinetics of methotrexate administered intrathecally, Lancet **1:**465, 1975.
63. Jaenke, R. S.: Delayed and progressive myocardial lesions after adriamycin administration in the rabbit, Cancer Res. **36:**2958, 1976.
64. Jensen, E. V.: Estrogen binding and clinical response in breast cancer. In Holland, J. F., and Frei, E., III, editors: Cancer medicine, Philadelphia, 1973, Lea & Febiger, p. 900.
65. Johns, D. G., and Bertino, J. R.: Folate antagonists. In Holland, J. F., and Frei, E., III, editors: Cancer medicine, Philadelphia, 1973, Lea & Febiger, p. 739.
66. Kennedy, B. J.: Mithramycin: therapy in advanced testicular neoplasms, Cancer **26:**755, 1970.
67. Kennedy, B. J.: Metabolic and toxic effects of mithramycin during tumor therapy, Am. J. Med. **49:**494, 1970.
68. Kennedy, B. J.: Ablative procedures in cancer

therapy. In Holland, J. F., and Frei, E., III, editors: Cancer medicine, Philadelphia, 1973, Lea & Febiger, p. 945.
69. Kennedy, B. J.: Hormonal therapies in breast cancer, Semin. Oncol. **1:**119, 1974.
70. Kennedy, B. J., and Yarbro, J. W.: Metabolic and therapeutic effects of hydroxyurea in chronic myelogenous leukemia, J.A.M.A. **195:**1038, 1966.
71. Kim, S. H., and Kim, J. H.: Lethal effects of adriamycin on the division cycle of hela cell, Cancer Res. **32:**323, 1972.
72. Kirschner, R. H., and Esterly, J. R.: Pulmonary lesions associated with busulfan therapy of chronic myelogenous leukemia, Cancer **27:**1074, 1971.
73. Krumbaar, E. B., and Krumbaar, H. D.: The blood and bone marrow in yellow cross gas (mustard gas) poisoning: changes produced in the bone marrow of fatal cases, J. Med. Res. **40:**497, 1919.
74. Lampkin, B. C., Nagso, T., and Mauer, A. M.: Synchronization and recruitment in acute leukemia, J. Clin. Invest. **50:**2204, 1971.
75. LePage, G. A., and Loo, T. L.: Purine antagonists. In Holland, J. F., and Frei, E., III, editors: Cancer medicine, Philadelphia, 1973, Lea & Febiger, p. 755.
76. Levine, A. S., et al.: Hematologic malignancies and other marrow failure states: progress in the management of infection, Semin. Hematol. **11:** 141, 1974.
77. Liegler, D. C., et al.: The effect of organic acids on renal clearance of methotrexate in man, Clin. Pharmacol. Ther. **10:**849, 1969.
78. Lippman, M.: Steroid hormone receptors and human malignancy. In Charyulu, K. K., editor: Hormones and cancer, Miami, 1976, Symposia Specialties, p. 205.
79. Lissauer, A.: Zwei Fälle von Leucaemie, Berl. Klin. Wochenschr. **2:**403, 1865.
80. Livingston, R. B., and Carter, S. K.: Single agents in cancer chemotherapy, New York, 1973, IFI/Plenum Data Corp, p. 25.
81. Lomen, P. V., et al.: Phase I study of 5-azacytadine (NSC 102816) using 24-hour continuous infusion for 5 days, Cancer Chemother. Rep. **59:**1123, 1975.
82. Louis, J.: The clinical pharmacology of hexamethylmelamine: phase I study, Clin. Pharmacol. Ther. **8:**55, 1967.
83. Lowenthal, R. M., et al.: Granulocyte transfusions in treatment of infections in patients with acute leukemia and aplastic anemia, Lancet **1:**354, 1975.
84. Mazia, D.: The cell cycle, Sci. Am. **230:**54, 1974.
85. McGuire, W. L.: Hormone receptors: their role in predicting prognosis and response to endocrine therapy, Semin. Oncol. **5:**428, 1978.
86. Mellencamp, E., and Wang, R. H.: The patient with nausea, Drug Therapy, p. 47, 1977.
87. Mendelsohn, M. L.: Autoradiographic analysis of cell proliferation in spontaneous breast cancer of C_3H mouse. III. The growth fraction, J. Natl. Cancer Inst. **28:**1015, 1962.
88. Meyskens, E. L., Tormey, D., and Neifield, J. P.: Male breast cancer: a review, Cancer Treat. Rev. **3:**83, 1976.
89. Mouridsen, H., Palshof, T., and Patterson, J.: Tamoxifen in advanced breast cancer, Semin. Oncol. **5:**131, 1978.
90. Neville, A. M., and Cooper, E. H.: Biochemical monitoring of cancer: a review, Ann. Clin. Biochem. **13:**283, 1976.
91. O'Connell, T. X., and Berenbaum, M. C.: Cardiac and pulmonary effects of high doses of cyclophosphamide and isophosphamide, Cancer Res. **34:** 1586, 1974.
92. Perlia, C. P., et al.: Mithramycin treatment of hypercalcemia, Cancer **25:**389, 1970.
93. Philips, F. S., et al.: Cyclophosphamide and urinary bladder toxicity, Cancer Res. **21:**1577, 1961.
94. Pinedo, H. M., et al.: The relative contribution of drug concentration and duration of exposure to mouse bone marrow toxicity during continuous methotrexate infusion, Cancer Res. **37:**445, 1977.
95. Primak, A.: Amelioration of cyclophosphamide induced cystitis, Cancer Res. **34:**1586, 1976.
96. Proceedings of the Symposium on The Metabolism and Mechanism of Action of Cyclophosphamide, Cancer Treat. Rep. **60:**299, 1976.
97. Proceedings of the Seventh New Drug Seminar on The Nitrosoureas, Cancer Treat. Rep. **60:**645, 1976.
98. Proceedings of The Second National Conference on Cancer Nursing, New York, 1977, American Cancer Society, Inc.
99. Roberts, J. J., and Pascoe, J. M.: Cross-linking of complementary strands of DNA in mammalian cells by antitumor platinum compounds, Nature **235:**282, 1972.
100. Rosencweig, M., et al.: Cis-diamminedichloroplatinum: a new cancer drug, Ann. Intern. Med. **86:**803, 1977.
101. Rosenoff, S. A., et al.: Alterations in DNA synthesis in cardiac muscle induced by adriamycin in vivo: relationship to fatal toxicity, Biochem. Pharmacol. **24:**1898, 1975.
102. Rundles, R. E.: Effects of allopurinol on 6-

mercaptopurine therapy in neoplastic diseases, Ann. Rheum. Dis. **25**:655, 1966.

103. Rutman, R. J., Cantarow, A., and Paschkis, K.: Studies in 2-acetylaminofluorene carcinogenesis III. The utilization of uracil-2-C^{14} by preneoplastic rat liver and rat hepatoma, Cancer Res. **14**:119, 1954.
104. Sallon, S. E., Zinberg, N. E., and Frei, E.: Antiemetic effect of delta-9-tetra-hydrocannabinol, N. Engl. J. Med. **16**:795, 1975.
105. Samuels, M.: Procarbazine in the treatment of advanced bronchogenic carcinoma, Cancer Chemother. Rep. **53**:135, 1969.
106. Samuels, M. L., Johnson, D. E., and Holoye, P. Y.: Continuous intravenous bleomycin therapy with vinblastine in stage III testicular neoplasia, Cancer Chemother. Rep. **59**:563, 1975.
107. Santen, R. J., et al.: Kinetic, hormonal and clinical studies with aminoglutethemide in breast cancer, Cancer **39**:2948, 1977.
108. Schabel, F. M.: The use of tumor growth kinetics in planning "curative" chemotherapy of advanced solid tumors, Cancer Res. **29**:2384, 1969.
109. Schabel, F. M.: Concepts for systemic treatment of micrometastases, Cancer **35**:15, 1975.
110. Schein, P. S.: The medical management of breast cancer, Georgetown Med. Bull. **28**:12, 1975.
111. Schein, P. S., et al.: Clinical antitumor activity and toxicity of streptozoticin, Cancer **34**:993, 1974.
112. Sherins, R. J., and DeVita, V. T.: Effect of drug treatment on male reproductive capacity: studies of men in remission after therapy, Ann. Intern. Med. **79**:216, 1973.
113. Sieber, S., and Adamson, R. H.: Toxicity of antineoplastic agents chromosomal aberrations antifertility effects, congenital malformations and carcinogenic potential, Adv. Cancer Res. **22**:57, 1975.
114. Skipper, H. E.: The cell cycle and chemotherapy of cancer. In Baserga, R., editor: The cell cycle and cancer, New York, 1971, Marcell Dekker, Inc., p. 358.
115. Skipper, H. E.: Kinetics of mammary tumor cell growth and implications for therapy, Cancer **28**: 1479, 1971.
116. Skipper, H. E., Schabel, F. M., Jr., and Wilcox, W. S.: Experimental evaluation of potential anticancer agents. XII. On the criteria and kinetics associated with curability of experimental leukemia, Cancer Chemother. Rep. **35**:1, 1964.
117. Stolinsky, D. C., Pugh, R. P., and Batemen, J. R.: 5-fluorouracil therapy for pancreatic carcinoma: comparison of oral and intravenous routes, Cancer Chemother. Rep. **59**:1031, 1975.
118. Stoller, R. G., et al.: Use of plasma pharmacokinetics to predict and prevent methotrexate toxicity, N. Engl. J. Med. **297**:630, 1977.
119. Stonehill, E. H.: Impact of cancer therapy on survival, Cancer **42**:1008, 1978.
120. Unpublished data from CTEP files, Cancer Therapeutic Evaluation Program, DCT, NCI.
121. Veenema, R. J., et al.: Bladder carcinoma treated by direct installation of ThioTEPA, J. Urol. **88**:60, 1962.
122. Waring, M.: Variation of the supercoils in closed circuit DNA by binding of antibiotics and drugs: evidence for molecular models involving intercalation, J. Mol. Biol. **54**:247, 1970.
123. Weiss, H. D., Walker, M. D., and Wiernik, P.: Neurotoxicity of commonly used antineoplastic agents (Parts I and II), N. Engl. J. Med. **291**:75, 127, 1974.
124. Woods, D D.: The relation of p-aminobenzoic acid to the mechanism of action of sulfonamide, Br. J. Exper. Pathol. **21**:74, 1940.
125. Yankee, R. A., et al.: The selection of unrelated compatible platelet donors by lymphocyte HL-A matching, N. Engl. J. Med. **288**:760, 1973.

15

Nursing care of the client receiving tumor immunotherapy

DEBORAH S. WHITE

Tumor immunotherapy is the science of introducing antigens or other materials into the body to stimulate the host's immune system to attack cancer cells. The first documented case of tumor immunotherapy used in humans was by Hericourt and Richet in 1895.[8] They raised antisera in dogs and donkeys and subsequently injected this material into 50 people who had malignant melanoma. Hericourt and Richet claimed many beneficial effects from this treatment but concluded that it was no better than any recognized form of cancer therapy at that time.[20]

In the early 1900's, many researchers performed animal experiments, taking a tumor from one animal and transplanting it into another animal. Rejection of the tumor was thought to be an antitumor effect. Tumor rejection indeed occurred, but it was later learned that this was a graft versus host reaction dependent on the genetic differences between the two animals and not representing true tumor immunotherapy.

Studies of tumor immunotherapy were then abandoned until syngeneic animal tumor systems and tumor-specific transplantation antigens (TSTA) were discovered. Since the early works of Hericourt and Richet, experiments in immunotherapy have been conducted, but the technical basis for significant advances (for example, specialized blood tests for antibody levels) did not exist.

SCIENTIFIC RATIONALE

The goals of tumor immunotherapy are few but cover a wide field of research. They are as follows:

1. To stimulate the immunologic system by active or passive immunotherapy to become competent in a tumor-bearing person
2. To generate tumor-specific immunity
3. As an adjunct to other forms of therapy in producing tumor regression

The two approaches to immunotherapy are (1) prophylactic and (2) therapeutic. Immunoprophylaxis is aimed at preventing the established disease. This is done in the normal population each year, for example, to protect against influenza. Tumor immunotherapy is applied in a similar preventive fashion in people who have undergone curative surgery but have a high risk of developing recurrent disease. The use of bacillus Calmette-Guérin (BCG) following surgery for melanoma is an example. To date no successful vaccine to prevent cancer has been developed. The most promising result in this area is the ability to prevent Marek's disease (a form of viral-induced avian lymphoma) in chickens.[22] Therapeutic immunotherapy is treatment given once a person has clinical evidence of a malignancy.

Certain general limitations apply to all cancer immunotherapy:

1. It is only effective against small bulk disease. With all forms of immunotherapy, the disease must be reduced to a minimal residual amount for the immunotherapy to work effectively. This may be accomplished by debulking surgery, chemotherapy, or radiation therapy.
2. Immunotherapy may theoretically enhance tumor growth, but according to the literature there have been few documented cases in humans. Deliberate tumor enhancement in humans obviously cannot be studied, but extensive testing in animals has been done since the 1950's.
3. It is difficult to standardize and measure the amount of some immunotherapeutic agents given. As will be explained further in this chapter, the dose of BCG varies greatly with each researcher as does the method of administration. Indeed, there is no method to measure the amount of the agent given, especially with BCG, which is administered intradermally. A dose of 3×10^8 organisms of BCG may be applied to the skin, but no measurement of the absorbed dose is possible.
4. We do not have a complete understanding of tumor immunobiology. We are still unsure of some of the biologic differences between normal and malignant cells and the mechanisms by which the body is able to distinguish between them.

TYPES OF IMMUNOTHERAPY

Immunotherapy may be classified into two main categories: active and passive. These two are further divided into specific and nonspecific therapies. Adoptive immunotherapy is a special category of passive immunotherapy (Fig. 15-1).

Active immunotherapy

Active immunotherapy refers to the administration of a specific antigen intended to develop an immune response (antibody or cellular response) in the host.

Polio and tetanus vaccines are familiar examples of active specific immunotherapy that are used in the general population. Likewise, in a cancer population, the person may be given a vaccine of modified tumor cells or tumor antigen to treat or prevent a recurrence of the disease. Cells derived from the person's own cells are autologous vaccines, whereas cells or antigens from another person with the same disease constitute allogeneic vaccines. Tumor cells are often modified prior to injection by techniques such as irradiation or neuraminidase treatment to render them nonviable or more antigenic.

Active nonspecific immunotherapy. Active nonspecific immunotherapy denotes the process whereby live bacteria or their products or chemical agents are used to stimulate the immune system. Agents in-

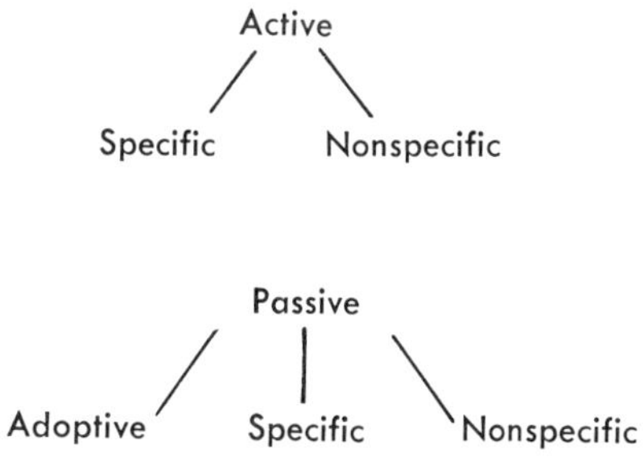

Fig. 15-1. Types of immunotherapy.

cluded in this class are BCG, *Corynebacterium parvum* (*C. parvum*), levamisole, and dinitrochlorobenzene (DNCB).

Passive immunotherapy

Passive immunotherapy may be accomplished by injecting antitumor sera, by giving lymphocyte transfusions from healthy donors, or by removal of immunosuppressive substances by techniques such as plasmapheresis. Plasmapheresis is taking blood from a donor, separating out the plasma in the blood by centrifuge, and finally reinjecting the packed cells into the donor in a saline solution. In this instance, the investigator is trying to remove the substances in the plasma that cause immunosuppression in the person being treated. A common example of passive immunotherapy is the treatment by injection of gamma globulin for accidental exposure to serum hepatitis. In general, passive immunotherapy has not been a very successful technique for inducing tumor remission.

Passive specific immunotherapy. Passive specific immunotherapy is the form of treatment in which people are injected with specific serum in an attempt to stimulate antitumor antibodies. In a few cases of Burkitt's lymphoma, people have been injected with sera from other persons in remission.[4] This procedure has been found to be moderately successful.

Passive nonspecific immunotherapy. The serum passive nonspecific immunotherapy is collected from normal individuals for injection into the cancer-bearing person as in the treatment of those afflicted with chronic lymphocytic leukemia who lack the ability to make normal amounts of effective antibodies. In noncancerous diseases, such as congenital hypogammaglobulinemias, the person cannot resist infection, so he is given pooled gamma globulin.

Passive adoptive immunotherapy. Passive adoptive immunotherapy requires the transferring of immunocompetent cells or their effector substances. Administration of "transfer factor" is an example of this and will be discussed in the section dealing with immunotherapy agents.

IMMUNOTHERAPY AGENTS

Many immunotherapeutic agents have been investigated or are now under investigation (Table 15-1). It is certain that in the future, research in this area will continue and intensify. Such agents are first tested in laboratory animals and then clinically tested on human subjects. Among the many that have reached clinical testing are BCG, *Corynebacterium parvum,* levamisole, and methanol-extracted residue of BCG (MER). These agents are probably the most thoroughly tested of all immunotherapeutic agents. They have been tested in multiple combinations, doses, and schedules, but studies continue to try to optimize this treatment.

Bacillus Calmette-Guérin

Bacillus Calmette-Guérin (BCG) was originally isolated by Calmette and Guérin at the Pasteur Institute in 1910.[25] It was not clinically tested until 1921 when it was used to vaccinate against tuberculosis. Forty years later it was applied to the control of cancer, owing to animal studies that have shown nonspecific stimulation of the immune system by agents such as BCG.

BCG, an attenuated bacterium, is considered to be an experimental agent in cancer therapy. At this writing it is still being vigorously tested by investigators at centers that have been licensed to do so by the Food and Drug Administration.

BCG has been prepared in almost as many ways as there are ways to administer it. The strain that is used by most institutions in this country is the Chicago Tice strain of 3×10^8 organisms (300,000,000 organisms) per vial

Table 15-1. Agents used in tumor immunotherapy

Agent	Usual dose	Applicable cancer
Bacillus Calmette-Guérin (BCG)	3×10^8 organisms	Melanoma, breast
Corynebacterium parvum (*C. parvum*)	5 mg/m^2	Melanoma, breast
Levamisole	200 mg/m^2/day	Lung, renal
Methanol-extracted residue of BCG (MER)	1 mg q2-4 wk	Leukemia, melanoma, lymphosarcoma
Transfer factor	Not applicable	Sarcoma, melanoma, breast, lymphoma
Immune RNA (I-RNA)	4-8 mg/wk	Melanoma, breast, sarcoma
Thymosin	50-250 mg/m^2	Leukemia, melanoma

supplied. This strain is lyophilized (that is, freeze-dried). Other lyophilized strains include Glaxo (60×10^6 organisms), Connaught (5×10^8 organisms), and Pasteur (6.2×10^6 organisms). There are approximately six other known lyophilized strains of BCG, with the number of viable organisms ranging from a count of 1.8×10^6 to 66.5×10^6.[12] The number of viable organisms varies widely, causing vast differences in the work of one researcher to that of another. To reconstitute the lyophilized BCG preparations for injection, nonbacteriostatic sterile water is added.

It should also be mentioned that BCG is sometimes used as a "fresh" preparation of 7×10^6 organisms, which has the limitation of the quick "dropping off" of viable organisms. The institutions using this strain need access to an airport or other method of fast transportation to preclude deterioration of the substance before it can be administered.

BCG, as discussed previously, comes in many preparations and is administered in a variety of ways and in various schedules. The multitude of variables with BCG noted by Carter[3]—"manufacturer, preparation, ratio of live to dead micro-organisms, viable cell count, route of administration, dose level, dose schedule and duration of treatment"—have caused wide differences in the results of research. (Viable cell count is the number of live organisms in the solution, although there may be many more total organisms in the vial. In immunotherapy, the live organisms are the only concern because those organisms are the ones that stimulate the immune system). However, there have been sufficient positive results to continue the quest for the ultimate therapy procedure.

BCG may be administered by the following methods:

1. Intradermal
2. Scarification
3. Aerosol
4. Intralesional
5. Intrapleural
6. Oral

The rationale for using so many different methods of administration for BCG is that the closer the agent can be administered to the lymphatics or tumor-bearing site, the more likely it is that immunostimulation will result.

Some recent trials of immunotherapy demonstrate the wide usage of BCG in clinical trials and the various methods and combinations. A recently cited study[14] on lung cancer therapy used one dose of BCG given postoperatively into the pleura with outstanding results. Further studies[5,11,13] using

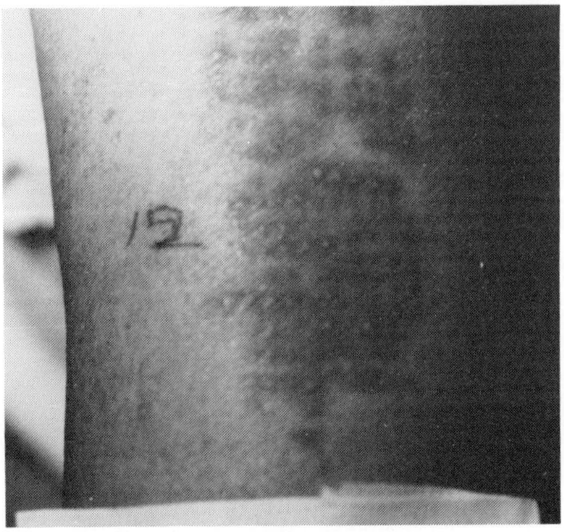

Fig. 15-2. BCG reaction.

BCG show that there is a definite role for immunotherapy in cancer therapy of most types. Particularly good results were shown in a study of sarcomas using BCG with allogeneic sarcoma cells.[16]

Side-effects observed with BCG usage are minimal when the agent is given intradermally. A majority of the people thus treated will respond with a significant amount of local irritation at the site of administration, which increases as the client becomes more sensitized with repeated injections. An example of such irritation is shown in Fig. 15-2. Itching and sloughing of the skin may occur, and occasionally a person may complain of general malaise lasting from 24 to 36 hours. On occasion, previously treated sites will flare up. These reactions may be minimized by administering diphenhydramine hydrochloride (Benadryl) or acetaminophen (Tylenol).

The chief side-effect of BCG administered orally, intralesionally, intrapleurally, or by aerosol is an influenza-like syndrome including chills, fever, malaise, nausea, and vomiting. These reactions may last up to 1 week following treatment. Fevers as high as 104° F have been observed, but temperatures of 101° F are more common.

When BCG is given directly into the lesion, the previously mentioned side-effects can be expected together with necrosis and sloughing of the injected lesion and eventual regression. On occasion, uninjected satellite lesions will also be affected by the injection and have the same sloughing action. Satellite lesions are those tumors that surround the primary site. People who have malignant melanoma frequently have numerous lesions. There is a large main lesion with multiple smaller lesions surrounding it. If the main tumor is injected with an immunotherapeutic agent such as BCG, some of the satellite lesions will also react to the treatment.

Occasional cases of hepatic dysfunction have been reported by Sparks and coworkers[26] following BCG treatment. Intratumor injection, Tine technique, and the injection of BCG with tumor vaccine were observed to produce this result. The persons in question all recovered either with treatment by isoniazid or spontaneously without the use of this drug. The cause of this side-effect is unclear.

Corynebacterium parvum

Corynebacterium parvum (*C. parvum*) was first shown to produce tumor resistance in experimental animals in 1958, and it was inferred that this agent might have some activity on cancer in humans.[17] *C. parvum* is a gram-positive anaerobe and is a vaccine of dead organisms. Unlike BCG, *C. parvum* is prepared by one company, Burroughs Wellcome. It is supplied in a vial of formalin-killed organisms in a concentration of 7 mg/ml. It is usually administered in a dose of 3 to 5 mg/m^2 of body surface area. *C. parvum* may be given subcutaneously or intravenously. When given subcutaneously, it is frequently mixed with small amounts (0.2 to

0.3 ml) of 2% lidocaine (Xylocaine) to prevent local irritation.

Side-effects of subcutaneous administration include redness, swelling, soreness at the site of injection, mild fever and chills, and occasional nausea or vomiting. There may be ulceration at the site. The side-effects usually last less than 24 hours, except for the swelling and ulceration, which may last a number of weeks. Reactions to *C. parvum* lessen with succeeding treatments.

When *C. parvum* is administered intravenously, the dose is computed in the same way, that is, 5 mg/m² of body surface area. It is given in an intravenous solution of 5% dextrose and water in quantities of 100 or more milliliters over a 1-hour period.

Intravenous *C. parvum* side-effects are more severe than those engendered by subcutaneous administration. People are likely to display fever, chills, and shaking, usually starting within 1½ hours after initiation of therapy and lasting from 3 to 36 hours. Temperatures may be as high as 104° F. Other common side-effects include nausea, vomiting, dizziness, and (occasionally) blurred vision and hypotension. The side-effects of IV *C. parvum* may often be minimized by prior administration of acetaminophen, diphenhydramine hydrochloride, and hydrocortisone sodium succinate (Solu-Cortef). Some investigators,[24] however, question whether such premedication may not cancel out any immunostimulant properties of *C. parvum*. During early trials of *C. parvum*, investigators found that some people were hypersensitive to either the bacterium or the preservative (thimerosal) in the agent, and in such persons *C. parvum* is contraindicated. The use of *C. parvum* should also be avoided in those known to have intracranial tumors. These individuals develop neurologic symptoms and an increase in intracranial pressure, which may be reversed by decompression or the administration of furosemide (Lasix).

Levamisole

Levamisole, an antihelmintic widely used in animals for treatment of worms, seems to restore inefficient cellular host defense mechanisms. The initial studies of levamisole for the treatment of cancer were started by Renoux and Renoux in 1971.[19]

Levamisole has been used as a prophylactic therapy against recurrence of lung, breast, and renal cancer with rather encouraging results. It has the advantage of being an oral preparation with few side-effects if given in doses of less than 200 mg/m²/day. Above that dose level, toxicities including nausea, vomiting, diarrhea, and neurologic disturbances may occur. It should also be noted that agranulocytosis has occurred in people treated with levamisole. The occurrence is higher in people who have rheumatoid arthritis. If unrecognized and untreated, this may be fatal, but when the drug was discontinued, the people recovered.[21]

The use of levamisole in cancer therapy is relatively new. Thus, it is still a phase II drug to be used only by those investigators who have been authorized to do so.

Methanol-extracted residue

Methanol-extracted residue of BCG (MER) is a particulate aqueous suspension that has been shown to be useful in prophylactic and therapeutic immunotherapy. MER is given intradermally or subcutaneously into the skin of the back and the proximal upper and lower extremities. It is very important that the sites be rotated, so that no one site receives a dose of more than 0.2 mg more often than every 2 to 4 weeks, as ulceration may otherwise occur. The usual dose is 1 mg divided into 5 to 10 sites of 0.1 to 0.2 mg. MER is fairly well tolerated if given every 2 to 4 weeks by this method.[9]

Side-effects of MER administration are mild fever and malaise lasting up to 24 hours after administration. There may be ulceration or inflammation at the site of injection. The side-effects appear more pronounced in persons exhibiting a positive purified protein derivative (PPD) skin test or in those who have been previously treated with BCG.

There are a few other immunotherapeutic agents that are being studied and should be mentioned briefly.

Miscellaneous immunotherapeutic agents

Transfer factor. Transfer factor, an extract of stimulated lymphocytes, is thought to be capable of transferring specific delayed hypersensitivity to other lymphocytes. Because this agent is highly specific, the only source is a person who has been in long-term remission. This is an example of an adoptive immunotherapy; its observed benefits clearly warrant further study.

Immune ribonucleic acid. Immune ribonucleic acid (I-RNA) is produced from the lymphocytes of animals that have been sensitized to the tumor antigen of the particular person by injection of tumor cells from that person. The I-RNA extract prepared from the lymphocytes of the animal is administered to the person intradermally in the lymph node areas (axilla, groin, or chest). It is given in single or divided doses of 2 to 60 mg/week but usually 4 to 8 mg/week.[19] Side-effects of this therapy include inflammation at the site of injection, but no other significant side-effects were noted. I-RNA is an example of passive adoptive immunotherapy.

Thymosin. A thymus extract called thymosin has also been used as an immunotherapy agent. It is a hormone preparation made from bovine thymus glands and is necessary for the maturation of T-lymphocytes. T-lymphocytes are required for cell-mediated immunity. This preparation is given intramuscularly or subcutaneously in 50 to 250 mg/m^2 of body surface area for a 7-day period with resulting increase in lymphocyte formation. Side-effects of this form of therapy are minimal and include only an occasional rash.[9] This is a passive adoptive form of immunotherapy. Its usefulness in cancer immunotherapy is uncertain at this time.

With all of the tumor immunotherapy investigational agents, as with anything else that is experimental, it is the nurse's obligation to get as much information as possible about the agent before administering it. Nurses are responsible for their own acts and should not rely on the physician's discretion when working in this area. Drug companies distributing the agent must make available all the information about the early trials of the drug on animals and any human trials. If there is any question, the drug company research department should be queried immediately. It also is the nurse's legal obligation to be sure an informed consent has been signed before administering any investigational agent.

NURSING CARE

Neoplastic disease in man is frequently accompanied by the inability of that person to respond to recall antigen skin testing or to a new contact delayed cutaneous hypersensitivity reaction antigen such as dinitrochlorobenzene (DNCB). It is unclear why the person cannot respond or is anergic, but theories state that it could be because of the immunocompetence preceding the neoplasm. The person should be tested for anergy with the previously mentioned types of antigens before starting therapy. The recall antigens usually used are those that 95% of a general population will have been exposed to in their lifetime. This list commonly includes: purified protein derivative (PPD) of tuberculin, streptokinase-streptodornase, histoplasmin, mumps, dermatophyton, tetanus toxoid, and *Candida albicans*. As illus-

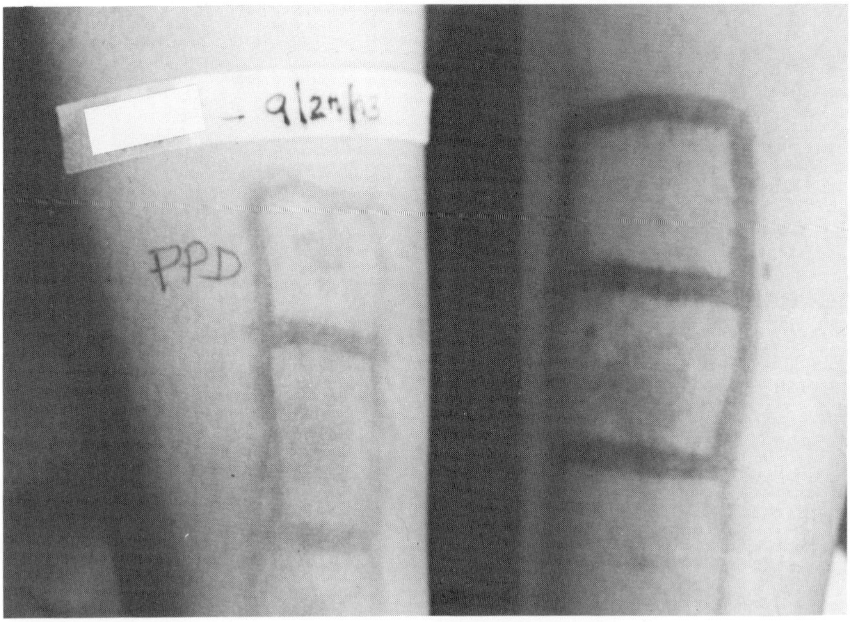

Fig. 15-3. Recall antigen skin tests.

trated in Fig. 15-3, the skin tests are placed on the forearms and outlined with a marker, so the person reading the tests knows where the antigens were placed.

The DNCB skin test is much different from the recall antigen testing. The DNCB is placed on the upper thigh in three doses at the initial testing. The highest dose is the sensitizing dose and is 2,000 μg; the other two doses are 100 μg and 25 μg. The solution is placed on the skin in a small ring to confine it to an area 15 mm in diameter, blown dry with a hairdryer, and the area marked so it can be identified properly at the end of the 48-hour testing time. All doses are applied in this same manner. The person should be instructed not to wash the area throughout this time. The person administering this test should wear gloves when handling the DNCB. This is a potent irritant when used for prolonged periods and will cause adverse skin reactions and even sloughing in the person administering the test if protective measures are not taken.

The reaction to the initial testing is erythema and induration as shown in Fig. 15-4. If there is no reaction within 14 days after the first testing, the 100 μg and 25 μg doses are again applied in the same manner. It is suggested that the opposite thigh be used on retesting, since testing again in the same area may cause the initial test to flare up. Any amount of erythema 48 hours after the challenge dose constitutes a positive test.

Recall antigens in doses of 0.1 ml are applied to the inner aspect of the forearms. As with the DNCB, these tests are read 48 hours later. In all cases except that of mumps antigen, 10 mm or more of induration constitutes a positive test; mumps is positive at 5 mm. The usual technique of intradermal skin testing is appropriate to the handling of the recall antigens. Skin testing is used as a treatment indicator to show increased im-

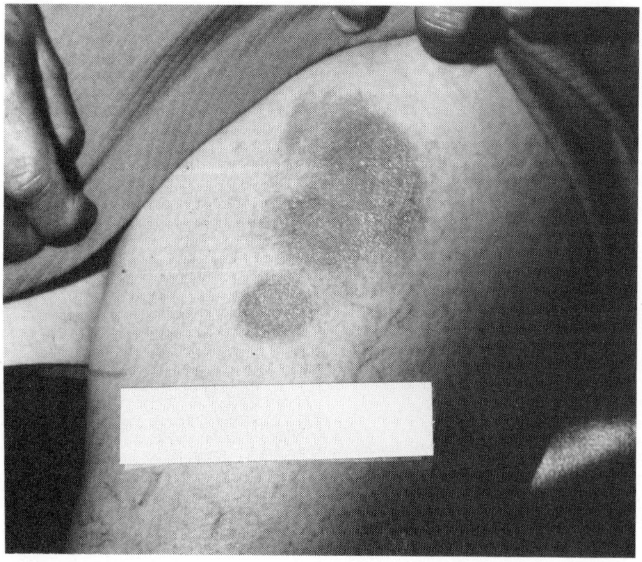

Fig. 15-4. Contact delayed cutaneous hypersensitivity reaction.

Table 15-2. Skin test comparison

Subject	PPD	Streptokinase-streptodornase	Dermatophyton	Mumps	Tetanus toxoid	*Candida albicans*	DNCB		
							2,000	100	25
Skin tests prestudy									
M. J.	−	+	−	+	+	−	−	−	−
R. K.	−	+	−	+	−	−	−	−	−
B. S.	−	+	−	+	+	−	−	−	−
J. K.	−	+	−	+	+	−	−	−	−
Skin tests after 6 mo therapy									
M. J.	+	+	+	+	+	+	+	−	−
R. K.	−	+	−	+	−	−	+	+	+
B. S.	−	−	−	−	−	−	−	−	−
J. K.	−	+	−	−	−	−	−	−	−

munity and is repeated approximately every 3 months while the person is being treated. As the person becomes more sensitive to the antigens, certain antigens will be discontinued from the antigen panel. Should the person become less sensitive, the physician should be made aware of this decreased sensitivity and do further tests to see if there is more disease present. In Table 15-2, all subjects were skin tested prior to starting therapy. Six months after the start of therapy their skin test readings indicated an increase in reactivity for subjects M. J. and R. K. and a decreased reactivity in subjects B. S. and

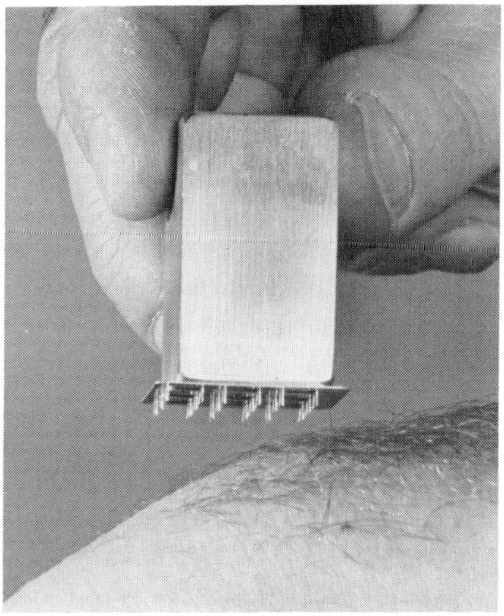

Fig. 15-5. Tine technique, 36-prong disc and magnet.

J. K. Further testing with x-ray examinations and scans showed recurrent disease in B. S. and J. K.; M. J. and R. K. maintained their sensitivity and have completed 2 years of treatment with no evidence of recurrent disease.

Because BCG is a live bacterium, it must be used with great care so that the person administering it has the least possible contact with it. Gloves ought to be worn while handling this material. An annual PPD skin test should be performed on all persons administering this agent. All instruments should be soaked in alcohol for at least 20 minutes before further processing. The syringes, the needles, the vials the agent is packaged in, the magnet, and the discs should all be soaked. The disposable equipment can then be discarded in the normal fashion, but the magnet should be wrapped and autoclaved.

As previously mentioned, BCG is administered many ways, although the intradermal route is most frequently chosen. The Tine technique, the Heaf gun, and scarification are three standard procedures for intradermal administration.

The Tine technique uses a 36-prong disc and magnet as illustrated in Fig. 15-5. The lymph node–bearing areas are the sites for treatment (axilla, chest, groin). After cleaning the site with acetone, the specified dose of the agent is applied to the skin, the area is stamped with the disc, and then blown dry with a hairdryer on cool setting to prevent heat from killing the bacteria. The person is asked not to wash this area for 24 hours.

People known to have reactions of severe itching and erythema are given a prescription for diphenhydramine hydrochloride (Benadryl), 25 to 50 mg orally as needed, following therapy. Because of the immunosuppressing characteristics of alcohol and aspirin-containing compounds, clients are advised to take acetaminophen for headaches or other problems requiring the use of these agents. The person is instructed to determine which compounds contain aspirin and to call the physician if there is any question, at which time suitable replacements can then be recommended. Persistent itching is treated by application of calamine lotion with diphenhydramine hydrochloride, alcohol, or any other soothing ointment or cream. Occasionally, for severe erythematous reactions, hydrocortisone cream, 1%, may be prescribed.

The Heaf gun is used in some institutions to administer the BCG intradermally. This equipment, as illustrated in Fig. 15-6, is probably most familiar to those people who have given tuberculosis (TB) tests for mass screenings. BCG administered with the Heaf gun is done basically the same way as with the Tine technique. The area to be treated is cleansed with acetone, 0.2 ml of the BCG solution is applied to the skin, and the area is injected approximately 15 times in the same 5 × 5 cm area with the Heaf gun. The area is

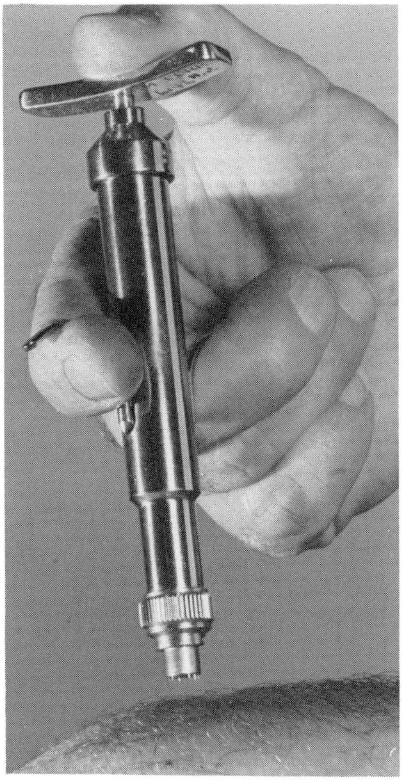

Fig. 15-6. Heaf gun.

then blown dry with the hairdryer on a cool setting. Precautions and side-effects are the same as previously described when the Tine technique is used.

The scarification method is also similar to the Tine technique. The area to be treated is cleansed and a needle (beveled cutting edge down) is used to scratch the area in horizontal and vertical lines to cover an area of 2 by 2 inches. This should be scratched hard enough to produce lines but not frank bleeding. The BCG is then applied to this area and blown dry with a hair dryer on cool setting. Ointment or cream may be applied, as with the Tine technique, to reduce irritation and itching.

Because family members fear cancer is contagious, they often avoid contact with the person. It is important to reassure them that physical contact cannot engender cancer in them. However, they should at the same time be cautioned against contact with the treatment site until the BCG has been cleansed from the site after the first 24-hour treatment period because of the potentiality for spreading live bacteria. As with many other treatment modalities, people react differently to side-effects. Discussing their individual reactions with them will help the person feel less like a "guinea pig." Making the individuals responsible for their own skin test readings has given some people a sense of being part of their own care. Mastering the reading of erythema and induration in millimeters gives a feeling of accomplishment to some people, and if a family member learns to read the test results, this lends family-involved care. Because the person is on an immunotherapy research protocol, every effort should be made to personalize the treatment and care.

C. parvum has side-effects that are quite different from those experienced with intradermal BCG. As explained previously, intravenous *C. parvum* causes flulike symptoms. The person is premedicated with diphenhydramine hydrochloride, 50 mg intramuscularly, two 325 mg tablets of acetaminophen, and hydrocortisone sodium succinate (Solu-Cortef), 100 mg IV push, to prevent severe reactions. Otherwise, the only other intervention is to provide supportive care. *C. parvum* given subcutaneously will not require any special nursing care unless there is ulceration, which is very rare. Should the site ulcerate, a culture of the area is taken. The person should be instructed to keep the area bandaged and clean. If the culture is positive for infection, appropriate antibiotics will be prescribed by the physician. People have discovered that applying ice to the injection site shortly afterwards reduces some of the swelling and discomfort. Freezing washcloths and applying them to the site may obtain the same results. After the initial treatment of *C. parvum,* the person will often choose to receive the injections only in the arms if swelling and pain in the leg injection sites have caused difficulty with walking and standing.

As an additional aspect of client teaching, some instructions are given on sunbathing. Many of the people on the immunotherapy protocols have a diagnosis of malignant melanoma. These people are warned not to have excessive sun exposure. The same applies for BCG-treated people. The BCG makes the treatment area photosensitive, and the areas should be protected from the sun by wearing a T-shirt or sunscreen. The people are given a list of sunscreens that are recommended by most dermatologists and are instructed to seek those containing para-aminobenzoic acid (PABA) in the ingredients because of its excellent screening properties.

At this writing cancer immunotherapy is still in the experimental stage.

Because of the experimental nature of virtually all forms of immunotherapy, it is necessary to keep records of a more detailed nature than would normally be required. The reason for this is easy to perceive. For example, suppose that a person on BCG therapy displays some side-effect. Knowledge not only of the dose level and method of administration but also of the lot number of the BCG sample involved might well provide information vital to the investigation of the drug, such as by suggesting the presence of some defect in the lot in question. It is information of this character that leads to the discovery of important results in applied science of any kind. Research is inclusive; the limit of the data recorded is set by the experimenter, and it is very difficult indeed to have too much information, especially when, as here, no particular result can be predicted. It is entirely likely that the work any one of us does will at some time be subject to a retrospective search. Nor should only the side-effects of the medication claim one's attention. Matters that may not seem consequent—client teaching, other medications given, vital signs, and so forth—should be recorded to make later analysis possible.

More work is needed to determine exactly what types of diseases are best treated by this form of therapy. Already it has been demonstrated as an effective adjunct in the treatment of sarcomas, lung cancer, leukemia, and melanoma. The same general nursing care that is used in other areas of cancer nursing also applies here, bearing in mind that this is investigational and that people need constant reinforcement of the positive aspects of immunotherapy.

REFERENCES

1. Allegra, J., et al.: Decreased prevalence of immediate hypersensitivity (atopy) in a cancer population, Cancer Res. **36:**3225, 1976.
2. Barrett, J. T.: Basic immunotherapy and its medical applications, ed. 2, St. Louis, 1980, The C. V. Mosby Co.
3. Carter, S. K.: Immunotherapy of cancer in man: current status and prospectus. In Southam, C. M., and Friedman, H., editors: International conference on immunotherapy of cancer, Ann. N. Y. Acad. Sci. vol. 277, 1976.
4. Fass, L., Herbmann, R. B., Zeigler, R., and Morrow, R. H.: Evaluation of the effect of remission plasma on untreated patients with Burkitt's lymphoma, J. Natl. Cancer Inst. **44:**145, 1970.
5. Guthrie, D., and Way, S.: Immunotherapy of nonclinical vaginal cancer, Lancet **2:**1242, 1975.
6. Harris, J. E., and Sinkovics, J. G.: The immunology of malignant disease, ed. 2, St. Louis, 1976, The C. V. Mosby Co.
7. Harvey, H. A., et al.: Immuno-chemotherapy with cyclophosphamide and *Corynebacterium parvum*—a clinical trial. In Crispen, R. G., editor: Neoplasm immunity: mechanisms, Proceedings of a Chicago Symposium, Chicago, 1975, Institute for Tuberculosis Research.
8. Hericourt, J., and Richet, C.: "Physiologie pa-

thologique" de la sérothérapie dans le traitement du cancer, C. R. Acad. Sci. **121**:567, 1895.

9. Hersh, E. M.: Modalities of cancer treatment: immunotherapy. In Clark, R. L., and Howe, C., editors: Cancer patient care, Chicago, 1976, Year Book Medical Publishers, Inc.
10. Hersh, E. M., et al.: Immunotherapy of human cancer. In Strollerman, G. H., editor: Advances in internal medicine, vol. 22, Chicago, 1977, Year Book Medical Publishers, Inc.
11. Lewis, W. R., et al.: Topical immunotherapy of basal cell carcinomas with dinitrochlorobenzene, Cancer Res. **33**:3036, 1973.
12. Mathé, G.: Cancer active immunotherapy. In Allfrey, V. G., et al., editors: Recent results in cancer research, vol. 55, New York, 1976, Springer-Verlag New York, Inc.
13. Mathé, G., et al.: Active immunotherapy for acute lymphoblastic leukemia, Lancet **1**:697, 1969.
14. McKneally, M. F., Mauer, C., and Kausel, H. W.: Regional immunotherapy of lung cancer with intrapleural BCG, Lancet **1**:377, 1976.
15. Morton, D. L.: Horizons in tumor immunology, Surgery **74**(1):69, 1973.
16. Morton, D. L., and Goodnight, J. E., Jr.: Clinical trials of immunotherapy, present status, Cancer **42**(5):2224, 1978.
17. Oettgen, H. F., Pinsky, C. M., and Delmonte, L.: Treatment of cancer with immunomodulators—*Corynebacterium parvum* and levamisole. In Terry, W. D., editor: Immunotherapy in malignant diseases, Med. Clin. North Am. **60**:511, 1976.
18. Physicians' desk reference, Oradell, N.J., 1978, Medical Economics Co.
19. Renoux, G., and Renoux, M.: Effet immunostimulant d'un imidothiazole dans l'immunisation des souris contre l'injection par *Brucella abortus*, C. R. Acad. Sci. [D] (Paris) **272**:349, 1971.
20. Roberts, J. A.: Immunotherapy in the treatment of cancer, Scot. Med. J. **22**:320, 1977.
21. Rosenthal, M., et al.: Levamisole and agranulocytosis, Lancet **1**:904, 1977.
22. Ross, L. J. N.: Antiviral T cell–mediated immunity in Marek's disease, Nature **268**:644, 1977.
23. Sakai, H., et al.: Thymosin-induced increases in E-rosette-forming capacity of lymphocytes in patients with malignant neoplasms, Cancer **36**(3):974, 1975.
24. Selker, R. G., et al.: Preliminary observations on the use of *Corynebacterium parvum* in patients with primary intracranial tumors: effect on intracranial pressure, J. Surg. Oncol. **10**:299, 1978.
25. Sparks, F. C.: Hazards and complications of BCG immunotherapy. In Terry, W. D., editor: Immunotherapy in malignant disease, Med. Clin. North Am. **60**:499, 1976.
26. Sparks, F. C., et al.: Complications of BCG immunotherapy in patients with cancer, N. Engl. J. Med. **289**(16):827, 1973.
27. Terry, W. D.: BCG in the treatment of human cancer, CA **25**(4):198, 1975.
28. Voisin, G. A.: Immunologic facilitation, a broadening of the concept of the enhancement phenomenon, Prog. Allergy **15**:328, 1971.

16

Cancer quackery: information, issues, responsibility, action

PAMELA K. S. PATRICK

The volume of publication, both pro and con, on various forms of cancer quackery strongly suggests that unproven treatments continue to adversely affect persons with cancer, their families, health care professionals, and the community. Adherents of certain unorthodox cancer treatments have taken to the political arena to seek legal and social sanction. Those who would attempt to ignore the serious issues presented by cancer quackery no longer can afford to remain uninformed. Nurses, in particular, must *learn* about quackery and then assume professional *responsibility* to take *action* that will retard or prohibit the impact that the use of quackery can have.

Prior to planning specific action, it is crucial that the parameters of the problem be outlined. A description of major forms of cancer quackery is followed by a discussion of significant issues emerging from the continuing controversy over unproven methods of cancer treatment.

INFORMATION: PARAMETERS OF CANCER QUACKERY

A variety of cancer quackery methods are available to the consumer, usually on a "black market" basis. While promoters of quack methods state that the client can only be "helped" by use of their products, more often the client and family are economically, medically, and emotionally victimized by the "helper."

Definition of quackery

Clarity on the definition of quackery can assist the nurse in recognition of the various forms it takes. Cancer quackery is:

> . . . the intentional misrepresentation and/or deliberate misapplication of diagnostic or treatment measures that impedes or delays the patient's entry into legitimate, constructive forms of cancer treatment.[7]

Key aspects of this definition are the phrases (1) "intentional and/or deliberate," and (2) "impedes or delays." The promoter of cancer quackery acts in an intentional, purposeful manner, often for financial profit. Those who promote quackery under the guise of "unproven methods," "unorthodox treatment," or "nonlegitimate therapy" can cause the person with cancer as much anguish as the designated quack: *time* is lost, and *time* is the crucial variable in the successful early detection and treatment of cancer. The person who is persuaded to use quackery, as well as the person who clearly chooses it, often eliminates the opportunity to benefit optimally from *proven* constructive cancer treatment.

Forms of cancer quackery

The available forms of cancer quackery are as diverse as the imagination of the originators. Quack methods of cancer treatment range from colonic purges, yogurt enemas, and injections of mineral oil to ozone generators, invisible surgery, and "miracle" drugs. These methods are costly both in terms of monetary outlay and needless human suffering. A brief summary of cancer quackery methods is presented here. Issues relating to specific methods and reasons for their continued use are discussed in a succeeding section.

Machines and devices. A wide assortment of machines, boxes, and "radiating" devices have been promoted as cures for cancer. In each case, the bizarre mechanical device was found to be *useless* in the diagnosis or treatment of cancer. For example, the cancer client might be instructed to (1) sit inside a zinc-lined box to absorb "orgone energy," (2) absorb "attuned color waves," or (3) wear a "Vrilium Tube" or "magic spike" to cure a cancer.[3,4] The inner mechanisms of many such devices are exceptionally simple and have absolutely no capacity to treat cancer.[2,10]

Devices continue to be used by a limited number of people with cancer but no longer represent a major form of cancer quackery. Cost to obtain a machine can range from $1 per day rental to $1,000 or more to purchase. Clearly, considerable financial burden can be created by such expenditures.

Chemicals and potions. Down through the ages, herbs, potions, and other medicines have been ingested to prevent and treat physical and emotional ills. In modern society, claims for "miracle drugs" and "breakthroughs" in the development of pharmacologic treatments for disease are often shared. In the case of cancer, there is an extremely diverse array of legitimate drugs used in the therapeutic management of cancer; that is, chemotherapy. The cancer quack also relies heavily on chemical approaches, none of which have any scientifically proven effectiveness against malignancies. It is this willingness to believe in "miracle" cures, drugs, and approaches—both for proven as well as nonproven methods—that partially supports the continued desire to use quack chemicals.

Some of the major cancer quackery chemical preparations are discussed in the following.

Hoxsey chemotherapy. Produced in pill and liquid form, this compound contains combinations of burdock root, red clover, cascara, licorice, stillingia root, buckthorn bark, and an assortment of other ingredients. This preparation and the accompanying diet provide no therapeutic benefit in the treatment of cancer.[2,6,7,32]

Krebiozen (carcalon). A second liquid preparation that continues to be promoted as a "cure" for cancer is krebiozen (also known as carcalon). Found to be composed of minute amounts of creatine monohydrate (a normal muscle constituent) and mineral oil, or solely of mineral oil, krebiozen possesses *no* curative potential for cancer.[2,6,21]

Laetrile (amygdalin). Mass produced in injectable and pill form, Laetrile continues to be the most popular chemical preparation promoted as a "cure" for all forms of cancer. Proponents claim it can prevent future as well as eliminate existing cancers.[32,36] Over the past several years, this extract of apricot, plum, and peach pits has been repeatedly investigated and consistently found to be devoid of any anticancer activity.[12,13,15,23]

Despite the preponderance of scientific evidence against the effectiveness of Laetrile, increasing numbers of people with cancer continue to use the compound. Reasons for this tenacious interest in Laetrile relate to the political and social issues arising from recent efforts to legalize its use. These issues are based on the fears many people have about cancer, dying, and death and are discussed in a succeeding section.

It appears that the controversy over Laetrile and its legalization as a sole or adjunctive treatment of cancer will continue in the face of overwhelming evidence of its uselessness. Because it is sought by consumers and their families, it is imperative that nurses become familiar with its use and availability.

Of the chemical cancer quackery approaches, Laetrile is by far the most dominant. Many proponents of the apricot remedy have sought to relabel it as a "nutritional supplement" or a vitamin (B_{17} Aprikern). The American Institute of Nutrition, however, clearly states that Laetrile is not a vitamin; instead it is classified as a toxicant.[9]

Despite the evidence stating that Laetrile is not an effective and proven treatment for cancer, the fervor over its nonlegal status continues. Recently, the National Cancer Institute agreed to a two-phase evaluation of Laetrile on humans.[13,15] The issues involved in conducting human trials are significant: (1) without a demonstration of proven anticancer activity in animals, human cancer subjects would need to be volunteers who could receive no further legitimate treatment; (2) these preliminary trials could involve only Laetrile, not a regimen prescribed by its proponent; and (3) if these trials produced no evidence of Laetrile's effectiveness, it would not resolve the issue; that is, proponents would continue to extol Laetrile's virtues. The risks to human life from both medical and humanistic viewpoints need to be carefully evaluated prior to institution of human clinical trials.

The method to be used in planning for human clinical trials has involved two phases: (1) A retrospective analysis of submitted case records in which Laetrile was thought to have had an objective beneficial effect. This analysis was conducted by a panel of 12 oncologists. Findings indicate that of 160 courses of treatment submitted for review, only six suggested a partial or complete response to Laetrile.[15] No definite conclusions can be drawn from these results regarding the anticancer activity of Laetrile. (2) A prospective clinical trial of Laetrile would involve several hundred people who have cancer. Such a test would most likely be carried out by the National Cancer Institute over a minimum of 1 year's time. Results would indicate the degree, if any, of the anticancer activity of Laetrile.

The clinical research sequence begins with tests on laboratory animals and culminates with trials on human subjects derived from a target population. If the controversy over Laetrile is ever to be laid to rest, this final phase of testing must be done. The ethical issues associated with such trials deserve an equivalent amount of attention.

• • •

Other quack chemical preparations promoted under the label of "drug" or "medicine" include Bamfolin (an extract of a species of bamboo grass), Carcin, CH-23 (prepared from plant toxins), Glover serum (obtained from human blood cultures and tissues), and Koch antitoxins.[2] Each of these, as well as many other quack drugs, is worthless in the treatment of cancer and other diseases.

Psychic and mystical methods. A number of cancer quacks rely on psychic or mystical methods to supposedly "treat" cancer and other serious illnesses much in the same way as ancient and modern shamans practiced. The elusiveness of these nontangible approaches serves two major purposes: (1) one's faith, hope, and belief in the method are the major criteria used by supporters to promote the methods, and (2) obviously, logical scientifically based arguments demonstrating the worthlessness of psychic methods are virtually ineffective when countered by nonconcrete arguments of faith in such techniques.

Seances, trances, and incantations are used by some purveyors of false cancer cures to invoke "mystical, universal powers" to cure malignancies. Magical injections may be administered after the trance is over.[26]

Chief among the cancer quacks using mystical approaches are the psychic surgeons located predominantly in the Philippines.[27,30] The psychic surgeon kneads, pushes, and manipulates a target body part such that the "tumor" is removed. During this process, the "surgeon" oozes a small amount of animal blood (contained in cotton or a small animal's spleen) over the "operative site" and then pulls the mass out. It is quickly disposed of by an assistant. Over several treatment sessions, psychic surgeons claim an ability to remove cancers from any body part without the need of making incisions.

Psychic surgeons have been investigated and consistently discredited,[27,29,30] yet desperate cancer clients continue to utilize this approach. The financial investment necessary to receive these worthless treatments is astronomical. The fears of cancer and the need for hope spur many to accept the outrageous claims made by the pushers of psychic surgery. It is this very fear and need for hope that provide the clues as to how the nurse can help the person with cancer avoid manipulation by the quack.

Nutrition and diets. Without doubt, high level maintenance and active support of the client's nutritional status is a key factor in the successful treatment of cancer.[31] Vigorous support of dietary intake is an integral part of any comprehensive approach to cancer therapy. However, adherence to strict, regimented, and at times bizarre diets has never been proved to be the sole cure for cancer. Despite this, the past decade has witnessed a phenomenal rise in the promotion of diet cures for everything from halitosis, to acne, to insomnia, to cancer.[1,11,19,25,28] By following diets consisting of raw foods, juices, and/or vitamins and carrying out such activities as (1) coffee, yogurt, or buttermilk enemas, (2) high colonic purges, or (3) episodes of fasting, the consumer is told that cure will result.

Many of the requirements for these nutritional approaches are contradictory to the dietary needs of people with cancer. Among the significant problems having potentially serious adverse impact on the body are the following[18,20]:

1. Prohibition of meat, fish, fowl, or dairy products: Lack of absorbable iron and calcium results in a higher frequency of iron deficiency anemia and a decrease in bone maintenance.
2. Cessation of animal protein intake: A primary source of vitamin B_{12} is animal protein. Basic biochemical processes can be interrupted without adequate B_{12} intake.
3. Increased intake of fruits containing cyanide: A low calorie, low animal protein, and high bulk diet of fruits (and vegetables) can be directly counter to the nutritional needs of the per-

son with cancer. In addition, high intake of cyanide (for example, Laetrile, apricot pits) poisons the body.

Each of these dietary alterations reduces the stability of the client's nutritional status. In addition, the physical requirements necessary to follow a rigorous enema or colonic purging regimen can be extremely fatiguing, thereby further reducing the body's capacity to combat the disease.

Information on quack nutritional approaches to cancer management is readily available in many health food establishments. The anxious and fearful client or concerned family member can purchase recipes and equipment (for example, superblenders) for cancer diets, receive suggestions on the benefits of various methods, and then buy the ingredients all in one location. The smooth and seemingly professional tone of books, pamphlets, and newsletters that promote dietary cancer treatment methods lends further superficial credibility to the approaches.

The forms that cancer quackery takes are diverse, creative, and above all, enterprising. Promoters are making financial profit by offering false hope for false cures. Why then do people continue to use known quack methods? This question can be answered by considering the major issues arising from the cancer quackery versus medical treatment controversy.

ISSUES: WHY CANCER QUACKERY THRIVES

Cancer quackery is a multibillion dollar industry in the United States.[5,16] The economic costs to clients and families are not reimbursed by third party payors. Emotional victimization by the quack produces equally tragic results: the client and/or family often feel guilty and responsible for a premature cancer death when legitimate therapy is abandoned in favor of quackery. Obvious physical trauma is caused when proven treatment is delayed or denied. Thus, the overall costs of cancer quackery to consumers, families, and society are excessive. With easy access to information on the worthlessness of quack cures, why then does quackery thrive? To answer this question, it is necessary to investigate the issues surrounding the cancer treatment controversy.

Whether to use or reject a quack cancer treatment is an *emotional* issue, not a *scientific* one. Empirical evidence is abundantly obtainable and available. The overriding issue has to do with the fact that clients and families are not getting their needs met by the current legitimate health care system. The scientific community continues to focus almost exclusively on efforts to repeatedly demonstrate the worthlessness of quack methods. *This has been accomplished*. In these efforts to show the mastery and accuracy of the modern scientific method, health caregivers have lost sight of the consumer's real message: "We want *more* than technical expertise; we want emotional involvement, caring, and trust that you will not abandon us when medicine has nothing more to offer." This is the underlying message of the following cancer quackery issues.

Freedom to make choices

Proponents of nonproven quack methods have taken up the battle cry of "monopolistic conspiracy," "governmental persecution," and "denial of constitutional rights" to politicize the controversy over legalization of such substances as Laetrile and vitamin B_{17}.[14,17,34] The issue is represented as a struggle of the "little guy" for freedom of choice in the face of powerful opposition of government and the medical establishment. In reality, federal agencies have been given the authority to regulate drugs and chemicals to ensure that products are both harmless *and* effective for their intended purpose. Deregulation, the demand of the Laetrile lobby, would be an abandonment of societal protection and would undoubtedly result in tragedy. The flag of freedom has been placed around Laetrile by its pushers. Research demonstrating its uselessness is rejected by these lobbyists because it is done by the "establishment."

Several states have legalized the use of Laetrile if prescribed by a physician. Recently, however, some of these states have begun to consider recension of this limited approval. Regardless of the legality of use within state bounds, it continues to be illegal to transport the ingredients for Laetrile manufacture interstate. Proponents who have been arrested for Laetrile smuggling have become folk heros to those who believe in the patriotic freedom of choice argument.

Amidst a general, nationwide climate demanding less government intervention, less taxation, and less centralization, the Laetrile movement has flourished. Cancer clients are prime targets for the emotionally laden propaganda of the Laetrile political lobby. Promises of cure coupled with manipulation of cherished beliefs about individual choice are powerful recruitment strategies used by the quackery proponents.

Organizational supports

A number of organizations have been created whose major purposes are to promote the use, sale, and selection of nonproven methods of cancer quackery. Three of these well-organized, national groups are: the National Health Federation, the International Association of Cancer Victims and Friends, and the Committee for Freedom of Choice in Cancer Therapy. Membership consists of persons with cancer, their families, interested persons, and people who fear they *might* "get" or have cancer.

These associations engage in a number of well-planned and executed activities: (1) lobbying in state legislatures for passage of bills to legalize unproven cancer treatment methods and to block legislation that would "constrict freedom," (2) publication of books, pamphlets, and bulletins proclaiming the curative powers of Laetrile, diets, machines, and so forth, (3) production of audiovisual media to be used in the promotion of cancer quackery, (4) recruitment of cancer clients via mailings, person-to-person contact while the client is still in the hospital, and terror tactics related to the "horrors of cancer treatment," (5) presentation of conferences, seminars, and conventions designed to lure clients and families away from reputable treatments, and (6) direction and guidance of cancer clients and families to Mexican, South American, or European quack clinics.

The quackery industry could not grow and prosper if it lacked the active, enthusiastic, and committed support of its parent organizations.

Medical model limitations

The traditional medical model places heavy emphasis on application of the scientific method to the treatment and cure of illness. In recent years, however, there has been increasing interest in the holistic approach to total health care. The holistic model emphasizes attention to all aspects of the person: physical, emotional, spiritual, social, and psychologic. An episode of physical dysfunction to some extent impacts on each of the other interconnected aspects of the individual's life. To attend only to the physical part is to ignore the holistic nature of the individual.

Attention to all aspects of the person requires a multidisciplinary approach in which the nurse, chaplain, physician, psychologist, and others participate in the promotion of *wellness*. While this philosophy may be discussed by members of the health care professions, it has not fully been implemented. Resistance to application of a holistic approach results in continuation of the physician's "godlike" position in relation to the consumer . . . the person with cancer. However, many health care service consumers are rebelling against this "one-up, one-down" relationship and want to be a participant in their health maintenance and treatment.

Unfortunately, the cancer quack has made client participation in the "treatment" process a key aspect of the helper-helpee relationship. Clients are encouraged to ask questions, are actively listened to, and are consulted. Clients who have dissatisfying interactions with physicians can openly express these feelings with the quack who not only takes *time* to listen and agrees with the client but also does not reject the client. The quack acknowledges the person and family for "taking action," for "being responsible," for "questioning." Many legitimate physicians and nurses either are not aware of the client's and family's need to talk, have not received specific communication or counseling skill training, or do not want to become involved to the extent the consumer wishes.

The quack meets this very basic consumer need to feel that the caregiver really cares and is involved in the outcome of treatment. Most physicians can express feelings of deep caring and involvement with co-workers, yet generally they do not convey this to the client. Consequently, some consumers turn to the quack when the level of dissatisfaction with the physician or nurse reaches intolerable levels.

Promises and guarantees

Perhaps the most glaring difference between the quack and the legitimate physician or caregiver occurs in the area of guarantees for cure. The cancer quack implies or guarantees that the nonproven approach works—it *will* cure the illness. No reputable physician would make such an outrageous claim. In addition, there is *no* governmental regulation of the quackery industry. There are absolutely no guarantees that a nonproven method will be *safe* to the consumer. Thus, the client is placed in a double jeopardy situation: the method is ineffective *and* may be unsafe or overtly harmful.

To prevent harm to the consumer of a product, the Food and Drug Administration has been charged with the responsibility of regulating the availability of medicines and substances that are taken into the body. Proponents of quack cancer cures seek to bypass this safeguarding agency and promote nonproven methods as cures. Quackery is administered and distributed without regard to established legal, ethical, and qualitative constraints; the drugs, machines, and diets are advertised and sold via underground networks or are disguised in such a way that legal regulatory technicalities are subverted. There is *no regulation* on quackery—the phrases, "anything goes" and "the buyer beware" are appropriate warnings for the person with cancer. The regulatory protection invested in a centralized agency (for example, the FDA) is available with *legitimate* treatments and is completely absent with false cancer cures. In addition, quality control, (for example, standards for purity and manufacture), effectiveness guarantees, pricing control, and consistent access are lacking with reference to quack methods.

While medical science and technology have made tremendous strides in reducing the mortality rate for certain kinds of cancer, it is neither realistic nor ethical to promise a client cure when the caregiver cannot guarantee a specific treatment outcome.

Yet, the client and family who desperately need to hear words of hope, reassurance, and concern may readily accept the false claims of cure propounded by the quack.

When approached by a seemingly sincere and legitimate "doctor" or spokesperson who clearly states that a particular method is curative, the person with cancer may eagerly seek out that method. Publications (characterized by quality production techniques in terms of printing style, layout, paper, and vocabulary) proclaiming the benefits of quack methods lend further credence to proffered guarantees. How is the consumer to discern the validity between these claims and those that sound equally justified made by the health care system? For many clients, the guarantee of cure tips the balance *away* from proven methods of cancer therapy.

Need for future hopes

Many people with cancer feel a sense of hopelessness about the possibility for cure or prolongation of life. Hope is a tomorrow word.[8] For the person who fears for today, loss of hope for tomorrow can produce profound despair. Whether caused by fears, myths about cancer, or the covert cues given by caregivers, the person with cancer may come to believe that he or she is a "hopeless" case. At times, the physician, nurse, or other helper is not aware of how their inner feelings of sadness about a poor prognosis for a client are communicated. If only these unspecified feelings are conveyed, the client tends to draw definitive negative conclusions about a limited future.

The cancer quack promotes hope for the present and future. Guarantees of "no cutting," "burning," or "mutilating" are made that ensure the person's physical integrity for the present. At the same time, promises for a future are also made. Despite the often overwhelming physical evidence to the contrary, the client and family need to *hope,* to have a chance for future tomorrows, and this is what the quack implies or promises regardless of the person's outward manifestations of illness.

Reduction of fears

Primary fears of many persons with cancer consist of dying, death, disfigurement, and side-effects.

Dying. For most people, a diagnosis of cancer is associated with dying—unpleasant dying. Fantasies of agonizing, unremitting pain and loss of control produce volatile fear in many people.

Death. A common equation is *cancer = death.* Despite the evidence that millions of people survive cancer, the fear that a diagnosis of cancer will result in premature death continues. (From a factual point of view, a significant percentage of cancer clients do die as a consequence of the disease.) This fear, however, may not only adversely affect treatment decisions but may also negatively influence the person's capacities to participate in treatment.

Disfigurement. Certain major forms of cancer require radical surgical intervention in order to dramatically increase chances for recovery. Fears about radical body image changes and methods of functioning can be overwhelming. Because the cancer quack guarantees that no such mutilation will occur, the vulnerable client may choose the nondisfiguring alternative as a means of reducing this highly threatening fear.

Side-effects. Stories about the "horrors of chemotherapy" or "radiation burning" abound. Friends of friends of friends relate information about the weeks and months of continuous vomiting, nausea, loss of appetite, loss of hair, or other negative consequences to these major forms of treatment. Yes, these side-effects do occur but not necessarily to the degree or severity that distorted third-hand accounts suggest.

Distorted reports of only the negative

side-effects are repeated and elaborated by those who push certain quackery methods. The person who is in the process of deciding whether or not to participate in a chemotherapy or radiation therapy program may be swayed by these ghastly accounts of misery. Yet, many, many people undergo these legitimate treatments and, with assistance, learn to manage adverse side-effects. The benefits seem to far outweigh the temporary experiences of discomfort.

Reaction to multiple losses

The person with cancer experiences and anticipates a number of losses over the course of an episode with this life-threatening disease. Chief among actual or anticipated losses are those that relate to control—control over one's destiny, health, future, and life choices. The nature of the cancer may determine a shortening of life span and, hence, a cutting off of future opportunities. Control over one's body and health also is affected; in a sense, the body may be viewed as a source of betrayal.

Socially and economically, the client may lose status in the employment context, as the leader in the family context, or as a decision maker in social contexts. Many people experience a gradual disenfranchisement of previously valued responsibilities as illness becomes more evident. While these losses may be realistic and predictable, their impact can be severe on the person's sense of worth.

A loss of freedom with consequent dependence on others may occur temporarily or can require a permanent adjustment. The fear that dependence may never be reduced can produce a feeling of helplessness and despair.

The pusher of cancer quackery strives to promote the client's independence and control. The very act of turning away from legitimate treatment and actively seeking out an unproven method suggests a reestablishment of control over one's destiny, of "taking matters into my own hands." Cancer quacks support these independence actions, while many in the traditional health care system promote dependence. Clients must feel that they are participants in care that can so greatly impact on them. Failure to do so adds another brick to the pavement leading to the purveyor of quackery.

Mythical, magical beliefs

It is not unusual to discover that belief in myths about cancer determined a person's decision to leave treatment and seek the services of a cancer quack. Myths that may influence clients or families in this manner include:

1. *Cancer is contagious:* "You might *get* cancer if you touch a cancer client."
2. *Cancer is always fatal:* Not true. Millions of people are alive and thriving after treatment for cancer.
3. *Cancer means pain:* Certain types of cancer are associated with varying degrees of physical pain. Conversely, many people do not ever experience severe pain, even if a terminal phase of living has begun.
4. *Cancer has a cure:* Quacks especially support the myth that a true cure for cancer has been found but is being withheld from the public by the "establishment."
5. *Cancer has no cure:* People who subscribe to this myth are likely to reject legitimate treatment as "useless" and may turn to the cancer quack.

These mythical beliefs are maintained by fear and misinformation. Adherence to these myths may impede a person's efforts to obtain diagnostic information and the treatment necessary to manage the illness effectively.

Advertisements and audiovisual media proclaim the healing powers of certain chemical preparations. The public is accustomed to hearing "miracle cure," "miracle drug," and so forth. It is not difficult, therefore, to believe similar claims made by the quack. The very technologic expertise that has dramatically improved health care may be distorted by the promoters of false cure.

Psychologic benefits

"Psychologic benefit" is currently a dominant theme of those who wish to legalize certain unproven methods of cancer treatment (such as Laetrile). The argument is based on two convictions: (1) consumers should have the freedom to use anything they wish to treat their disease, and (2) a "terminal cancer client" can receive psychologic benefit from maintaining hope in a nonproven method. The second argument has face validity; if a person knows that traditional treatment cannot alter the course of the disease and wishes to try a nonproven method, the health care professional is hard pressed to deny the implied right. The caregiver knows that the unproven method is ineffective in the treatment of cancer yet may acknowledge the client's need to hope. The cancer quack eagerly supports the person's need to hope, try, and "never give up." The emphasis is on creating a false hope and not supporting the person in examining fears, feelings, and emotional responses.

The issues presented in this section encompass reasons why a person with cancer, or someone who fears a cancer diagnosis, would use a false cure. Each issue gives rise to a potential solution to the cancer quackery problem. Nurses, as well as other health care professionals, *must* attend to the intensity with which these issues are debated in order to recognize points of intervention.

RESPONSIBILITY AND ACTION: THE NURSE'S ROLE

Discussions on the impact of cancer quackery have occurred with greater frequency in nursing over the past few years.[6,7,22,36] Knowledge of the underlying dynamics of a problem precedes interventive efforts. Now that the nursing profession knows the "what, how, and why" of cancer quackery, it is time to identify the profession's degree of responsibility and commitment to resolving the issues that support the problem's continued existence.

Nurses are viewed by health care consumers in roles of expert, teacher, intervener, and behavior model. In the area of cancer quackery, the nurse can actualize each of these roles in an attempt to reduce the tragic losses incurred when quackery is used.

Communication

The *key* to reduction in the client's need for cancer quackery is *communication.* When the person with cancer is undergoing legitimate treatment and suddenly decides to drop out in order to use a quack method, communication has seriously deteriorated between caregiver and consumer. If the lines of communication are open, honest, empathic, and frequently used, the nurse and physician will be aware of the client's fears and need for hope.

Honesty and straightforward interaction between client and caregiver need not be characterized by brutal, insensitive confrontation to be so classified; it does need to be accurate and caringly carried out. Purposeful attention to the client's emotional, social, spiritual, and psychologic needs must accompany accomplishment of physical care goals, that is, the holistic approach.

Communication also may involve a greater degree of self-disclosure than nurses are accustomed to. Sharing one's feelings and goals (personal or client related) reduces barriers between human beings engaged in a struggle for life. Clients are capable of giving care as well as receiving it. Learning to actively listen, reflect, and convey understanding of the client's feelings can be accomplished through self-awareness training, classes on communication skills, and study of counseling skills.

Nurses must also be willing to assume responsibility for ensuring that resources are available to the client and family for discussion of potentially sensitive topics. When topics related to sexuality, spirituality, or dying arise, the nurse needs to feel prepared to discuss feelings, thoughts, or fears associated with these subjects. If the nurse feels unqualified to do so, a specific attempt can be made to keep the topic open while other health team members are consulted and/or the nurse seeks the assistance necessary to allow more effective intervention. Clients need to know that sensitive topics are legitimate areas for consideration.

Information

One very common complaint of clients is a fear that physicians or nurses withhold information or don't tell "the whole truth." Clients can be thoroughly informed about diagnosis, treatment, and prognosis if this is done in a sensitive manner. (In fact, informed consent is an ethical and legal requirement.) Sensitivity refers to careful assessment of the person's *level of understanding and readiness to hear and integrate* what is said. Clarification is essential. For example, the caregiver's *message* may be, "We are not able to *cure* your disease," but the client may hear, "*Nothing* can be done for me."[35] In fact, much can be done for the person in terms of pain management, emotional support, comfort, and rehabilitation to the limit of one's potential.

It may be necessary to break up information blocks into smaller quantities that are delivered in a gradual manner using *lay terminology*. In this way, each portion of information is added to a solid base of understanding. Even under these circumstances, however, clients may need to hear key information over and over again. For example, when first told all the facts and requirements associated with chemotherapy, the client takes in a portion of the information. On each subsequent visit, the nurse needs to assess the person's level of understanding and need for a repetition of information previously given. Teaching the client is *not* a "one shot deal."

Readiness and availability to answer clients' questions can also reduce dissatisfaction with the health care system. Clients may be unclear as to the specificity of question content. In this situation, the nurse needs to be able to pursue the topic until the question is defined and then obtain the appropriate answer using care team resources.

Emotional support

Clients are people. They, as well as the caregiver, respond positively to emotional involvement and support. Support includes a willingness to discuss painful issues and feelings, not shrinking away from the intense demands for interpersonal contact, and an acknowledgment that one's *humanness* is the greatest gift that can be shared with a fellow human who is suffering, despairing, or seeking answers to unanswerable questions. Faced with one's finiteness and mortality, the person with cancer and the nurse confront feelings that are usually suppressed and hidden. Whether the client survives or not, significant changes in values, philosophy, and attitude toward living may occur. The nurse can facilitate this enhanced self-awareness by supporting the search for answers and exploration of values. The nurse can actively support the client's *healthy* parts and abilities to seek the highest level of wellness possible.

To be supportive, the nurse needs support. It is this area of staff emotional support that is often neglected by health care institutions. Perhaps the lack of staff support promotes less involvement with clients, which in turn produces the client's feeling of abandonment. This negative, self-perpetuating cycle can be disrupted by implementation of staff support groups, one-to-one counseling, and group therapy experiences. As the nurse receives nurturance, it is then realistic and possible to give emotional nurturance to the person with cancer as well as family members.

Decision making

Increasingly, persons with cancer, as well as other health care consumers, seek to participate in the decision-making process related to their care and treatment. Clients must be informed prior to giving consent for treatment. However, clients may feel that the decisions have already been made when they are asked to sign a consent form. In this area, nurses have much to offer by way of teaching, assessment of understanding, advocacy, and sequencing of treatment.

Teaching. Explanations of diagnostic tests and treatment components can be simplified and explained to the client and family. Remember, while the nurse may *assume* that the client understands expectations for cooperation, this cannot be determined unless the nurse overtly assesses comprehension. In addition, the test or treatment generally is a "first" for the consumer—the nurse may have carried out the procedure countless times. The nurse, then, needs to remember the client's viewpoint and carry through with explanations—making no *assumptions*. Nurses can use audiovisual media, printed matter, and the discussion group format to ensure that clients understand the information presented.

Assessment of understanding. Many persons with cancer are anxious when first told about the suggested course of treatment. The nurse can return to these topics and offer an additional explanation and an opportunity to ask additional questions. An affirmative head nod *does not* justify an inference of understanding.

Advocacy. Often the nurse is aware of questions the client is hesitant to ask a physician. The nurse can support the client in questioning or can voice the questions for the client. The client needs to know that he or she has rights and that no punitive consequences will occur if these rights are asserted.

Sequencing of treatment. Once the client has decided to begin a treatment program, decision making continues to be an important element in the care process. The client can be encouraged to participate in the timing of certain aspects of treatment. For example, the convenience of the institution may be served by scheduling treatments at certain times. However, the client's convenience might be better served by a more personalized schedule constructed by client, nurse, and the particular hospital department.

• • •

The person with cancer is often able to make decisions that relate to care, yet nurses must *actively promote* such *involvement* for it to occur. A sense of involvement, regardless of the level of complexity, reduces feelings of powerlessness and dependence.

Nonjudgmental attitude

When discussing cancer quackery with a family or client, the nurse's attitude must be nonjudgmental. This can be difficult when personal beliefs are antiquackery. For the client to be willing to question, receive information, and then make an informed decision about use or nonuse of a quack method, the nurse's nonjudgmental attitude is essential.

Once a client has used an unproven method to the detriment of overall progress, the nurse's nonjudgmental acceptance of the person can support return to legitimate treatment. Feelings of guilt, self-blame, and anger may surface and need to be accepted by the caregiver. Time lost to delay can never be regained. Thus, the client needs to know that the nurse and other caregivers will do all that is possible despite the detour into quackery.

Education and community awareness

For the nurse to knowledgeably interact with the client in reference to quackery, it is vital that the helper receive education on the topic. That has been one purpose of this chapter. While the nurse keeps up-to-date with the newest developments in cancer care, it is equally important to keep abreast of changes in quackery approaches. Maintaining one's knowledge base through self-educative efforts is one aspect of the nurse's professional responsibility.

People with cancer and their families also need to be educated about the dangers of cancer quackery. Teaching about quackery does *not* mean that the nurse is "putting ideas into the client's head" that will result in use of unproven methods. Receipt of information reduces ambiguity, mystery, and the unknown. As clients are trusted and supported in making informed choices, the *need* to seek unproven alternatives will be decreased.

Nurses are leaders in the health professional community. In this role, the nurse can assume a degree of personal responsibility for being educated on community, state, and national efforts to legalize potentially harmful unproven cancer treatments. Involvement may consist of writing letters to legislators, supporting spokespersons by one's presence at hearings or conferences on quackery, and overtly proclaiming one's position as a concerned health professional in relation to quackery.

The public needs to be educated so that the "myths of mystery" about cancer and its treatment are dispelled. Nurses are in key positions to educate in the workplace, at home, with neighbors, at churches, and in other community settings. Mobilization of interest in this health problem is another aspect of the nurse's educative role. Often by working through others, the nurse can achieve highly effective outcomes in educating the public on the danger of cancer quackery.

SUMMARY

Cancer quackery is a health problem that will not just fade away. It is a clear and present danger to people with cancer, their families, and the community as a whole. Delay and interruption of effective treatment occurs when the person with cancer turns to unproven and ineffective remedies. Regardless of the reasons for this behavior, the nurse has a crucial role to play in reducing the quack's threat to quality care. As health care professionals *implement* a philosophy of involvement, caring, and a belief in promotion of qualitative living regardless of the severity of illness, the consumer will have little desire to have those needs met by the quack.

REFERENCES

1. Airola, P. O.: Cancer causes, prevention and treatment: the total approach, Phoenix, 1972, Health Plus Publishers.
2. American Cancer Society: Unproven methods of cancer management, New York, 1971, American Cancer Society, Inc.
3. American Medical Association: Facts on quacks: what you should know about health quackery, Chicago, 1971, American Medical Association.
4. American Medical Association: Mechanical quackery, Chicago, 1965, American Medical Association.
5. Brody, J. E.: Personal health: dangerous lure of cancer quacks, New York Times, July 13, 1977.
6. Burkhalter, P. K.: Cancer quackery, Am. J. Nurs. **77**:451, 1977.
7. Burkhalter, P. K.: Cancer quackery: what you need to know. In Burkhalter, P. K., and Donley,

D. L., editors: Dynamics of oncology nursing, New York, 1978, McGraw-Hill Book Co.
8. Cassell, E. J.: Laetrile—when the patient asks, Hosp. Prog. **12**(8):11, 17, 1977.
9. Commentary: Laetrile (vitamin B_{17})—a statement by the National Nutrition Consortium, J. Am. Diet. Assoc. **70**(4):354, 1977.
10. Crawford, J.: Cancer quackery flourishing trade, Rocky Mountain News, Denver, October 11, 1974.
11. DeVries, A.: Therapeutic fasting, Los Angeles, 1963, Chandler Book Co.
12. DiPalma, J. R.: Laetrile: when is a drug not a drug? Am. Fam. Physician **15**(1):186, 1977.
13. Dorr, R. T., and Paxinos, J.: The current status of Laetrile, Ann. Intern. Med. **89:**389, 1978.
14. Edson, L.: Why Laetrile won't go away, The New York Times Magazine **41:**44, 103, 1977.
15. Ellison, N. M., Byar, D. P., and Newell, G. R.: Special report on Laetrile: the NCI Laetrile review, N. Engl. J. Med. **299**(10):549, 1978.
16. Faw, C., et al.: Unproved cancer remedies: a survey of use in pediatric outpatients, J.A.M.A. **238**(1):1536, 1977.
17. Golden, F.: Freedom of choice and apricot pits, Time **54:**109, 1977.
18. Goodhart, R. S., and Shils, M. E., editors: Modern nutrition in health and disease, Philadelphia, 1974, Lea & Febiger.
19. Haught, S. J.: Has Dr. Max Gerson a true cancer cure? North Hollywood, Calif., 1962, London Press.
20. Herbert, V.: The nutritionally unsound "nutritional and metabolic antineoplastic diet" of Laetrile proponents, J.A.M.A. **240**(4):1139, 1978.
21. Holland, J. F.: The krebiozen story: is cancer quackery dead? J.A.M.A. **200:**125, 1967.
22. Isler, C.: The fatal choice: cancer quackery, R.N. **37**(9):55, 1974.
23. Jukes, T. H.: Laetrile for cancer, J.A.M.A. **236**(11):1284, 1976.
24. Kelley, W. D.: New hope for cancer victims, Grapevine, Texas, 1969, Kelley Research Foundation.
25. Kirschner, H. E.: Live food juices, Monrovia, Calif., 1957, H. E. Kirschner Publications.
26. Loyd, F. G., and Irwin, T.: How quackery thrives on the occult, Today's Health **48:**21, 87, 1970.
27. Nolen, W. A.: Healing: a doctor in search of a miracle, Greenwich, Conn., 1974, Fawcett Publications.
28. Nolfi, K.: The raw food treatment of cancer and other diseases, Manchester, 1973, The Vegetarian Society.
29. Psychic surgery, Time **92:**92, 1968.
30. Rogers, P.: Faith healers of the Philippines, Honolulu Star Bulletin C-1,2, May 24, 1974.
31. Shabert, J. K.: Nutrition and cancer. In Burkhalter, P. K., and Donley, D. L., editors: Dynamics of oncology nursing, New York, 1978, McGraw-Hill Book Co.
32. Smith, R. E.: New traffic in cures for cancer, Saturday Evening Post **241:**62, 1968.
33. Soffer, A.: Worthless but harmless drugs can be deadly, Chest **69**(3):331, 1976.
34. Wetherell, R. C., Jr.: Does prohibition of Laetrile interfere with freedom of choice, Chest **70**(3):407, 1976.
35. White, L. P.: Death and the physician: mortui vivos docent. In Feifel, H., editor: New meanings of death, New York, 1977, McGraw-Hill Book Co.
36. Whitney, R. P.: Is Laetrile worse than no hope at all? R.N. **41:**54, May, 1978.

V

NURSING CARE OF THE CLIENT WITH ADVANCED CANCER

17

Control and comfort: caring for the client who has advanced cancer

LISA BEGG MARINO

Clients with advanced cancer are defined as those clients having disseminated or widespread disease. Generally, these persons have been treated previously with some form of definitive treatment but have suffered a recurrence of their cancer, or they were initially seen with widespread disease. Regardless, most of these clients will still be undergoing some form of active treatment designed to provide them with significant control or even cure of their cancer. This group of clients is a very large one, characterized by numerous challenges and opportunities for professional nursing care. These opportunities revolve around a central concept of comfort, which is nurse directed. The concept complements the physician's goal of control and thereby provides more comprehensive care to this population of clients.

SCOPE OF THE PROBLEM

The Division of Cancer Treatment of the National Cancer Institute maintains statistics on the stage of clients' cancers relative to cancer treatment interventions. Using 1977 statistics as an example, the report states that 700,000 new cancers (exclusive of skin and in situ cervical cancer) were diagnosed, 500,000 of which were diagnosed as localized cancers and 200,000 of which were widespread. Of the 500,000 with apparently localized cancer, 220,000 clients have invisible microscopic disease that can be expected to develop into recurrent disease. Some of these latter clients received adjuvant therapy, generally chemotherapy, which eradicated the microscopic disease. Others proved refractive to adjuvant therapy or never received additional therapy following the definitive treatment.[2] Combining the two groups, the 220,000 clients with microscopic disease and the 200,000 clients with disseminated cancer, forms a larger group of 420,000 clients *each year* who probably will have, or who already do have, advanced cancer. Ironically, because cancer treatment is more successful, this group of clients has been *increasing* in number. Previously, when fewer treatment options were available, the client was initially treated, and if recurrence developed, death was more likely to occur. Now, greater numbers of clients with residual or recurrent disease are living for longer and longer periods. They are generally receiving some form of cancer treatment, may be experiencing symptoms directly related to their disease state, and can possibly benefit from professional nursing interventions.

SCIENTIFIC BASIS FOR TREATING ADVANCED CANCER

Research on the advanced stages of cancer has yielded valuable information relative to treating clients in all stages of the disease. Knowledge about the mechanisms of metastasis, cell kinetics, and the responses to therapy can be useful to the clinician treating cancer, regardless of its stage. Characterizing advanced or metastatic cancer into four main groups aids in the plan of therapy: delayed metastasis occurs after the primary tumor has been removed and a period of no apparent disease exists until recognition of recurrence; locoregional disease is present with the strong likelihood of metastasis developing within a short time; poor prognostic factors are present at the time of primary tumor removal; metastasis is present when no primary tumor can be identified.[4] Most scientists have noted that metastatic tumors can respond quite differently to treatment than did the primary tumor. It has been postulated that the difference exists because every step in the metastatic process is highly selective. Only a small number of cells are shed from the primary tumor and of these only a small proportion can be expected to survive and grow into clinical metastasis. The preferential growth of these tumor cells is now known to be more important than whether they spread via the blood, lymph, or other means. Host factors, host cells, and the tumor cells all need to interact for metastasis to occur. In the end, the host's homeostatic mechanism may be the determining factor; if it can withstand this attack, no clinical metastasis will become evident, and if the host is deficient, metastasis will occur.

This knowledge has given the physician more opportunities to treat cancer over all possible stages and has led to a major shift in attitudes. Previously, physicians approached cancer treatment more or less as curable versus incurable. As discussed in Chapter 11, treatment was sequential: surgery only if the tumor was presumed curable, radiotherapy principally for metastatic disease, and chemotherapy for far-advanced cancers. Because of limited knowledge, many clients were not given complete benefit of these modalities. Now, with the successes achieved through multiple modality cancer treatment, therapy is more control oriented. The concept of control as opposed to cure allows the physician many more opportunities to aid clients. Physicians can treat clients aggressively throughout the various stages of cancer and continue to treat them when there are high-risk situations, first recurrence, second recurrence, and so forth. Physicians can offer hope to clients even when the limited concept of cure is not possible by concentrating on controlling their cancer. A physician may not be able to cure a client with metastatic breast cancer, but it is possible to control the bone metastases and even the liver and brain metastases for a period of time so that the client can continue to live. This concept of control has also opened up opportunities for nurses to intervene, since many of these clients have needs based on problems they are experiencing because of the stage of their disease. The treatment course is protracted, requiring major adjustments on the part of the client and family. The remainder of this chapter will discuss the client-family needs and the nursing interventions that are appropriate for them.

CHARACTERISTICS OF CLIENT POPULATION

In terms of characteristics, clients with advanced cancer are quite heterogeneous.

Cullen[3] has been one of the few nurses to ascribe discrete characteristics to this population of clients. In her paper, she utilized three phases to describe clients who had metastatic or disseminated colorectal cancer. In Phase I were those clients who had early recurrence of their cancer, residual disease, or controlled minimal disease; Phase II clients had progressive disease or disease controlled after a moderate amount of progression; Phase III clients had end-stage, extensive cancer. As one might expect, the needs of clients with advanced cancer can vary substantially, but there are some needs that are common to many clients; they will be discussed later in the chapter.

Aside from the variety of symptoms and needs of this client population, heterogeneity exists relative to age and developmental stages. Just as cancer in general can affect people of all ages, many of them go on to have disseminated cancer. This stage of cancer presents problems to many of those affected, but it is particularly difficult on the elderly. Maintaining mobility; preserving skin integrity, nutrition, and hydration; and conserving energy can all be special problems for the elderly.[5] Additionally, clients in the older age groups frequently have concomitant diseases that complicate their health situation and any treatment for cancer. Since over 50% of all cancer clients are beyond the age of 65, this represents a sizable subset within the number of clients with advanced cancer.[8]

CONCEPT OF COMFORT

The primary responsibility of the physician caring for the client with cancer is to control the disease process. Nurses aid physicians in this goal, but since this is medical practice and not nursing practice, nurses may not always achieve professional satisfaction by concentrating exclusively on activities directed toward this aim. Rather, focusing on providing comfort to the client can offer satisfying opportunities to nurses, complement the medical goals, and provide needed resources to the client and family.

Comfort is defined broadly as the minimizing of psychobiologic distress[6] and represents what I consider to be the major need in all cancer clients, but particularly so for those clients with advanced cancer. It is recognized and acknowledged that other needs exist, but comfort represents *the major need and also the concept that unites all the nursing interventions aimed at this population of clients.* This philosophy permits the nurse many more therapeutic tools with which to intervene and provides the client and family with more resources as they cope with what is happening to them.

Psychologic comfort

The psychologic component of comfort rests mainly with aiding the client and family to continue valued activities and relationships. This concept requires that the nurse be available to the client and family as they continue to live their lives by adjusting to meet an altered physical capacity caused by changes in the client's disease state. These changes may be related to the cancer itself, to the therapeutic interventions, or to refractiveness to these interventions that will eventually lead to the client's death. Clients' psychologic states are dependent to a large degree on how well they adapt to these physical changes that accompany cancer. For example, physical limitations, regardless of their cause, that prevent the client from performing valued roles are anxiety provoking experiences. The mother who cannot "do," the father who cannot "support," and the child who cannot "play" will have difficulties in adjusting to their new states. Nurses can provide valuable service to clients and open up opportunities for their own professional satisfaction by aiding clients to make the adjustments that will permit them to continue these valued activities or, in cases where physical limitations make this impossible, lessen the anguish they will experience as they grieve for these losses. Relative to this latter aspect, the nurse supports the clients by indicating a desire to continue to work with them. One of the major expressed fears of all cancer clients, particularly those in the advanced stage, is that they will become so burdensome that family, health care providers, and friends will abandon them. The nurse can minimize these fears a great deal by maintaining support and contact with the cancer client and indicating that communication will be kept open. Communication is also important to the client with cancer because of the isolation that almost invariably occurs. It is generally acknowledged that isolation affects all parties, the client, the family, and the health care providers, because of the societal stigmas associated with cancer. People are still uncomfortable in dealing with these diseases, and this discomfort generally manifests itself by isolating the major source of this discomfort, namely the client. The nurse can do two important things to aid the client: first, set an appropriate example by continuing to interact openly and honestly with the client, and second, do whatever is necessary to promote increased communication between the client and significant others, other health care providers, and people the client wishes to interact with. Aggressiveness on the part of the nurse allows the client to be less of an initiator in this regard. This professional action permits the client to benefit from the interactions while not having to expend the energy to promote their occurrence. The client's psychic and physical energy is better spent fighting the spread of cancer.

When isolation is coupled with a loss of future sense, the client may be dealt with as "an object and not as a sentient, responsive individual."[1] This development is more likely to occur if it is perceived that the client is succumbing to cancer and control of future events no longer rests with the client. Because of functional limitations, items such as property and money have already been disposed. The American culture is so future oriented that persons with only limited futures can be easily bypassed. There is little the nurse can do to change these attitudes, but continuing to relate to clients as thinking, feeling persons can reinforce some state of dignity and control over what is happening to them.

Along this same area, spiritual comfort can be very important to some clients, and their wishes and beliefs need to be respected by all health care providers. During this stage of cancer when physical limitations may increase, many clients and their families find great solace from religion, so the nurse should respond supportively to requests to see clergy or to discuss their feelings.

Physiologic comfort

The physiologic dimensions to the concept of comfort in clients with advanced cancer include numerous activities such as hygiene; activity, rest, and sleep; safety; nutrition; elimination; oxygenation; sensory needs; and pain. Each of these will be discussed in detail. One study confirms that advanced cancer clients experience physical discomfort more than clients in the earlier stages.[7]

Hygiene. Hygiene includes such needs as mouth care, hair grooming, and skin care. The first two items are usually treatment related because chemotherapy can cause stomatitis and alopecia and radiation therapy to the head and neck can do likewise. Relative to stomatitis, it is important to determine whether its development represents the beginning of severe toxicity. Many of the antimetabolites and antitumor antibiotics cause stomatitis before severe myelosuppression appears. Stomatitis can also appear by itself as a consequence of the treatment effects on rapidly dividing normal cells. Regardless of its cause, stomatitis needs to be treated because it can interfere with the client's ability to eat. Mouth care must be given routinely, preferably with a diluted hydrogen peroxide rinse. The mouth should be rinsed thoroughly at 2-hour intervals, dentures should be removed, and lidocaine (Xylocaine) viscous or acetaminophen (Tylenol) elixir can be given prior to meals to enable the client to eat without pain. Along with these measures, the diet should be altered so that bland foods predominate, hot liquids are avoided, and cold liquids are used to help soothe the oral passages. If a client is prone to develop stomatitis, the nurse should offer instruction and encouragement in the practice of good oral hygiene so that secondary infections can be avoided and nutrition maintained. If the client is too weak to undertake this care, family members can be taught how to provide mouth care and food preparations so that the client can remain as comfortable as possible.

Alopecia, or hair loss, can result from both radio- and chemotherapies for the same reason as stomatitis. Hair follicles are rapidly dividing cells and are affected by these treatments. With chemotherapy, most of the agents responsible for hair loss are known, since they are principally the plant alkaloids, alkylating agents, and some of the antitumor antibiotics. There has been some preliminary information that scalp tourniquets or devices to lower the surface temperature can reduce hair loss from intravenous agents. With radiotherapy, hair loss cannot be prevented. In cases where it is anticipated that hair loss will occur, the nurse can do the following: prepare the client for the expected loss and suggest that a wig be purchased before the hair loss occurs and reassure the client and family that the loss is temporary, with regrowth occurring after the chemotherapy ceases and after a period of recovery from radiotherapy. To delay the hair loss, the nurse can suggest that the client keep the existing hair short, wash it with a pH-balanced shampoo, and rinse it thoroughly. Since hair loss represents an obvious sign of disease, its importance to the client's self-image should not be minimized. The nurse should carefully assess the client's perceptions in this regard and adjust interventions and support accordingly.

Skin care needs can be disease related or secondary to treatment. For example, earlier detection of breast cancers is reducing the likelihood of discovering a breast cancer that has already ulcerated through the skin. Skin reactions caused by treatment with radiation or fistula formation can occur but are more likely to occur when the client is debilitated. Stomal care following a colostomy or ileal conduit is very important since skin breakdown can cause great discomfort to the client and reduce the ability to live a normal life. Careful dressing changes help clients reduce their discomfort, and palliative radiotherapy for ulcerated lesions is generally an effective way to reduce problems. Skin care can be taught to family members so that further problems can be avoided. With skin problems, prevention is preferred to treating problems once they have developed, so client instruction can help both the nurse and the client.

Activity, rest, and sleep. As with some of the previously mentioned client needs, activity, rest, and sleep needs can be affected by the disease process, or they can be secondary to cancer treatment. Cancer, particularly if it becomes refractive to treatment, will slowly drain the client's strength and cause progressive debility. Adjustments in schedules help to preserve the client's strength to continue to participate in valued activities and relationships. In this regard, it is particularly important for the nurse to validate what the *client* considers to be valued because the nurse's own values may distort assessments. Once there is agreement, the nurse can be a helpful buffer to the client as negotiation with family, friends, or employers takes place. Secondary gains from any illness also work to help the client cut back and preserve energy levels. Fatigue can also occur as a result of cancer treatment so that the nurse's ability to manipulate the care system to permit the client needed rest is challenged once more. Many times, frequent laboratory tests can be cut back to conserve energy, or if they cannot be, negotiations with the hospital or outpatient facility to minimize the wasted time and efforts can be partially successful in conserving the client's resources. The nurse can also be helpful to family members in terms of supporting them since they serve as a buffer to the client so that social contacts can better match the client's reserve of energy.

It should be noted here that *inactivity* is not being encouraged, but rather a sensible level of activity that the *client* wishes to pursue. In fact, activity and mobility need to be *encouraged* within the client's physical state so that conditions such as hypercalcemia can be minimized. Hypercalcemia, a life-threatening condition, can develop in clients with advanced breast cancer. Activity helps to reduce its incidence, and if hypercalcemia does develop, activity can help to control the pathologic process. Relative to hypercalcemia, pathologic bone fractures can accompany this condition so it is important for the nurse to work with the client's physician to determine a safe plan for ambulation.

Safety. Problems of safety can be attributed to the disease itself or, again, secondarily to its treatment. These problems occur frequently in clients who suffer metastases to their brain from some primary site such as the lung or breast, and they can manifest themselves through memory loss, visual disturbances, and motor dysfunction. Since these problems are obvious to clients and everyone else, clients become upset and concerned over this loss of functioning and control over their lives. The nurse can do a great deal here by supporting them, providing them with a safe environment, and working with them to preserve functioning for as long as possible. For example, memory loss is frightening to clients and their families, so helping them to retain information can increase functioning. Having a calendar posted, reviewing recent events with clients, and encouraging them to take notes on important events gives them some control over what is happening to them. All these actions are helpful, but since the losses in functioning are so profound, the nurse should expect acute grief to take place. This is particularly so for the family, as conditions may deteriorate to a point where the client does not recognize family members.

Visual disturbances and motor dysfunction present obvious safety problems that may be difficult to deal with except to provide guidance to the client during periods of activity. Again, these problems represent obvious signs of disease progression that will generally trigger both fear and despair. The nurse can be instrumental to the client by providing consistent support.

Safety problems that develop as a result of cancer treatment are numerous. Myelosuppression resulting in a higher risk of infection and bleeding are common to clients undergoing chemotherapy or radiotherapy that includes major bone marrow sites. Risks are increased because most of these clients receive their therapy as outpatients. This means that both the physician and nurse need to instruct the client and family about what is important and then closely monitor them for any occurrence of problems. Clients need to be taught how to interpret their blood counts so they will understand their vulnerable periods. This is one of the better examples that reinforces the importance of encouraging the client's and family's participation in the treatment being given. For chemotherapy to be effective, myelosuppression must take place so a delicate balance between therapeutic intent and toxicity must be maintained. With radiotherapy, ports are developed to shield as much of the bone marrow as possible, but when treating large areas such as the pelvis, myelosuppression is common. The radiotherapist closely monitors the client so that treatment can be temporarily stopped if severe suppression occurs. This fact may alarm the client and family, so the nurse should reinforce the temporary nature of the interruption and the reasons it became necessary.

Nutrition. Nutrition in general is attracting more attention from the public and scientific sectors as a possible contributing factor to the etiology of cancer. While this aspect continues to be debated, no debate is necessary for demonstrating the importance of nutrition to the advanced cancer client.

Nausea and vomiting secondarily related to treatments or progression of disease are quite common. Unfortunately, the client may be unable to maintain an adequate nutritional state because of this, so further disability occurs. Sometimes, nausea and vomiting can be minimized by carefully scheduling meals in relation to radio- or chemotherapeutic treatments. Other times, as in the case of taste sensations directly related to chemotherapy, only adjustments in the type of food consumed can be altered, not the primary source of the problem. Smaller, more bland meals are helpful as is utilizing preferred homemade foods. The nurse needs to determine what foods are important to the client and work actively with both the client and the food preparer. Chapter 25 discusses nutrition and the cancer client in detail.

Elimination. Problems with elimination can be related to progression of the cancer, as with obstructions, or secondary to treatment, as with neurotoxicity from vincristine causing a paralytic ileus or diarrhea following radiotherapy to the pelvis. Surgeries such as ileal conduit and colostomies are lifesaving procedures, but the adjustments required on the part of the client are substantial. Both of these procedures are best dealt with by careful preoperative evaluation to determine the best location for the stoma. Once acute needs pass, there is ample need for client education so that the all too frequent "client is cured but becomes a social recluse" theme does not occur. These problems are dealt with in detail in Chapter 30.

Oxygenation. Problems with oxygenation develop because of the progression of cancer or because of problems resulting directly from treatment. Respiratory function may be severely compromised by the presence of malignant pleural effusion or ascites. Anemia may diminish the oxygen carrying capacity of the blood. Pulmonary fibrosis from previous radiation therapy or from a chemotherapeutic agent called bleomycin is more difficult to treat because a significant decrease in functional capacity is generally experienced.

Positioning the client and working with the medical staff to relieve symptoms is important in minimizing disease-related problems. For the client whose problems develop directly from treatment, adjustment may be complicated by the fact that a cure may have taken place. The client then finds out a major functional impairment has occurred, thereby diminishing the benefits incurred by the cure.

Sensory. Sensory problems generally develop directly because of disease progression, with the exception of neurotoxicities caused by chemotherapy. One of the better examples is that of cord compression owing to a tumor. This serious complication of cancer can occur with a variety of solid tumors as well as the lymphomas. The client usually complains of a sudden onset of weakness and numbness in the extremities and incontinence. Once confirmed, an emergency laminectomy is usually performed to relieve the obstruction and preserve functioning.

Pain. Pain is probably one of the most misunderstood subjects concerning cancer. Contrary to common assumptions, pain is not a problem for most cancer clients. True, there is a subset of clients for which pain is a serious problem, but the numbers are not large. However, because pain can be so misinterpreted and frustrating to the health provider, Chapter 18 addresses cancer pain in detail.

CONCLUSION

This chapter has discussed the needs of clients with advanced cancer. The concepts of control and comfort have been suggested as models for medical and nursing interventions with those clients: control more accurately reflects the medical capability of cancer treatment and comfort is a broader concept under which a variety of needs can be met. Also central to comfort is open and honest communication. Generally speaking, the client is compromised in some fashion, therefore, assertive nursing actions to provide them with support and fulfillment of their needs is a major focus of practice and one that can provide professional satisfaction to the nurse.

Because clients with advanced cancer have such special needs that are so great in number, Chapters 18 through 21 will address key aspects of care. Chapter 18 presents a comprehensive discussion of pain in cancer; Chapter 19 discusses communication; Chapter 20 discusses the problems of coping that a cancer health care provider must deal with; and Chapter 21 presents a nurse-coordinated model in home care for children who are dying. Each of these chapters builds on earlier discussions and is included to give the professional nurse additional information and encouragement to work with these clients because, in spite of these clients' progressive disease, they are attempting to live to the fullest and could have their burdens lessened by skilled and empathetic nursing care.

REFERENCES

1. Brennan, M. J.: The cancer gestalt, Geriatrics **25**(10):96, 1970.
2. Committee Publication No. 96188: Hearings before the Select Committee on Aging, House of Representatives, June 19-21, 1979.
3. Cullen, P. P.: Patients with colorectal cancer: how to assess and meet their needs, Nursing **6**(9):42, 1976.
4. Gilbert, H. A., and Kagan, A. R.: Introduction to metastases, Semin. Oncol. **IV**(1):1, 1977.
5. Mummah, H. R.: Oncologic nursing of the aged. In Kellogg, C. J., and Sullivan, B. P., editors: Current perspectives in oncologic nursing, St. Louis, 1978, The C. V. Mosby Co.
6. Oncology Nursing Society and American Nurses' Association: Outcome standards for cancer nursing practice, Kansas City, Mo., 1979, American Nurses' Association.
7. Schneider, L.: Identification of human concerns by cancer patients. In Kellogg, C. J., and Sullivan, B. P., editors: Current perspectives in oncologic nursing, St. Louis, 1978, The C. V. Mosby Co.
8. Zislis, J. M.: Rehabilitation of the cancer patient, Geriatrics **25**(3):150, 1970.

18

The nursing management of pain

ADA K. JACOX and ADA G. ROGERS

"I'm not afraid of dying; I'm afraid of the pain; I don't want to suffer." These words have been expressed by many people who have cancer. Despite the many advances that have been made in the treatment of cancer, there are still those who feel that cancer is an incurable disease accompanied by intractable pain, ending only in death. If this sounds extravagant, it is not.

In this chapter, the concept of pain is examined generally as a framework for discussing the various kinds of pain associated with cancer and cancer treatment. Following that is a discussion of pain assessment and general approaches to the alleviation of pain, including biologically oriented and psychosocially based interventions. Finally, the nurse's role in assessment and alleviation of pain associated with cancer is addressed.

OVERVIEW OF PAIN AND PAIN ASSESSMENT

Pain is perhaps one of the clearest possible examples of the mind-body relationship, in which a phenomenon is acknowledged as having both biologic and psychosocial aspects. A definition of pain by Sternbach[43] reflects the relationship. Pain is "an abstract concept which refers to (1) a personal, private sensation of hurt; (2) a harmful stimulus which signals current or impending tissue damage; (3) a pattern of responses which operates to protect the organism from harm."[43] Because it is a "personal, private sensation," only the one experiencing it really knows its intensity and nature. Others must infer the presence of pain and its characteristics from the person's verbal reports and from observation of the person's behavior.

The subjectivity makes assessment difficult for both the client and the person making the assessment. All of us have attitudes toward pain and how we should respond to it. The nurse who believes, for example, that people should experience as little pain and discomfort as possible may have difficulty understanding a client who believes that measures should be taken to reduce pain only when it is very severe. Neither attitude is right or wrong, but they reflect some of the variation in people's beliefs regarding how pain should be expressed and handled.

This work was supported in part by NIDA Grant DA-01707, NCI Core Grant CA-08748, and Division of Nursing Grant NU-00467.

Additionally, what one person views as very painful, another may experience as only mildly discomforting. In one study, for example, the sensations associated with a surgical incision site while turning the first few days postoperatively were defined by 70% as painful, while 20% said that turning produced only discomfort, and 10% said it produced neither.[20]

The second and third elements in Sternbach's definition of pain emphasize the notion that pain is a warning of current or impending tissue damage to which the person must respond. The warning can signal anything from a fleeting pressure sensation to destruction of the organism. Interpreting pain associated with common experiences such as touching a hot stove or bruising an arm is not difficult. But to interpret and respond to unfamiliar painful sensations from within the body is not so easy, especially for someone with a very limited understanding of what lies beneath the skin. All of these and many other factors make pain and its interpretation difficult for both the client and the health care provider.

GATE CONTROL THEORY OF PAIN

While there have been numerous theories regarding pain, one that has been developed during the past 15 years by Melzak and others is the gate control theory.[28-31] One of the most useful aspects of this theory from the nurse's point of view is its assumption that pain is not only a neurophysiologic phenomenon to be explained solely in terms of a certain intensity of stimulus always producing the same amount of pain sensation in persons. Rather, the gate control theory proposes that cognitive and emotional factors influence how pain is perceived and responded to, thus providing a basis for understanding pain as a mind-body problem.

The gate control theory accepts the idea of neurophysiologic specialization but proposes that there is some modulation of impulses in the dorsal horn of the spinal cord. The theory postulates the presence of T cells, or transmission cells, in the dorsal horn that transmit impulses through fibers in the anterolateral spinal cord into two major brain systems. The gating mechanism in the spinal cord controls the amount of peripheral nerve fiber input that is transmitted to T cells. The gating mechanism is influenced by input from two sources: afferent peripheral nerve fibers and efferent pyramidal and other central control fibers. Small and large peripheral fibers have opposing facilitating and inhibiting effects on the input to the T cells. Thus, T cell input is a function of (1) balance of small and large fiber activity and (2) brain activity. Brain activity can influence the input from peripheral fibers at the earliest synaptic levels.

Impulses are transmitted from the T cells into both the neospinothalamic brain system and the paramedial ascending system. Sensory input into the neospinothalamic system provides part of the basis for the sensory-discriminative aspect of pain. Input into the paramedial ascending system, which activates the reticular and limbic structures, produces the unpleasant affective quality associated with pain and motivates the organism to act to stop the pain. Both of these systems, in turn, are influenced by higher central nervous system processes. Corticifugal influences act on the sensory-discriminative system, and neocortical and limbic forebrain structures act on the brain stem reticular formation to influence the motivational-affective system. Melzak and Casey[29] suggest that, because of its interconnections with all sensory and associated cortical areas and its connections with reticular and limbic structures, the frontal cortex may be especially significant in mediating between cognitive activities and the motivational-affective features of pain.

The central control activities provide the basis for cognitive evaluation of input in terms of past experience, psychologic state, the meaning of the pain-producing situation, and similar factors. Cognitive functions may act either on both the sensory and affective dimensions or primarily on the motivational-affective dimensions.

This brief overview is not intended as a complete description of the gate control theory, rather it is intended to indicate the basis for the assertion that cognitive activities interact with neurophysiologic events in the perception of and reaction to pain. This interaction occurs both before and after peripheral nerve input activates the sensory and motivational systems. The gate control theory provides a good framework for understanding the mechanisms through which cognitive and emotional factors operate in the pain experience.

SELECTED FACTORS INFLUENCING THE PAIN EXPERIENCE

Pain threshold and tolerance

Two other terms commonly used in discussions of pain are "pain threshold" and "pain tolerance." *Pain threshold* refers to the intensity of the noxious stimulus necessary for the person to perceive pain. *Pain tolerance* refers to "the duration of time or the intensity at which a subject accepts the stimulus above the pain threshold before making a verbal or overt pain response."[43] These two dimensions of the pain experience are not necessarily related, nor is there a clear relationship between either threshold or tolerance and the likelihood that the person will complain of pain. The wide variation among threshold, tolerance, and readiness to complain of pain add greatly to the complexity of the perception of pain.

Chronic versus acute pain

Another useful distinction in types of pain is the differentiation between acute pain and chronic pain. Acute pain is associated with a condition that lasts for a short period of time such as a few minutes or a few weeks. Examples of acute pain are the initial sensation experienced in burns or traumatic injuries, incisional and other pains experienced postsurgically, and slamming one's finger in a door. Generally, the source of the acute pain can be quickly determined and alleviated.

Chronic pain, in contrast, is variously defined, but generally is considered as pain that extends beyond a 3-month period. The pain may last for several months, several years, or a lifetime. While the cause of the chronic pain may be understood, its treatment often is considerably more difficult than treatment of acute pain, since a balance must be achieved between reducing the pain to an acceptable level while still permitting the person to carry on, as far as possible, a normal life. Chronic pain may come and go or be constantly present, depending on the condition with which the pain is associated. Another term used with regard to chronic pain is "intractable pain." This usually refers to an inability to obtain pain relief through various treatments and may be as much a reflection of the health care providers' inability to find an effective treatment as it is a characteristic of the pain itself.

Individual perceptions of pain

As noted in the preceding, past experience, attitude toward pain, personality characteristics, cultural expectations regarding how one should deal with pain, and a host of other factors all influence how a person experiences pain. Only a few of these will be considered here.

Clearly, an important factor that influences how a person experiences pain is the origin or type of pain and the meaning this has for the person. Mark Zborowski, an anthropologist who has studied pain, noted that "depending on the nature of their illness, they [clients] are more or less concerned about the immediate as well as symptomatic significance of this pain and the future effects of their illness.[50] Once the source of an acute pain, for example, is known and effective treatment instituted, the person often can put the pain aside and get on with life. Clients who experience several days of pain following a cholecystectomy may be sufficiently relieved to be finished with the excruciatingly painful attacks that preceded the surgery that the pain and discomfort associated with the postsurgical period may be relatively easy to deal with. It is quite another matter, however, for a person with rheumatoid arthritis, for example, to put the thoughts of pain behind when the nature of the disease is such that when one period of pain is over the person may expect another bout in other joints of the body. Clearly, the *condition* with which pain is associated is a major influence in how a person deals with it.

Other factors that may influence how pain is experienced are age, personality characteristics, sex, cultural group identification, and previous experience with pain. There is a vast literature dealing with how each factor influences pain, and much of the literature is contradictory in its findings. What is clear, however, is that there are a multitude of psychosocial and cultural factors as well as physiologic factors that influence how a person perceives and responds to pain. As Chapman[9] notes, just as the physiology of vision cannot explain the appreciation of a painting, the physiology of pain cannot explain how it is experienced by a person.

PAIN AND CANCER

Pain associated with cancer and cancer treatment cannot be easily distinguished from other aspects of the cancer experience nor from the person's total life experience. As has been repeatedly noted, psychologic characteristics play a profound influence in the development of cancer, its progression, and a person's response to it. As the literature indicates, however, the precise way that psychologic factors influence the development or progress of cancer is not clear. There are studies that show various psychosocial precursors to specific types of cancer, and it is also known that the experience of having cancer can have a profound impact on a person's psychologic condition.

Additionally, as any experienced cancer clinician knows, symptoms do not present themselves neatly one at a time nor can they be dealt with separately. Pain is frequently confounded with psychologic symptoms such as anxiety, depression, and guilt. One study,[11] for example, indicated that more than half of the clients admitted to a cancer research unit showed moderate to high levels of depression, and 30% had increased levels of anxiety. Similarly, pain may be interrelated with other symptoms that have a more direct physiologic basis such as fatigue, nausea, vomiting, and so forth. A person who is unable to sleep and becomes excessively fatigued, for example, may have much more difficulty in tolerating pain. The fatigue, in turn, may be associated in part with the depression that commonly accompanies cancer. Treatment of the depression may help to alleviate *both* the depression and the fatigue associated with it and subsequently make it easier for a client to handle the pain. Thus, even though this chapter is a discussion of pain in cancer, a clinician must keep in mind that pain is not an isolated phenomenon but must be dealt with as part of a whole complex of symptoms.

Incidence of pain in cancer

While there is general acknowledgment of the fact that pain accompanies many kinds of cancers in various stages, there is little in the literature to indicate what the usual pain patterns associated with various kinds of cancer and cancer-related problems are. This lack of information was reflected in a request for research proposals from the National Cancer Institute in the fall of 1978. The request was for persons interested in developing and testing a methodology that would permit a determination of the incidence and natural history of pain in people with cancer. As noted in the request, "Out of the large number of presentations and workshops considering various cancer pain problems, experiences, and treatment efforts, there has evolved a consensus that no data base exists from which to determine the true magnitude of the cancer pain problem."[34]

Reflecting again how pain is confounded with other aspects of the disease, Cole notes that:

> Pain is rarely extremely severe in most cases of cancer, but general discomfort is often present. Pain can be constant and excruciating in some forms of sarcoma and neoplasms of the pancreas, but it is a general discomfort of an ill-functioning organ, with the anxiety, both personal and in many cases financial, together with the general debilitation, that magnifies this discomfort into pain.[10]

Estimates of the incidence of pain in cancer vary widely. Luce and Dawson[26] suggest that about one third of people with cancer have significant pain. Saunders,[40] on the other hand, found that over 70% of institutionalized clients required strong analgesics for pain relief and 10% did not obtain satisfactory relief.

Ramon Evans,[13] director of a pain clinic at Toronto, Canada, noted that approximately 80% of all clients treated at the clinic had intractable pain associated with malignancy. Surveys done at Memorial Sloan-Kettering Cancer Center in 1975 and 1977 indicated that 38% of those hospitalized had pain that required analgesics. Of these, 50% had pain due to bone disease, primary or metastatic.[14]

Lloyd and co-workers[25] report on clients with cancer who were referred to a pain relief clinic. Table 18-1 is modified from their analysis of 295 people with malignant disease who were admitted to a pain relief unit at Abbington Hospital in Oxford, England.

These clinicians were dealing with clients who had experienced pain of 1 to 3 months duration that was not relieved by conventional methods. As nearly as they could determine, approximately 38 of every 1,000 persons in the Oxford region who were diagnosed as having cancer of the cervix were referred to the pain relief clinic for treatment. This is slightly less than 4% of all persons with cervical cancer and was the type of cancer pain most commonly referred. In contrast, only one person in 1,000 with ovarian cancer was referred. Other types of carcinoma in which more than 1% of diagnosed persons had sufficiently severe pain to be treated in the pain clinic were cancer of the

Table 18-1. Referrals to the regional pain relief unit*

Types of carcinoma	Incidence of pain referral per 1,000 cases diagnosed in the region†
Lung	12.7
Breast	12.2
Cervix uteri	38.2
Rectum	16.5
Bladder	18.3
Prostate	11.8
Pancreas	13.8
Colon	5.4
Stomach	3.4
Kidneys	11.9
Corpus uteri	4.5
Ovary	1.3

*Modified from: Lloyd, J. W., et al.: Practitioner **220:**453, 1978.

†Oxford Regional Health Authority: 1972 is the most recent complete year available at the Regional Cancer Registry and there has been no significant alteration in the incidence of these tumours since 1966.

bladder, rectum, pancreas, lung, breast, kidneys, and prostate. While people seen in pain clinics comprise a very small minority of those with cancer generally, these figures do give some indication of the percentage of clients with various kinds of cancer whose pain has been unable to be relieved by conventional measures.

Cartwright and others[8] noted that 87% of people with cancer have pain at some time during the terminal stage of illness. There is little evidence given to substantiate his estimate, however.

Additional information on the intensity of cancer pain is supplied in a study done by the late Mary Stewart at a large midwestern university hospital in 1975.[44] In a study of 40 people in advanced stages of cancer, eight were followed through to their deaths, with regular communications by them of the amounts of pain that they were experiencing during the last several weeks of their lives.

Of the eight clients, there were four women and four men. Their average age was 41, with a range of 20 to 64 years. Their time in the study ranged from 5 to 72 days with an average of 25 days. For half the clients, pain measurements were obtained up to the day before death. Others were unable to complete the pain measurements for a period of from 2 days to 3 weeks before their death because of lethargy or other incapacity. The measurement used was a scale ranging from 0 to 100, with 0 being no pain and 100 being the worst possible pain imaginable. The average pain experienced during the final weeks of their life was 66.92. The average worst pain experienced by them during this time was 81.6. Half reported pain levels of between 80 and 100 at least half of the time during the last few weeks before their deaths. None indicated a level of pain below 50. All had medications ordered for pain relief, with the vast majority being on an as necessary basis. These brief results indicate that at least in this one fairly typical university hospital those experiencing pain associated with their malignancy may experience intense amounts of unrelieved pain during the final weeks of their lives.

In summary, the estimates of incidence of pain in cancer vary widely, and there is little systematic evidence regarding pain and pain patterns associated with cancer. There is agreement that in the early stages of cancer there may be little or no pain. The pain that is experienced generally is that associated with treatment of the cancer, such as short-term acute postoperative pain following excision of a tumor. The cancer itself seldom causes pain in stage I, the localized or initial stage. In stage II, the regional involvement or intermediate stage, there may be more pain, and frequently there is pain associated with stage III or the advanced stage.

Many of the estimates of pain incidence are based on clinicians' experience. Considering that such estimates depend in part on the setting in which clients are treated, the kinds of people seen, the clinicians' values and beliefs, and so forth, it is understandable that the estimates are highly variable. It would be a useful contribution for nurses to conduct and participate in studies systematically describing the nature and extent of pain associated with cancer.

Causes of pain in cancer

Pain may be due to the disease itself, to a treatment or procedure related to the illness, or to a condition unrelated to the cancer. In the following, these sources of pain are dealt with separately.

Bone pain. As noted earlier, one study[14] indicated that approximately 50% of the pain experienced by hospitalized clients is the result of bone disease, either primary or metastatic. When bones are involved, this may lead to pathologic fractures. If the lesions are in the vertebrae, it may cause collapse of the body of the vertebra thus leading to compression of the nerves and roots and the spinal cord. Cord compression may also be caused by a soft tissue mass within the spinal cord. These lesions have often been missed even by neurologists, since x-ray examinations, bone scans, and neurologic examination may fail to demonstrate the disease process until it is too late. In clients who are complaining of severe back pain that increases on lying flat, who may also report a feeling of pins and needles or numbness in the upper or lower extremities, or who may be having urinary problems, one must suspect the possibility of an impending cord compression. The diagnosis can be made by doing a myelogram. If these symptoms are ignored, the end result is paraplegia, which in many instances may not be reversible even with treatment.

Obstruction. Intestinal obstruction, another complication seen in clients with advanced cancer of the pancreas, colon, uterus, and ovaries, will manifest itself by the client complaining of severe abdominal cramping, nausea and vomiting, constipation, or diarrhea.

Involvement or obstruction by a tumor of a hollow viscus such as the esophagus, stomach, gallbladder, urinary bladder, or ureters, will cause severe burning along with sharp or dull pain.

The blockage of blood vessels or lymphatics or the stretching of pain-sensitive tissues often is described as a pressure, pulling type of pain, although other descriptive terms may be used.[36]

Neurologic involvement. Involvement of peripheral nerves, plexus or root, is seen in clients with tumor invading the brachial plexus, lumbar plexus, or sacral plexus. Radicular pain is the presenting complaint.

Central nervous system disease such as carcinomatous meningitis and brain tumors are often missed because pain may not be significant. These clients may complain of a slight headache, low back pain, dizziness, nausea, or may show signs of behavioral changes such as paranoia, visual hallucinations, disorientation, and confusion. The symptoms may become more pronounced when clients are receiving potent narcotic analgesics. In many cases, the narcotics will be blamed for this behavior and the underlying disease missed.

Inflammatory problems. Infection, inflammation, ulceration, and fistula will cause pain. It is sometimes surprising to hear physicians dismiss these as causes of pain, especially if the client has no evidence of active disease.

Pain caused by treatment. The surgical excision of tumors will produce acute postoperative pain to be dealt with in much the same way as any postoperative pain. In addition, the surgical removal of primary tumors of the breast, lung, and head and neck may cause pain in the incisional area after the healing of the incision. These are called postmastectomy, postthorectomy, and postradical neck surgery syndromes. The clients will complain of burning, numbness, or "a funny feeling" months after the surgery. Phantom-limb pain after the amputation of extremities may continue for years. This should not be confused with *phantom-limb sensation,* which is the experience of feeling that an amputated part is still a part of the body.

Radiation therapy may cause fibrosis or necrosis, which will produce pain even though there is no evidence of the original disease. In the last few years, it has been demonstrated that radiation may induce peripheral nerve tumors in areas that had been irradiated. These treatment-produced cancers can also give rise to pain.

Chemotherapeutic agents such as vincristine have accounted for peripheral neuropathy that may incite pain for approximately 2 months. The aftermath of herpes zoster will create a postherpetic syndrome that may cause months of suffering.

One or more of these factors for pain can be found in an individual client and each must be treated adequately in order to provide the maximal relief.

Prior pain experiences. An additional factor to consider in trying to assess the cause of specific pains in people with cancer is the observation made by many clinicians that a person who has experienced some kind of pain prior to the onset of cancer may later misattribute that same pain to the cancer. Miller notes, for example, that a person who has had occasional backaches prior to the onset of cancer may, after learning of the diagnosis of cancer, be afraid that the backache represents a metastasis to the spine.[32] An important point to remember is that all pain experienced by a person with cancer is not necessarily attributable to the cancer or the cancer treatment. It may be caused by a preexisting condition or another condition that develops subsequent to the onset of cancer. This, of course, even further complicates the assessment of cancer pains.

Pain assessment in cancer

Lack of standardized terms. The problem of the difficulty in pain assessment because of the subjectivity of the experience was noted earlier. Clients often have difficulty describing what they are experiencing even though they may want to do so because of a general lack of ability to articulate or express what they are feeling.[15] They may not have the vocabulary to be able to communicate to the health professionals in a way that makes identification of the source of pain clear. In addition, Black and Chapman note that there is no standard taxonomy of pain, "but the terms used force the clinician to condense a constellation of problems related to human suffering into a single diagnostic category with a single therapy."[3] There are literally dozens of words that can be used to describe pain. A few of these are "flickering, pulsing, beating, flashing, boring, stabbing, cutting, pinching, gnawing, crushing, pulling, wrenching, hot, scalding, itchy, stinging, sore, aching, hurting, taut, splitting, exhausting, sickening, frightful, punishing, vicious, wretched, blinding, troublesome, intense, radiating, piercing, numb, squeezing, tearing, freezing, nagging, agonizing, and so forth."[30]

In spite of the numerous causes of pain and ways to describe it, there are some general guidelines that can be useful in assessing the origin and other characteristics of a person's pain. Table 18-2 was developed by Johnson to summarize the major characteristics of pain as they are related to the source of pain.

Major sources of pain. As Table 18-2 indicates, specific types of pain seem to produce relatively consistent sensations that are described in similar terms. The table indicates three major sources of pain. Cutaneous pain is well localized and commonly has an initial sharp sensation followed by a dull burning sensation that lasts longer. Deep somatic pain is poorly localized, described as boring and dull, and often occurs with inflamed joints. Visceral pain also is poorly localized and, depending on its cause, may be dull and aching or very sharp.

Location and intensity. In attempting to determine the source of pain, some important characteristics to note are its location and intensity, the words used by the person to describe the quality of the pain, and the chronology of the pain, including its onset, what precipitates it, and the kinds of variation in intensity and quality.[23]

One practical suggestion made by Twycross in identifying the kinds of pain being experienced by a person is to use a body chart to explain graphically the sources and

Table 18-2. Characteristics of pain as commonly related to source of pain*

Source	Location	Intensity	Quality	Chronology
Cutaneous	Well localized	Correlates with intensity of stimulus	Bimodal sensation may occur; sharp, tingling, stinging; abnormal surface sensations may occur	Correlates with stimulus changes and tissue damage; may be steady or throbbing in inflamed tissues
Deep somatic	Poorly localized; may localize with tendon, periosteum, ligament pain; may be referred to body surface	Correlates with intensity of stimulus and with movement of involved area	Vague, aching, boring, dull; cutaneous tenderness may accompany	May be steady or change in character with stimulus change or movement; correlates with stimulus changes
Visceral	Poorly localized; may localize as duration extends; may be referred to body surface	May be severe with colic; may increase if not relieved; correlates with intensity of stimulus	Vague, dull, aching, burning; if continues, may become sharper; if due to obstruction, may be gripping, cramping, twisting	Obstructive pain generally occurs in cycles; untreated pain may mount; correlates with stimulus changes

*From Johnson, M.: Assessment of clinical pain. In Jacox, A. K., editor: Pain: a sourcebook for nurses and other health professionals, Boston, 1977, Little, Brown & Co.

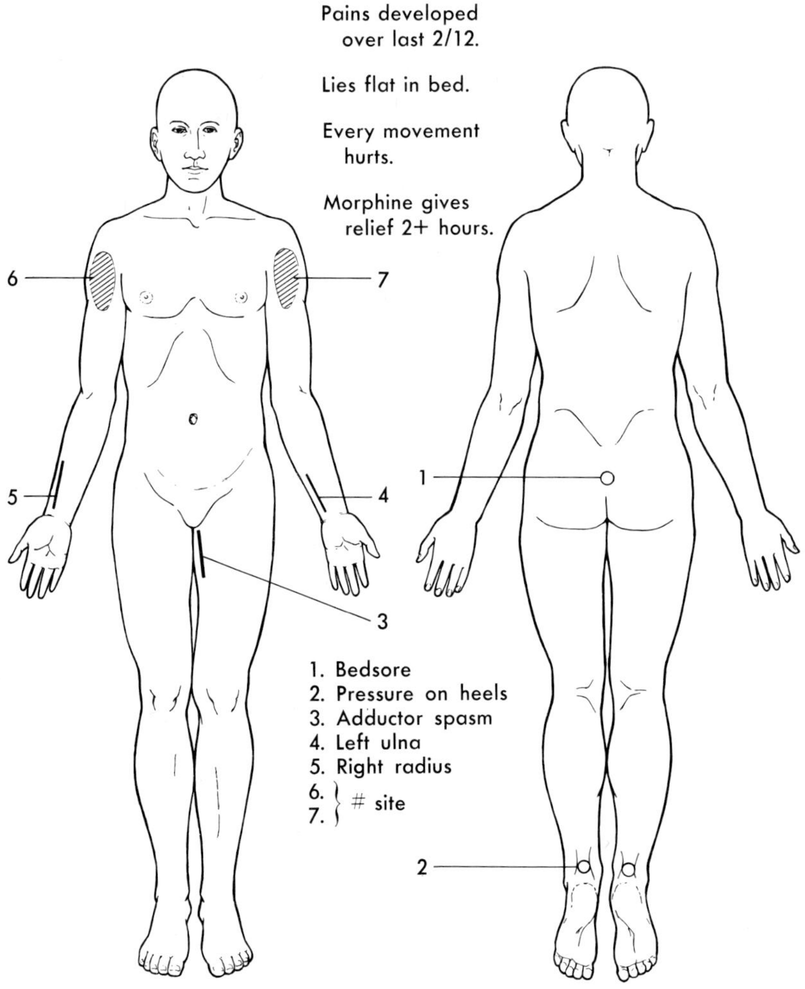

Fig. 18-1. Body chart. # = Site of pathology. Body chart used to record pain data relating to 65-year-old man with cancer of the prostate gland. (Modified from Twycross, R. G.: J. Med. Ethics **4:**112, 1978.)

nature of the pains[47] (Fig. 18-1). A careful and systematic pictorial description of the location of various pains done at periodic intervals can be useful in assessing progress in dealing with certain kinds of pain and in reminding both client and clinician that pain may be of various origins.

Another observation with regard to pain assessment in people with cancer is that for many clients an increase in the intensity of pain is to them an indication of the progression of the disease. While this may be true in some cases, it is not in many others. Because of this tendency to associate increasing pain with progression of the disease, clients may be reluctant to admit to themselves or others the presence or severity of pain. One anecdotal example comes from a study in which one of the authors (A.J.) was involved. In an attempt to learn how clients discriminate between the words "pain" and "discomfort," a research assistant was asking a convenience sample of hospitalized clients to indicate on one scale of 0 to 10 how much pain the person was experiencing at the time and on a second scale from 0 to 10 how much discomfort. One woman with cancer had indicated to another nurse 10 minutes before that she was experiencing no pain at all because, as she related, the physician had just put her on a new course of treatment that she was hopeful would control the disease. However, while she indicated to the research assistant that she was feeling no pain, she indicated that her discomfort level was 10, or "as uncomfortable as I could possibly be." This seems to be a fairly clear example of the need in some clients to deny the pain in the hopes that it will deny the disease itself. It also is an indication of the need for nurses to use multiple words in addition to pain in trying to determine what kinds of unpleasant sensations a person is feeling and also to attempt to learn what the pain means to a client.

Attitudes of health professionals. Another factor to remember in assessing pain is that the attitude of the health professional toward pain may influence the assessment of the client's pain. Thomas Hackett, a psychiatrist, noted a series of prejudices that characterize physicians but likely apply equally to nurses.[17] Hackett notes that one problem in assessment of pain is that clients experiencing chronic pain are expected to display the same behaviors as those experiencing acute pain. This of course is not a reasonable expectation since many clients who have chronic pain learn to control the expression of their symptoms. A second prejudice is the belief of health professionals that in order to hurt, pain must have an organic basis. "Following the tradition of Virchow, we must see cellular pathology before we trust the symptoms. In other words, the cell is more reliable than the person. While I would not claim this to be untrue in all cases, it is in many . . ."[17]

Hackett identifies as a third bias health professionals' tendency to undermedicate clients because of an often unreasonable concern for iatrogenic addiction. Although this attitude of health professionals has been somewhat modified in the past few years with the advent of the hospice concept and wider acceptance of a more humane approach to relieving clients from unnecessary pain, it still exists widely.

The attitude of health professionals and others toward pain complaints is illustrated in a study done in 1972 in which clients were asked to indicate whether or not they liked to discuss their pain with others.[22] In a sample of 30 clients experiencing pain associated with cancer, 17 indicated that they did not like to talk about their pain. Of these, more than a third said the reason for not wanting to talk about it was that there was some social stigma attached to complaining. Examples of some of these responses are: "I rarely discuss it unless someone asks me." "I'm not one of those hypochondriacs." "No one likes a complainer."

In summary, pain assessment is a complex process that involves knowledge of the numerous sources of pain, ability to elicit accurate and understandable pain descriptions, and acknowledgment of one's own attitudes toward pain. The accurate assessment of pain is necessary to informed action for pain alleviation.

INTERVENTIONS FOR CONTROLLING PAIN

As noted earlier, many people realize that pain may indicate the presence of disease, and in clients who have had cancer, the onset of pain may cause intense anxiety and fear. Is this the beginning of the end? Will they be able to treat it? These questions are constantly tormenting the client who may not be able to verbalize these fears. Health professionals must be aware of what pain means to the client, and an effort should be made to relieve the pain as quickly as possible. This may be attempted through use of biologically based interventions such as interruption of the pain pathways and psychosocially based interventions such as relaxation techniques and hypnosis or some combination of these. In this section, biologically based techniques are considered first, followed by a discussion of psychosocially based interventions for pain relief.

Biologically based techniques

Interruption of pain pathways. Although clients may accept the temporary relief of pain with the use of analgesics, they prefer the more definitive approach of treatment of the disease. Because the permanent alleviation of pain may assure them that the cause of the pain has been treated successfully, people who continue to experience pain may seek further surgery, radiation therapy, or chemotherapy.[36] It is not unusual to find people who have received all these definitive modalities for whom the pain continues unrelentingly.

Depending on the client's condition, prognosis, and benefits derived, the interruption or modification of pain pathways may be considered. The most commonly used interventions are nerve blocks, cordotomy, acupuncture, and noninvasive techniques such as transcutaneous nerve stimulators. The client must be prepared for the possibility that any of these methods may prove unsuccessful, for nothing is a panacea in the management of pain.

Nerve blocks. In many hospitals and pain clinics, nerve blocks are preferred even before the use of narcotics. Bonica has stated that his own personal experiences during the past 35 years and the experience reported by others suggests that skillfully administered in properly selected clients, nerve blocks are among the most effective methods of relieving cancer pain. On the other hand, these procedures improperly applied result in failure and, at times, serious complications.[5] To avoid or determine the possibility that adverse effects can occur, diagnostic nerve blocks using a short-acting anesthetic agent such as lidocaine, which lasts only a few hours, should be done first. This will also determine the specific nociceptive or pain pathways, the distribution and focus of pain, and it will give the client the opportunity to experience the numbness that occurs and the possible side-effects. There are many clients who find that the numbness or other adverse effects such as dysfunction of bladder and rectal sphincter and limb-muscle weakness can be more disturbing than the actual pain. In some instances, these diagnostic blocks alone may decrease burning cancer pain and muscle tension pain.

Neurolytic agents used in promoting longer relief by destroying nociceptive pathways are alcohol (hypobaric) and phenol (hyperbaric) solutions. Some anesthesiologists prefer phenol because it diffuses less readily than alcohol, it has less effect on tissues adjacent to the nerves being blocked, and it appears to give a longer lasting block.[16]

Since a list of all types of blocks would be considerable, only a few will be mentioned.

Type of block	Site of cancer
Stellate ganglion block (local anesthetics)	Metastatic breast (pain in area of affected side)
Alcohol celiac (splanchnic plexus block)	Pancreas, stomach, liver and bile ducts, gallbladder

Type of block	Site of cancer
Intrathecal phenol block	Cervix, rectum, colon, bladder, kidney, bone, lung pleura, mediastinum
Subarachnoid and extradural blocks (alcohol or phenol)	Rectum, cervix, bronchus, breast, colon
Cranial nerve block (alcohol or phenol)	Head, face, and neck

Cordotomies. Like nerve blocks, cordotomies, open or percutaneous, have adverse effects similar to those of nerve blocks and are not always successful. Therefore, the adverse effects must be weighed against the benefits derived from these procedures. Even when they are successful, pain may recur in several months.

In an open cordotomy, a laminectomy and a complete unilateral transection of the anterolateral quadrant of the cord are made. This is usually done at the upper thoracic or cervical levels and will relieve only the lancinating, toothache-like pain carried by the anterolateral ascending system or the lateral spinothalamic tract. This is a major surgical procedure and it may not be tolerated well by many cancer clients, especially since there is a high incidence of weakness of one side of the body and bladder dysfunction.

Percutaneous cordotomy entails the interruption of the anterolateral quadrant of the cord by the insertion of a coagulating probe in the upper or lower cervical level in the spinal cord under x-ray control. This procedure seems to offer the same amount of pain relief as the open cordotomy with fewer adverse effects even when done bilaterally.[39]

Acupuncture. Acupuncture received a great deal of attention a few years ago; because of this, a pilot study was done at Memorial Sloan-Kettering Cancer Center in clients who had pain caused by cancer. The results were disappointing. Bonica has stated that he has reviewed the American literature and could not find that anyone was using acupuncture, and therefore there are no statistics. He also pointed out that in his 3-week visit to the People's Republic of China he was surprised to find that this was one of the few areas in which the Chinese do not use acupuncture. Bonica concluded that apparently the Chinese had tried it and it is no longer used.[4]

Transcutaneous nerve stimulator. A transcutaneous electrical nerve stimulation (TNS) device consists of a battery-generated, solid-state compact pulse generator connected by cables to transmitting electrodes placed on the skin and held in position by straps, adhesives, or tapes. The client controls output of the pulse generator and most units also have controls for intensity, rate, and pulse duration of waveform. Peak current amplitudes vary from less than 1 milliampere to more than 100 milliamperes. The electrodes are placed on the skin over the site of the pain. In some instances placement is made distally.

Adverse effects have been minimal and have involved skin reaction and burns at the electrode sites. TNS should be avoided in those clients with demand cardiac pacemakers. Further, health providers should avoid placement of the electrodes over the carotid sinuses to avoid vagovagal reflexes, and the use of electrodes should be avoided in clients during the first trimester of pregnancy. All clients should be warned to avoid sudden movement of the pulse generator controls to avoid a "startle" response that could have adverse consequences during operation of a motor vehicle or a potentially dangerous piece of machinery.[7] Results of the success of TNS vary depending on the type of pain and the enthusiasm of the reporter. In pain caused by cancer, the success rate has been low; however, there have only been a few reports thus far published. Ventafridda[48] states that in treating clients with chronic pain syndrome of cancer origin, the long-term usefulness of the stimulating device is quite limited. He notes that "even if a high percentage of patients initially respond well to the method of pain modulation, the success rate declines rapidly. After a month or so, it continues to be effective in only a small percentage of patients."[48] At Memorial Sloan-Kettering Cancer Center, the results have been similar.

Central gray stimulation. A new technique for the relief of pain is the electrical stimulation of the periaqueductal (PAG) or the periventricular gray (PVG) matter in the brain. Although thus far only a few clients with cancer pain have been treated with this technique, limited experience has shown that it may be an effective way of relieving intense cancer pain.

The technique (PVG) used by Richardson[35] involves two steps: (1) the insertion of a single, four-contact, pulldown, platinum electrode through a coronal burr hole on the side opposite the more intense pain, using a Trent Wells sterotactic instrument under local anesthesia. Final positioning and locking of the electrodes is done after stimulation testing determines adequate pain relief and minimal side-effects. For the next 2 weeks, periodic testing is done for effectiveness and side-effects before step 2, the internaturalization of the system. (2) This is done under general anesthesia and entails the implantation of a receiver in the pectoral area and connected to the two most effective electrode contacts through a mastering connector in the parietal area. Internal settings in the transmitter allow variations of pulse width, frequency, and maximum voltage. These are selected during the period of testing. The client achieves stimulation by slowly increasing the variable voltage until no side-effects are felt. This is carried out for approximately 10 to 30 minutes every 2 to 4 hours each day.

Analgesics. When all efforts to control disease or pain have failed, the one method left that will provide some measure of relief is analgesics. The failure of analgesics to control pain has been due primarily to the *inadequate knowledge of the pharmacology of analgesics and the misconceptions and attitudes of those health care professionals who are involved in the care of people who have pain caused by cancer.*

Analgesics are readily available, easily administered, comparatively safe, and most of their adverse effects are reversible.[33] In the last several decades, controlled clinical trials of analgesics have provided meaningful data as to their relative potency and side-effects, enabling practitioners to manage pain more effectively with the proper use of analgesics.[18]

Analgesics have been classified by many as nonnarcotic or narcotic, mild or potent, addicting or nonaddicting, with certain analgesics specified for use only in acute pain and others only in chronic pain. Unfortunately, these classifications have contributed more to confusion than to enlightenment in dealing with pain owing to cancer. Every client is unique, and studies of relative potency, biotransformation, absorption, and elimination have shown that the response to analgesics can vary considerably from one individual to another.[24] Therefore, every client cannot be expected to respond the same way to an analgesic or to a particular dose of an analgesic.[38] In determining the proper analgesic and the adequate dose of an analgesic for a client, the following factors have to be considered.

1. Is the client having acute or chronic pain?

2. What route of administration is the most suitable in this particular situation?
3. What is the client's condition and prognosis?
4. Has the client been receiving analgesics? If so, what analgesics, dose, and route, and for how long?
5. Is the client sensitive or allergic to analgesics?
6. What other drugs is the client receiving?
7. Is the client in the hospital or at home?

It is difficult to specify in detail the multitude of factors that must be considered when using analgesics for pain relief. What follows are some general points to consider, together with some specific examples to illustrate a representative set of situations that health professionals may encounter.

Situation 1. There is no direct relationship between type of pain experienced and size or route of dosage. The client with acute pain, for example, may require a large dose of a potent analgesic such as morphine, 20 mg IM intramuscularly. Conversely, the client with chronic pain may be adequately controlled on an intermediate analgesic, for example, Percocet-5, one tablet (oxycodone, 5 mg, plus acetaminophen, 325 mg) every 3 hours by or around the clock (ATC).

Situation 2. The client is vomiting or unable to swallow and thus is unable to take oral analgesics. The client's platelets are only 48,000, which means that he will not be able to be given analgesics intramuscularly (IM), subcutaneously (SQ), or by rectal suppository. In this situation, the only route available is intravenously (IV). The therapeutic IV dose is usually one half of the IM dose titrating up and down as needed. Intravenous narcotics will have a peak effect in approximately 15-50 minutes. Duration of effect, however, will be shortened. Tolerance to narcotics given by this route will develop very quickly within 2 to 3 days, requiring that the dose be increased every 2 to 3 days.

Tolerance will develop to narcotics given intramuscularly in approximately 2 weeks. Tolerance to oral narcotics will develop more slowly. Physical dependence goes hand in hand with tolerance; therefore, a client receiving narcotics for several weeks must gradually be tapered off the narcotics when the pain has subsided.

Situation 3. The client's prognosis is guarded, but not terminal, with condition listed as poor. The client is dehydrated, electrolytes are unbalanced, and blood urea nitrogen (BUN), lactic dehydrogenase (LDH), and calcium are all elevated above normal. The client is vomiting, short of breath, tremulous, disoriented and confused, and complaining of severe pain that is not being controlled with meperidine (Demerol), 75 mg IM every 3 hours. Since the client's BUN is elevated, meperidine should be avoided. Recent blood level studies have shown that repeated administration of meperidine to clients with compromised renal function may lead to the accumulation of the toxic metabolite, normeperidine, thus producing central nervous system excitation ranging from apprehension to tremors and seizures. Measurement of the plasma normeperidine levels in clients who have received repeated doses of meperidine suggests that the level of normeperidine is related to the different degrees of these side-effects.[45] Recent studies have shown that this can also occur after repeated doses of meperidine in clients without renal dysfunction.[24] The elevated LDH suggests that the client may have lung disease, which may account for shortness of breath, disorientation, and confusion. The elevated calcium may also be causing disorientation and confusion. All drugs that cause sedation should be avoided. The client is vomiting and is receiving prochlorperazine (Compazine), 10 mg IM. The tremors have been interpreted as anxiety. The client is also receiving diazepam (Valium), 5 mg IM. Prochlorperazine and diazepam should be discontinued. Trimethobenzamide (Tigan) or hydroxyzine (Vistaril) can be used instead for the vomiting. Since the client is no longer receiving meperidine, tremors will decrease; the client may be less disoriented and confused when prochlorperazine and diazepam are discontinued. Morphine, 5 mg IM every 2 hours, or hydromorphone (Dilaudid), 0.75 mg IM every 2 hours, may control the client's pain without compromising the breathing.

Situation 4. The client has been taking levorphanol (Levo-Dromoran), 6 mg orally every 4 hours for the past 2 months. In the past few weeks, duration of effect has lessened. The client's pain returns in 2½ hours; this is the first sign of the development of tolerance. The dose will have to be increased and, in many cases, the time interval decreased. In this situation, physicians are reluctant to increase the dose. They may be sure the client is becoming a drug addict and may also fear that the client will have respiratory depression with the increased dose. Tolerance is a pharmacologic effect of all narcotics, and it is not synonymous with addiction or drug abuse. Tolerance can develop to other drugs as well as to narcotics and to other effects of the drug such as respiratory depression. There is cross-tolerance to other narcotics; however, this is not complete.[37] In some instances, it may be advisable to switch to another narcotic or add an antipyretic-type analgesic (aspirin or acetaminophen). Since this class of drugs acts on a different mechanism than narcotic analgesics (aspirin inhibits prostaglandin synthesis),[42] the effect will be additive. A narcotic antagonist such as pentazocine (Talwin) should not be administered, since this will produce a withdrawal syndrome in clients who are physically dependent on narcotics.

Situation 5. This client has developed a rash when she has taken aspirin, codeine, and morphine. Percocet and meperidine make her vomit; however, she can tolerate propoxyphene hydrochloride (Darvon) and acetaminophen (Tylenol). Unfortunately, these drugs do not relieve her pain even when given together. Since propoxyphene hydrochloride (Darvon) is closely related to methadone (Dolophine) and methadone is more potent, it would be the narcotic chosen.

It is important to check all drugs that the client is taking. Tranquilizers such as diazepam may increase sedation, disorientation, and confusion if the client is also taking potent narcotics. Diazepam will increase depression in the client already depressed. Instead of using tranquilizers, antidepressants such as amitriptyline (Elavil) may be more beneficial. Amitriptyline used at bedtime has provided better sedation, and in phantom limb, decreases in sensation and pain have been noted. Combination drugs containing aspirin should be avoided in clients taking steroids. This will increase the danger of gastrointestinal bleeding. Antipyretics should not be given if the fever curve is being watched. Physicians may forget that Darvocet-N 100, Tylox, and Percocet contain acetaminophen and that Percodan contains aspirin. Clients with liver disease should avoid taking acetaminophen and phenothiazines. These drugs may cause liver toxicity.

When a client is hospitalized, analgesics can easily be given regardless of the route. A client who is at home, however, may present a different problem. Oral analgesics can be easily administered, but if the client is vomiting or unable to swallow, the administration of parenteral narcotics may be needed. This may be difficult unless there is 24-hour nursing coverage. Many family members may be reluctant to learn how to give an injection. In some communities, hydromorphone may be available by rectal suppository. The dose required to produce the same analgesic effect as 10 mg of morphine IM is not known.

• • •

The preceding situations and many others that occur make the management of pain through use of analgesics difficult. These situations are meant to illustrate the many factors involved in the selection of the proper analgesics. The use of a fixed combination of drugs or doses may not be feasible, nor is there a magic formula that applies to all clients. Not even the "Brompton Cocktail" can achieve this. In fact, Twycross does not advocate the use of the Brompton Cocktail any longer. In recent studies, he has concluded that oral morphine in tap water produces the same analgesic effect as the Brompton Cocktail without the side-effects of the Brompton Cocktail. He concludes "The Brompton Cocktail is, therefore, merely a traditional way of prescribing oral (dia) morphine. It is not the panacea nor does it possess magical properties. In practice a combination of drug, non-drug, and common-sense measures are necessary to achieve maximum benefit."[46]

Mechanisms of action of morphine and electrical stimulation. Recent research in pain and pain alleviation has suggested that the body has the ability to produce its own pain-reducing mechanisms. This section presents some of the recent findings.

The understanding of the mechanism of action of morphine is based on recent research that has made it possible to identify a portion of the outer surface of certain nerve cells that attract and hold morphine molecules. These sites are called *opiate receptors*. When morphine combines with an opiate receptor, the structure of the receptor changes and produces a biochemical alteration in the properties of the nerve cell. To produce analgesia, the drug administered must fit the receptor site and activate the receptor. Since opiate receptors have been found in the spinal cord, brain stem, thalamus, and limbic system and are concentrated in each relay station along the pain pathway, pain impulses may be intercepted or modified at one or more of these relay stations, thus preventing the pain impulses from reaching the cerebral cortex. Morphine acts via the opiate receptor to short-circuit pain impulses.

The discovery of naturally occurring morphinelike substances (endorphins in the pituitary, enkephalins in different parts of the nervous system) tends to parallel the distribution of opiate receptors. Evidence now indicates that the enkephalins are neurotransmitters of specific neuronal systems that mediate the integration of sensory information concerned with pain and emotional behavior. When the enkephalin neuron is activated, it releases enkephalin onto the opiate receptor, and, like morphine, the message is short-circuited.[42] Data suggest that electrical stimulation of specific areas of the brain (PAG, PVG) and the nervous system (TNS) induces the release of enkephalin. At first, it was thought that the TNS blocked pain by the "gate control theory." We do not know what physiologic mechanism is involved in the activation of the enkephalin neurons. A better understanding of this system may explain the differences in pain tolerance and pain behavior, help in the development of new analgesics, and increase our knowledge of pain mechanisms.

The role of the nurse in the management of pain through analgesics. Nurses

Table 18-3. Commonly used analgesics

Drug	Route	Dose (mg)	Time interval	Equivalent to	Comments
Acetaminophen	PO	600	q4 hr	Aspirin, 600 mg	In large doses may cause liver toxicity; less
(Tylenol, Datril, Tempra, Nebs)	Rectal	600	q4 hr	Morphine, 2 mg IM	anti-inflammatory action
Aspirin	PO	600	q3-4 hr	Morphine, 2 mg IM	Do not use with steroids, blood dyscrasies
Codeine	PO	30-60	q3 hr	Aspirin, 600 mg	No ceiling effects, short acting
	PO	200	q3 hr	Morphine, 10 mg IM	
	IM	120	q3 hr	Morphine, 10 mg IM	
Hydromorphone	PO	7.5	q3 hr	Morphine, 10 mg IM	Short acting, quick onset of action
(Dilaudid)	IM	1.5	q3 hr		
	Rectal	?*	q3 hr		
Levorphanol	PO	4	q4 hr	Morphine, 10 mg IM	Longer acting, accumulative effects may cause
(Levo-Dromoran)	IM	2	q4 hr	Morphine, 10 mg IM	sedation, hallucination, disorientation, confusion, respiratory depression
Meperidine	PO	50	q3 hr	Aspirin, 600 mg	Short acting, quicker onset, should not be used in
(Demerol)	PO	300	q3 hr	Morphine, 10 mg IM	clients with renal dysfunction
	IM	75	q3 hr	Morphine, 10 mg IM	
Methadone	PO	20	q4 hr	Morphine, 10 mg IM	Longer acting, accumulative effect causes sedation,
(Dolophine)	IM	10	q4 hr	Morphine, 10 mg IM	confusion, respiratory depression

Morphine	PO	60	q4 hr		Standard narcotic
	IM	10	q4 hr		
	IV	5	q2-4 hr		
Oxycodone	PO	5	q3 hr	Morphine, 2 mg IM	Short acting, quick onset of action, in combination only: Percodan (with aspirin, phenacetin, caffeine), Percocet (with 325 mg acetaminophen), Tylox (with 325 mg acetaminophen)
Oxymorphone (Numorphan)	IM	1	q4 hr	Morphine, 10 mg IM	Long acting
	Rectal	10	q4 hr	Morphine, 10 mg IM	
Pentazocine (Talwin)		30	q3 hr	Aspirin, 600 mg	Narcotic antagonist, causes abstinence syndrome in clients physically dependent on narcotics: psychotoemetic effects, contraindication in cardiac abnormalities
	PO	180	q3 hr	Morphine, 10 mg IM	
	IM	60	q3 hr	Morphine, 10 mg IM	
Propoxyphene hydrochloride (Darvon)	PO	65	q3 hr	Aspirin, 600 mg	Similar to methadone, weak narcotic
Propoxyphene napsylate (Darvon N)	PO	100	q3 hr	Aspirin, 600 mg	Absorbed slower than propoxyphene hydrochloride, fewer side-effects (Darvocet-N 100 in combination with 650 mg acetaminophen)

*No studies have been done to determine optimal dose.

should be able to predict when analgesics may be necessary and to assess their effectiveness. To do this the nurse should become acquainted with the relative potency of the commonly used analgesics. Although there have been several equianalgesic lists published, there have been discrepancies. Table 18-3 is based on double-blind, controlled studies conducted by the Analgesic Studies Section at Sloan-Kettering Institute for Cancer Research over the past 28 years or other investigators using a similar method.[2,18,19,38,49]

In reviewing the equianalgesic list, it may be surprising to find that the ratio between oral and parenteral analgesics varies considerably from one narcotic to another. This should be noted when narcotics are offered, especially when clients are being switched from parenteral to oral narcotics. Clients should be made aware that oral narcotics will have a *slower* onset of action than parenteral and that they will need to take them *before* the pain becomes severe. Most clients tend to wait too long before asking for or taking analgesics. They have stated that they "don't want to take that much" or they "may be afraid of becoming addicted." This fear is usually perpetrated by the attitude of some of the health care professionals who believe the same. Clients should be encouraged to take analgesics on a regular basis to promote better analgesia with a less potent narcotic and fewer side-effects and less anxiety and fear, which usually increases the severity of pain. The nurse can be instrumental in teaching clients these techniques as well as in allaying fears of addiction. It is interesting to note that only approximately 1%[27] of all clients receiving narcotics will abuse narcotics after the cessation of pain and yet, in many instances, the fear of addiction is the one factor that will deter many physicians from prescribing narcotics in appropriate doses and many nurses from admininstering narcotics on a regular basis. In clients who have pain owing to cancer, few indeed have abused drugs. As soon as the pain starts to decrease, the intake of narcotics diminishes. In clients with recurrent cancer in the advanced stages, abuse is of no consequence. The one humane effort left is the adequate control of pain so that clients may die with dignity. Nurses who are dealing with these clients must understand the necessity for eliminating pain and suffering with whatever means are at their disposal. All efforts must be directed toward this goal. The nurse must truly be the "angel of mercy" in these instances.

Psychosocially based interventions

Elsewhere in this book is a chapter concerned with psychiatric treatment for problems associated with cancer. If the premise is accepted that cancer is a problem involving both the mind and the body, this has implications for interventions both for the cancer itself and for the pain associated with cancer.

There are two ways in which psychosocially based interventions in cancer can be considered. One kind of intervention is directed at cure of the cancer itself, and hence the pain and other symptoms associated with it. The second set of interventions is directed at alleviation of symptoms produced by the cancer or cancer treatment, including the symptom of pain.

An example of one of the most well-known and controversial attempts to cure cancer at least in part through the application of psychosocial interventions is the work of the Simontons.[41] They combine the use of imagery with traditional biologically based treatments for cancer. Mental imagery is an introspective process that is accompanied by visual images. It is also referred to as visualization, seeing with the mind's eye, or inner vision.[1] O. Carl Simonton, a radiation oncologist, and Stephanie Mathews-Simonton, a cancer counselor, encourage clients to accept some personal responsibility for their illness and its cure. They encourage clients to realize that mind and emotions and their body act as a unit and cannot be separated.[41] The technique that the Simontons use is to teach their clients a combination of relaxation and visualization. ". . . it is a basic relaxation technique in which the patients are told to visualize their disease, their treatment, and their body's own immune mechanisms (we call them white blood cells to make it simple) acting on the disease. We tell them to do this three times a day, every day."[41] The approach involves clients' imagining their bodies fighting the cancer and eventually overcoming it. The Simontons have reported case studies in which they have illustrated the alleged success of their technique in effecting a cure of the cancer. They are presently involved in additional studies to test this on a more widespread and systematic basis.

Another approach aimed at curing cancer and the symptoms associated with it is suggested by Brown and co-workers.[6] Building on the idea that psychologic factors are involved in the etiology of cancer, they suggest that clients who participate in psychotherapy may sufficiently change their cancer-prone personality and, further, the life span may be increased for those clients who already have cancer. They note a study conducted on cancer clients in which half of those who participated in supportive psychotherapy were alive at the end of 5 years and none of those who refused to participate in the therapy were alive at that point.

Finally, there are a number of clinicians and researchers who have reported the use of psychosocially based interventions to treat the pain and other symptoms associated with cancer. Dempster and co-workers,[12] for example, report the use of hypnotism to provide support for clients during the radical treatment of malignancies. Acknowledging the physical discomforts that frequently accompany radical cancer therapies, such as drawing blood, obtaining bone marrow specimens, and similar procedures, the authors suggest that the discomfort of these procedures can often be reduced by hypnotherapy. They report cases where hypnotherapy decreased the anticipatory anxiety associated with treatment and generally helped clients deal with the prospect of death.

There are a number of cognitively based interventions that have been used with persons experiencing pain associated with conditions other than cancer. Some of these studies have been with experimentally induced pain, such as subjecting a person to electric shock or intense heat. Other studies have been done on persons with clinical pain. While few studies have had cancer clients as subjects, there is need for clinicians and clinical investigators to be creative in their use of pain-alleviating interventions with cancer generally. Therefore, even though the interventions have not been used to treat cancer pain, they are summarized here briefly.

Use of these interventions to increase either pain threshold or pain tolerance can be grouped into two broad categories: one in which the effort is centered primarily within the person experiencing the pain and the other in which someone other than the person experiencing the pain tries to increase the threshold or tolerance. Examples of the first category include giving the person information that will reduce anxiety associated with pain and thus reduce the pain, reinterpreting sensations to encourage the person to view the experience more positively, giving the person control over when and how much pain will be experienced, and using biofeedback to help the person regulate his own responses. Examples of the second category are distraction, hypnosis, social modeling, and operant conditioning. A summary of each of these methods and a report of the studies using them is available elsewhere.[21]

One of the authors (A.K.J.) was involved in a study in which one group of clients with pain associated with advanced cancer was randomly assigned to learn a series of relaxation techniques while a second group was assigned to receive the usual nursing care.[20] The technique involved a tape recording of a series of exercises in which the clients progressively tensed and relaxed muscles throughout their body. While there were no significant differences in the amount of pain and anxiety experienced by the clients in the experimental group and those in the control group over the entire course of the study, there were some interesting reactions among the clients who received the relaxation therapy. Some clients found the relaxation methods very useful in reducing primarily their anxiety and in some clients their pain. They reported continuing to use the relaxation techniques following discharge from the hospital. Other clients, in contrast, found the relaxation techniques to be more anxiety producing than reducing. For these clients, it was speculated that asking them to actively visualize and focus on parts of their bodies that were deteriorating through disease produced a negative psychologic effect. A conclusion of the study was that the use of relaxation techniques and similar methods that require the client to take an active role in *responding* to the illness must be undertaken with great care and with an exploration of how people generally may respond to the content of the procedure.

Finally, the recent advent of hospices in this country is explicit acknowledgment of the need to treat cancer pain and other symptoms within a generally supportive atmosphere. One of the objectives of the hospice is to anticipate and reduce the pain and anxiety rather than expect clients to suffer unnecessarily. An extension of the hospice idea is that of the home care program that has been carried out by members of hospices as well as by community health nurses.

CONCLUSION

Many nurses, professionally and personally, have seen clients or loved ones suffering needlessly because of the mismanagement of pain owing to cancer. In the past several years, there have been attempts to rectify this, but those attempts have not been universal. The education of health care professionals in this area has been sadly neglected. Since nurses are the health professionals most frequently and consistently in contact with people with cancer, it seems reasonable to expect them to become significantly more involved in the assessment and management of pain. This is particularly essential in the person who has pain owing to cancer. Although pain may not be a sign or symptom in the early stages of cancer, it frequently will be the first sign or symptom in those with metastatic, recurrent, or advanced cancer. Therefore, it is necessary to diagnose the cause of pain correctly. This may be difficult since the pain may be due to the disease itself, the treatment of the disease, or a condition totally unrelated to the cancer. Unfortunately, failure by a health care provider to accurately identify the source of pain may result in its being called "psychogenic" and dismissed. In such cases, people have been referred to psychiatrists, and months later the reason for their pain becomes apparent.

There is need for nurses and others who work with cancer clients to understand the basic principles of pain assessment and alleviation and to be able to apply these to clients with cancer. This chapter has described pain assessment and management generally, with illustrations representative of the numerous complex situations that may be encountered by clients with cancer and those who care for them.

REFERENCES

1. Achterberg, J., and Lawlis, G. F.: Imagery of cancer, Champaign, Ill., 1978, Institute for Personality and Ability Testing.
2. Beaver, W. T., et al.: A clinical comparison of the analgesic effects of methadone and morphine administered intramuscularly, and of orally and parenterally administered methadone, Clin. Pharmacol. Ther. **8**:415, 1967.
3. Black, R. G., and Chapman, C. R.: SAD index for clinical assessment of pain. In Bonica, J. J., and Albe-Fessard, D. G., editors: Advances in pain research and therapy, vol. 1, New York, 1976, Raven Press.
4. Bonica, J. J.: Therapeutic acupuncture in the People's Republic of China, J.A.M.A. **228**(12):1544, 1974.
5. Bonica, J. J.: Introduction to nerve blocks. In Bonica, J. J., and Ventafridda, V., editors: Advances in pain research and therapy, vol. 2, New York, 1978, Raven Press.
6. Brown, S. B., et al.: Psychological factors in the etiology of lung cancer, Va. Med. Mo. **102**:935, 1975.
7. Burton, C.: Transcutaneous electrical nerve stimulation to relieve pain, Postgrad. Med. **59**:6, 1976.
8. Cartwright, A., Houckey, L., and Anderson, J. L.: Life before death, London, 1973, Routledge.
9. Chapman, R.: Psychologic and behavioral aspects of cancer pain. In Bonica, J. J., and Ventafridda, V., editors: Advances in pain research and therapy, vol. 3, New York, 1979, Raven Press.
10. Cole, R.: The problem of pain in persistent cancer, Med. J. Aust. **1**:682, 1965.
11. Craig, T. J., and Abeloff, M. D.: Psychiatric symptomatology among hospitalized cancer patients, Am. J. Psychol. **131**:1323, 1974.
12. Dempster, C. R.: Supportive hypnotherapy during the radical treatment of malignancies, Int. J. Clin. Exp. Hypn. **24**:1, 1976.
13. Evans, R. J.: Intractable pain associated with malignancy, Appl. Theor. **12**:21, 1970.
14. Foley, K. M., et al.: Pain in patients with cancer: a quantitative appraisal, Proc. Am. Soc. Cancer Res. **19**:356, 1978.
15. Fordyce, W. E.: Behavioral methods for chronic pain and illness, St. Louis, 1976, The C. V. Mosby Co.
16. Goldiner, P. L.: The role of neurolytic agents in the treatment of pain caused by malignant disease, J. Thanatol. **2**:729, 1972.
17. Hackett, T. P.: The pain and prejudice. Why do we doubt that the patient is in pain? Med. Times **99**:130, 1971.
18. Houde, R. W.. The use and misuse of narcotics in the treatment of chronic pain. In Bonica, J. J.: Advances in neurology, vol. 4: Pain, New York, 1974, Raven Press.
19. Houde, R. W., et al.: Clinical pharmacology of analgesics. 1. A method of assaying analgesic effects, Clin. Pharmacol. Ther. **1**:163, 1960.
20. Jacox, A. K.: Pain alleviation through nursing interventions. Final report of grant NU-00467, Division of Nursing, 1976, Department of Health, Education and Welfare.
21. Jacox, A. K.: Sociocultural and psychological aspects of pain. In Jacox, A. K., editor: Pain: a sourcebook for nurses and other health professionals, Boston, 1977, Little, Brown & Co.
22. Jacox, A. K., and Stewart, M.: Psychosocial contingencies of the pain experience, Iowa City, 1973, University of Iowa School of Nursing.
23. Johnson, M.: Assessment of clinical pain. In Jacox, A. K., editor: Pain: a sourcebook for nurses and other health professionals, Boston, 1977, Little, Brown & Co.
24. Kaiko, R. F., and Houde, R. W.: Relationship between methadone plasma levels and analgesia in cancer patients (abstract), Pharmacologist **18**:178, 1976.
25. Lloyd, J. W., et al.: The pain of cancer, Practitioner **220**:453, 1978.
26. Luce, J. K., and Dawson, J. J.: Quality of life, Semin. Oncol. **2**:323, 1975.
27. Marks, R. M., and Sachar, E. J.: Undertreatment of medical inpatient with narcotic analgesics, Ann. Intern. Med. **78**:2, 1973.
28. Melzack, R.: The puzzle of pain, New York, 1973, Basic Books, Publishers Inc.
29. Melzack, R., and Casey, K. C.: Sensory, motivational and central control determinants of pain: a new conceptual model. In Kenshado, D., editor: The skin senses, Springfield, Ill., 1968, Charles C Thomas, Publisher.
30. Melzack, R., and Targenson, W. S.: On the language of pain, Anesthesia **34**:50, 1971.
31. Melzack, R., and Wall, P. D.: Psychophysiology of pain, Int. Anesthesiol. Clin. **8**:3, 1970.
32. Miller, T. R.: Psychophysiologic aspects of cancer, Cancer **39**:413, 1977.

33. Mines, S.: The conquest of pain, New York, 1974, Grosset & Dunlap, Inc.
34. Request for research grant applications: RFA, a pilot study of cancer pain, NIH guide for grants and contracts, vol. 7, no. 13, Bethesda, Md., 1978.
35. Richardson, D. E., and Akil, H.: Pain reduction by electric brain stimulation in man. Part II. Chronic self-administration in periventricular gray matter, J. Neurosurg. **47:**18, 1977.
36. Rogers, A.: Pain and the cancer patient, Nurs. Clin. North Am. **2:**4, 1967.
37. Rogers, A.: Drugs for pain, Proceedings of the American Cancer Society Second Conference on Cancer Nursing, May, 1977.
38. Rogers, A. G.: Pharmacology of analgesics, J. Neurosurg. Nurs. **10:**4, 1978.
39. Rosomoff, H. L.: Bilateral percutaneous cervical radiofrequency cordotomy, J. Neurosurg. **31:**41, 1969.
40. Saunders, C.: The management of terminal illness, Hosp. Med. **1**(4):317, 1967.
41. Simonton, O. C., and Simonton, S. S.: Belief systems and management of the emotional aspects of malignancy, J. Transpersonal Psychol. **1:**29, 1975.
42. Snyder, S. H.: Opiate receptors and internal opiates, Sci. Am. **236:**44, 1977.
43. Sternbach, R. A.: Pain: a psychophysiological analysis, New York, 1968, Academic Press, Inc.
44. Stewart, M. C.: Pain-drug study. Unpublished report of study of incidence of pain in cancer, supported by Grant No. NU-00467, 1976.
45. Szeta, H. H., et al.: Accumulation of normeperidine, an active metabolite of meperidine in patients with renal failure or cancer, Ann. Intern. Med. **86:**738, 1972.
46. Twycross, R. G.: Bone pain in advanced cancer. In Vere, D. W., editor: Topics in therapeutics, ed. 4, Turnbridge Well, 1978, Pittman Medical.
47. Twycross, R. G.: The assessment of pain in advanced cancer, J. Med. Ethics **4:**112, 1978.
48. Ventafridda, V., et al.: Transcultural nerve stimulation in cancer pain. In Bonica, J. J., and Ventafridda, V., editors: Advances in pain research and therapy, vol. 2, New York, 1978, Raven Press.
49. Wallenstein, S. L., and Houde, R. W.: Clinical evaluation of relative potencies of anileridine, meperidine and morphine, J. Pharmacol. Exp. Ther. **122:**81, 1958.
50. Zborowski, M.: People in pain, San Francisco, 1969, Jossey-Bass, Publishers.

19

Communication approaches to effective cancer nursing care

RUTH McCORKLE

Some of the greatest challenges that nurses face are the dilemmas associated with the interpersonal communication with persons who have cancer and their family members. This chapter will deal with the basic concepts that need to be taken into account by professional nurses when establishing a nurse-client relationship.

THE THREAT OF CANCER

There are many events that may be perceived as threatening to a person and his or her relationships with others. The individual's perception of the event as threatening requires an interpretation by the person about the significance of the stimulus situation. This interpretation process is called appraisal by Lazarus.[16] A stimulus may be perceived as threatening to one individual and nonthreatening to another. The threat is not simply out there as an attribute of the stimulus; it depends on the person's appraisal of the stimulus for its threat value, which in turn depends on the person's beliefs about what the stimulus means to that person.

When an event such as an illness occurs that is perceived as personally threatening, stress occurs that manifests itself in a period of disequilibrium. A crisis results when an individual's homeostatic mechanisms are overpowered by disequilibrium. During this time, the individual finds him or herself faced with a problem that is of basic importance because it is linked with fundamental instinctual needs and is not quickly solved by normal problem-solving mechanisms.[8]

An illness associated with a cancer diagnosis may have an additional effect on the person's perception of what is happening. The meaning of that diagnosis is a personal experience for each of those persons in whom it occurs, and there is general agreement that many people believe a diagnosis of cancer means they will die.

> In the reaction of the patient to the news he has a cancer, the significant event is a major change in the patient's relation to himself. The lesion, often minor in size and almost silent as a site of pain or distress, becomes in the most important way a symbol, and the catastrophic reaction which can be observed is a manifestation of the inner prospective relation of the reciprocal aspects of self. The meaning of the lesion-symbol is death, and this meaning radically disrupts the balance of current self with future self upon which all of our orientations are based.[22]

In addition, cancer is dreaded by most because of projected fears of pain, body changes, deterioration, increased physical and social dependency, abandonment, and death itself. Thus, when a cancer diagnosis is made, it becomes an unusually stressful experience that disrupts a person's most well-established lifelong patterns of behavior.

Delay and awareness

For the majority of people who develop cancer, it is a new experience for them. They may or may not have had a previous experience of knowing someone with cancer. If they have known someone, chances are the type of cancer and recommended treatment will be different.

Whether a person has known someone with cancer or not, nearly everyone delays taking any action for at least a short time when they first recognize the symptoms of a breakdown in the health of their own body. If the threat is perceived as organized fear, the person will seek medical help. But if the threat remains disorganized, then the person may go to the extreme of denying the existence of any warning signs or symptoms in order to emotionally survive. Some delay is expected and permits a person to adapt to the threat and to realize his or her defenses for coping with it.[4] Prediagnostic delay may be due to denial, especially when a client has someone to help foster and encourage denial. Ironically, it may be a physician who encourages the client to false security because of the difficulty in diagnosing cancer or its unexpected occurrence within a certain age group. Denial is a protective mechanism that is used repeatedly in everyday life. It is a selective process whereby the informational content of certain internal and external stimuli is unacknowledged. When denial occurs, overwhelmingly threatening thoughts or facts are not allowed to reach the person's conscious awareness, and to all intents and purposes, they do not exist for the person.[17] It is important to remember that the distinctive quality of denying and denial is its occurrence in relationship to certain people, not all people. The purpose of denial in cancer is not simply to avoid the threat of a diagnosis but to protect and prevent the loss of a significant relationship.[26]

The consequences of prolonged delay with cancer can be devastating, and yet there are people who wait until their disease becomes far advanced before seeking help. No matter what the stage of disease when the person seeks help, the nurse must be alerted to the person's fears and value systems. The initial encounter with a person who has mobilized him or herself for help must be the beginning of an ongoing assessment. This assessment process is of the person's ability to take what is happening into account and the person's particular susceptibilities to hear and understand what to expect and how to behave. Once a person has sought constructive action designed to eliminate the threatening symptoms, health care professionals must look at both short- and long-term plans with the intent of minimizing and preventing a recurrence of the threatening event or symptoms. Help is provided to the alarmed person by sharing and transmitting information to obtain the mutual views of health care providers and the client. It is at this point that if the person's alarm is not lessened, anxiety prevails.[4]

Bard[4] has identified anxiety as a formidable barrier between the person with cancer and the people with whom he or she relates. He found anxiety interferes with the person's ability to hear, to understand, and to remember; therefore, it causes distortions and shifts on emphasis of what is said. For communication to be effective, efforts must be made to lessen disruptive anxiety. More frequent than not, lessening anxiety occurs when attention is focused on how messages are conveyed rather than what is said. The medical priority of immediate intervention of the person's disease needs to be balanced carefully with the psychosocial care of the person as a human being who is experiencing a life-threatening illness. The person's cancer needs to be treated and cared for in the context of the person, his value system, and his relationship with others.

Abrams,[2] a medical social worker, systematically studied 30 clients with cancer to determine their patterns of communication and the pattern changes at different stages of the illness. She described the clients' verbal communication with their physicians at three stages: (1) initial, (2) advancing, and (3) terminal. In the initial stage when the diagnosis was confirmed and treatment instituted, communication between the client and physician was direct and truthful. Clients initiated questions about what was happening, and the physician felt comfortable in responding. When interviewed, clients were aware of their medical situation and reasons for treatment.

In the advancing stage, clients realized that their cancers had not been eradicated and that further medical therapies were indicated to suppress their progressive disease. Communication became measured, weighed, and guarded. The key difference was between what the client presently asked as contrasted with earlier questions. Frequently clients asked everyone in the health care system about the diagnosis and prognosis, but they seldom confronted their physicians for this information. There was a slow insidious change that occurred in the physician-client relationship primarily owing to a nagging fear of abandonment that the clients handled by becoming the "good and accepting client." In the terminal stage when the client's disease was irreversible, verbal communication was minimal. In this stage, clients progressed from a state of anxiety and controlled agitation to a state of calmness. Communication was limited to the client's report of an intensification of symptoms rather than a discussion of the disease process per se. Specifically, Abrams[2] found there was no need to question the client's awareness of what was happening because it was apparent that a client who had deteriorated to the point of dying knew it without being told. She concluded that professionals need to seek guidance from the client because it was the client who offered the clues to how much, how little, or how often he wished to discuss his prognosis.

Glaser and Strauss[13] studied whether or not hospitalized clients, the majority of whom had cancer, were aware of their dying. They identified four types of awareness contexts between clients and personnel: closed awareness, suspected awareness, mutual pretense awareness, and open awareness. In the open context, the client's initial response to disclosure was described as depression. Most clients with time moved into another stage of the response process, either denial or acceptance. The degree of awareness was not absolute. From time to time there was selective openness and receptiveness. Often enough to be considered typical was the finding that denying the facts about certain symptoms of a disease took place mostly among people who had recently become symptomatic and not as much with those persons who had lived with their disease for a long time.

Telling

There are numerous references[12,21,25] on whether cancer clients should or should not be told their diagnosis and prognosis. There is general agreement that the argument against telling is associated with the anticipation of profoundly disturbing psychologic effects.[18] These disturbing psychologic effects have been investigated in some detail.* The crucial issue here seems not to be the verbalization of the word "cancer" but how

*See references 1, 3, 5, 10, 11, and 20.

that person is helped to manage what is happening at the moment and its consequences.

Feder[10] found that the question of whether to tell the client the truth was unimportant, but how the client felt and reacted to the threatening disease and how the people caring for him reflected their knowledge for the client's benefit was more salient. All 100 clients he interviewed preferred to speak about what was happening to them in their everyday affairs such as their symptoms rather than directly about their illness. Once the physician committed himself and gave the client an opportunity to talk, a relationship developed that permitted a necessary and beneficial release of the client's tensions. Feder found the greatest threat seemed to be not so much that of death but rather of pain, helplessness, rejection, and progressive isolation. He encouraged physicians to listen to clients because clients need to share their experiences; they are too often unsure that they are going to find someone with whom to do it. Feder's observations led him to conclude that by avoiding an open relationship and by not offering opportunities for emotional discharge, physicians may be encouraging mechanisms unfavorable to the client's resistance to the disease.

Telling is rarely an urgent question. The intent of establishing a diagnosis is to identify a reason for the client's existing symptoms and concerns, not to undermine the person. The actual conveying of messages to a person about his diagnosis and future needs to be an ongoing process. If a physician chooses not to tell a client a cancer diagnosis, the client soon becomes aware that something is amiss as his family and friends are poor actors. In the event of advanced cancer, persistent symptoms and ineffective treatments soon reveal the true nature of the disease long before the physician may be willing to discuss the situation with the client. Under these circumstances, the messages received by the client include feelings of disinterest, avoidance, and fear that what is happening is so dreadful that it cannot be discussed.

According to Krant,[15] knowing is integrated with sentiment, interpretation, symbolism, will, courage, and style. Nurses can play a unique role with clients when knowing is open, shared, and supported. This type of knowing can help a person take into account the personal meaning of the cancer to himself and mourn the threat of the loss of a loved and secured environment. Knowing by sharing can occur only with time.

Uncertainty

All stages of cancer are overshadowed by degrees of uncertainty. There is no question that some treatment protocols recommended and implemented for certain cancers have a stronger scientific base than others. Doubt may occur when the histology of a specific tumor or stage of disease is unclear. This seems to be particularly true in cancers where advances have been limited, that is, lung cancer. Where the type and stage of cancer are clear, the treatment may still remain controversial among physicians as illustrated by the continuing debate of appropriate treatment for women with breast cancer, that is, surgical intervention versus radiation therapy after the removal of the lump.

The importance of the meaning of uncertainty lies in how much of the circumstances of a given client's situation and the available alternatives are discussed with a client by his physician. Few clients are aware that they have choices available to them about diagnostic procedures and treatment modalities that would result in varying short- and long-term effects. For example, a woman who elects radiation therapy in place of a mastectomy will need to make daily short visits to a clinic over 4 or 5 weeks as compared to a more intensive recovery from major surgery where hospitalization is needed. Some women are never told that there are other options if the recommended medical treatment is unacceptable in their particular situation.

A major dilemma in decision making for clients occurs when they come face to face with a sense of urgency to make a decision about a situation in which they have had little or no experience and in which they have been given inadequate information as to what to expect. Uncertainty that results from lack of the provider's responsible behavior to inform the client of the disease, its effects, and treatment options should never occur but it does. Helping clients to understand what is happening to them and what they can do about the cancer reduces uncertainty. As stated in the previous section, informing people takes time and can never be accomplished by seeing the client only once. A series of contacts are needed to allow the client and health care provider freedom to share their concerns, validate their feelings, and clarify their goals. There are many aspects of cancer diseases and treatment modalities that are certain; it is these aspects that health care providers must make explicit when indicated by the client's questions or behavior.

Another dilemma occurs in cancer care because there are, in fact, many aspects of cancer that remain unknown and uncertain. Davis[9] coined the phrase "in limbo" for clients who were beyond the initial stage of disease, on active treatment, and living with a cancer with no predictable known end in sight. Unlike the previous type of uncertainty, these clients were knowledgeable about their illness and treatments. They were sensitive to and capable of interpreting symptoms and experiences in terms of favorable or unfavorable medical signs, indicating they had the necessary clues for thinking about and visualizing the course of their illness. They had to learn to manage to live 1 day at a time, fully aware that each day may be the beginning of their final decline.[9]

One approach that increases a person's ability to cope with the uncertainties surrounding a cancer in which the actual length of survival is unknown is to provide an ongoing mechanism for monitoring the client's symptoms and activities. If frequent client contacts are not feasible, then a 24-hour call system needs to be instituted so the client has immediate access to care if concerns arise. Uncertainties cannot be eliminated, but they can be managed. Nurses can play key roles in reducing the uncertainty of the situation by remaining available and creating a secure environment for the client where whatever occurs will be faced together.

NURSE'S SPECIALIZED COMMUNICATION KNOWLEDGE

In this part of the chapter, the focus is on the specialized knowledge that the nurse must have to communicate effectively with clients. Communication is the essence of everything a person does in life. Thayer[24] defines communication as the basic phenomenon that occurs when a person "takes something into account." The basic phenomenon is ultimately an intrapersonal one. It is a process whereby the person attributes meaning or significance to raw sensory data that he or she takes into account. The process never occurs between people only within. Similarly, in the nurse-client relationship, the basic processes of human communication occur in the individuals involved.

On this interpersonal level, the emphasis is on how given individuals affect each other through intercommunication and thereby mutually regulate and control each other.[24] Any human communication situation involves the production of a message by someone and the receipt of that message by someone.

Preconditions for intercommunication

There are certain basic factors relevant to an adequate understanding of the processes of human communication. Considered here are a set of conditions that are unique to intercommunication. For intercommunication to occur, at least one of the individuals involved must have a conceptual model (conscious or nonconscious) that a relationship exists. In the health care system, common relationship factors such as status and prestige may influence a nurse-client relationship. For example, clients may view the nurse as an expert and themselves as a novice, or they may see themselves as inferior in position to the nurse.

A second precondition necessary for intercommunication to occur is that at least one of the persons in the relationship has either some need to be communicated *with* or some intention to be achieved through communicating *to* the other. It is also necessary that the individuals involved in the intercommunication follow certain minimum rules and perform certain roles. These rules are so basic that many people take them for granted; for example, the rules that English is spoken to clients who understand only English and that clients be able to hear what is spoken. Performing a certain role is following a rule. In nursing, there are specific guidelines established for evaluating one's professional behavior in a given client situation to delineate the nurse's role.

A fourth and final precondition to be considered here is language. When two people want to communicate, they need some mutual acceptance of standardized symbols such as words. There are other conditions that underlie communication, but these are the necessary ones the nurse needs to examine if intercommunication does not occur. Communication will occur on some level, but successful intercommunication will not occur if these preconditions are not met.[24]

Communication strategies

It is generally accepted that the majority of human communication is instrumental or purposeful in that people hope to accomplish some end even though there are times when people simply enjoy what they take into account for the pleasure of doing so.[7,24] In short, people communicate to influence or to persuade others.

Rogers[19] defines communication as a process by which an idea is transferred from one person (a source) to another (a receiver) with the intent to change the former's behavior. Usually, the first person wants to alter the second person's knowledge of some idea, create or change the person's attitude toward an idea, or persuade the person to adopt the idea as part of his or her regular behavior. This process is especially applicable when describing a nurse-client relationship. The nurse purposefully plans communication so that the messages received by the client will produce certain efforts. This plan, called a communication strategy, is a design for changing human behavior on a large-scale basis through the transfer of new ideas. A strategy is the unit of communication management. A strategy is effects oriented. The nurse looks at what communication consequences are needed, and then plans how to attain them.

An important part of determining the effects produced in communication is to examine the nature of feedback. Feedback is a response by the receiver (client) to the source's message, which the source (a nurse) may subsequently use to modify further messages. Therefore, feedback is a special kind of message in that it concerns the effect of a previous message (from nurse to client). From the nurse's perspective, feedback may be thought of as messages conveying "knowledge of communication effectiveness." Feedback is one way of looking at the source as a receiver. Feedback emphasizes the mutuality of effective communication and is an essential part of planning and implementing strategies.[7]

Nurses strategize most of the time, but their degree of awareness about their behaviors varies. In cancer nursing, nurses need to bring into consciousness their strategizing skills. One way to do this is for nurses to systematically document the different types of strategies used and the effects that result. This increase in awareness will allow nurses to see those approaches that they are most successful with and those strategies that they need to abandon or revise. Another important part of strategizing is that nurses share their assessment of what is needed and plans with others. Most nurses are reluctant to ask other nurses or professionals for their advice and feedback. Collaboration and consultation are essential ingredients in cancer care.

Expectations

The concept of expectations is crucial to human communication. All human communication involves prediction by the source and receiver about how other people will respond to a message. Every person carries around with him or her an image of his receiver. Each participant of a nurse-client relationship has certain expectations of the other participant. The nurse carries around an image of the client and vice versa. The nurse takes the client into account when producing a message, anticipates the possible responses of the client, and tries to predict them ahead of time. These images affect the nurse's message behaviors. Similarly, clients have expectations about nurses.

Communication breakdowns frequently occur in a client-nurse relationship because one or both participants have unrealistic or false expectations of the other person. One method of limiting the number of communication breakdowns is to make explicit how each member is expected to behave. Another method is to allow for degrees of flexibility in the relationship and provide opportunities for the participants to clarify and validate their own and each other's behavior and intentions.

Contracting—the art of negotiation

One special type of intercommunication in a nurse-client relationship is the art of negotiation. Negotiation is a process in which the objective of both participants is to find a compromise that is mutually acceptable. By definition, a compromise, although mutually acceptable, gives each side less than the best possible outcome. It is assumed that negotiation does not make any sense unless a conflict of interests exists. However, the conflict of interests per se is not a sufficient reason for negotiation to occur. In other words, a negotiation becomes desirable only if a conflict of interests is activated and begins to generate social conflict.[6]

Negotiating with clients who have cancer is a necessary part of care, especially for those clients in whom the disease is no longer curative. Clients want to improve, and nurses want clients to improve, but each person may have different views as to how to achieve the client's improvement. To assess the situation and determine in what ways improvement can be achieved and under what conditions, both the nurse and client will have to give and listen to one another. They will negotiate and compromise.

One part of the process of negotiation is the establishment of a nurse-client contract. Contracts can be informal or formal agreements. A contract explicitly specifies the work to be done by both parties and the time frame for achieving it. In cancer nursing, it is a priority that clients be involved in their own health care, especially assuming an active part in the decision-making process affecting their day-to-day living. The use of a contract helps the client and the nurse to be accountable for the effort and time invested in their relationship.[23]

The overall purpose of the contract is to establish a framework in which the client has control of choice about intervention. Contract negotiation has as its cornerstone freedom of the client to accept, reject, or modify information or services offered by the nurse. "The emphasis in contract negotiation is on collaboration in relation to goals and objectives for change, specification of the target system, role expectations and ongoing role definition, anticipated time frame, ongoing evaluation, and contract negotiation as an ongoing process."[14]

CHALLENGING SITUATIONS

All behavior is communication and therefore influences and is influenced by others. The behavior of both the nurse and client in their relationship is related to and dependent on the behavior of each participant and the other people they "take into account," that is, other health professionals and family members. Situations that are not frequently presented in the literature because there are no easy answers to the complex problems that clients with cancer experience and the circumstances that surround their situations will be described in the following. The examples presented are client-nurse situations that have occurred and continue to occur. The behavior of the nurse needs to be examined for process as well as outcome.

Acting out

In situations where clients are described as difficult or acting out, it is important for the nurse to understand the client's disease state and treatment effects. Understanding a client's behavior by differentiating between the recurrence or progression of a tumor, the side-effects of specific treatment protocols, or identification of a long-standing coping mechanism can be extremely difficult.

• • •

Thelma was 44 years old when she was operated for lung cancer. She knew something was wrong for months prior to her pneumonectomy because she could not get rid of a chronic cough and cold. After surgery, she returned home to be with her husband and two teenage children. Both children were involved in their own activities and had little understanding of the seriousness of their mother's illness. Thelma remained asymptomatic for 18 months. During that time, her son graduated from high school and moved out of state to work.

One afternoon after Thelma's daughter, Mary, arrived home from school, Thelma had a seizure that neither of them expected. Thelma was yelling at Mary to pick up things in her room when she fell to the floor and had what Mary described as "uncontrollable jerking motions." Mary thought she had caused this reaction in her mother, and it was not until months later that the home health nurse learned of the child's guilt.

Thelma was hospitalized and a brain tumor was diagnosed. Two days later Thelma had a partial parietal lobectomy, and the cancer was found to be metastatic from the lung. Again, she did well for several months until she developed pain in her right chest. She was diagnosed with osteolytic lesions to her ribs. Once her pain was controlled, she lived over a year with episodes of acting out behavior. Thelma was able to live and die at home because of the nursing care she received.

Thelma's acting out behavior was directly related to the recurrence of her brain tumor. She had periods of being irritable, belligerent, and paranoid. Her behavior was antagonized by her daughter's and husband's avoidance of her. Neither of them understood what was happening and thought they were not doing things right. Mary, at the age of 15, had to assume the shopping, cooking, and housekeeping duties. She had always been taken care of and suddenly found herself responsible for the safety of her mother. Thelma was not eager to be dependent on others and struggled as she gradually lost her ability to drive, cook, and shop.

The home care nurse saw Thelma weekly throughout her illness. She had obtained a history about Thelma and her family's established coping patterns. She knew the strengths of this family and the areas where they needed assistance. The nurse established a contract with each member of the family. Negotiation was not possible until each member understood what was happening to Thelma and how her illness affected them. Part of their contracts included the right to know what was happening; this was especially important to Mary because up to this point she had been protected from her mother's diagnosis.

As Thelma's intracranial pressure increased, her behavior became explosive with verbal accusations and physical violence. Her behavior was managed by medications and consistent approaches by all who came in contact with her. Thelma's symptoms were closely monitored by the nurse so medication dosages could be altered. Thelma was maintained on multiple drugs: phenytoin (Dilantin), phenobarbitol, haloperidol (Haldol), benztropine (Cogentin), dexamethasone (Decadron), hydroxyzine (Vistaril), and methadone. At times she also needed furosemide (Lasix), digoxin, and a potassium replacement.

The last 6 months of Thelma's life, she needed a nurse with her every day. Many times both the family and the nurses became discouraged because they did not know how much longer they could carry on. Thelma needed repeated explanations, at times, of why she was behaving the way she was. Similarly, her family needed the same explanations, and they were taught to reinforce the same answers to her questions. Support sessions were arranged weekly so everyone involved in Thelma's care could express their feelings.

The priority of care from everyone's perspective was the establishment of a secure environment where Thelma was accepted and would be safe and those around her would not be harmed by her. At times, it was necessary to set limits with Thelma and this was possible by renegotiating the contract. The success of this case came about with the fulfillment of the contract to see this client and her family through the entire process. With help, Thelma was able to fulfill her own goal to die at home.

Living with guilt

Once clients seek medical care to relieve their distress, they very often search for a reason for their misfortunes. Two general classifications of causes are described by clients. The first is characteristic of an external cause such as an inescapable environmental agent or a bad break owing to fate, God, or other human beings. The latter reason can be especially stressful to nurses if they find their clients criticizing the physician for what has happened to them. Some nurses find themselves defending the physician before they realize that the clients need to express their feelings and blame others.

The second characteristic of a cause concerns clients internalizing their feelings and blaming themselves. They see themselves as personally failing or sinning in some way that has caused the disease. They have a devalued sense of self-esteem. Clients that are characterized by either of these feelings of guilt present challenging situations for the nurse.

• • •

Marilyn was 36 years old when she had her fourth child. She and her husband were happily married; they had bought a farm several years ago and were working hard to make ends meet. One day when Marilyn was taking a shower she noticed a lump in her breast. It was right in the middle of harvest so she did not take it into account as being more important than getting the meals on the table for the work crew and driving the farm truck for her husband. Several months passed until one night her husband felt the lump when they were having intercourse. Marilyn reassured him that her obstetrician had told her women frequently have changes in their breasts, especially after having a child. He accepted her response temporarily, and both of them agreed that with the first break in their work Marilyn would see a different doctor.

Six months passed before Marilyn found time for herself. She had delayed because she had to get the children ready for school, their clothes in shape, and the fall canning done. When she finally went to the doctor, a simple mastectomy with radiation therapy was recommended because her cancer had metastasized to her lungs and vertebrae. Both Marilyn and her husband, Paul, were overwhelmed by feelings of guilt. Paul became severely depressed and blamed himself. Marilyn was bitter and felt her obstetrician should have followed her more closely and recommended treatment sooner.

A home nursing care referral was made for Marilyn after her chest incision broke open during her radiation therapy. Her lesion remained open, draining, odorous, and extremely difficult to keep clean and dry. Marilyn lived over a year and a half before she died. She was able to remain at home with supplemental nursing care. The same home health nurse worked with the family throughout this process. Dressing changes needed to be done at least three times a day and two people were needed to do the task. Paul and three of the children were taught how to change the dressings so at least two of them could help at a time. It was important for the nurse to be aware that self-blame and blame of others are common effects found in people with cancer and their family members. The nurse arranged times together and separately for Marilyn and Paul to openly talk and discuss their feelings. The nurse encouraged each of them to work out their feelings of resentment by hypothesizing what would have happened if things had been different and what things meant to them at the time.

The major objective of the nurse came to be to work on both Marilyn's and Paul's images of themselves; neither of them thought they were worthy of help or the attention of others. They thought they were rightly being punished for their own failure to seek help sooner. The nurse behaviorily communicated to Marilyn and her family by seeing them through her disease that they were worthy of her attention and that they were important as human beings. It was also important that the nurse maintained contact with Paul for a period of time after Marilyn's death in order for him to live with his guilt and accept it. Paul's guilt did not disappear, but with time it became less important and he was able to plan a life with his children. He had learned to live with his guilt by making the most out of his time with Marilyn before she died. They each spent as much time as possible together sharing the things they had decided to do as a family. The nurse helped Paul identify how much he had accomplished with Marilyn as a husband and father so he could complete his grieving.

The badgering family

Cancer is a disease that not only affects the person who is diagnosed with it but also affects the person's family. How the disease affects the family depends on which family member becomes ill. For example, an illness occurring in the husband or father affects the other family members differently than if the cancer strikes the mother or child. All family members struggle with the meaning of how the person's cancer impinges on their lives individually and in relation to each other. What appears to be an overwhelming situation from a nurse's perspective may be in reality not so bad for the client and vice versa.

• • •

Kate was 56 years old when she was diagnosed with lung cancer with metastasis to her supraclavicular nodes. She and her husband, Johnny, had remained childless throughout the 32 years of their marriage. Johnny owned his own business and they lived a very comfortable life. Both Kate and Johnny adored each other and had established a long-standing dependent relationship on each other. Kate took care of the house, prepared the meals, and entertained Johnny's friends regularly. Over the years, Johnny managed his business from their home so they could be together as much as possible. Kate selected what Johnny would wear each day, and Johnny would suggest what Kate should wear.

As Kate's cancer progressed, she became fatigued, weakened, and depressed. Her malaise was confounded by a series of radiation treatments and chemotherapy injections. Kate was no longer interested or able to participate in many of the activities she and her husband had enjoyed for years. Johnny had difficulty accepting the changes in Kate's appearance and weight. He was adamant that Kate's condition would improve if she would eat. A home health referral was made to see what nursing interventions could be planned to help improve Kate's nutritional status. The nurse found Johnny refused to discuss the implications of Kate's disease and insisted that Kate's physician treat her with the latest protocols on the market. In contrast, Kate was a quiet, pleasant woman who talked only when spoken to because her voice had become so husky that she spoke in a whisper. As the nurse watched Johnny and Kate talk with each other, she wondered why Kate tolerated Johnny's demands and described Johnny as badgering Kate.

Each intervention that the nurse planned with Kate was not acceptable to Johnny. He had no patience with Kate's eating six small meals a day or taking a nap before a meal. Johnny wanted Kate to sit at the table with him at their usual time and with their usual servings. The nurse became increasingly frustrated with Johnny's interference and decided she needed to consult with someone who could advise her. The nurse arranged a client care conference with her supervisor, a clinical specialist, and two other staff nurses. The outcome of the conference was to support this family in the context of their relationship as it had always been as long as Johnny's demands were acceptable to Kate. The nurse had a professional responsibility to validate this plan with Kate. Johnny's behavior was interpreted as denying what was happening to his wife because his recognition of her premature death would mean multiple losses to him that he could not manage. Periodic care conferences were held over the 3 months while home care was needed for Kate.

An additional nurse saw Johnny separately twice a week to help him describe what was happening to Kate. The nurse would clarify Johnny's misconceptions by initiating additional aspects of Kate's behavior to Johnny without interpreting that Kate was dying. Gradually, Johnny was able to clarify for himself the meaning of the changes in Kate. Kate told the nurse that Johnny meant well by his attempts to help her. Kate knew that Johnny had always been a person who got what he wanted and that this was one situation where he could not buy her health back or be in control of annihilating what was threatening their relationship. The nurse had to assess both the client's and husband's needs and find a balance in meeting both, since the wife's primary need was to see her husband's needs met.

All participants in this situation had different ideas as to what they expected. Johnny expected Kate to eat and improve. Kate expected to die but was unsure what would happen to Johnny. She had no concerns about herself. The nurse expected to help Kate with her acceptance of dying. Each of these three persons needed time to work together to become aware of each other's expectations and to work toward common goals.

Nonpersuadable physician

Cancer care requires the services of multiple providers working together to assist clients to live their lives as fully as possible. In medicine, there are on occasion some physicians who write orders for their clients without taking into account whether the order is realistic for the clients to follow or whether there are unusual hardships placed on the clients if they comply. The nurse is seen by these physicians as a person who is responsible for seeing that the client follows the orders, not as a person who questions them. Nurses who find themselves in this type of situation are often left unsupported to challenge the physician or they learn to survive by placing the burden of noncompliance on the client.

• • •

Carl was 68 years old when he was diagnosed as having prostatic cancer with metastasis to his pelvis. Carl lived alone and very much wanted to continue to be as self-sufficient for himself as possible. He found it increasingly difficult to bear weight on his bones because of the pain. His doctor had placed him on Percodan and instructed him to take the pills only when necessary. During Carl's last hospitalization for radiation therapy, a home nursing referral was made.

When the nurse made her initial assessment of Carl in his home, her immediate response was to ask Carl's physician for a longer acting narcotic to regulate his pain because it had helped so many other clients. Instead, she decided to call the physician, inform him of her assessment, and review his plan of care. The nurse used this strategy because she had previous experience with this physician and he had not responded to any of her suggestions before. This time she was determined to have a stronger base of observations to recommend changes in care before making suggestions to the physician. This was an ideal situation for her to improve her communication strategies with this physician because even though the client was in pain and needed relief, his situation was not one that required an immediate change in intervention.

After the nurse established the pattern of pain and the intensity of pain with the client, she recommended that he take his Percodan on a schedule consistent with his pain pattern. The client was also instructed to keep a log to record the degree of relief obtained, including his ability to eat, sleep, and do things. In Carl's situation, he needed three tablets every 2 or 3 hours in order to get relief; therefore, the nurse felt she had to attempt to obtain a longer acting drug such as methadone.

The nurse arranged to see the physician vis-à-vis to review what he had ordered and what the effects had been over the 4-day period. The nurse told the physician she very much wanted to work with him to help this client, but the drug he had ordered was ineffective. The nurse was prepared for the physician's response because she had reviewed with the client what his priorities were and reviewed with a pharmacist the range of medications that could be used. The nurse knew that the physician would have no patience or time to hear her entire assessment so she asked for what the client had identified as most important, pain relief, and showed the physician the client's pain relief record. The nurse asked for a change in the narcotic, but the physician refused. She then asked for a drug that would potentiate the effects of the Percodan as advised by the pharmacist, and the physician reluctantly agreed. She also made arrangements to meet with him in 1 week to review the patient's reactions and status. The drug ordered was hydroxyzine (Vistaril), 25 mg orally every 6 hours.

Carl's ability to ambulate and get around his house improved. It is difficult to know whether it was the addition of the medication or the effects of the nurse's commitment with Carl to see him regularly and to discuss options for coping with his limitations that accounted for his improvement. One option always available to a client such as Carl is to see another physician. For clients like Carl, unfortunately, this is rarely considered an option because of the trust the person has that his physician is doing everything possible.

• • •

Generally, the majority of clients have physicians who work collaboratively with all disciplines, including nurses, to assist the client in achieving the best quality of living with a chronic disease.

THE NURSE'S MULTIPLE RESPONSIBILITIES

In the client situations presented in the preceding section, the nurse had multiple professional responsibilities. The major component of clinical care in cancer nursing is providing direct care to people. In providing care, the nurse's primary responsibility is to the client. The essence of care is the establishment of a nurse-client relationship. Implied in the formation of a relationship is the concept of time and the process of intercommunication.

The nurse continually needs to assess the client, the situation, and her own reactions. The nurse brings to the relationship a broad base of knowledge and skills and varying degrees of experience with similar situations. The task for the nurse becomes one of selectively and constructively using that knowledge to find out what clients need, how she can help clients, and how clients can help themselves.

In chronic care where situations are not urgent, clients can be guided by the nurse communicatively to explore, reflect, and find their own solutions to coping with the problems of daily living. Often in their relationship with clients, nurses are uncomfortable listening and being with clients without doing physical tasks for them. Nurses need to identify in what ways they are uncomfortable and purposefully work on improving their skills in these areas so that their uneasiness is not interfering with their abilities to take things into account. Nurses need to validate and clarify their observations with their clients and provide opportunities for the clients to do the same with them. When interventions are planned by the client and nurse jointly, the nurse is responsible for obtaining feedback from the client and evaluating the care in order to integrate the effects into their ongoing relationship.

In cancer care, the nurse has a responsibility to prepare clients for the uncertainties and potential consequences of their cancer and treatment effects. The nurse behaves based on the assumption that all clients have a right to be informed and that the nurse is responsible for identifying under what conditions and in what circumstances verbal messages about the disease and its implications are conveyed. In the past, nurses have been criticized for initiating talk about sensitive areas of potential complications if the client's responses were perceived as disturbing to the client or as disrupting others. Channels of criticism about the nurse's behavior may come from the client, the family, the physician, the nurse's supervisor, or other nurse colleagues. In those clients who do not exhibit acting out behaviors such as angry outcrys or depressive retreats, the nurse's actions go unnoticed. The success of the nurse's intercommunication with the client should not be judged by the presence or absence of criticism but rather whether a relationship is established that allows both participants to question and challenge each other to grow. Nurses in cancer care are responsible for providing opportunities for clients to explore their feelings about what is happening to them and for creating an environment that allows clients to behave and act out in their own way. Extreme client behaviors indicative of destructive ways of coping need to be identified and a plan designed by both clients and nurses to help clients use their energies for more constructive efforts that will benefit them. Somehow nurses themselves must assume the responsibility of standardizing this aspect of care for all clients regardless of the client's behavior. Nurses must be willing to be accountable for their actions and the provision of continued care.

In addition to the nurse's responsibility to the client, the nurse has a responsibility to inform, plan, and establish a feedback mechanism with the other health care professionals involved with the client's care. This responsibility is especially important in facilitating and coordinating care with physicians. Because of the diversity of the nurse's role and the amount of contact with clients, nurses are the logical persons in the health care system to coordinate care among the multiple providers involved in the management of cancer. Nurses and physicians both have an important role to play in assisting clients with making informed decisions about complex problems.

Equally important with the nurses' other responsibilities are their responsibilities to themselves. Taking care of themselves involves finding a balance in their time for themselves with time for work. At work, the client's needs must have priority over the nurse's needs, and similarly nurses need time away from work when their needs have priority. Responsibility involves the process of keeping up with the advances in cancer care. It involves the realization that as nurses, they do not have to have all the answers for the client and family, but they have to have the knowledge of where and how to get the answers and the ability to ask for help. It involves the development and use of support systems for themselves.

Today and in the future, nurses must be prepared for these multiple responsibilities, since clients with cancer are living longer with the advances in therapies. Cancer nursing requires nurses who are sensitive to others, flexible in their approaches, knowledgeable about people's behavior, and capable of taking risks. It requires nurses who have had opportunities to confront their own life experiences and who have developed a pattern of coming to terms with those experiences in order to rely on those established patterns when needed. Most of all, cancer nursing requires nurses who are capable of establishing and maintaining a relationship with clients in order to help them manage their day-to-day problems of living with cancer by intercommunication.

REFERENCES

1. Abrams, H. S.: Psychological responses to illness and hospitalization, Psychosomatics **10**:218, 1969.
2. Abrams, R. D.: The patient with cancer—his changing pattern of communication, N. Engl. J. Med. **272**:317, 1966.
3. Abrams, R. D., and Finesinger, J. E.: Guilt reactions in patients with cancer, Cancer **6**:474, 1953.
4. Bard, M.: The Psychological impact of cancer and cancer surgery. In Proceedings of the American Cancer Society's National Conference on Human Values and Cancer, American Cancer Society, Inc., p. 24, 1973.
5. Bard, M., and Sutherland, A. M.: Psychological impact of cancer and its treatment, Cancer **8**:656, 1955.
6. Bartos, O. J.: Process and outcome of negotiations, New York, 1974, Columbia University Press.
7. Berlo, D. K.: The process of communication, San Francisco, 1960, Rinehart Press.
8. Caplan, G.: An approach to the study of family mental health, U.S. Public Health Rep. **71**:10, 1956.
9. Davis, M. Z.: Patients in limbo, Am. J. Nurs. **66**:746, 1966.
10. Feder, S.: Psychological considerations in the care of patients with cancer, Ann. N. Y. Acad. Sci. **125**:1020, 1966.
11. Finesinger, J. E., Shands, H. C., and Abrams, R. P.: Managing emotional problems of cancer patients, Cancer **3**:19, 1953.
12. Fitts, W. T., Jr., and Randin, I. S.: What Philadelphia physicians tell patients with cancer, J.A.M.A. **153**:901, 1953.
13. Glaser, B. G., and Strauss, A. L.: Awareness of dying, Chicago, 1965, Aldine Publishing Co.
14. Hall, J. E., and Weaver, B. R.: Distributive nursing practice: a systems approach to community health, Philadelphia, 1977, J. B. Lippincott Co.
15. Krant, M. J.: What does the patient know? In Proceedings of the American Cancer Society's National Conference on Human Values and Cancer, American Cancer Society, Inc., p. 48, 1973.
16. Lazarus, R. S.: A laboratory approach to psychological stress. In Grosser, G. H., Wechsler, H., and Greenblatt, M., editors: The threat of impending disaster, Cambridge, Mass., 1964, The M.I.T. Press, p. 43.
17. Mastrovito, R. C.: Cancer: Awareness and denial, Clin. Bull. **4**:142, 1974.
18. Oken, D.: What to tell cancer patients, J.A.M.A. **175**:1120, 1961.
19. Rogers, E. M.: Communication strategies for family planning, New York, 1973, The Free Press.
20. Rothenberg, A.: Psychological problems in terminal cancer management, Cancer **14**:1063, 1961.
21. Seelig, M. C.: Should cancer patients be told the truth? Mo. Med. **40**:33, 1943.
22. Shands, H. C.: The informational impact of cancer on the structures of the human personality, Ann. N. Y. Acad. Sci. **164**:885, 1969.
23. Sloan, M. R., and Schommer, B. T.: The process of contracting in community nursing. In Spradley, B. W., editor: Contemporary community nursing, Boston, 1975, Little, Brown & Co.
24. Thayer, L.: Communication and communication systems, Homewood, Ill., 1968, Richard D. Irwin, Inc.
25. Weisman, A.: The patient with a fatal illness: to tell or not to tell, J.A.M.A. **201**:152, 1967.
26. Weisman, A. D.: On dying and denying, New York, 1972, Behavioral Publications.

20

Dealing with our own grief

CORINNE ANN SOVIK

You are a staff nurse on duty. You receive a call from Mrs. Walker, a 49-year-old woman in her final stages of metastatic breast cancer. She may die in the next few weeks.

When you enter her room she reaches out with tear-filled eyes and asks you if she is dying. You sit next to her and hold her hand. She begins weeping and clutches your hand and you respond by holding her tighter.

You begin instantly to think to yourself, "She is dying but how do I tell her without frightening her? I don't even know what she has been told. . . . What if I say the wrong thing?"

Mrs. Walker interrupts your thinking by asking, "Why won't someone just tell me what's happening to me. I don't want to die. Can't you, can't someone, make me feel better?"

You look deep into Mrs. Walker's eyes and feel helpless in not knowing what to say and maybe hopeless because you know there is no treatment to cure her or to help her now. Your loss for words and your sense of sadness for this woman overwhelm your ability to respond as tears well up in your own eyes.

As in the traumatic situation above, the nurse's task in caring for dying clients is difficult and emotionally draining. Death is overwhelming. It evokes emotions that often prove as painful for the nurse as for the client and family.

To best help the client, the nurse must learn to solve the personal, professional, and institutional problems encountered while caring for terminal clients. For our own sakes, as well as for our clients', we must ensure our own well-being. We must learn to cope with the stress so that we do not lose control while performing important tasks or "burn out" and leave the profession. When we feel comfortable in dealing with our own feelings, we will then gain the unending satisfaction of knowing we have helped clients and their families.

We can develop this ability to cope by (1) becoming aware of our own feelings, (2) understanding our fears, (3) separating our feelings from those of the client and staff, (4) identifying clinical situations that potentiate negative feelings, and (5) establishing support systems for ourselves.

INTROSPECTION—BECOMING AWARE OF OUR OWN FEELINGS

The only way nurses can cope with dying clients is to realize that we *are* human beings with real emotions. By examining honestly and rationally our feelings about death, religion, and life after death, we can use our own experience to understand, assess, and care for the dying client.

To begin to understand our feelings about death, we should take some time to ponder the following questions. First, we should think about childhood experiences with death.

- What was my first personal involvement with death?
- At what age was I first aware of death?
- When I was a child, how was death talked about in my family?
- How can I best describe my childhood concepts of death?[3]

Questions like these enable us to examine our perceptions of our personal past experiences. We can begin to analyze how we reacted and felt about death and how that influenced us as we grew. By examining these childhood experiences, we can identify some of the influences that brought us to our current thoughts and feelings about death.

To explore another perspective of our feelings about death, consider:

- How much of a role has religion played in the development of my attitude toward death?
- Do I believe in life after death?
- Regardless of my belief in the hereafter, what do I wish about?[3]

Death is a mysterious concept in life. Our perceptions of what happens to our bodies, our intellects, and our souls are influenced by our religious background.

Often people do not turn to religion until a psychologic need arises. For example, when people experience a crisis, they may begin to think about God to try to make sense of the situation. Therefore, to identify our own beliefs before a crisis occurs, either personally or with a client, may help us cope with future crises. Also, because the role of religion is changing in our society, many people have not developed a strong identification with a particular faith. Identification, or the lack of it, may add confusion at a time of crisis.

Introspection will also enable us to separate our own personal beliefs from those of others. The difference, for example, between the Jewish and the Presbyterian perspective is vast. The nurse must be aware of these differences and how they influence clients' views of their own death. We must be careful not to project or impose our religious concepts onto other persons, in particular, those who have a religion that works for them.

Now consider your present concept of death.

- What has most influenced my present attitude toward death?
- What does death mean to me right now?
- What is most frightening about my own death?
- Can I describe my own feelings about dying?[3]

Thinking about death seems foreign to beginning nurses who are in their early 20's. This is the period of our lives when we plan for a lifetime ahead. In America, a "death denying" culture, it seems more appropriate and relevant for a 60-year-old person to be concerned about death than a 20-year-old. Because a person has lived longer, death may be perceived as closer at hand. New practitioners must overcome societal inhibitions and encourage themselves to consciously think about death and dying.

The process of self-awareness and sensitivity to our own feelings about death is an ongoing process that builds and changes as we continue to experience and grow. We need to appreciate that we cannot resolve all that introspection reveals at one time.

FEARS

Sometimes, the anxiety experienced in dealing with dying clients stems from our inability to recognize the specific factor that provokes uncomfortable feelings. Often, the factor is one of our own fears.

Because everyone will die someday, nurses experience many of the same fears that clients do. These fears often include the following:

1. Fear of the unknown
2. Fear of sorrow
3. Fear of loss of identity
4. Fear of loss of the future
5. Fear of loneliness
6. Fear of suffering and pain
7. Fear of loss of family and friends

Beyond these personal fears, nurses experience fears that result from the professional role. By focusing on fear, an emotional response to a specific, perceived danger, we may be able to alleviate the generalized anxiety. By identifying some of the problems that we are afraid of dealing with, we can prepare ourselves to solve them.

Fear of causing pain

Nurses fear making a mistake and performing a destructive act rather than a helpful one. If a nurse is in error, he/she may be devastated, and begin to feel guilty. For example, a nurse might question, "If I had checked the IV sooner, maybe the potassium would not have infiltrated and caused so much edema." In this situation the nurse may be feeling insecure and is questioning his or her own competence. Reflection on what actually occurred will clarify the situation. If the nurse was extremely busy with an emergency, she or he could not have watched the IV. In this case, the edema could not have been avoided, and the nurse was expecting too much of himself or herself. On the other hand, if the nurse was not particularly busy, she or he should have been more observant and avoided the mishap.

When a mistake occurs, one must analyze why it happened and how it could have been prevented. We must accept responsibility for our errors, work hard to prevent and to correct them, and keep in mind that we generally do the best job that we can. As we continue to practice, our self-confidence will grow and this fear will lessen. When feeling insecure, we should work along with an experienced nurse who can review and check our rationale and plan of care.

Nurses also fear not being able to give enough emotional support to a client, thus causing psychologic pain. When we are under great stress, our abilities to give emotional support to our clients decrease. Stress on the job develops from encountering successive emotionally demanding situations without a break. If one of our clients has just died, we will not be able to give as much to the next client we see. Physical exhaustion, emergency situations, and charge duties add stress. We must be aware of our physical and psychologic limitations so that we do not overextend ourselves. When overextended, we cannot do a good job and are prone to feel guilty. By recognizing our limitations and needs, we can get help from other members of the health care team. By communicating with the members of the team and by coordinating all those involved with the client's care, we can assure that the client's needs are met as completely as possible.

Fear of causing death

Nurses fear making an error in judgment that results in death. Because we are human beings and subject to mistakes, this fear is something nurses have to live with. Often when feeling insecure, this fear can seem even more prevalent.

For example, a nurse might question, "Maybe I should not have given the extra prescribed dosage of morphine to Mr. Frank who died last night. I knew he was dying, his blood pressure was low, and he had shallow respirations. But I knew from the past that morphine was the only drug that relieved him and he was crying in pain."

The nurse's ambivalence stems from not understanding the total purpose behind her action. If the goal was to keep Mr. Frank, who was unsalvageable, as comfortable as possible, and the approach had been decided by the physician, team, and family that this was to be accomplished through the use of morphine, then an error in judgment did not occur. On the other hand, if the status of the client at the time of administration was not expected, then an error may have occurred, particularly if the client died as a result of the drug. If one is aware of the purpose of the orders, there is less chance for ambivalence or error.

The fear of causing death may stem from lack of knowledge, time to think, or confidence in a particular situation. If one does not feel comfortable in performing a procedure or administering care such as assisting in a cardiac arrest or passing a nasogastric tube, then the person should not do it. One should always ask for assistance, for example, observe how the cardiac arrest or emergency team works before taking on the responsibility of joining in or request that an experienced nurse be present when attempting to perform a new procedure. Furthermore, if the rationale for any procedure, drug, or plan is not clear, do not carry it out until it is understood.

There is always the chance for an error that we all have to deal with. However, the likelihood is far less if we try to consciously think through and anticipate our actions.

Fear of loss of control

Nurses fear losing control, breaking down and crying, and not knowing how to respond to a situation. We also suffer in the situation when we do lose control. Identifying situations where we might lose control and planning strategies may help us to cope.

Lack of knowledge or confidence in responding to clients' questions and emotional states. Often we question our actions in various situations as we retrospectively and prospectively review encounters. Consider the phases a cancer client goes through: prediagnostic, diagnostic, treatment, dying. At each phase the nurse may not know how to respond to the client. For example, in the prediagnostic phase a client may be unaware of the implications of being "worked up" for cancer. Nurses may become anxious if they do not know when the client will comprehend the situation and how the client will react at the time. Also, anxiety may stem from uncertainty about the nurse's response, for example, "Should I be the one who alludes to the fact that the client probably has cancer, and is this more stressful than if the physician does it?"

By logically assessing the physical and emotional state of the client and becoming aware of our own feelings we can more appropriately respond to the client's questions and reactions. When we are knowledgeable, also, of the philosophy of the team and institution responsible for the client's care, we will become more secure in our approach. This knowledge can be acquired through seeking input from staff members who are more familiar with the principles of care. Nurses, then, will feel more comfortable in responding because they will know they are backed by the team. Also, responses to the client will be consistent if everyone concurs and is aware of the general plan.

Another example of lack of knowledge as to the appropriateness of a response may be seen in the following situation. Consider a nurse who has been working with a client and family for months. The client has just died and the nurse has been in the room with the family through the death. The nurse is holding the 16-year-old daughter who is weeping and the nurse realizes that she, too, is crying. The daughter continually repeats, "Don't go, Mommy. Oh, please, don't leave me." The nurse is unable to respond to the daughter because of her own sadness and begins to feel she has lost control. Depending on the situation, it may be appropriate for the nurse to acknowledge feelings of grief and to share the daughter's grief by an outpouring of her own emotions.

However, if the nurse feels overwhelmed by the interaction and cannot function, then the nurse cannot help the daughter. Nurses may not be able to respond appropriately if they have not been working through their grief throughout the client's illness. If the grief had been worked through, then tears may not have been the best or most appropriate response. However, each situation is unique, and the most appropriate response depends on the total circumstances and backgrounds of all who are involved. By analyzing the problems and by trying to solve them as they occur, we will learn to cope with difficult situations.

Inability to recognize negative feelings. As people die, they lose energy, vitality, strength, and responsiveness. They begin to think less quickly and accurately as they literally lose control of their bodies and minds. Our society places a strong emphasis on the development and maintenance of self-control from early childhood to adulthood. Urinary and fecal incontinence, for example, are experienced during the latter stages of dying. If it becomes difficult for the nurse to keep a client clean because of fecal incontinence, the nurse may experience repulsion. The nurse may also feel frustrated, and the situation may lead to despair and feelings of personal defeat. To prevent these feelings from becoming overwhelming requires identifying them as they occur. Perhaps if we are frustrated or desperate, we may need to talk with another nurse about how difficult it is to constantly watch the client who is continually incontinent. We may even need to ask for help in changing the client.

Assessing our feelings not only enhances our adjustment to the client's status but also enables us to respond appropriately. We must be conscious that as nurses we function as the primary if not sole contact with society for the hospitalized client. Our reaction may be taken as a reflection of how the rest of society, specifically family and friends, will view the client. If the nurse responds negatively to the client, then the client may think that his family will respond negatively.

An increase in the number of losses or threat of losses either in our personal or professional lives. Losses either in our personal or professional lives can interfere with our ability to maintain control. For example, if there is a death in our family, divorce, or financial difficulty, or if we are caring for many dying clients at the same time, we may have trouble maintaining composure. By recognizing that these problems intensify the already difficult task of nursing dying clients, we will not be so harsh on ourselves if we do lose composure. By understanding and working through our own problems, we will be more capable of handling individual situations on the units.

The ability to cope decreases as the number of stressful encounters and emotional situations increases. As the number of demands on the nurse increases, responses to the various stimuli may become entangled. It, then, becomes difficult to decifer which behavior is in response to which stimulus. These behavioral responses may become confused, exaggerated, and intensified, leading to inappropriate responses to the client. At this point, the nurse needs to seek help in desensitizing herself in order to continue to function effectively.

Inability to recognize past unresolved grief. Nurses may associate one of their clients with a person from their personal life. Perhaps the 28-year-old woman who has leukemia reminds you of your sister who died of the disease 2 years ago. These associations are common and natural. Professional responsibility in dealing with this situation involves recognizing how you are relating to the client. Nurses have to avoid expressing unresolved grief. If nurses find themselves withdrawing and feeling that "I can't deal with it" or find their behavior nonproductive, they must then arrange for another nurse to undertake the care of this client.

Fear of loss of identity

The fear of loss of professional identity often creates additional coping difficulties. For example, a nurse has been working to build rapport with a client for a number of days. The nurse has encouraged verbalization from the client and finds that progress is being made. The nurse is off duty for 1 day and returns to the nursing unit the following morning to find that the client has talked with the social worker and has discussed every detail that the nurse had hoped to promote. How does this make the nurse feel? Does the nurse feel inadequate, as if she or he is the wrong person for the client to discuss his or her feelings with? In this situation it is most difficult to perceive oneself as the facilitator who stimulates a client to verbalize his or her feelings. It is difficult to recognize that you cannot be "everything to everyone." However, the help you have provided in these situations is essential for improving the client's total well-being.

Negative feelings can be avoided in this situation by communication. It is vital to continually share the assessment, plan of care, expectations, and outcomes with the significant team members. This enables all to define their specific role with the client. If two roles tend to overlap, as seen in the case of the social worker and the nurse, the two professionals need to work together for the benefit of the client.

Fear of loss or lack of support

Throughout our nursing careers we develop support systems within our settings to help us cope on a daily basis. We generally have one or a few close associates with whom we ventilate our feelings and consult on a personal and professional level. As the work situation changes, nurses may fear losing their support and finding themselves having to cope alone. Who will nurses turn to on the day their client dies if their confidant, another nurse on the unit, spouse, or roommate is unavailable. "Who will console me?" they may ask "after I have spent all my energy taking care of another client." How well we support our clients is directly proportional to how well we are emotionally supported.

Staff often turn to their own family and friends to express their feelings. It is worthwhile to caution here that people who are not directly related to a particular client may not fully understand or appreciate the situation and may not be able to provide the insight we need. Also, continual discussion of our professional experiences can become draining on our personal relationships. For these reasons support should be sought within the system where we function as nurses.

Understanding how we react to our experiences, both personal and professional, takes a lifetime of introspection. This process is a struggle of inward and outward feelings and expression that may be exhausting, frightening, and frustrating, but normal and necessary. As we grow, our needs, fears, and perceptions change. Introspection can help us reevaluate our feelings, behaviors, and coping strategies.

SEPARATION OF OUR OWN FEELINGS FROM THE CLIENTS'

Throughout our experiences we need to understand how our feelings differ from those of the client. This is imperative in developing an effective nursing role, mainly to separate our feelings from the client's so as not to misinterpret what emotion is coming from whom. An example is projecting our feelings onto a client, which not only confuses or misleads the client but also leads staff's responses to the client in an inappropriate manner.

CLINICAL SITUATIONS

The emotional components of dealing with a cancer client in the clinical setting are complex. The emotions and behaviors of not only the nurse and the client but also the physician, social worker, other nurses, dietitian, other physicians, client's family, friends, and clergyman, come into play.

At some point a member of the team, usually the physician, informs the client that she or he is dying. The knowledge of impending death creates a crisis for the cancer client. All concerned, the client, family, and the health care team, must then adapt to perceiving the future in new terms.

Perception of time of death[2]

Even though it is understood that we all live with the potential for death at any moment, we project ahead and anticipate life. When it has become apparent that the client is going to die, the actual time or point of death is projected by all persons involved. For example, the physician who makes the diagnosis of cancer may believe that the client will live approximately 6 months. The nurses involved, because they have seen three clients with the same disease die in the past year, may believe the client has 5 months to live. The client's husband may think of his wife as a strong woman and a "fighter" and predict that she will live 8 months. Perhaps a new intern may have seen a number of clients with the same disease survive 9 months because of chemotherapy. Projection of the time of death differs to accommodate each individual's needs and past experiences as seen in Fig. 20-1.

For example, a comatose, emaciated client dying from metastatic cancer is about to suffer a cardiac arrest. Should the client be resuscitated? Perhaps the nurse does not feel that the client should be resuscitated because he or she sees a dying client who will not survive the process. The husband, feeling his wife would not want to give up, pleads for resuscitation. The intern on call feels that the client has not had time to respond to the treatment and should be given every chance to live.

What becomes obvious here is that each person's perceptions and feelings involved are different and unique. Conflict arises because the expectations of or the point of death are not the same. Each individual concerned with the client will then react and approach the client with a different attitude. The behavioral patterns of the staff may create an atmosphere that is confusing for the client. This confusion interferes with the client's preparation for death.

Similarly, the practitioner's preparation for the death of the client is interrupted. For example, the nurse may feel helpless if he or she is ordered to resuscitate a client whom he or she perceives would not survive. The nurse may feel angry with the physician who carries out the resuscitation because she or he feels he is exposing the client to a fu-

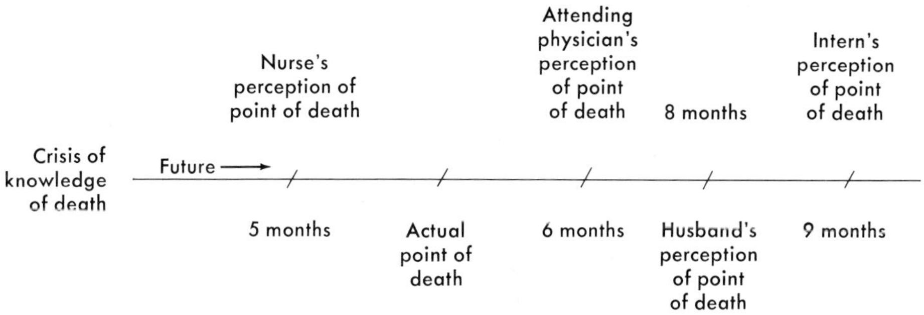

Fig. 20-1. Individual differences in perceptions of death.

tile and invasive procedure. These feelings cause the nurse to divert his or her emotional energy from preparing personally for the client's death. In this situation, then, time and emotional energy are wasted.

This situation is less likely to occur if all health care team members expect the client to die at the same time. Communication among staff leads to a better understanding of how to deal with the client. Sharing ideas and feelings will ensure that consistent messages are conveyed to the client. By sharing similar expectations for the client's death, all team members can comfort the client and ease the process of dying.

Personality conflicts with clients[4]

Coping mechanisms and individual personality traits of clients may evoke responses in nurses that they need to be aware of. Nurses must recognize that they may experience personality conflicts with clients that may or may not be related to the trauma of the disease.

On one end of the spectrum there is the "difficult client" and on the other is the "good or respected client." The "difficult client" may be a person that we personally do not like because she or he exhibits unacceptable behavior. The client, for example, may refuse to cooperate and accuse staff of being malicious or inept. The client may maintain apathetic, hostile, or reproachful behavior. Or perhaps the client may become hysterical, noisy, or even shop around for unrealistic cures.

Generally staff appreciate clients who neither create scenes nor cause emotional strain. The "respected client" may be one who faces illness or hospitalization with composure, is not demanding of caregivers, and cooperates with staff members. Such clients evoke admiration and sympathy. On the other hand, it is difficult to admire a client who behaves in a manner that makes us uncomfortable. It is even more difficult to sympathize and interact. Instead, staff may judge the client and lose sight of why he or she is behaving in this way and why the client makes us feel uncomfortable.

For these reasons the nurse needs time to discuss in private each client's personality characteristics and mannerisms that provoke distressing situations. Such discussion can reveal areas of conflict and result in constructive suggestions for alleviating conflict.

Application of theories of Kubler-Ross[5]

Nurses can use the framework outlined by Kubler-Ross to analyze their feelings about a dying client. Kubler-Ross's five stages were originally designed to explain the feelings of the client about his or her own death.[1] With slight modification, Kubler-Ross's analysis applies quite well to nurses' feelings. It is important to note that the application of these stages are not absolute nor do nurses necessarily have to experience any one in particular or in any specific order.

Denial. The first reaction to knowledge of impending death is denial. The client may say "no, not me . . . it can't be true." The nurse's response could be similar: "I'm sure the biopsy will be negative. He's just too nice a guy." Many times practitioners will maintain distance from the dying client so that they will not experience their own feelings about death. Some nurses go as far as avoiding the dying client as much as possible. Denial should be a temporary defense, a buffer to unpleasant or unexpected news. The client has time to work through this period and mobilize coping strategies. The practitioner, however, must move on owing to demands of the job to the next task, often without immediate time to deal with feelings. Thus, nurses must actively find time to deal with their feelings so that they can move on.

Anger. According to Kubler-Ross, anger is the next stage. The client asks, "Why me?" Nurses may ask "Why him; he has two children, he's in love with his wife, he's moved into a new home and is so happy." Caregivers may express their anger on their peers, physicians, x-ray department, or the client. They may also feel helplessness in spite of the advanced state of medical science.

Bargaining. Bargaining is the third stage. The client may state "If I can just see my daughter take her first step and walk over into my arms." The nurse may feel, "I'll care for him, keep him pain-free, and give him what he needs. Just don't let him die on my shift. I can't take it; I'm too drained."

Depression. The fourth stage, depression, serves to prepare the client for the impending loss of love objects. Caregivers may struggle with the loss of their newly acquired relationship. Difficulty is seen when they share in the life of a person who is about to lose everything that is precious to him. Nurses at this point need time to sit and discuss their feelings, to feel the presence of someone who cares, and to have time to concentrate on impending events. It is vital to keep in touch with one's feelings and to have control in order to continue intervention as a caregiver. In the same way that nurses encourage clients, practitioners also need to review the meaning of the client's life and, perhaps, recall their clients in the past who have died, and question their own inner meaning. Nurses must intervene to support one another. We need to listen to our colleagues as they encounter this situation—listening to their fears, doubts, and worries. As practitioners, we need each other for help, so that we can reach out to the client.

Acceptance. The final stage, according to Kubler-Ross, is acceptance. "It's almost a void feeling. It is as if the pain has gone, the struggle is over and there comes a time for the final rest before the long journey."[1] Nurses may perceive that when their clients are in a stage of acceptance, both the nurse and the client may feel that the pain is almost over and both may become devoid of feeling. Often, for the client and caregiver, reaching acceptance of the impending death provides strength to see the end. Acceptance is usually developed through formulating and clarifying one's own feelings of death and dying and gaining knowledge about the feelings of oneself. It allows the nurse to care for the client effectively. For example, the nurse can focus on simple pleasures for the client, such as giving a client an ice cube and suggesting the cool and quenching feeling as the water trickles down, allowing for diversion and sensitivity to the client's physical needs or wants for the moment.

If, on the other hand, nurses are unable to work through these stages, they may be unable to accept the death of their clients. If they cannot accept the death of their clients, they may have trouble caring for them effectively. This applies, too, if nurses have unresolved emotions. Possibly, they may find acceptance at a later time, perhaps with another client or family.

SUPPORT STRUCTURES

As members of the professional team, we need to first understand how to support ourselves and, second, how to support our colleagues. We need to incorporate support systems within the working environment. One way may be by setting aside time once a week to meet with a peer to verbalize feelings of joy, plans, accomplishments, fears. "Psyche rounds" led by a clinical specialist can provide an important forum for discussing interventions and evaluations, as well as feelings, encounters of staff, and relations with clients. Through such "psyche rounds" staff may begin to express needs, especially the need for support in dealing with the dying in the terminal phase.

Becoming sensitive to staff in working situations can benefit all. For example, the team leader or charge nurse who is aware that one of the nurses on the unit is working with a dying client may lighten her client load. This will allow the nurse more time to deal with his or her own feelings and tend to the client's needs. Another example may be seen when a primary nurse is relieved of some tasks, such as bathing the client, so that he or she may have more time to spend working with the family.

Often the term "closet comfort" is used to describe the relationship between two nurses who confide their feelings. By developing this type of relationship with another health care practitioner, a continual exchange and growth may take place involving the genuine qualities and limitations of each one.

Institutions might assign one nurse or practitioner to every unit as a resource person. This consultant would be available to team members to aid in dealing with their own needs and those of the clients.

CONCLUSION

Unfortunately, there is no recipe or manual to dictate the process of grieving. Individuals can only be aware of their feelings and understand their reactions and behaviors. Each situation as it is encountered adds to the learning experience.

The professional needs to recognize the inherent stresses in different clinical situations. For example, intensive care units, renal units, and cancer units all are stressful, unique to their own client populations. If the creation of some assistance to afford support for nurses undergoing "constant grieving" is made available, the likelihood for physical and emotional debilitation is avoidable. If measures are not taken, the professional may become ill, or "burn out," because the nurse as a human being can reach a saturation point and no longer be able to work through experiences. This usually causes the nurse to leave the position.

With each client relationship, each individual, and each death the nurse is involved with, a unique and different experience prevails. Thus, with each new encounter, the nurse expands personally and becomes an even greater, more sensitive caregiver.

REFERENCES

1. Kubler-Ross, E.: On death and dying, New York, 1969, MacMillan Inc.
2. Pattison, M. E.: The experience of dying, Englewood Cliffs, N.J., 1977, Prentice-Hall, Inc.
3. Schneidman, E. in consultation with Parker, E., and Funkhauser, G. R.: Resource pamphlet, New

Haven, Conn., 1977, Education Center for Dying, Death and Bereavement.
4. Schoenberg, B., et al.: Loss and grief: psychological management in medical practice, New York, 1970, Columbia University Press.
5. Sonstegard, L., et al.: The grieving nurse, Am. J. Nurs. **76**(9):1490, 1976.

ADDITIONAL READING

Gow, C., and Williams, J.: Nurses' attitudes toward death and dying, a causal interpretation, Soc. Sci. Med. **11**:191, 1977.

Harper, B.: Death: The coping mechanism of the health professional, Am. Health Care Assoc. J. **3**:42, 1977.

Howard, E.: The effect of work experience in a nursing home on attitudes toward death held by nurse aides, Gerontologist **11**:54, 1974.

Kubler-Ross, E.: To live until we say good-bye, Englewood Cliffs, N.J., 1978, Prentice-Hall, Inc.

Mildred, E.: Health professionals as survivors, J. Psychiatr. Nurs., vol. 15, 1977.

Quint, C. J., and Strauss, A.: Nursing students, assignments, and dying patients, Nurs. Outlook **12**:24, 1964.

21

Nurse-coordinated care of the child with advanced cancer

IDA M. MARTINSON

The role of the nurse has developed over time in response to the needs of society. The strength of the nursing profession is its ability to grow and adapt to meet the changing health needs of individuals as well as the family unit.

With continued advances in diagnosis and treatment, some life-threatening diseases are becoming memories merely recorded in textbooks. However, disease caused or aggravated by heredity, changing life-styles, and environment as well as chronic disease processes continue to create health care needs and demand attention. The care of the client at the end stage of life has always been part of the nurse's role. The increasing recognition of the impact of death on the individual, the family, and on society as a whole makes it imperative for nurses to examine their roles in providing care for the dying client.

Acute care health institutions are no longer considered the only appropriate facilities for persons with terminal diseases. Care of the dying in their homes and in hospice settings has been seriously considered and studied.

This investigation was supported by Grant CA-19490, awarded by the National Cancer Institute, Department of Health, Education and Welfare.

IDENTIFICATION OF NEED

The identification of need is an exceedingly appropriate direction when one considers the goals of the dying client and family compared to the goals of the acute care facility. Hospitals focus on providing curative, restorative care. Modern technology, up-to-date treatment protocols, and well-trained professionals work within a framework with cure or restoration as a goal. Using this approach, institutions are meeting the needs of numerous sick and dying people.

However, clients with end-stage disease, for whom cure-oriented therapy has been attempted and failed, do not fit into the curative framework of delivery of health care. Such an approach to care is not helpful; it is expensive and can be exceedingly demanding and frustrating to the client and the family.

Hospice concept

The hospice concept of care includes a home care program for dying clients and a special inpatient facility for those clients who, for whatever reason, cannot be cared for at home. Whether or not at home, dying clients and their families require specialized care. Professionally, nurses are suited for providing this care. These units, with a team of health professionals including a physician, nurse, social worker, clergy, lay volunteers, and others, can be utilized to suit a variety of needs as outlined in the "Standards for terminal care."[5]

These standards are specifically oriented to those client populations where cure of cancer is impossible. The focus then is found on palliative or supportive treatment, the control of pain, and providing support to the client and family.

The cases where multiple discharges are involved can, in fact, be more effectively dealt with through a more limited core of health professionals. Nurses, who may consult with other experts as needed, can deal with the client's and family's broad needs. Supervising care, providing physical care, and taking the time to listen to the individual and family go hand-in-hand. When clients are at home, it makes especially good sense economically if one person makes home visits and assists the family with their needs. Viewed in this framework, the nurse's role emerges as the matrix of such care.

Adding additional importance to this flexible model is the fact that although some 3,000 children die from cancer each year in the United States, these children are so geographically spread out that special facilities that could attend to their special needs are of no value. However, having nurses available to coordinate this care makes a much more individualized and comprehensive care plan quite feasible. The following list identifies factors that make this nurse-facilitator model both feasible and desirable.

1. Availability of nurses.
2. Nurses are knowledgeable about the expertise of the other health professionals and seek their expertise as well.
3. Nurses have always facilitated care in both hospital and nonhospital settings.
4. Nursing care includes comfort care.
5. The major needs of the dying client are nursing oriented.

Principal among these factors are nursing's demonstrated ability to work with the multiple health disciplines. This can be readily shown by considering the number and variety of health workers the general duty staff nurse encounters during a normal 8-hour shift. These are the full-range physicians, dietitians, physical therapists, social workers, hospital administrators, and so on. These same disciplines, as well as a full range of community-based professionals, are required in caring for dying children.

The concept of nurse-directed care with the nurse responsible for the coordination of this care is a new image, and the following is a discussion of the background, implementation, and early findings of a nurse-directed and coordinated program of care for children with advanced cancer.

HOME CARE FOR THE CHILD WITH CANCER PROJECT

Background

Initial plans for the Home Care for the Child with Cancer project began in 1972 after recognition of the need to aid the parents of children who were dying from cancer. The parents became the primary health care providers so that the child could be monitored at home. This innovation was satisfying to both the parents and the children. This situation contrasts strongly with the traditional approach of protecting the parents from difficult situations. In the nurse-coordinated approach, the nurse can provide valuable services by supporting the parents during their intense involvement with their child. Separation and the sense of helplessness may well be diminished.

The parent-support meetings that further

identified these needs were initially attended by several couples. One parent, a father of a 6-year-old child who was diagnosed with leukemia the previous year, worried how he would respond if his daughter asked if she was dying. Once the group began to establish itself, considerable emotional support was given to the other parents. Morale improved as well as the sharing of common concerns. Most of the discussion periods centered on the general course of childhood leukemia. The parents did not want to be "kept in the dark," rather they wanted to know what to expect and how the question of when to discontinue "curative" treatment would be presented and dealt with. Serious questions such as with whom does the decision lie regarding cessation of treatment were discussed. Some parents shared what to expect when death was near. There was no question this topic was anxiety provoking, but the parents requested the topic be addressed. This need for specific information is a common focus for many self-help groups.[1]

The total group met over a period of years before it disbanded when the local Candlelighters group was formed. The "need to know" was partially satisfied as was the mutual caring the parents expressed to each other. The stresses placed on the parents were substantial; however, it appeared nurses could affect care and so the research project on home care continued.

Program description

The University of Minnesota School of Nursing undertook the Home Care for the Child with Cancer Project as an alternative care setting for children with cancer where medical cure-oriented therapy is no longer effective. During a 24-month period, 58 families had a child die from cancer while participating in the project. Of these 58 families, 46 or 79% cared for their child at home through the death event itself. The remaining children, who were hospitalized for their deaths, spent considerable time at home as part of the program and several were hospitalized for only a few hours before their deaths. These figures contrast strongly with a survey of the location where children with cancer died prior to initiation of this study. A survey record of all children living in Minnesota who died of cancer during a 2-year period identified only six children who died at home.

About one half of the children in the project lived in the Minneapolis – St. Paul, Minnesota area, while the other half lived in cities and rural areas throughout Minnesota and neighboring states. The 58 referrals included 31 or 53% from the University of Minnesota Hospitals and 27 or 49% from nine other hospitals. A total of 23 different physicians referred children to the project; 15 or 63% were affiliated with the University Hospitals, and 9 or 38% were affiliated with other hospitals.

Ages of the children who died at home were a mean of 9.2 years, a median of 8.5 years, and ranged from 1 month to 17 years. The children who died in the hospital had a mean age of 9.8 years, a median of 10.5 years, and ranged from 3 to 17 years of age.

Types of cancers in the 58 children included leukemias, lymphomas, and solid tumors.

Hollingshead's[2] index of social position that combines occupation and education of the head of the household to a single index was used to measure social class of the household. All classes were represented with about one third in classes I, II, or III and two thirds in the lower classes, IV and V.

The Hollingshead two-factor index is a sociologic measure based on education and occupation to determine the socioeconomic position on which may be considered "social class." Utilizing this index allows some comparison to be made across family units.

The actual place of death in the home for the 46 children was a bedroom for 15 or 33%, and the living room, family room, or similar area in the center of household activity for the others.

Length of involvement in the project from first contact to the child's death was a mean of 38.9 days, a median of 20.5 days, and ranged from 1 to 256 days. Fifteen children were involved for less than 1 week, 11 for 1 to 4 weeks, 16 for 1 to 3 months, and 4 for over 3 months. Difficulty in predicting when a child in the terminal stages of cancer will die and also differences among physicians as to when a child should be referred for home care are reasons for this wide range in duration.

The child's parents provided the primary care in the home and a nurse facilitated the care as needed. The nurse was on call to make a home visit or for telephone consultation 24 hours a day, 7 days a week. Direct professional nurse involvement with the 46 children who died at home entailed a mean of 13.4 visits, a median of 8.5 visits, and ranged from 1 to 104 visits per child. The mean length of time per home visit was slightly over 2 hours and varied greatly. Some visits extended for several hours; such long visits were often at the time of death. Telephone conversations between the nurse and family members entailed a mean of 22.7, a median of 15.5, and a range of 0 to 101.

Process of referral

Admittance to the study was based on the physician's judgment that the child had only a limited time to live so that hospitalization with all its disruptions were no longer imperative from the medical standpoint. If the referral did not come from the child's physician, contact was made with the physicians to determine whether or not they concurred. These two mechanisms represented the only ways a child could be admitted to the study.

Once the preliminary discussion took place with the physician, informed consent was obtained and the home care nurse visited the parents and the child. Each family had its own "primary" nurse who would have overall responsibility for the services to be rendered as well as a backup nurse to provide these services when the primary nurse was unavailable.

During the initial visit, the nurse made an assessment of the child and informed the parents as to the care that the child would require and what to expect as the cancer progressed. Encouragement was given by the nurse so as much of the care as possible could be delivered by the family with the nurse acting as a support person, a liaison and advocate for the family. The nurse involvement was continuous and did not stop until several weeks after the child died.

Characteristics of home care nurses

The role of primary nurse was shared by two, three, or even four nurses in a few instances. A total of 58 different nurses served as primary or coprimary nurses to the 58 children. Home care of a critically ill child was a new experience for most of the nurses. All but four of the nurses were RN's; half had baccalaureate degrees. The time since receiving the RN for the 54 registered nurses ranged from 1 to 44 years. These nurses' backgrounds ranged from doctorally prepared nurses to nurses with no academic degree. Additionally, the setting from which the nurses came varied in that some nurses were retired, others hospital based, and some functioned as public health nurses in their communities.

Project objectives

A principal concern of the study was to determine if home care was desirable and feasible as an alternative in the care of children with cancer. Central to this question was discerning the needs of these families and children and how they could best be met. While beginning work was done in 1972 on this model of nurse-directed and nurse-coordinated care, the subsequent years have, with increased financial support, allowed for more development of the role.

Assessment of needs

Needs of parents. Parents' needs and the nurses' role in providing for these needs were assessed in six areas of concern. They were (1) the parents' desire to care for the child, (2) the change in focus from cure-oriented to comfort care, (3) the need for privacy, (4) emotional support for parents and child, (5) pain control for their child, and (6) liaison with the physician, pharmacists, and health care agencies.

Needs of child. The childrens' needs were assessed according to four major categories. These included their desires for (1) home care versus hospital care, (2) the comforts of the home environment, (3) the emotional and physical closeness of the family, and (4) the need for symptom control.

It becomes evident that home care for dying children is desired by the child. During hospitalization, children can be quite demanding and persistent in obtaining an answer to "When can I go home?" When time is at a premium, as in terminal illness, this is an important question. One mother wrote about her desire that the home care alternative be made available to everyone who wants it and included this statement: "My son just gave me his affirmative statement that a kid ought to die where he wants to!"

At home, the children enjoy the "comforts" of home. The family, friends, pets, toys, food—all the constants of their lives—are there to help them live each day until the moment of death does come. In one family, the child received daily communication from her classmates in the form of letters, cards, and drawings. While she felt too weak to be visited in person, she appreciated so much their acts of kindness and continued concern. A child who was struggling with nausea and the resulting poor fluid intake was assisted by his parents and siblings in choosing from his favorite dietary preferences. One child requested his mother's pie crust; his mother was grateful that they could be at home so that she could make the pie crust when he desired it. In another family, the primary nurse described the situation in the home for the dying child and her notes state: "No one was put out of their room. The family continued to live in their usual areas. She slept in her bedroom. During the last week or so, the living room was used. They weren't bothering her and she wasn't putting them out of any place." In contrast to the dismal and depressed atmosphere that many outsiders had predicted, in most cases the feeling of these home environments was warm, loving, and comfortable.

At home, the family has the opportunity for multiple interactions with the child and the ability to maintain emotional and physical closeness to the child. The family can spend more time with the dying child, and at home family members are more available to support and comfort each other. The sometimes lengthy separation of hospitalization is avoided at a time when family unity is needed. The parents are available to answer the siblings' questions and to talk with and be with the child. Our staff has heard repeatedly from surviving family members that the experience of their child dying at home helped their family develop a more realistic acceptance of death.

Symptom control for the children is possible in the home environment. The families are able to monitor and assess their children's needs on a continuing basis and, with support from the health professionals, meet these children's needs. Parents have voiced the desire to care for the child themselves. The findings of our project indicate it is quite possible for parents to assume the caregiving activities with the nurse acting as the principal resource for information, teaching, and support. This direct caregiving by parents has emotional and physical benefits for both parents and child, as well as for participating siblings. Indeed, many parents cite being able to provide better individualized care for the child as a main reason for taking the child home. Observing these interactions demonstrates that health care providers cannot compete with the quality of care these parents provide for their children, with professional support as needed.

With the 58 families included in the project, specialized equipment and supplies have not been required extensively. Of the 46 children who died at home, 5 required oxygen, 4 required suction machines, and 4 required intravenous equipment. However, 25 required no equipment at all. Hospital furnishings, such as wheelchairs, were used by 14 children and a hospital bed by 7 children. It is interesting to note that some children might have been more easily cared for with a hospital bed, but the child rejected the bed because of its association with the hospital.

In facilitating the family's care of their child, it is vital to recognize the change in focus from cure-oriented care to comfort care. The traditional views regarding nutrition and activity may no longer be necessary. The principal rule becomes meeting the child's desires and needs in whatever manner possible. Many of the children in the project were out of bed, walking, playing with siblings, and eating regular meals during the last week of life.

Parents and families often voice a need for privacy during this phase of a child's illness. The home care nurse can assist the family in this area and support them in assuring their privacy during this time. As one nurse stated, "A lot of friends would come to the house and charge in whenever they wanted to. I felt sorry for the family. While trying to be generous, the parents also wanted to have their child alone. The last few days, I was really kind of relieved when they put a sign on the door, 'No Outsiders.'" The nurse may help by interpreting the family's needs to others, including neighbors and extended family.

The tremendous emotional and psychologic burden of living with, and caring for, a dying child, hospitalized or at home, are obvious. These parents have a great need for emotional support. They need to talk and be listened to, reassured, and comforted. The nurses' success as family supporters has been appreciated by the families in the project. Many of them mention the major function of the nurse as "just being there whenever I needed her—to talk, listen, to hear her say that everything was going as well as could be expected."

In addition to the teaching of direct physical care and providing emotional support, families expressed the desire to be taught signs of impending death, probable symptoms such as Cheyne-Stokes respirations, and appropriate courses of action. This information can be readily provided by nurses with their background in physiology and practical experience with such conditions. Even though many of the complications often do not occur, families have stated that they were grateful for the preparation for potential problems and the eventuality of death.

Pain control is of principal concern to anyone involved in care of the child dying from cancer. Within the study, only eight of the 46 children who died at home did not require any prescription analgesics. With the nurse's teaching regarding positive and negative effects of analgesia, dosage, and administration, the parents became quite competent in judging the need for varying levels of analgesia and drug administration.

In the area of pain control and medication, the physicians were most necessary. The physician determined medication choice, dosage limits, and boundaries in administration. However, the nurse and the family were most capable in determining efficacy, dosage requirements, and need for supplemental medications. For example, one nurse, after telephone consultation with the physician, decreased the methadone dosage for a child because the parents perceived the pain had decreased. The need for a change in dosage or a new medication can be dealt with by the nurse in consultation with the physician. Family members also learn to administer medications by injections.

In this care model, the physician serves as a consultant to the nurse. Decisions are made by combining the physician's knowledge of diagnostics and therapeutics with the nurse's intimate picture of the client's highly individualized responses and specific needs. Only a few home visits were made by physicians.

Nursing interventions

Type of nursing interactions employed. In terms of documenting the amount of time these children needed, contacts were divided into two categories: direct services and facilitative services. Direct services were defined as nurse visits to the home, telephone calls between the nurse and the family or child, and visits to the clinic or the hospital.

The second category, facilitative services, included such activities as telephone calls made on behalf of the family to secure some service. This category also included any activity that could be carried out without the family's involvement.

Families and children often need a liaison or advocate between themselves and the physician, pharmacist, and health care agencies. The nurse, familiar with medical terminology, procedures, and schedules, can act on the family's behalf to save them from confusion, misunderstanding, and wasted time away from their child.

In terms of responding to parental and child needs, two important interventions are employed with these families. One is that of "parental control" and the other is "limiting the uncertainty."

Nurses, because of their professional knowledge, skills, and experience, would be able to manage the situation of a dying child and keep everything "under control." However, the parents of a dying child should have the opportunity to be in control. The nurse is challenged to assess the parents and enable them to function as the primary caregivers, "in control" of their child's last days. Parents' confidence in their own abilities needs to be developed by the nurse. The parents may well be giving excellent care but believe that they are not. The nurse should compliment the high quality of care given by the parents while recognizing the lack of parental confidence in the care.

The nurse could encourage parental confidence by explaining to the parent how a specific care procedure is to be done and then letting the parent do it. For instance, suctioning has been taught to parents with little or no difficulty. It is essential that parents realize the nurse's professional support is available at any hour. Families must be encouraged to call or request a visit by the nurse whenever they feel they need help or advice. During the 6 years of this study, an unnecessary phone call has been a rare exception.

Support may also be offered by preparing the parents for complications that may occur, such as hemorrhage, infection, coma, or changes in respirations.

The second intervention, limiting the uncertainty, is necessary to alleviate the parents' fear of the unknown. When anxious parents have no idea of what to expect, the explanation of all the possibilities is reassuring to them. With limits on uncertainty, they have a better understanding of the situation. For example, an anxious parent might call the nurse for instructions concerning the problem of bleeding from the gums. The nurse might simply say that bleeding could increase and explain measures to control the hemorrhaging or that the situation might return to normal without emergency intervention. This would limit the uncertainty for the parent by establishing end points of a continuum of possibilities.

Findings of project

Essentially, what this project proposed was that nurses are capable of managing the care of end-stage clients and supporting the family. The concept of nurse-directed care is not a foreign one, although relatively new. Nurses now manage the care of well adults and children, normal women and their pregnancies, and newborns. Indeed, readily available consultation and backup are essential, but the nurse can effectively serve as the primary care manager with clients with a normal state of health. Death can be seen as a normal event once the course of disease is medically irreversible. Fig. 21-1 illustrates the skills the nurse must bring into this area to successfully coordinate care.

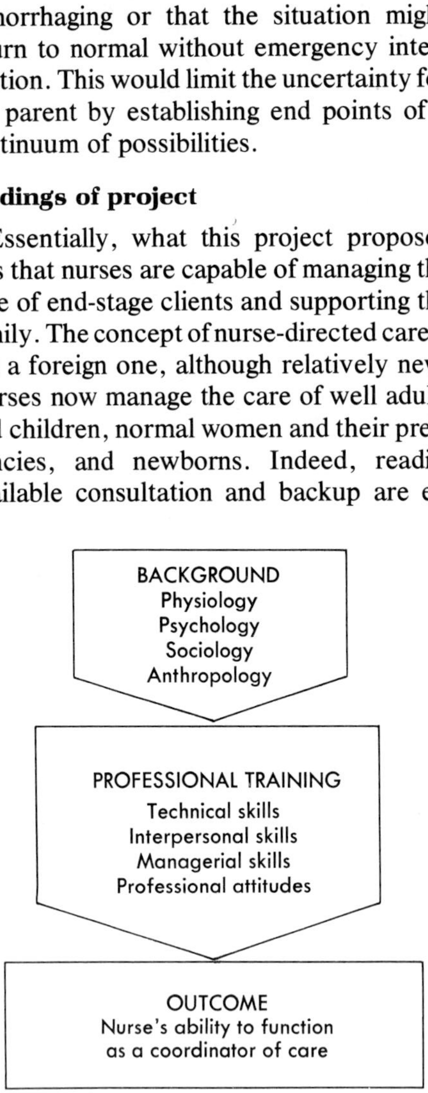

Fig. 21-1. Nurse-coordinator model.

Appropriateness of nurse-coordinator model

The nurse's ability to function as a coordinator of care is based on a combination of skills. First, the nurse draws knowledge from the biologic and behavioral sciences to form a theoretical basis for interventions. Second, the nurse possesses skills to perform care procedures, individually and collectively, as well as the ability to relate to multiple segments of the health care system. These two components merge to allow the nurse to coordinate complex care.

The project staff support the concept of the interdisciplinary health team as a predetermined group of professionals available to the nurse for consultation. However, the use of several professionals from differing backgrounds, each dealing with the family at this crisis period, may be emotionally wearing on the client and family, confusing, and inefficient as well as costly.

Cost factors. Aside from the psychologic, emotional, and sociologic benefits to the family, the question of cost-effectiveness of home care is a valid one. The home care research study has found the average cost of child dying at home is under $1,000, compared to a control group of children dying in the hospital at a cost of about $13,000.[3] Breaking these figures down, the mean dollar cost of their hospital care was $443 per day. Fully two thirds of this amount was accounted for by two items: laboratory tests constituted 38% or $168 per day, while room and board, including nursing services, totalled 29% or $128 per day.

In contrast, home care was substantially less expensive as can be seen by the cost of a home visit by the nurse at $45 per visit, resulting in a mean daily cost of $25. Additionally, laboratory tests were generally not done and room and board were supplied by the parents in the home.[4]

Given the similarity between the goals of caregiving appropriate for home care and the hospital setting, it can be questioned whether hospices need to be physician directed. Care for dying children is within the scope of nursing practice, using the physician for backup and consultation. Consumer satisfaction with the Home Care for the Child with Cancer project has been gratifying, and nurse management is certainly cost-effective.

CLINICAL IMPLICATIONS

Change of attitudes on the part of parents

The clinical implications of the success of this study are numerous. While parents of such children do not tend to react positively all the time to the hospital staff providing care to the child, this study found that parents recognized the valuable services rendered by the home care nurses and expressed appreciation to the interviewing staff during a follow-up interview 6 months after the death of their child. These parents recognized the support the nurse or nurses had given them as well as minimizing discomfort for their child.[4]

Minimizing the child's discomfort. This latter aspect, minimizing the child's discomfort, is important from a humanistic perspective as well as an ethical perspective. For example, if the child and his or her parents had no alternative to hospitalization, the child would be hospitalized for long periods. This would deprive the child from participating in any normal sense; unduly strain the mother, who generally was the primary care provider; create separation between the child and his or her parents; as well as separate the mother from the rest of the family. Support to the child and the parents would be difficult because of the inherent difficulties hospital settings create when "cure" is no longer possible. The feelings of helplessness on the part of the parents could be substantial, as hospitalization promotes an increased use of technology and laboratory tests.

Ability to readily respond to the child's needs. Likewise, the parents have more control over the home situation as opposed to the hospital setting. They can respond more individually to a loss of function on the part of the child or better assist the child to maintain valued activities.

Need for privacy. Privacy is crucial during the last days of the child's life. Death of a child is inherently a family matter, and allowing the child to be at home provides a "closed" setting in which the family members can interact. Outsiders should be kept out, thus preserving the strength of the child as well as the parents and other siblings.

CONCLUSION

In the future, alternative settings need to be explored and expanded. Both the home and in-house hospice can provide humanized, cost-effective, high-quality care for clients at the end stage of life. The need for a very flexible nonhospital role for the home care nurse was discussed earlier. Hospital nurses, who are most familiar with physical crises and death situations, may be uncomfortable in the home without the familiar support systems of the hospital. Public health nurses, on the other hand, are more comfortable working in the home and at ease using community resources but may not be used to handling crises that occur with a critically ill child at home. This seems to suggest that a different orientation is needed to prepare nurses for successful home care experiences. Perhaps this could be accomplished through expanded basic nursing education in this area or specialized assistance from a community home care service, possibly based in a hospice.

Home care may not be the most appropriate alternative to a child dying of cancer, but it was effective in over 90% of the project children and deserves continued implementation and testing by nurses everywhere.

ACKNOWLEDGMENT

I express my appreciation to D. Gay Moldow, R.N., M.S.W., Research Associate, for help in the preparation of this manuscript.

REFERENCES

1. Adams, J.: Mutual-help groups: enhancing the coping ability of oncology clients, Cancer Nurs. **2**(2):95, 1979.
2. Hollingshead, A. B.: The two-factor index of social position, Yale University, 1957, A. B. Hollingshead.
3. Martinson, I. M., et al.: Home care for children dying of cancer, Pediatrics **62:**106, 1978.
4. Martinson, I. M., et al.: Facilitating home care for children dying of cancer, Cancer Nurs. **1:**41, 1978.
5. Wald, F. S., et al.: Assumptions and principles underlying standards for terminal care, Am. J. Nurs. **79:**296, 1979.

ADDITIONAL READING

Martinson, I. M.: The child with leukemia: parents help each other, Am. J. Nurs. **76:**1120, 1976.

Martinson, I. M., editor: Home care for the dying child: professional and family perspectives, New York, 1976, Appleton-Century-Crofts.

Martinson, I. M.: Why don't we let them die at home? R.N. **39:**58, 1976.

Martinson, I. M.: Alternative environments for care of the dying child: hospital, hospice or home. In Sahler, O. J., editor: The child and death, St. Louis, 1978, The C. V. Mosby Co.

Martinson, I. M.: Loss of a child: two case studies. In Kjervik, D., and Martinson, I., editors: Women in stress: a nursing perspective, New York, 1979, Appleton-Century-Crofts.

Martinson, I. M., et al.: When the child is dying: home care for the child, Am. J. Nurs. **77:**1815, 1977.

VI

MAJOR CLIENT NEEDS OR HIGH-INCIDENCE PROBLEMS

22

The spectrum of care for clients with cancer

LISA BEGG MARINO

In earlier chapters, various aspects of cancer care were discussed. Some of these chapters are more oriented to the dynamics of cancer nursing practice, while other chapters focus more directly on clinical problems or needs. All the previous chapters are designed to prepare the reader for the following group of chapters that focus attention on certain functional or clinical areas of need. However, before these chapters can be discussed, the reader is asked to focus on general aspects of cancer and cancer nursing practice. Knowing the range of tumors, their large numbers, and the characteristics of clients who are affected is needed to appreciate why and how problems can occur. Discussion of psychologic care, ethics of practice, and client-family teaching, as well as nurse burnout and nursing research can help the nurse to broaden the base of practice and to work toward the generation of new knowledge. Although nurses have been caring for cancer clients for many decades, major concepts pertaining to the appropriate roles for nurses as well as major client and family needs have undergone substantial revision within the last decade. Because cancer nursing is changing so quickly, coupled with the changes in cancer health care, refinements and outright expansion of responsibilities will continue for some time. This trend is a positive one in that most of the client-family needs would not have appeared before cancer treatment advances were achieved, which resulted in greater long-term survival. However, as profound as these cancer treatment advances have been, they have not been entirely positive. For example, the morbidity associated with many forms of cancer treatment is substantial. This consequence has troubled many oncologists and has reinforced the need to develop equivalent treatment regimens that produce an acceptable level of effectiveness while reducing the resulting morbidity. This medical goal is commendable and should be encouraged and aided by nurses everywhere. However, there are a wealth of other needs that can be addressed, many of which are appropriate for nurses to pursue. These needs form the basis for this chapter as well as the next section in its entirety.

DOCUMENTATION OF CLIENT AND FAMILY NEEDS

It is generally acknowledged that the multiple diseases commonly referred to as cancer are catastrophic in their nature and place the client and family under severe stress. The threat of illness, diagnosis, and treatment and their consequences all place the client in varying degrees of disruption. Many of these disruptions stem from the fatalistic perceptions of cancer that still persist, but a large number of disruptions occur secondary to the pathologic process, its diagnosis, and treatment requirements. Regardless of their cause, the clients and the entire social network in which the client participates is disrupted. For example, consider what it may mean to a family to learn that their child has cancer. The child's immediate family, extended family, and friends are all affected in some fashion because of the value we place on our children and the crucial time frame in which the child is in terms of growth and development. Similarly, morbidity as a direct consequence of the disease itself or secondarily owing to treatment can adversely affect the client, family, and their entire social network by limiting interaction because of physical limitations or a perceived inability to function with others. An example of morbidity related to cancer treatment can be clients who successfully underwent a curative colon resection with colostomy. The cancer was eradicated, but because of fears of offending others or embarrassing themselves owing to odors or spillage, these people do not return to their former preoperative life-styles. Instead, because of real or perceived fears, they become social recluses. Since this may not have been their pattern of behavior, this situation could be considered morbidity from cancer treatment. This situation also represents a good opportunity for nurses to intervene so that adequate education in self-care and appropriate support can be given to minimize or completely prevent such morbidity.

Many more needs can exist with the client and family. Not all clients have all of the needs that will be discussed later in this chapter, but awareness on the part of the nurse for possible needs in these areas makes it more likely that these needs will be met appropriately.

IMPORTANCE OF NURSING CARE IN CANCER

Throughout the chapters of this book, there have been numerous comments as to the appropriateness of nurses in rendering care to this population of clients. This action is explicit and intentional because of the growing awareness of the stress that is inherent with cancer as well as the potential problems that can be caused by the sophistication of diagnostic and treatment procedures. Additionally, many more clients are surviving their cancer, and so needs that would have never appeared are appearing now. The potential need areas or problems are varied and can be present in all clients regardless of whether they are at high risk for cancer, undergoing diagnostic or therapeutic procedures, or in the advanced stages of illness. Additionally, these needs are not limited to a particular cancer site or an individual's developmental stage, but rather the nurse should be sensitive to the possibility that all of these needs may be present in any cancer client. The difference may be represented in *degrees* of need, with one or two needs being more central. For example, sexuality is a need in all persons, including cancer clients. A person's sexuality may be threatened by a long-term illness such as cancer, especially if the cancer involves a major body part that represents a great deal to that person's concept of his or her own sexuality. Nurses, because of their visibility and skills and the fact that many clients perceive them to be nonthreatening, can do much to validate with clients what their illness means to them, support them as they grieve, and aid them to adapt as much as possible to their altered state. With this type of goal in mind, each potential need will be discussed along with suggestions for appropriate nursing interventions.

A beginning core of needs and the appropriate nursing action was recently published by the Oncology Nursing Society and the American Nurses' Association. This document, called the *Outcome Standards For Cancer Nursing Practice,* was developed jointly by these two organizations to provide nurses with guidelines for improving the care of these clients.[1] Publication of these standards also formally acknowledged nursing's responsibilities in the care of cancer clients.

OVERVIEW OF NEEDS

There are thirteen major potential needs or problem areas that have been identified for cancer clients. They are: comfort, morbidity, growth and development, prevention and early detection, information gathering, coping, nutrition, infection control, sexuality, elimination, changes in body image, safety, and oxygenation. These needs correspond somewhat with the previously cited *Outcome Standards For Cancer Nursing Practice* because I established the Oncology Nursing Society committee that developed these standards at the same time preliminary plans for this book were being made. These standards and the needs identified in this book differ in some respects, with Table 22-1 listing those areas of agreement or difference. The primary differences are that there are 10 standards, each of which is considered separately and given equal "weight," while the needs identified in this text cover some additional areas and consider certain needs to be more global than some of the others. For example, Chapter 17 discussed the needs of clients in the advanced stages of cancer with their principal need of comfort being identified. Persons in this stage of illness have a great many physiologic and psychologic comfort needs as well as many

Table 22-1. Comparison of needs or problem areas as discussed in *Outcome Standards For Cancer Nursing Practice*[1] and this text

Needs or high-incidence problem areas identified in this text	**Needs or high-incidence problem areas identified in *Outcome Standards For Cancer Nursing Practice***
Unifying needs or problem areas	High-incidence problem areas
Comfort	Comfort
Information gathering	Information
Morbidity	Coping
Coping	Prevention and early detection
Specific needs	Nutrition
Prevention and early detection	Protective mechanisms
Growth and development	Sexuality
Nutrition	Elimination
Infection control	Mobility
Sexuality	Ventilation
Changes in body image	
Elimination	
Safety	
Oxygenation	

other needs such as nutrition, sexuality, safety, and changes in body image. Likewise, comfort is not an exclusive need to clients in advanced stages but may also be important to many other clients in varying states of wellness or illness.

Unifying needs

There are four needs or problem areas that are considered to be more global, serve to unify the other needs, or are especially important areas on which nursing should concentrate.

Comfort. The concept of comfort as a need in cancer clients was extensively discussed in Chapter 17. It will be briefly reviewed here. Comfort has been defined as the minimizing of psychobiologic distress, which means that there is a psychologic component as well as a physiologic component.[1] The psychologic component can be exemplified by aiding clients in disclosing their diagnoses and what it means to their children. How cancer affects communication has been discussed many times in this book, but this fact cannot be reinforced too much. It is a stressful experience to be a person with cancer. The social stigmas that prevail with cancer carry over to the client. Children are not immune to these perceptions, and so it is difficult for the parent to disclose that they have cancer and that it might mean disability or even death. Helping the client decide what and how to tell children can be a valuable professional activity. Supporting them during the disclosure event is also important as is being available to answer questions that may arise. If the client is willing to disclose this information, the tension and fears that might have been present are minimized as the children once again become involved in the important life events of their parents. It should be noted that some ambivalence may be observed in the children because greater responsibilities may be forced on them by the illness of their parent. Household duties, an afterschool job to help meet financial obligations, and altered school plans may be required. In these cases, the nurse can be very helpful by reinforcing the universality of these feelings and by working with the family to explore alternatives if they wish.

Another example in the area of physical comfort measures can be demonstrated by the man who places his value as an employee on his physical skills. He finds out that he has cancer with some debility resulting. He can no longer work in his former capacity. Sometimes it may be a straightforward case of not having a job, but many times an employer will make an attempt to adjust the affected employee's responsibilities to better meet his new physical state. Exploring with clients, male or female, if this is a possibility and helping them to negotiate for these changes or reinforcing the importance of attempting to meet clients' needs to the employer are all important and professional activities the nurse could pursue. Relative to maintaining working positions after a diagnosis of cancer, the nurse should be sensitive to the fact that many clients do not wish to continue their employment. Because nurses get caught up in the "work ethic" attitude that is common in the United States, they *assume* the client wants to return to work. This may not always be the case, so nurses should be careful they do not allow their own values to dictate care. It is far better to determine what is important to clients and then direct interventions toward *their* goals.

Along with considering comfort as a separate need, it can serve to unify an entire nursing strategy for many cancer clients. For example, the woman who has had a breast biopsy that has been confirmed to be cancerous may be quite anxious. Her needs may be multiple, with comfort being the most important need as well as serving to unite all other needs such as information gathering, prevention and early detection, coping, morbidity, sexuality, and changes in body image. To exemplify, the client may need general support during these anxious days (comfort) as well as adequate information on which to base any decisions (information gathering). While the woman is considering her options, the nurse needs to continue to maintain communication so that questions can be correctly answered and a plan to deal with discovery of this breast cancer is completed (prevention and early detection). This need is particularly important when the cancer is in the breast because of its highly emotional nature and the multiple controversies that are still evident within the medical community as to how to best treat these cancers. In the long term, these controversies will probably produce improved treatments for breast cancer; however, in the short term, they only heighten the woman's anxiety because she does not know who and what to believe and unfortunately cannot delay a decision for the lengthy period it will take to resolve these medical controversies. The nurse can be extremely helpful by being available to the client as a key resource so that the decision can be made on how the woman wishes to proceed.

Promoting the client's adaptation can be met by a consistent approach that strives to compartmentalize the crisis so that the client can solve the problems needed to successfully cope. Morbidity is a major problem area in breast cancer because most surgeries are mutilating and result in diminished physical functioning on the part of the client. Research is attempting to demonstrate if more limited and thus less morbid procedures give an equivalent survival rate. It is still too early to be sure, but given the current surgical procedures, adequate client and family teaching can help to minimize morbidity associated with breast surgery. For example, clients should be taught exercise plans once the surgeon ascertains safety; then simply stressing the importance of protecting the affected arm from injections and other punctures can prevent or minimize additional problems. Needs relating to sexuality when cancer is found in the breast can be major, since many women and much of the American culture place great sexual value in the female breast. The nurse cannot change perceptions but can reinforce how important the client is as a person and that her value includes more than her sex appeal. These same statements are also true for the real or perceived changes in the client's body image.

Information gathering. Information gathering has been stressed as a vital need for the client and family throughout this book. It will be discussed here further to encourage the nurse reader to expand interventions in this area.

The client's need for information is particularly important in seeking medical aid, deciding on the preferred therapy option, ascertaining the prognosis so that personal matters can be arranged, and determining the response to therapy. These situations are but a few examples of client advocacy in which the nurse can facilitate care.

This need is also considered to be a unifying one because it is central to just about every other need. For example, if nutrition is considered to be a need with a client, information gathering about what the client's food habits are, preferred times to eat, methods of coping, and capability to make changes are all needed before an adequate nutritional plan can be developed. Information gathering is also important in terms of infection control because the client and family can be taught important hygiene measures or methods of minimizing the client's risk of infection. Since much of cancer treatment, particularly radio- and chemotherapies, is given on an outpatient basis, it is doubly important that the entire cancer team instruct everyone concerned about protective measures. Nurses, because of their strong teaching ability, are the ideal health care providers to lead these efforts.

Morbidity. Morbidity is defined as a negative change in the physical or psychologic functioning of the client, which is a direct result of disease or its treatment. Because of the pathologic process and the treatments that are employed for a diagnosis of cancer, morbidity is a major problem area. Morbidity associated with the disease process can be represented by such consequences as anorexia and fatigue owing to the presence of a cancer. These symptoms are common to many cancers, particularly those in the gastrointestinal tract. Physical morbidity owing to cancer can also be represented in the deterioration that develops as a consequence of primary or metastatic brain tumors. The loss or impairment in motor functioning limits the client's ability to move about a great deal and can cause serious safety problems for everyone concerned. The nurse can work actively with the medical team to devise a safe plan for ambulation and then work closely with the client and family to implement it.

Psychologic morbidity associated with cancer has been discussed many times through examples such as negative perceptions in the client's self-image, limitations on social interaction because of some fear related to rejection by others, or being a physical burden.

Morbidity from some form of cancer treatment is a major problem today. Increased awareness of the problems that result from treatment have led to a concerted effort to reduce these occurrences. Examples such as amputations to cure sarcomas; diversionary procedures such as colostomies for colorectal cancer; and nausea, vomiting, diarrhea, myelosuppression, and alopecia all caused by chemo- or radiotherapies greatly limit the person's ability to remain functional.

Morbidity as a major problem that combines with other specific needs can be represented by the amputation of a child's leg because of osteogenic sarcoma (morbidity) so that normal growth and development through participation in play experiences are hindered. It has been cited previously that many forms of cancer treatment, particularly surgery, produce significant morbidity that affects the client's needs such as sexuality, elimination, oxygenation, and changes in body image. Since many of these changes are permanent, the nurse should expect profound grieving to occur because the client is suffering a loss. Many times the individual's perceptions make for an even greater loss, but at a minimum there is some feeling for the lost body part. Showing the client and family that adjustments can be made is helpful. For example, clients who have lost their larynx may be skeptical that they will ever be able to communicate verbally again. Having them visit someone who has learned esophageal speech and who has made a successful adjustment can offer important encouragement at a time of overwhelming anxiety about their future. This combination of approaches, acknowledgment of their loss, and the fact that grieving must take place, coupled with encouragement that the loss can be minimized is the essence of professional cancer nursing practice.

Coping. Since the diagnosis of cancer is universally acknowledged as being stressful, the client and family are forced to deal with this stress and manage it as best they can. It has been mentioned previously that individuals' past experience with crisis or their perception of what is happening to them and the available supports are important factors in determining how well or how poorly a person will be able to cope with a diagnosis of cancer. For example, a person's manner of coping will determine how he or she will respond to possible prevention or early cancer detection measures. Chapter 4 discussed the delay in diagnosis, which is still commonly encountered today even though significant advances have been obtained with publicity being frequent. Still, the vast majority of people delay for some period of time before acting on their suspicions, with many people delaying for many months. A certain amount of delay is both normal and expected as the person attempts to integrate these fears and become capable of formulating a plan for acting on the problem. Further delay develops out of extraordinary fears or needs that may have to do with changes in body image, sexuality, or elimination, for example.

Specific needs

Prevention and early detection. Prevention and early detection as a specific need for cancer clients centers mainly on obtaining information and the utilization of this information. The former point centers principally on client and family education to inform the public of known cancer risk factors so that they can decide if they wish to act on this information and alter their lifestyle or seek further evaluation. It has been stressed many times in this book that nurses are appropriate and effective client educators. One of the most crucial needs in all of cancer care is that of making the client and family aware of the truth so they can decide for themselves how they wish to proceed. So often, health care providers are tempted to evaluate the situation within their own value system. Unfortunately, the situation is more complicated than that. Why people continue self-destructive behaviors and ignore proven causal relationships is proving to be quite complex. Much effort and financial support are being directed to a better understanding of this phenomenon so that cancer incidence can eventually be reduced. Nursing, because of its long and strong interest in preventive care, can do much to help explain what is occurring and how to affect some positive change on the part of those at high risk for cancer.

Along the same theme, many people can benefit from early detection programs that are aimed at high-risk populations. Finding out how to better meet individual needs so that greater utilization of services can be achieved would be an important first step. Moreover, those clients who need further evaluation and possible treatment can benefit from skilled nursing care. This care is directed at minimizing their stress as much as possible by the identification of the best way to explain the pathology and to aid them in decision making. This professional attitude and approach is really an ethical basis of practice that was discussed in Chapter 5. Since this area is undergoing rapid and profound change, it represents both a challenge and a series of opportunities for nurses to enhance the care being rendered to the client and family.

Growth and development. Growth and developmental changes or disruptions that occur because of a diagnosis of cancer can affect an individual throughout any age or stage of development. These disruptions and the resulting requirements for change are most profoundly seen in children who have cancer. Here you have all the negative characteristics of cancer, the stigma, the threat of death, the morbidity, at a time of rapid physical and psychologic change that is stressful in itself. Coupled with a diagnosis of cancer and even with conscientious health care providers, problems may not be completely solvable. For example, a child who has acute leukemia will undergo extensive treatment that will probably produce a remission of the disease. If this does occur, the child is essentially normal and can pursue play activities without any restrictions. However, during the illness phase, the child is gravely ill and thus unable to pursue these childhood activities. This means that the development that would be likely to occur through play experiences and interactions with other people may not occur or may be delayed. Health care providers are certainly aware of the importance of play and attempt to structure times so that play is optimized, but if the child is too weak or because of myelosuppression must be kept apart from other children, play and interactions with other children may not occur. Therefore there is a loss or delay in the development of the child. Likewise, growth may be retarded by the treatments, such as growth retardation from radiotherapy to bony regions or possible untoward effects of surgery or chemotherapy. The nurse may not be able to do anything about these effects, but aiding the family to obtain correct and complete information and supporting them in their decision can help the child. This same approach is helpful in maximizing children's developmental processes by acknowledging their personhood, answering their questions, and accepting their fears. Offering support and minimizing the disruptions by actively working with the parents, community resources, and the child's school officials are important nursing activities.

Nutrition. Nutrition is a basic need for all people and is extremely important in terms of cancer etiology and treatment. Nutrition is also a complex problem in terms of the differing individual perceptions of its importance and the difficulty in teaching new dietary habits. Both of these activities are time consuming, require the professional to be capable of assessing the current situation and making adjustments as needed, plus conscientiously following through with counseling the client and family. Many of the health care providers could fill the role, but the nurse has the greatest overall skills to aid the client and family with this potentially frustrating and debilitating problem. Proper nutrition may make the difference between a good quality of life and one that is inadequate. The nurse, by maintaining an ongoing relationship with the client and family, can work to enhance food and fluid intake, thereby enhancing the client's level of energy.

In terms of nutrition's role, if any, in cancer etiology, nurses can complete careful history taking that might identify information as to a possible relationship between diet and cancer. Also, the nurse can help explain interim, possibly conflicting, reports on this relationship. Many times, the public becomes confused or discouraged with the large number of detailed, technical reports and so a nurse can serve a very useful purpose by being a client educator.

Infection control. Infection control is a major goal in all forms of cancer treatment. From the surgical incision to the skin lesions associated with immunotherapy to the myelosuppression caused by radio- and chemotherapies, these client needs require the nurse to be an instructor in self-protective care and an observer for problems that could develop. Since it is widely recognized that cancer clients are compromised in terms of immunologic functioning from the pathologic process itself and secondarily from the treatment, infection control is a vital need. Nurses can provide information to both the client and family on the importance of maintaining skin integrity, prevention of trauma, awareness of possible sources of infection, and supportive interventions that can be instituted. Many of these activities require at least a minor change in life-style, so it is important for the nurse to maintain contact with the client and family so that feedback can be given, alterations made, and general encouragement offered to continue these protective measures.

The nurse as an observer can be crucial in terms of identifying problems early before they become a serious threat to life, since much of cancer treatment is given on an outpatient basis. Reinforcing the significance of these problems and the value of "checking in periodically" can be helpful to everyone. If the client or a family member has a question about some development, it is far better that they be encouraged to call so that correct information and monitoring will be possible. Much of the morbidity and mortality associated with modern cancer treatment is associated with infection control specifically and to the larger concept of protective mechanisms. The protective mechanisms are composed of the immune, hematopoietic, integumentary, and sensorimotor systems. The nurse is perceived by the client to be more approachable and does possess the knowledge and skills to positively affect the client's outcome.

Sexuality. Sexuality is one of the more obvious needs of cancer clients. Unfortunately, it is also one of the more neglected. This fact can be partially explained by the sheer effort that is consumed on the part of the client, family, and health care team to care for the client. When one deals with literally a life-or-death situation with the threat of death continually present, worries about an individual's sexuality may seem to be insignificant. However, this need is being recognized as being very important because of the increasing numbers of persons who are surviving after the diagnosis of cancer. Sexuality or sexual identity is a significant aspect of the quality of life. Unfortunately, along with being preoccupied with rendering general care, many health care providers are uncomfortable in discussing individuals' perceptions of their sexual functioning and expression. Because this is such an important need and the nurse is oriented to meeting client needs, a serious attempt should be made to actively work with the client to achieve optimal functioning in this area or to help arrange for the appropriate consultation so that the client can achieve a high level of functioning.

Treatments that almost always produce alterations in a client's sexual identity and functioning should be given greater weight, but *all* cancer clients should be assessed for sexuality needs so that those persons who are uncomfortable in discussing their perceptions can be actively dealt with in a nonjudgmental and supportive approach.

Changes in body image. Changes in body image are examples of commonly acknowledged problems in cancer care but can also be neglected on the part of the health care provider. The major way the health care provider neglects this important need is to assume that the client does not need to grieve for the lost or changed body part. When body image is discussed with cancer, grief is acknowledged, but little recognition to the degrees of grieving necessary for adjustment is given. Grieving for the lost breast, perceived unattractiveness owing to a diversionary procedure, or alopecia from chemotherapy will be related to the client's placement of value on this part or obvious sign of disease. This latter aspect is being recognized as being very important because it can label the client as "sick." Nursing's attempts to minimize treatment-induced changes can be helpful to the client as can reinforcing value as a person. However, the nurse should be cognizant that grieving needs to occur before any meaningful adjustment can be made so that sanctioning the client's right to grieve is important. Continuing to provide support to both the client and family is an important professional intervention because many people are too embarrassed to openly grieve or want to show how strong they can be. The perception of the "ideal" client is reinforced by supporting behavior that promotes the "compliant" client rather than the one who acknowledges the loss by sorrowful expression. Likewise, offering support to clients as they work through family dynamics as they relate to the clients' "new" self can be very important to clients and promotes family support and interaction.

Elimination. Elimination is another basic human need that can be adversely affected by cancer or secondarily by cancer therapy. Alterations in elimination may include fecal and urinary diversions, fistulas, diarrhea, constipation, bladder insufficiencies, incontinence, or fecal or urinary obstruction.[1] Nursing has made major strides in working to better meet clients' needs in this area. Nurses have recognized the varied perceptions elimination holds for different people and the fact that problems in this area can profoundly affect the client's quality of life. For example, nurses are the predominant group in enterostomal therapy and routinely consult with surgeons preoperatively to determine the best location for the stoma. Nurses also serve as observers to detect treatment-related toxicities such as neurotoxicity, which can adversely affect the client's elimination. Client and family teaching as to self-care and ways to protect the self are routinely done by nurses. Nurses are very aware of the disruptions that can occur because of changes in elimination and so can actively work with clients and their families to minimize these disruptions and promote a high level of self-care. This allows clients to better integrate these changes based on *their* value system, *their* perception of what is happening to them, and what *they* need in the way of assistance to successfully adjust.

Safety. Safety has both a psychologic and physiologic component and represents one of the latest awarenesses of client and family needs. Safety can be compromised by the cancerous process or secondarily by treatment. Regardless, these changes represent further disability of the client and usually evoke increased anxiety on the part of the client and family.

In terms of disease-related safety problems, the nurse can concentrate on developing safe care plans with the physician so that functioning can be preserved to the greatest extent possible while further problems can be avoided as much as possible. A good example is the woman with metastatic breast cancer who has pathologic fractures and needs a very carefully planned ambulation strategy to prevent further fractures while still maintaining function to continue valued activities.

Safety needs that are related to cancer treatment are numerous, with most of them centering on drug-related changes or potential problems. Steroids and chemotherapeutic agents require close monitoring by the nurse and careful client and family instructions so that problems can be prevented or at least minimized.

Oxygenation. Oxygenation is another important need for all humans that can be adversely affected by cancer or its treatment. Respiratory insufficiency caused by the presence of disease or secondarily caused by radio- or chemotherapies frequently limits the client's life-style. The nurse can work with the medical team to provide as much support and comfort to the client as possible. The nurse can be observant for possible oxygenation problems caused by the cancer itself such as anemia in the client. Working with the client to identify normal schedules and developing revised schedules that provide for more rest and sleep are important to clients regardless of their stage of disease.

Teaching self-care to the client or supportive management of their compromised state is important because it may make it possible for the client to be maintained outside the hospital. Since many oxygenation needs appear later in cancer's course, the quality of life may also be improved.

GENERAL FORMAT FOR SECTION

The following eight chapters in this section deal with some of the needs previously cited. These needs represent important areas that nurses caring for cancer clients should be aware of so that care can be enhanced. To discuss these needs further, each chapter concentrates on one need and goes into detail utilizing a major cancer site. For example, growth and development are important needs to children that can be adversely affected by the diagnosis of a cancer. Cancer in children is a leading cause of death before age 15, so combining the need and the representative cancer can help the reader integrate the content of this book. Most of the following eight chapters have a similar format in that overall incidence and characteristics of the particular cancer site open the chapter and are followed by a discussion of overall client needs and then concentrate on one specific need. Table 22-2 lists the chapter(s) and the major need that is discussed. Some of the unifying needs were more appropriate earlier in the book and these are also listed in the table. Case studies are used liberally in each chapter so that the reader can see practical approaches that may be utilized.

It should be stressed that listing a client need with one cancer site has been done for *learning purposes only* and does not seek to promote a singular attitude as to the presence of these needs. For example, earlier in this chapter the need of sexuality was discussed and it was mentioned that sexuality is a basic need of all humans. For some, it has greater meaning because of individual perceptions or the fact that cancer affects a body part that has increased sexual conno-

Table 22-2. Client needs and problem areas with chapters in which they are discussed

Client need	Chapter(s) that discusses need/problem area
Unifying need or problem area	
Comfort	17, 18, 21
Information gathering	3, 5, 6
Morbidity	24
Coping	4, 7
Specific needs	
Prevention and early detection	9, 10
Growth and development	23
Nutrition	25
Infection control	26
Sexuality	27, 30
Changes in body image	28
Elimination	30
Safety	29
Oxygenation	22

tation. The same is true for all the other needs. Nurses should be assessing *all* clients for *all* possible needs and then developing a care plan based on the nursing process or problem-solving manner.

CONCLUSION

This chapter has listed 13 major needs that are common to clients who have cancer. Some of these needs have been documented by the ONS and ANA through their *Outcome Standards For Cancer Nursing Practice*. The difference between what has been discussed in this chapter and the ONS/ANA standards is that certain needs or problem areas are considered to be more universal or unifying than others. The example of comfort as an umbrella concept was put forth.

The important points to remember are that nurses have begun to identify major client characteristics and corresponding areas of need. This knowledge will continue to be refined, but for the present it serves as a guideline for the nursing care of this population of clients and a fertile area for nursing research. This chapter and the remaining eight chapters in this section are intended to inform and stimulate nurses to more completely assess their clients so that more comprehensive care can be rendered.

REFERENCE

1. Oncology Nursing Society and American Nurses' Association: Outcome standards for cancer nursing practice, Kansas City, Mo., 1979, American Nurses' Association.

23

Children with cancer: a developmental approach

MARY MORROW and HARRY L. WILSON

Cancer in children in the United States, although rare, is second only to accidents as the major cause of death in children after the first year of life.[1,3] The overall annual incidence of new cancer cases is approximately 20 per 100,000 children.[1] Until recently, the diagnosis of cancer meant the eventual death of the child. However, through clinical research and well-organized national treatment programs, remarkable advances have been made. Cures in the sense of long-term, disease-free survival have been achieved for many victims of these devastating childhood diseases. For example, acute lymphocytic leukemia was once thought to be universally fatal. Of the children who have this disease now, more than 45% remain disease free for 5 or more years.[10] These children are probably cured. Even if cure is not achieved, however, current treatment for childhood cancer results in longer survival, better control of active disease, and an improved quality of life.

Childhood cancers are different from adult cancers. Most adult cancers are of epithelial cell origin and are often associated with exposure to toxic environmental agents.[14,18] Childhood cancers do not have such clear causal relationships, and environmental and nutritional factors do not seem to be involved in their etiology. A few childhood malignancies, like retinoblastoma and Wilms' tumor, may have a hereditary basis.[17] In general, however, the cause of childhood cancer is unknown. Below is a list of common childhood cancers in order of their relative frequency:[1,18]

1. Leukemia
   a. Lymphocytic
   b. Myelocytic
   c. Monocytic
2. Central nervous system tumors
3. Lymphoma
   a. Hodgkin's disease
   b. Non-Hodgkin's
4. Neuroblastoma
5. Soft tissue sarcomas
   a. Rhabdomyosarcoma
   b. Fibrosarcoma
   c. Undifferentiated sarcoma
6. Wilms' tumor (nephroblastoma)
7. Bone tumors
   a. Osteogenic sarcoma
   b. Ewing's sarcoma
8. Retinoblastoma
9. Germ cell tumors
   a. Teratoma

10. Liver tumors
    a. Hepatoma
    b. Hepatoblastoma

These malignant tumors are of four general types: embryonic tumors (blastomas), lymphoreticular disorders (leukemia and lymphoma), connective tissue malignancies (sarcomas), and brain tumors.

Traditionally, cancer therapy has been directed toward local control of disease. Increased understanding of the natural history of solid tumors in children has shown that systemic spread by subclinical micrometastases is probably present at the time of diagnosis. Systemic spread renders local extirpative surgery and radiation inadequate for cure. Clinical researchers discovered that systemic chemotherapy helps eliminate micrometastases, thereby increasing the possibility of cure. Surgery and radiation therapy provide local control; chemotherapy treats systemic disease. The multimodal approach to cancer therapy was developed by pediatric oncologists to treat leukemia, and this approach has subsequently been successfully applied to other childhood cancers. Multimodal therapy has resulted in remarkable improvements in cure rates for solid tumors as well as leukemia and has become the hallmark of effective cancer treatment for children.

A multidisciplinary team of medical and surgical specialists from oncology, radiotherapy, pathology, neurology, dentistry, pediatric surgery, and other surgical subspecialties, such as opthalmology and orthopedics, is essential for comprehensive management of multimodal therapy. No one medical specialty can anticipate and manage the complex medical problems that arise during the treatment of the child who has cancer. Large medical centers facilitate optimal multidisciplinary interaction and are the best setting for pediatric oncology treatment. Because the incidence of childhood cancer is low, major pediatric oncology centers throughout the country have organized themselves into large study groups that share and coordinate information. Statistically significant data gained through these study groups have resulted in major advances in the understanding and management of these diseases. In the course of this chapter, acute lymphocytic leukemia and Wilms' tumor will be presented as examples of childhood cancers for which organized studies have yielded significant advances.

A diagnosis of cancer produces an ambivalent situation in which there exists the possibility, but not the certainty, of cure. Apprehension about cure will remain for many years. Cure is realized only through a lengthy and diligent process of demanding and complex therapy, followed by years of observation of the child. Cancer is a harsh intruder into any individual's life; for the developing child, it is an insult with the most profound impact. Treatment involves the whole child, not just the cancer. "Caretakers"—physicians, nurses, social workers, dietitians, child life specialists, and chaplains—provide for the many needs of the child with cancer. They must recognize the impact of this disease on the intellectual, emotional, and social, as well as the physical, growth of the developing child.

The "Concepts of Therapy" section will discuss details of therapy for childhood cancer. The "Developmental Approach" section will discuss the impact of cancer and its therapy on the child's development.

CONCEPTS OF THERAPY

Surgery

Surgery is often the first therapeutic procedure performed on the child who has cancer. The basic concepts as discussed in Chapter 12 are the same. For most of the malignant childhood tumors, complete resection improves the chances for cure. If complete tumor removal is not possible, safe debulking often enables other modes of therapy to be more effective. However, certain tumors, such as neuroblastoma, are often difficult to resect because of extensive vascularity, friability, and local tissue infiltration. In such cases, surgery is performed to confirm the diagnosis, and treatment consists of radiation, chemotherapy, or both. Any aggressive attempt to resect extensive or widespread tumor may endanger the child's life and is often unnecessary with current curative programs of radiation and chemotherapy. In some cases, surgery may be used to assess a tumor's response to therapy, and any remaining tumor may be resected. For childhood lymphomas, surgical resection is inappropriate because of the high probability of systemic involvement. Treatment relies on chemotherapy and radiation; however, surgical biopsy is essential to determine the kind of lymphoma. If Hodgkin's disease is diagnosed, then an exploratory laparotomy with splenectomy may be necessary for adequate staging of the disease. Surgery is often essential for accurate diagnosis of childhood malignancies and plays a major role with radiation and chemotherapy in treating cancer in children.

Chemotherapy

The paradox of cancer chemotherapy is that treatment intended for good also does harm. Chapter 14 details the pharmacokinetics, toxicities, and nursing interventions associated with this therapy. Chemotherapy agents help cure cancer by killing or injuring individual cancer cells, but these drugs are not selective and therefore also damage normal cells. The goal of cancer chemotherapy is to administer drugs that kill or injure the greatest number of cancer cells and do the least harm to normal tissues. Table 23-1 lists some examples of drugs currently used for the treatment of childhood cancer. Frequent side-effects are indicated. Individual agents can also cause unique side-effects including cardiac damage (doxorubicin), pulmonary fibrosis (bleomycin),

Table 23-1. Side-effects of certain chemotherapeutic agents commonly used in treating childhood cancers

	Effect				
Chemotherapeutic agent	**Local tissue damage and ulceration if extravasation occurs**	**Dose-dependent nausea and vomiting**	**Irritation and ulceration of oral and gastrointestinal mucosa**	**Hair loss**	**Bone marrow depression**
Actinomycin D	X	X	X	X	X
Doxorubicin (Adriamycin)	X	X	X	X	X
Cis-platinum		X			X
Cyclophosphamide	X	X	X		X
Cytosine arabinoside		X			X
Methotrexate		X	X		X
Nitrogen mustard	X	X	X	X	X
Vincristine	X			X	

renal and oto-toxicity (cisplatin), hemorrhagic cystitis (cyclophosphamide), anaphylaxis (L-asparaginase), neurotoxicity (vincristine), and immunologic and metabolic disturbances (prednisone). Parents and, as appropriate, the child should be fully informed of the potential risk of chemotherapy and of the precautions and observations necessitated by its use. Although the basic principles of cancer chemotherapy are the same for the child as for the adult, potential long-term side-effects also must be considered in the physically immature child.

Because children successfully treated by chemotherapy are living into adulthood, late onset complications of chemotherapy should be considered at the time therapy is planned. Many of the problems that result from chemotherapy take years to develop and still await discovery. Some recently identified long-term effects from cyclophosphamide and nitrogen mustard include possible sterility and increased risk of a second malignancy. The future consequences of cardiac damage from adriamycin or pulmonary injury from bleomycin, even when cumulative dosages are kept within theoretically tolerable limits, are unknown. Future liver dysfunction from certain drugs may become a serious problem. Caretakers should carefully explain to parents and, when appropriate, the child that toxic effects from chemotherapy may occur years later and that potential clinical problems have yet to be identified.

Radiation therapy

Radiation therapy, like chemotherapy, injures normal cells while it destroys cancer cells. Although the radiation beam can be directed to a specific area of the body with sets of shields that protect other areas, all tissues within the specified treatment area (the radiation port) will be affected by the beam. The goal of radiation therapy is the administration of radiation that will kill as many cancer cells as possible and will do the least damage to normal tissues. Chapter 13 discusses in detail this modality of treatment.

Because radiation ports are so carefully defined, the child must be perfectly still during radiation treatments. Although these treatments do not involve injections or other painful procedures, young children are often unable to hold still for the short times required. To ensure that radiation is delivered safely and effectively to the proper port, clinicians often must sedate the child. Radiation therapy requires frequent, sometimes daily, clinic visits for a set period of time. The duration of treatment depends on the specific disease, the total dose required for treatment, and the child's ability to tolerate radiation. Daily visits may become a strain on child and parents alike. The large and forbidding radiation machines may frighten the child. With kind, friendly, and attentive technicians and therapists, the child is usually able to adjust to this new experience.

Complications from radiation therapy depend on the part of the body being treated, the total body area involved, and the total dose received. Serious side-effects are more likely if the child has received or is receiving chemotherapy along with radiation treatments. Several side-effects that occur from radiation are similar to those from chemotherapy. When bones such as ribs, vertebrae, or long bones are included within the treatment ports, bone marrow depression may result. Children are often given rest periods from radiation treatment so that the bone marrow can recover. When the gastrointestinal tract is involved in the radiation port, nausea, vomiting, and anorexia are potential side-effects. With cranial vault radiation, hair loss and headaches may occur.

Radiation therapy has other side-effects that are different from those of chemotherapy. When the jaw or mouth area is radiated, potential damage to the teeth must be anticipated. Pretreatment with fluoride helps to protect the teeth. When the mouth, jaw, or throat are within the radiation port, mucous membranes may become dry and sore, and the child may have difficulty swallowing. The skin in radiation treatment areas may develop a burn similar to sunburn. Total daily dosages must be planned carefully to lessen the risk of burning the skin.

When vital organs such as the heart, lungs, liver, and kidneys are included within radiation ports, high-dose radiation can cause severe damage. Every attempt must be made to shield these organs when they have received their maximum "tolerable" dose. Often the treatment of a body area that is affected by cancer is limited by the maximum safe dose for normal tissue within the radiation field. When the dose needed for cure exceeds the safe levels of exposure for normal tissues, treatment objectives must be reevaluated.

Because the child's physical growth is incomplete, his or her tissues are more vulnerable to radiation injury than those of adults. Radiation to bones can disrupt and limit normal growth. The resulting shortening and deformity of bones can produce unequal limbs and scoliosis. To prevent scoliosis, radiation to the spine is performed symmetrically whenever possible.

If radiation to the ovaries or testes is necessary, sterility can result. For the child who has not yet attained puberty, radiation to the gonads can disrupt sexual maturation. These children should be followed carefully for problems with growth and sexual development; if necessary, supplemental hormonal therapy should be given. Abdominal radiation is required for many tumors; when possible, the ovaries should be surgically moved to avoid unnecessary exposure.

The thyroid is also susceptible to dysfunction following radiation exposure, and hypothyroidism is a common complication of radiation therapy to the neck. Low-dose radiation has also been shown to increase the risk of thyroid cancer.[15] Other second malignancies will be a significant future problem for the child receiving radiation therapy. The likelihood of sarcoma in the areas of high-dose radiation increases with the length of time after exposure. The young child cured of cancer with a long life expectancy thus is at great risk. Because of the potential complications of radiation therapy in childhood, every attempt is made to use the lowest possible dose and the smallest port to treat malignant disease.

Modes of therapy

Acute lymphocytic leukemia. Acute lymphocytic leukemia is the most common childhood cancer.[1] The term "leukemia" was first used in 1827 to describe a disorder of the blood.[8] The word actually means "white blood" and refers to the puslike appearance of blood found at autopsy of individuals with leukemia. This disease results from an abnormal proliferation of malignant white blood cells within the bone marrow. The malignant cell population replaces normal marrow cells, and in acute lymphocytic leukemia, these malignant cells are called lymphoblasts.

The initial symptoms of leukemia result from the replacement of normal marrow cells by malignant lymphoblasts. This replacement decreases the number of normal cells in the blood. If the red cell count is low, the child may have symptoms of anemia such as pallor, weakness, and fatigue. If the platelet count is low, the child may suffer from nosebleeds or bruise easily. Frequently, because of an abundance of circulating malignant lymphoblasts, the total white cell count may be high when the normal white cell count is low. In this situation, the child can be vulnerable to infection. The proliferation of lymphoblasts in the bone marrow can also result in diffuse bone pain that may be mistaken for symptoms of juvenile rheumatoid arthritis. Often fever is present as an initial symptom, not necessarily as a sign of infection but as a manifestation of leukemia.

Leukemia was once regarded as a universally fatal disease. It is a systemic disease where use of systemic chemotherapy has dramatically improved prognosis. Periods of disease control have been prolonged and cure rates have increased. Organized, cooperative clinical studies among pediatric oncology centers throughout the country have been crucial in advancing the understanding of this disease and improving its therapy.[21]

Clinical researchers discovered that vincristine and prednisone rid the child's bone marrow of malignant cells and allowed the return of normal marrow elements. The disappearance of malignant cells from the blood and bone marrow is called remission. Researchers found, however, that obtaining remission usually did not cure the child of leukemia for two important reasons. First, leukemic cells appeared in other body areas even when the blood and bone marrow were free of disease. These other areas, referred to as "sanctuary sites," shelter leukemic cells from the full effects of systemic therapy. The central nervous system proved to be the primary sanctuary site for leukemic cells. Second, researchers discovered that if systemic chemotherapy were discontinued shortly after remission was obtained, the disease would soon return to the bone marrow. Through cooperative studies, pediatric oncologists have designed therapy programs that (1) induce systemic remission, (2) provide special treatment for the central nervous system sanctuary site, and (3) maintain remission. Table 23-2 shows an example of a current therapy program for acute lymphocytic leukemia.

The induction phase is designed to eliminate detectable leukemic cells in blood and bone marrow, thereby producing systemic remission. In addition, intrathecal methotrexate is given to combat any potential central nervous system leukemia during induction. The central nervous system phase of treatment is designed to eliminate any undetected leukemic cells that may have escaped the effects of induction therapy. Treatment in this phase involves cranial vault radiation and intrathecal methotrexate. Pediatric oncologists routinely give central nervous system treatment to prevent central nervous system involvement even if there is no evidence for central nervous

Table 23-2. A protocol for lymphocytic leukemia

Induction phase (duration, 4-6 weeks)	**Central nervous system phase (duration, ~3 weeks)**	**Maintenance phase (duration, ~3-5 years)**
Vincristine—IV	Methotrexate—IT	6-mercaptopurine—PO
1 dose weekly × 4-6 dosages	1 dose weekly × 3 dosages	Daily
Prednisone—PO	6-mercaptopurine—PO	Methotrexate—PO
Daily × 28-42 days	Daily	1 dose weekly
L-asparaginase—IM	Prednisone—PO	Vincristine—IV
1 dose 3 × per week for 9 dosages	Daily in tapering dosages × 1-2 weeks	1 dose monthly
Methotrexate—IT	CNS radiation	Prednisone—PO
1 dose on days 0 and 14	Daily for ~2 weeks	Daily × 5 consecutive days each month

system disease. This second phase of therapy takes approximately 3 weeks, during which time systemic remission must be maintained. The risk of bone marrow relapse is lessened by use of oral 6-mercaptopurine.

When the first two phases of treatment are complete and tests reveal no evidence of leukemia in bone marrow or central nervous system, maintenance therapy is initiated to prevent return of overt disease and to kill any undetectable leukemic cells. The longer a child with leukemia remains in remission, the better the child's chance for cure. Maintenance therapy usually continues for at least 3 years. During this time, the child undergoes routine monitoring of blood and bone marrow, and drug dosages are adjusted to preserve adequate blood counts as well as to prevent the return of leukemic cells. Periodic studies are also necessary to assess other toxic side-effects of chemotherapy.

Although the advances made in the treatment of acute lymphocytic leukemia have enhanced survival rates, many children with this disease will not be cured. The etiology of leukemia and the reasons for recurrence are still unknown. If leukemia does recur, either in bone marrow or central nervous system, the chances for eventual cure are greatly diminished. Relapses are treated with appropriate reinduction therapy, but subsequent periods of remission usually grow shorter and shorter. Currently, national study groups are searching for causes of multiple relapse. Statistical analysis of children with leukemia has indicated that those children who have high white blood counts at the time of diagnosis appear to be at high risk for future relapse.[5] Children older than 10 years when diagnosed also have a poorer prognosis than most younger children. Prognosis may be related to newly defined histologic subtypes of acute lymphocytic leukemia. For the child diagnosed between the ages of 3 and 10 years with an initial low white blood cell count, risk of relapse is low and 5-year disease-free survival and probable cure is approximately 80%. However, overall 5-year disease-free survival rates for acute lymphocytic leukemia are still about 45%.[10] By identifying those children who are at higher risk of relapse, it is possible to use more aggressive induction and maintenance regimens. Because high-risk clients are likely to develop central nervous system involvement, current maintenance protocols include periodic intrathecal methotrexate to continue central nervous system prophylaxis. The struggle to improve therapy for acute lymphocytic leukemia continues through the efforts of the organized study groups.

Several of the principles discovered for the treatment of leukemia—systemic treatment, prophylactic treatment, and maintenance therapy—have been successfully applied to other childhood cancers. Although childhood solid tumors might not appear to be systemic disease, their metastatic patterns indicate that micrometastases are probably present at diagnosis. The application of systemic treatment to solid tumors has decreased the incidence of metastasis and has improved survival rates for children with these diseases. For leukemia, prophylactic central nervous system treatment is often given when there is no detectable disease, and maintenance therapy is given even though the child is in remission. These practices have proved very effective in decreasing the incidence of central nervous system leukemia and in maintaining remission. In the treatment of solid tumors, the use of systemic chemotherapy when no apparent cancer is present is called adjuvant therapy. Adjuvant chemotherapy has been successfully used to prevent metastases in other childhood cancers after primary tumor resection is performed.

Wilms' tumor. Wilms' tumor or nephroblastoma is another childhood cancer for which prognosis has been greatly improved because of a nationally organized study. Wilms' tumor, a malignant solid tumor of primitive kidney tissue, is frequently diagnosed in early childhood. This embryonic tumor spreads by direct extension or by vascular and lymphatic metastases. The most common metastatic site is the lungs, and pulmonary metastases may be present at diagnosis. This tumor grows as an enlarging abdominal mass and may cause nonspecific symptoms of weight loss, abdominal pain, and malaise. Tumor growth destroys and displaces normal kidney tissue and interferes with kidney function. If the tumor occurs in both kidneys, there is the risk of renal failure. When the tumor arises in the right kidney, it can extend into the liver in such a way that complete surgical excision is impossible. In the past, the prognosis for this disease was poor. Standard treatment with surgery alone, or radiation alone, was often inadequate and would only cure children with limited disease. However, the chemotherapy agents vincristine and actinomycin D had previously been shown to be effective against this tumor and further use of these agents was considered.

To better understand this cancer and to develop effective therapy, clinical researchers in several institutions organized the National Wilms' Tumor Study Group in 1969.[2] First, researchers established a staging system based on the extent of the disease at the time of initial diagnosis. The following shows a current staging system for Wilms' tumor:

Stage I: Tumor is limited to one kidney, and the kidney is completely resected.

1. The surface of the renal capsule must be intact.
2. The tumor must not be ruptured before or during removal.
3. There must be no residual tumor beyond the margins of resection.

Stage II: Tumor extends beyond the kidney but is completely resected.

1. The renal vessels outside kidney substance can be infiltrated or contain tumor thrombus, but the tumor must be completely removed.
2. There must be no residual tumor beyond the margins of resection.

Stage III: Residual nonhematogenous tumor is confined to the abdomen. Any one or more of the following can occur:

1. The tumor has been biopsied or ruptured before or during surgery.
2. There are peritoneal surface implants.
3. There are involved abdominal lymph nodes.
4. The tumor is not completely resectable because of local infiltration into vital structures.

Stage IV: There are tumor deposits beyond stage III, for example, lung, liver, bone marrow, brain.

It was assumed that the more extensive the disease, the worse the prognosis. Clinical research was coordinated among the study's participants, and several treatment regimens were evaluated. The study revealed that a multimodal program of extirpative surgery followed by systemic chemotherapy and appropriate radiation therapy improved cure rates even in children with widespread disease.

As the study progressed, it became apparent that the extent of the disease was not the only major prognostic factor. The histologic subtype of the tumor showed close correlation with prognosis. The importance of histologic subtype was demonstrated by cases in which children with widespread disease but favorable histology did well in treatment, while others with limited disease but unfavorable histology did poorly. Further research clarified the nature of the extent of disease and its relationship to prognosis. For example, a large tumor or tumor that had

Table 23-3. A Wilms' tumor treatment protocol

Days														Months												
0	**1**	**2**	**3**	**4**	**5**	**7**	**14**	**21**	**28**	**35**	**42**	**49**	**56**	**3**	**4**	**5**	**6**	**7**	**8**	**9**	**10**	**11**	**12**	**13**	**14**	**15**
Stage I (favorable histology)																										
S																										
	A	A	A	A	A						AAAAA			AAAAA			AAAAA			AAAAA			AAAAA			AAAAA
						V	V	V	V	V	V V		V	V V			V V			V V			V V			V V
Stage I (unfavorable histology) and stages II, III, IV																										
S																										
	RT																									
	A	A	A	A	A																					
						V	V	V	V	V	V V															
														AAAAA			AAAAA			AAAAA			AAAAA			AAAAA
														V V			V V			V V			V V			V V
												ADR				ADR			ADR		ADR			ADR		

AAAAA—Actinomycin D, IV (1 dose daily for 5 days); ADR—doxorubicin (Adriamycin), IV (1 dose); V—vincristine, IV (1 dose); S—surgery according to stage; RT—radiation therapy according to stage.

spread to abdominal lymph nodes was found to correlate with poor prognosis. Researchers used these factors from initial diagnosis to determine which children had good or poor prognoses and adjusted therapy accordingly.

Although aggressive multimodal therapy has improved overall cure rates for Wilms' tumor (75% disease-free survival for 5 years), complications of therapy became more apparent.[4] Children are particularly vulnerable to future complications of radiation therapy, and ways have been sought to minimize the need for radiation. A goal of the Wilms' tumor study has been to utilize prognostic factors to determine appropriate therapy. Children with poor prognosis receive more aggressive therapy to maximize their chances for cure. Those with better prognoses receive less aggressive therapy so that future complications of treatment are minimized. Table 23-3 shows a treatment program for Wilms' tumor that has been planned according to stage and histologic subtype of disease. Children with stage I disease and favorable histology are treated with only two chemotherapy agents, actinomycin D and vincristine. This therapy is the least aggressive in the Wilms' tumor program because researchers have determined that the possibility of cure in this case is neither diminished by the elimination of radiation therapy nor improved by the addition of doxorubicin (Adriamycin) as a third agent. However, doxorubicin improves cure rates for those with more extensive disease or with unfavorable histology. Children with stage II, III, or IV disease, as well as those with unfavorable histology, are treated with surgery and multiagent chemotherapy. Radiation therapy is adjusted individually according to the extent of disease.

Currently, the Wilms' tumor study is attempting to determine whether the duration of treatment for children with stage I disease can safely be reduced from 18 to 6 months. This study is also exploring the feasibility of decreasing the use of radiation therapy and modifying chemotherapy schedules in children with more extensive disease. The Wilms' tumor study continues to refine therapeutic regimens so that optimal cure rates are achieved and future complications minimized. As these discussions of leukemia and Wilms' tumor have shown, cure rates and control of childhood cancer have greatly improved through the cooperative efforts of pediatric oncology centers. As further studies continue, more progress will be made in the understanding and treatment of these diseases.

Process of therapy

Cancer treatment requires that the child submit to a demanding and arduous therapeutic process. Numerous time-consuming laboratory studies, as well as repeated physical examinations, are necessary to monitor the course of the disease and the effects of therapy. Painful procedures such as blood tests, intravenous infusions, spinal taps, and bone marrow aspirations are often required. Caretakers should be aware of the stress that cancer therapy causes and should provide explanations that the child can understand. Parents will also need assistance to cope with the difficulties of therapy.

In pediatric oncology, outpatient care with home support is encouraged so that time spent in the hospital is greatly reduced, and the child is better able to pursue usual age-related activities. However, good outpatient care requires that the family make repeated clinic visits. In addition, they must have appropriate knowledge to conduct home care safely. Parents need to be aware of common side-effects and complications of therapy and know when to seek medical assistance. Caretakers should provide information and instruction so that parents will be knowledgeable and confident in caring for their child. Oral chemotherapy is routinely given at home. Families with more experience undertake even more intricate chemotherapy procedures by performing subcutaneous or intramuscular injections or giving intravenous chemotherapy through a preplaced heparin lock. Caretakers should encourage the family to carry out home care functions but should not overwhelm them with responsibilities beyond their capabilities.

In light of the numerous toxic effects of therapy, careful observation of the child by caretakers and parents is required. Often it is difficult to prevent some of the more common complications of therapy, but knowledgeable anticipation of problems can prevent significant disruption of the child's life. Common complications for which the family and child must be prepared include an increased susceptibility to infection, problems with low blood counts, hair loss, and various gastrointestinal difficulties. The inherent immunosuppressive effect of many childhood cancers and the direct effects of chemotherapy result in an increased susceptibility to certain fungal and viral infections. Of particular concern are childhood diseases like chickenpox and measles. With a decrease in normal immune function, the occurrence of such diseases can be life-threatening. Parents must be informed of this risk and seek to prevent the child's exposure if possible. For example, the child may have to stay out of school during outbreaks of specific diseases like chickenpox. If the child is exposed, preventive hyperimmune globulin should be given and the child watched for early symptoms. If the disease occurs, hospitalization is often necessary.

When bone marrow toxicity decreases the total white blood count and the absolute neutrophil count, the child becomes prone to serious bacterial infections. Although attempts are made to adjust chemotherapy dosages and radiation schedules, some periods of low blood counts cannot be prevented. Certain measures are taken to lessen the risk of infection when the child is neutropenic. The strictness of these measures and the time when they are initiated vary at different institutions. Protection of the hospitalized child can range from complete reverse isolation to simple room confinement. Home protection for the child is also variable. The child may be required to stay out of school and away from crowds, and the parents instructed to report promptly any fever or sign of infection. If fever occurs, the neutropenic child should be hospitalized, appropriate cultures taken, and antibiotics started until the nature of the fever is determined. The length of such hospitalizations can vary from a few days to several weeks depending on the type and severity of the infection.

When bone marrow toxicity reduces the platelet count, the child will be susceptible to bleeding and bruising and should avoid activities in which there is the risk of trauma, such as contact sports. Bleeding from low platelet counts can be difficult to control and may require hospitalization and platelet transfusion. Especially dangerous is the risk of bleeding into the central nervous system.

Hair loss, a frequent side-effect of therapy, does not endanger the physical well-being of the child. However, such loss may have a strong psychologic impact, particularly for the older child and adolescent. Caretakers should not underestimate the emotional stress of hair loss and should be prepared to help the child and parents cope with this problem.

The oral ulceration that follows use of certain chemotherapy agents can be painful and interfere with proper nutrition. Ulceration may also involve the esophagus and stomach. Persistent ulceration increases susceptibility to superimposed infections, such as oral moniliasis. If the ulceration is severe, the *Candida* infection may spread and become systemic and life-threatening. The parents and child should understand this risk so that importance of good mouth care will be clear. The child should brush frequently with a soft bristle brush and rinse with mouthwash. Hydrogen peroxide rinses are also used for oral ulceration; nystatin (Mycostatin) is applied if oral moniliasis occurs.

Although children usually have less difficulty with nausea and vomiting than adult clients, certain chemotherapy agents will cause these effects. Often the child suffers nausea and vomiting for a period of about 24 hours after drug administration. Some children may have temporary anorexia after which they will resume usual eating habits. If a general decrease in appetite occurs in conjunction with oral ulceration, the child may have difficulty eating and lose weight from poor nutrition. The dietitian, an important member of the oncology team, can assist parents and caretakers in planning and adapting the child's diet so that optimal nutrition is achieved. Usually nutritional problems in children with cancer will not be severe unless the disease is resistant to therapy and the child becomes terminal. Good nutrition, however, improves the child's tolerance of therapy and increases resistance to the complications of serious disease.

Philosophy of care

Caretakers should be aware of the profound emotional impact that cancer has on both child and family. Early discussions with the family of a child who has cancer should focus on the extent and type of cancer, the therapy that will be required, and the possibilities for cure. The explanations used should strike a balance between encouraging hope for cure while establishing realistic expectations of serious disease. While long-term prognosis depends on the type and extent of the cancer, hope should never be discouraged. It should be emphasized that the goal of therapy is cure. The family should be informed that the child's response to therapy over time will be a crucial factor for the eventual outcome of the disease.

Childhood cancer and its treatment require that parents and child make a firm commitment to intense therapeutic regimens. This commitment includes accepting potential complications and side-effects and tolerating repeated painful procedures. Parents and child will need to devote much time to clinic visits and therapy-related activities and will have to become knowledgeable about the disease and its treatment.

Each child and family are unique in their reactions to the extraordinary experience of childhood cancer. However, caretakers should anticipate certain feelings and responses common to most families. Initially the child and family will express feelings of shock, fear, anger, denial, and sadness. As the child settles into a treatment program and seems to be doing well, a growing mood of cautious optimism develops. Complacency may even be evident. Despite this relative calm, caretakers should encourage frequent discussions with the child and family about any concerns that they may have.

To meet the complex developmental, emotional, and social needs of the child and family, an interdisciplinary pediatric oncology team of social workers, chaplains, child life specialists, physicians, and nurses is essential. This spectrum of expertise allows the parents and child access to a broad range of information and provides them with assistance for psychosocial as well as medical aspects of care. The pediatric oncology team also facilitates communication with other health care personnel and the community (for example, school, scouts) concerning the child and family. The team approach also enables its members to support each other through the emotional strain involved in caring for the child with cancer.

The caretaker's approach to family and child is a crucial factor for easing the adjustment to therapy. At the time of diagnosis, caretakers, child, and family embark on a long and intense relationship. The child and family usually relate primarily to one or a few caretakers, but eventually they will know all members of the team. It is essential that these relationships have an atmosphere of honesty and trust. The child and family must be able to express feelings, seek emotional support, ask questions, and acquire the knowledge necessary to carry on through treatment. From initial diagnosis and throughout the course of therapy, caretakers must be a constantly available source of support and knowledge for both family and child.

The hospital atmosphere should be adapted to the needs and well-being of the children and families who must spend their time there. Consistency of care is one way in which a comfortable environment is created. When hospitalizations are necessary, having the child return to the same unit is reassuring for child and family. Whenever possible, parents should be allowed to stay with the child if they wish. The presence of family members, siblings, and friends also helps ease long and frequent clinic visits. Routine clinic visits, rather than prolonged hospital stays, are encouraged because children make better developmental progress at home. Yet, frequent clinic visits are time consuming for family members and may require considerable travel. For this reason, many centers provide families with convenient clinic times and overnight facilities. The clinical environment should be made as comfortable as possible for child and family without compromising efficiency of care.

Play is an important component of the child's experience while in the hospital or clinic. Under the direction of a professional child life specialist, play can be planned in accordance with the child's developmental needs. Play for the child with cancer not only provides recreation, but helps the child act out and thus lessen the fear, pain, and anxiety associated with cancer therapy. The child life specialist's observations and interactions with the child and family are an important component in assessing the child's developmental progress and general well-being. The child life specialist is an important member of the oncology team and is often a primary caretaker with whom the child closely identifies.

When the child's disease is under control or in remission, anxieties lessen and clinic visits become more routine. Yet, the fear of a relapse or recurrence remains. This fear becomes more apparent at times of reevaluation of disease or when another child with similar disease has had a relapse. When such fears occur, the family may need to review with caretakers their child's disease status and again discuss prospects for the future. If relapse or metastasis has occurred, the psychologic impact often is greater than that experienced at original diagnosis. Recurrence or spread of disease indicates a lack of therapeutic responsiveness and usually implies poor long-term prognosis. Attempts at cure through alternative therapeutic regimens may be pursued, but the chances for cure will be diminished. At the time of a relapse, both child and family must again face the fact that the child will possibly die from the disease. The tragic impact of relapse was expressed by one mother of a 7-year-old boy who had leukemia in remission for 2½ years and who had just relapsed: "You just forget, damn it. You forget everything that they told you about leukemia. He has done so well. He has not been sick since his diagnosis. We've become so used to coming to the clinic, so sure that he would be cured." Parents will express strong feelings of anger, sadness, and depression if their child relapses. Parents and the older child with cancer will often feel cheated. They did everything they were supposed to do; they went through all the pain and difficulties of treatment, and yet it did not work. How unfair it all seems. Caretakers must understand such feelings and be prepared to help the parents and child deal with these feelings so that they will be able to cope with further therapy.

After multiple relapses or continued spread of the disease when conventional therapeutic regimens have failed, the question arises as to whether experimental or research drugs should be used. Experimental agents are never utilized without appropriate consent from child and family. Such decisions must be weighed carefully. The potential palliation offered by a new drug must be balanced against the disruption and discomfort it may cause the child. A further consideration is whether therapy should be stopped altogether. These are difficult issues, both ethically and medically, and are issues that must be considered individually to take into account the child's medical condition as well as the needs and feelings of family and child.

DEVELOPMENTAL APPROACH

Overview

The child with cancer struggles to mature amidst the upheaval of serious disease and complex therapy. To help the child progress, caretakers must understand child development and be sensitive to the individual child. The emotional and intellectual strengths of the child should be reinforced to help him or her adjust to the rigors of therapy. Caretakers must communicate with the child on a level he or she can understand. They should recognize the perceptions and fears of the child at various developmental stages and plan their approach and explanations accordingly.

The following sections highlight the main developmental characteristics for each of five stages of childhood—infant (birth to 1 year), toddler (1 to 3 years), preschooler (3 to 6 years), school age child (6 to 12 years), and adolescent (12 to 18 years). A specific childhood cancer is discussed in conjunction with the stage in which it frequently occurs. The discussion then focuses on how cancer and its therapy affect the child at that stage of development. Specific ways are offered for caretakers to aid the child during cancer therapy. Although certain aspects of child behavior, concerns of the family, and effects of therapy are presented within specific age groups, they often apply to other developmental stages. Certainly each of the diseases discussed can occur at other ages.

Each child with cancer is unique, and the interplay of the disease and therapy with the child's developmental process is complex. As the following discussion shows, however, there are many problems common to all children with cancer. By having familiarity with these problems, caretakers can plan ways to help each child cope with the difficulties of his or her disease. Caretakers should also be able to adapt their care to meet the unique needs of each child.

Infant—birth to 1 year

Unfortunately, the infant is not exempt from the devastating impact of cancer. Malignancies that occur during infancy often arise during fetal development. Cancers in infancy include retinoblastoma, neuroblastoma, nephroblastoma (Wilms' tumor), and leukemia. Retinoblastoma is a malignant proliferation of primitive neural tissue of the eye. Early signs of retinoblastoma include the infant's inability to fix on an object, persistent strabismus, or a white spot within the eye. A possible genetic predisposition for this disease warrants close observation of the retinoblastoma victim's uninvolved eye and the eyes of other family members.

Diagnosis of retinoblastoma requires thorough examination of the eye and appropriate staging of the disease to determine local extent of tumor and central nervous system or systemic involvement. Bone marrow aspirations and spinal taps are painful but important diagnostic procedures. Treatment often includes surgical removal of the eye, radiation therapy, and sometimes chemotherapy.

Cancer and its therapy not only interfere with the delicate growth of the infant but also disrupt his or her psychologic development. At a time when most infants are at home, the infant with cancer spends a great deal of time in the clinic enduring painful and upsetting treatment. To help the infant adjust to these experiences, all those involved with the infant's care should understand the infant's physical and emotional needs and communication modes.

Developmental needs. The infant's basic needs are simple: food, comfort, oral satisfaction, environmental stimulation, and self-exploration and expression. The main developmental task is the acquisition of trust.[7] Infants learn to recognize persons who meet their physical needs, and they build trust through repetitive and consistent interactions with those who provide care and comfort. A gentle touch and a soft tone of voice enhance the acquisition of trust. Holding and cuddling convey love and security, and gentle tickling and stroking provide pleasant stimulation and excitement. Infants respond to and communicate with the adult world in many nonverbal ways. They show tension and discomfort by crying and thrashing about. They display pleasure and contentment by smiling, cooing, and showing interest in their surroundings. When planning cancer therapy for the infant, all of these developmental aspects should be kept in mind.

Problems relating to cancer treatment. Cancer therapy often requires that the infant be still for certain periods of time. Immobilization deprives the infant of the experience and pleasure of free movements, wiggling, rolling over, and sucking. Intravenous infusions used to administer chemotherapy and to treat infection or dehydration often necessitate immobilization for several days. With ingenuity and attention, caretakers can protect infusion sites while minimizing the extent of immobilization. During prolonged immobilization, periods of play should be planned to allow free movement and close contact with parents and caretakers. Visual and audio stimulation should be provided even though physical activities are constrained. When the infant is unable to take nourishment, a pacifier should be provided for sucking.

Performing painful procedures on an infant is an unpleasant task, made more difficult because the purpose cannot be explained to the recipient. To finish the task quickly, caretakers tend to hold the infant tightly and proceed with few comforting actions. The caretakers' anxiety over inflicting pain may interfere with recognition of the infant's needs. Although it is impossible to assess the infant's perception of pain or the future psychologic consequences of pain, caretakers should recognize the potential negative effects of repeated painful experiences. Procedures should be performed in a gentle and caring manner, with reassuring words and comforting touches. The infant's perception of a calming touch and soothing voice may lessen any psychologic trauma from the pain. Sharp and loud tones should be avoided, and sudden and startling moves should be minimized. The infant should be held firmly but gently with periodic stroking and should be spoken to calmly throughout the procedure. Immediately following the painful experience, the infant should be held, comforted, and provided with a bottle or pacifier.

Parents should be invited to accompany their infant during procedures. The nature and purpose of the procedure should be carefully explained to them. However, seeing their child in pain is stressful, and they should decide whether they wish to be present during the procedure or to wait and comfort their child afterwards. Caretakers should be aware of conflicting feelings over such a choice and reassure the parents regardless of their decision.

Common parental feelings. Parents are confronted with enormous problems when cancer and its therapy interrupt the usual experiences of raising a child. For the infant with retinoblastoma, parents may face the additional emotional strain imposed by the surgical removal of their child's eye. Although parents realize that the infant usually will adjust to the loss of one eye, they have understandable difficulty accepting this loss. Every effort should be made to use a temporary prosthesis as soon as possible to lessen the unpleasant cosmetic effect and to allow proper growth and remolding of eyelid tissues. Often parents feel guilty about their inability to protect their child from disease and may feel responsible for the harm that befalls their child. Caretakers should acknowledge feelings of guilt and assure the parents that they are not responsible for their child's disease. Careful explanation about the nature of the disease and reasons for treatment will strengthen the parents' confidence in their own nurturing skills as well as help them anticipate and understand problems the infant will experience during therapy. Caretakers should make themselves readily available to parents and answer all questions that may arise. Caretakers can provide invaluable support to help parents cope with the emotional stress of their child's disease and treatment.

Parents will particularly need assistance to maintain adequate nutrition for the infant with cancer. A dietitian is most helpful in coordinating nutritional care with problems of therapy. Parents will need advice about routine and special diets and aid with the management of periods of anorexia. Although vomiting following therapy is not as frequent for the infant as for the older child, some vomiting may occur along with poor sucking and feeding. The infant's greater fluid requirement and dynamic metabolic state increase the risk of dehydration. Parents should be informed of this risk and the need to notify caretakers if their infant is unable to tolerate oral feedings. Intravenous fluids may be required to maintain hydration.

Infants' perceptions. Despite cognitive immaturity, infants are able to perceive and make associations with the events of therapeutic procedures. For example, one infant girl with leukemia was started on therapy at 6 months of age. Her treatment included intravenous infusions, bone marrow aspirations, and spinal taps. After a few months, she showed recognition of the clinic environment and familiarity with her caretakers. Although fretful on arrival at the clinic, she would soon become content and play with her family in the play area. She was cautious and withdrawn with new people, but when approached by her caretakers, she would usually relax, smile, and sometimes even enjoy being held. When her parents brought her into the examining room, she would again become anxious. Once in the room, she was usually playful throughout the physical examination. If the IV cart was brought into the room, however, and action and discussion focused on a forthcoming intravenous infusion, she would become anxious, resistant, and agitated even though no attempt had been made to carry out the procedure. This child anticipated a therapeutic event through perception of the activities, language, and equipment that preceded it. If taken to the treatment room where bone marrow aspirations and spinal taps were performed, she would become agitated, cry, and reach for someone to hold her. When the procedure was finished, she was quickly taken from the room. Gradually she became calm, but a long time had to pass before she allowed the caretakers to approach her.

This child's behavior demonstrates that infants are able to perceive what is happening during therapeutic procedures. They can learn to distinguish between painless and painful procedures and to recognize the events that precede each and the caretakers that are involved. Even though a specific procedure performed by this infant's caretakers did upset her, she still had a good relationship with her caretakers and readily played with them in the early part of the visit. She could relax with them in a neutral environment but became agitated when preparations for a painful procedure were made. Consistency of care—that is, doing the procedure the same way with the same people—enables an infant to anticipate therapeutic events. He or she can learn that, although a painful procedure will be performed, he or she will be treated with care and given comfort afterwards. Knowing this, the infant can develop trust in the relationship with the caretakers.

Toddler—years 1 to 3

Developmental needs. Armed with newly acquired skills and a developing verbal ability, the child between the ages of 1 and 3 years advances from the relative calm and dependency of infancy to a tumultuous period of environmental exploration. However exciting this adventure, the toddler is quickly confronted with the demands and restrictions imposed by the social and physical constraints of the adult world. Necessary limits must be set to protect the child against falls, burns, and ingestions and to preserve the local environment from the often disruptive activities of the toddler. Social constraints, like toilet training and table manners, place further demands on the toddler. During the conflict between growing capabilities and imposed restrictions, the toddler struggles for a sense of autonomy.[7] The toddler often protests strongly against imposed restraints. Although the toddler's communication skills are rapidly improving, he or she has yet to acquire sufficient reasoning ability to understand the necessity for constraints imposed by the adult world. At this age, behavior is based more on repetition and constancy than reason. In the struggle for environmental mastery, the toddler often establishes and clings to a repetitive style for activities such as preparing for bed, eating, or bathing. The rituals created by this behavior give the toddler a sense of familiarity and control over activities that he or she may not yet understand.

Neuroblastoma, a solid tumor that frequently occurs at this age, is a malignant embryonic neoplasm of primitive neural tissue that probably arises during fetal development. This disease often appears as a large asymptomatic mass in the chest or abdomen. When in the chest, the tumor usually arises from the sympathetic ganglia of posterior mediastinal tissues; in the abdomen, it can originate either from sympathetic ganglia or from the adrenal gland. This tumor has a propensity for metastasis to bone and can cause bone pain or limit mobility of the extremities. Other systemic symptoms associated with neuroblastoma may include weight loss, anorexia, unexplained fevers, or persistent diarrhea. Treatment of neuroblastoma may vary from surgery alone to a combination of surgery, radiation therapy, and chemotherapy. Unfortunately, when widespread, this disease is often refractory even to the most aggressive therapeutic regimens.

Problems relating to cancer treatment. The many disruptions and restrictions imposed by a cancer like neuroblastoma and its therapy should not be allowed to interfere with the toddler's developing sense of autonomy. Caretakers should be aware of the toddler's growing abilities and developmental struggles. The toddler's exploratory energy and enthusiasm should be incorporated into the treatment program. Curiosity about clinic equipment and facilities can be satisfied by allowing supervised exploration. Painful procedures present a difficult challenge to the toddler and create frustration for the caretakers. The toddler is able to anticipate and protest painful events but is unable to understand their necessity or stop their occurrence. Caretakers must remember that no matter how annoying, protest and resistance are a healthy response from a toddler seeking mastery over events.

Painful procedures performed on the toddler should be done in a consistent and predictable fashion. Providing simple but accurate explanations in a comforting manner will inform the toddler of the order of events and allow him or her a sense of control. Simple descriptions, such as "washing you off . . . ready to stick . . . hurt now . . . almost done . . . ," not only provide information but also acknowledge the child's right to know and to protest. Such descriptions are not used to silence objection but to lessen fear. Discussion of painful events as they occur is a positive response to the child's protest; it conveys that he or she has been heard. The limited duration of the procedure should be emphasized. After the procedure is over, the child should be comforted and reassured that the procedure is finished. The application of a Band-Aid or bandage can be used to symbolize the end of a procedure. Toddlers soon recognize the significance of a Band-Aid and often enjoy carrying several around. During the course of the procedure, and at its end, the toddler learns to repeat, "Done now, done now" both to question whether the treatment is over and to declare happiness at its completion. The child should always be encouraged by statements such as, "You were good, you did a good job." This bolsters self-esteem and reinforces trust at a time when the child is denied control.

Parents should be allowed to accompany their child during painful procedures. The presence of a parent often provides security and can diminish the mystery and fear surrounding a painful event. Because observation of a painful procedure can be stressful, the parents' ability to cope with the emotional strain involved must be assessed. If the parents choose not to participate, the caretakers should constantly assure the child that the parents are close by and will soon return.

Toddlers' perceptions. When the same caretakers consistently interact with the toddler, he or she comes to know them as caring adults and learns to trust their actions. This trust helps ease the fear and uncertainty inherent in painful procedures. A 2½-year-old boy who had been under treatment for neuroblastoma for several months had become accustomed to one physician who performed all his painful procedures. When a new physician was introduced, the child cooperated with the physical examination and the taking of history. When preparations were made for an intravenous infusion, he began to cry, complain, and move about. After a specific vein for the injection had been chosen, his cries suddenly changed from protest to demand. He began pointing dramatically at the chosen site and called loudly for his regular physician by name. This incident illustrates several points about this toddler's ability to integrate events of cancer therapy into a struggle for autonomy. This child knew the difference between nonthreatening procedures—history taking and physical examinations—and a painful event—intravenous infusion. He was secure enough with the predictability of the clinic routine to allow a new caretaker to initiate care, but when the possibility of pain was imminent, he demanded the caretaker he trusted. This example shows that the toddler seeks control even amidst difficult and painful phases of treatment. He seemed to be saying, "I don't want this, but if I have to have it, get me the physician I trust."

Despite careful attention to the toddler's need for control and autonomy, he or she will suffer many frustrations from the various impositions of cancer therapy. Play can relieve many of the tensions and anxieties associated with treatment. Play areas provide safe, nontreatment places for the toddler to relax and to become involved in self-expressive activities. The integrity of these areas should not be threatened by their use for treatment-related events like blood drawing. By playing with safe medical instruments, such as plastic syringes or appropriate medical models, toddlers become familiar with them. Thus, some of the mystery and fear associated with their actual use during medical procedures is alleviated.

Common parental feelings. Although toddlers are frightened and frustrated by therapy, they cannot comprehend the significance of having cancer. Parents of the toddler are not only burdened with the stress of their child's therapy, but they are also fearful of the outcome of the disease. Because of their stress, parents often have difficulty providing their child with appropriate guidance. The caretakers should encourage the family to use gentle but firm discipline to help the child attain the necessary skill and self-control for social activities such as table manners and toilet training. Parents and caretakers alike have a continuing obligation to care for the child as a whole developing person and not simply to focus on problems related to the treatment of disease.

Preschooler—years 3 to 6

Developmental needs. The preschooler's rapidly improving reasoning abilities and language skills enable him or her to have a greater understanding of the world. Because these abilities are still new and undergoing growth and change, misconceptions and misapprehensions about the world lead to the fantasies and fears that are a prominent component of the preschooler's thinking. Along with maturing mental capabilities, the preschooler's physical skills and coordination are improving. The combination of developing mental and physical proficiencies produces increased self-awareness, and preschoolers begin to view themselves as unique and separate individuals. Because of increased self-awareness, preschoolers recognize their own vulnerability and have fears that often focus on bodily harm. They become actively curious about the adult world and recognize its inherent power over their lives.

Preschoolers often use play to act out their understanding and fantasies about the world. Their curiosity about adult activities is often manifest in mimicry of adult behavior. Play and the attendant interactions with peers are the first steps toward socialization. New physical skills are employed in self-expressive activities such as drawing and painting. Interactions with imaginary characters allow the child some control amidst an imposing world and provide an outlet for fears and fantasies.

Freud labeled this period, from ages 3 to 6, the genital stage because the child's discovery of personal sexuality becomes a key part of expanded self-awareness.[9] Freud also noted the occurrence of the oedipal phenomenon as the child observes the adult world and yearns for the power and privilege of adults.[9] Erickson referred to these struggles as being the conflict of initiative versus guilt.[7] With increased skill and self-awareness, the preschooler acquires new capabilities for action, but because of feelings of guilt over thoughts and impulsive behavior, fear of adult reaction and punishment occur. Often the child's fears and fantasies about adult reprisal focus on bodily harm, as exemplified by the "castration complex."[9] Preschoolers fluctuate between feelings of power and security derived from newly acquired skills and feelings of helplessness and anxiety derived from recognition of the power of adults over them. Adult controls evoke frustration and fear, yet adult approval is very important.

Rhabdomyosarcoma, a solid tumor that occurs in preschoolers, is a malignant tumor of primitive connective tissue. This tumor may arise from connective tissue elements anywhere in the body and has characteristics of skeletal muscle. It most frequently occurs in the neck, extremities, and head, particularly in the orbits. Because this tumor originates as a mass in soft tissues, local pain and deformity are early problems. As with other childhood malignant tumors, rhabdomyosarcoma, although appearing as a local lesion, is actually a systemic disease. Systemic spread is frequent and chemotherapy is used to control potential metastases. Bone marrow examination should be done to determine marrow involvement. Head and neck rhabdomyosarcoma carry the risk of central nervous system extension; therefore, spinal taps and central nervous system imaging studies are performed. Therapy involves surgery for diagnosis and local tumor excision. Complete removal of the tumor is frequently impossible. Radiation therapy is used to improve control at the local site because of extensive and indefinite tumor margins. Diagnostic evaluations, surgery, chemotherapy, and radiation injure and insult the child with rhabdomyosarcoma.

Preschoolers' perceptions. Preschoolers' fears and fantasies about bodily harm can lead them to interpret painful and intrusive procedures as punishment for vague or unknown transgressions. The child's sense of self-control and power to act in the world is attacked on two fronts: therapeutic regimens interfere with the child's assertions of power and control, and intrusive procedures heighten the child's fear of punishment and bodily damage. To avoid misconceptions, caretakers should acknowledge the preschooler's fear of punishment and provide information to countervail this interpretation. Preschoolers are able to understand that medical treatment and procedures are to help make them better and not to punish them. Discussion with the preschooler before and during any procedure should be more detailed than that used with the toddler. Information should be presented in a calm, reassuring way that is neither confusing nor alarming. Preschoolers understandably resist and fear painful procedures. Often while crying and protesting they will ask questions that focus on why it is being done, what part of the body is involved, when it will be over, what needle will be used, and who will do it. Explanations should include an accurate account of events and note when any pain will be experienced. These specific explanations are intended not to silence protest but to help eliminate surprise and dispel any sense of punishment. Stating that the procedure must be done to help the child get better will reassure him or her that fault or bad behavior is not involved. Specifying what is or is not being done to various parts of the body serves to diminish fear of damage to other body areas.

Often preschoolers will attempt to cooperate with procedures in order to attain adult approval. One way to enhance this cooperation is to encourage verbal protest in place of physical resistance. The caretaker can say, "Yell loudly or cry all you want, but try to help us by holding still." With the physical cooperation of the child, the procedure is more easily and quickly performed. Such cooperation also allows the child a sense of control. As familiarity with caretakers and treatment regimens develops, the preschooler may even attempt to help with a procedure. However, such resolve often weakens or fails, particularly when the procedure is difficult or initially unsuccessful. Caretakers can lessen any feelings of guilt by assuring the child that he or she is not the cause of procedural failures. Even if the child's cooperation fails entirely, it is important that he or she be told, "You tried and did a good job." Often parents will feel frustrated and embarrassed by their child's performance. Caretakers should tell parents that the child did the best that he or she could and that the child should not be blamed for difficulties with the procedures.

Problems associated with cancer treatment. By recognizing the preschooler's developmental struggles and intellectual abilities, caretakers can help the child understand the necessity for therapy in spite of its pain and intrusiveness. For example, over several months, caretakers had worked to explain reasons for treatment and to enlist the cooperation of a 4½-year-old boy who had rhabdomyosarcoma. During one clinic visit, he endured the start of his intravenous infusion with only a small amount of crying. After his infusion was begun, he watched preparations for another intravenous infusion in a 4-year-old girl who had leukemia. Shortly before the insertion of the needle in her vein, he turned to her and announced, "Just say 'ouch, ouch, ouch' and then it will be over." He paused and proceeded to say, "You will get your medicine in that tube." Although close to tears, she nodded at him with comprehension. The boy's statements demonstrate a significant understanding of the procedure. With proper explanations and support, preschoolers can understand that painful procedures are done to make them better. Another 4½-year-old boy became quite nauseated each time he received intravenous chemotherapy for his Wilms' tumor. One day in the clinic he said somewhat angrily to his doctor, "If you are supposed to be making me better, why do you give me medicine that makes me sick?" This child had identified the central contradiction in cancer therapy: one must use chemotherapeutic drugs with harmful effects in order to cure cancer. The caretaker explained to the child that he had an illness that made him sick and that the medicines were given to try to make him better. He was told that the medicines had to be strong, and that if he felt sick, it was because the medicines were working. The child appeared to accept this explanation without difficulty.

The preschool child with cancer often confronts caretakers with perceptive questions about disease and treatment. Honest, simple, and specific explanations are necessary to maintain the child's trust. The child should not be overburdened with detailed information or abstract concepts. Parents also must deal with the preschooler's many questions and may need advice and help from the caretakers to respond in an appropriate manner to their child. Parents may find that the preschooler is aware that being sick can be used to weaken parental authority and avoid punishment. For instance, a 3-year-old girl with rhabdomyosarcoma stated to her mother, "I can do anything I want, can't I? Because I'm sick!" Other preschoolers have pointed out to their parents that they could not be spanked when their platelets were low. Parents who are dealing with their own fears and anxieties about their child's illness may need guidance in managing their child's attempts at manipulation. Parents should be encouraged to use reasonable discipline with their child. Caretakers should also encourage parents to enroll their child in nursery school or kindergarten as long as the medical situation permits.

As with other age groups, play provides the preschooler with a way to work out conflicts and anxieties related to cancer therapy. The increased intellectual and motor development of the preschooler enables him or her to mimic the adult world. Caretakers can provide safe medical equipment for the child to use when he or she acts out clinic experiences. While a child is undergoing cancer therapy, play often reflects with remarkable accuracy clinic procedures such as spinal taps, bone marrow aspirations, and intravenous infusions. The child may mask, glove, and arrange needed equipment on a tray before performing these procedures on a doll. The child's words during this play often echo what has been heard from caretakers during actual procedures: "Sorry, I missed your vein. I will have to try again" or "Try to hold still now." Play such as this allows the child a sense of control over the environment and can be an outlet for the frustration inherent in cancer treatment. The child should be allowed to enter into play activity by his or her own initiative. During play, which reenacts painful procedures, the child may occasionally show glee and enthusiasm while inflicting pain on a doll. This enthusiasm could be subject to many interpretations, but it is important to remember that by acting out therapeutic events and asserting control, the child will be better prepared to deal with the impositions of actual procedures.

School age—years 6 to 12

As the preschooler enters the school age years, he or she displays flickers of advancement and shadows of regression. There is no clear demarcation of developmental characteristics for the child during this transition. The caretaker's assessment of the young school age child's developmental capabilities should be based not on number of years but rather on specific behavioral and intellectual characteristics of the child.

Developmental needs. The child in the school years gains independence and individuality and experiences the challenge of a new social environment. These years are distinguished by improved and refined physical skills and intellectual abilities that enable creative self-expression through art, writing, music, and drama. The child uses his or her growing capabilities to function competently within the school milieu and to participate in activities like sports that require both individual skill and social interaction. Erickson viewed this period as one of "industry" because the child strives for a sense of worth through personal and social accomplishments.[7] The concentration on learning new skills often gives the school age child a look of contentment and complacency. Freud thought that this complacency was a result of the calm between the sexual inquisitiveness of the preschooler and the sexual tensions of the adolescent; therefore, he designated this stage the "latency period."[9] The school age child is able to separate from parents for long periods of time and can develop lasting relationships with peers and nonfamily adults. As the child's social world expands, his or her independence from the family grows. With increasing intellectual experience and wider social contacts, the child becomes more curious about other people and the world at large. Moral values of right and wrong become important, and the child embraces an often rigid moral code that he or she expects others to follow.

Lymphomas are malignant disorders of lymphoid tissue that occur during the school years as well as during adolescence and adulthood. Although these diseases are referred to as solid tumors, they often behave like systemic diseases. The child's presenting symptom is frequently an enlargement of various lymph node groups. There may also be systemic symptoms such as fever, fatigue, weight loss, anorexia, or pruritis. If mediastinal lymphoid tissue is involved, the child may develop respiratory distress. Based on histologic subtype, lymphomas can be divided into two major groups: (1) Hodgkin's disease and (2) non-Hodgkin's lymphomas. During childhood, the most common types of non-Hodgkin's lymphoma are Burkitt's lymphoma and lymphoblastic lymphoma. Surgical biopsy is necessary for accurate diagnosis of the type of lymphoma. Often a biopsy from a peripheral lymph node is sufficient, but sometimes a thoracotomy is necessary if a mediastinal mass exists without other node enlargement. Bone marrow aspirates and biopsy, as well as numerous radiologic studies, are essential for adequate evaluation of disease. Childhood non-Hodgkin's lymphomas are considered to be systemic disease from their onset, and therapy requires a rigorous combination of local radiation and aggressive systemic chemotherapy. Unfortunately, the rate of cure for non-Hodgkin's lymphoma has been low, but current therapy shows promise of an improving outlook.

Hodgkin's disease, on the other hand, has good cure rates, but the extent of disease must be accurately determined to plan appropriate therapy. A surgical laparotomy with splenectomy is often necessary to adequately determine the extent of disease. Hodgkin's disease is categorized into four stages, ranging from minimal disease confined to one lymph node group, stage I, to widespread disease with spread to nonlymphoid tissues, stage IV. Stage I and stage II disease have been successfully treated by radiation therapy. Stage IV disease requires aggressive multidrug chemotherapy for cure. For certain stage II and many stage III disease clients, radiation therapy alone may be inadequate and a combination of radiation and systemic chemotherapy is currently being used.

Life-threatening disease represents a harsh challenge to the school age child's developing sense of self and independence. Not only is self-worth brought into question by the nature of the disease and its therapy, but newly acquired confidence in socialization may become threatened. Caretakers must be aware of the many developmental disruptions created by cancer and carefully reinforce the school age child's strengths and skills. With appropriate explanations and support, the school age child will be able to adapt to clinical routines in much the same way that he or she adjusts to school. The child can become surprisingly comfortable with various clinic settings, and the open curiosity and active questioning of this age can be used to encourage the child to become an active participant in the medical care.

Children's perceptions. The developing mental capabilities of school age children enable them to understand and talk about their disease. They are quick to name the disease and to describe accurately many of its facets. They come to recognize various medications and associate specific side-effects with specific drugs. They quickly learn the routines for various procedures like blood counts and spinal taps. They show an interest in their own blood samples and bone marrow aspirates and may wish to view these samples through a microscope. They enjoy explaining their disease and its treatment to new staff, uninitiated peers, and schoolmates. They may even ask to take slides or samples to school for discussion.

Because the school age child is able to comprehend the necessity of cancer therapy, the painful procedures required are tolerated with reluctant familiarity. To develop knowledge and understanding, gain cooperation, and lessen fears, caretakers must take the time to explain to the child details of the procedures that will be done. Caretakers can give the child some sense of control by allowing him or her to make certain decisions about the conduct of care. For instance, while a procedure should not be postponed indefinitely, the child may be allowed to decide at what point during the clinic visit it will be performed. Often the child can select which vein will be used for an intravenous injection or what site will be prepared for bone marrow aspiration. The child may wish to designate which family member will be present during the procedure. Although some school age children want their parents to be present, others will not. In an effort to appear brave and unconcerned, a 10-year-old boy with Hodgkin's disease stated: "My parents just can't take watching these things." School age children may ask permission for a sibling or friend to accompany them and are often receptive to having new staff observe them. Although they will be proud of their ability to tolerate many of the painful aspects of treatment, such procedures can still create anxiety. School age children can become quite anxious if the procedure is done by an unfamiliar caretaker or is done at an unexpected time.

School age children tend to develop their own routines for dealing with fear and pain. Some children tense their bodies and hold their breath; others squeeze an object or hand during painful moments or say: "Tell me when you're going to put the needle in so I can yell." Caretakers should cooperate with the child's method of coping and should provide an atmosphere in which the child feels free to cry, to get angry, or to be upset when procedures do not go easily. Frequent praise for the child's cooperation helps bolster his or her self-confidence.

Problems related to cancer treatment. The school age child is apt to be upset by various complications of chemotherapy, such as nausea, vomiting, or hair loss. Often, the child may anticipate nausea and vomit before any chemotherapy has actually been given. The anticipation and vomiting can be upsetting and may depress the child. Caretakers can ease the discomfort when vomiting occurs by helping the child find ways to deal with the problem. Some children may wish to lie down and rest quietly; others will prefer some type of distraction such as playing a game or reading a story. Children should be allowed to eat or not as desired; they soon learn which pretherapy state best lessens nausea. Caretakers should see that adequate intravenous hydration is provided and that antiemetics are used when appropriate and desired.

Hair loss during school years can seriously injure the child's self-image and disrupt the process of socialization. Because of the child's growing self-awareness and self-consciousness, hair loss can contribute to a feeling of embarrassment. At this age, children with visible differences are potential targets of ridicule. Caretakers should be sensitive to the child's feelings of awkwardness and help him or her to obtain wigs or other head coverings. Caretakers are significant adults in the child's life, and their easy acceptance of his or her change in appearance can be reassuring. Caretakers should emphasize to the child that hair loss is an expected, but temporary, result of therapy. Classmates and friends are more likely to accept hair loss when they understand why it happens. It is therefore helpful to allow friends and siblings to accompany the child to the clinic so that they can get an idea of clinic events. This insight will help them understand the many differences in life-style of the child with cancer; hair loss, therapy-induced malaise, and extended school absences will become less mysterious to the child's peers.

In the clinic, school age children quickly become acquainted with each other. They enjoy playing games together and express interest in each other's therapy programs. They often talk to each other about their experiences in the clinic. School age children are receptive to adult attention and frequently enjoy talking to other clinic personnel, including secretaries and laboratory technicians. These interactions foster continued socialization and encourage a more relaxed and pleasant clinic environment.

Independence and socialization of the school age child will be fostered if he or she participates in as many normal activities as feasible. Because school age children function within the social context of school and after school activities, people in the school and community who work with the child, such as teachers, coaches, and scout leaders, should be informed about the child's condition. School teachers and administrators should understand that even though the child has cancer normal school activity usually can be followed. When appropriate, restrictions imposed by the disease or treatment should be clarified. Often such restrictions are minimal, for example no contact sports or strenuous physical activity during periods of low platelet count, enforcement of protective measures against specific infections like chickenpox or measles, and withholding routine live virus immunizations. School personnel should be kept informed about necessary absences related to medical care or hospitalization, and cooperation should be sought to make up any missed schoolwork. Often caretakers will need to communicate directly with school personnel to help parents with these issues.

The school age child can comprehend the seriousness of cancer and its treatment and has some awareness that his or her life could be in danger. Although the school age child primarily is concerned with immediate problems, it is not unusual for questions about prognosis and the possibility of death to be asked. Such questions should be answered honestly but without overwhelming the child with excess information. One 7-year-old boy with leukemia in remission asked if he was going to die. Apparently, classmates at school had told him that children with leukemia die from the disease. He was given an honest answer by his caretaker, "While it is possible that the disease might make you sick enough to die, you are doing well and, unless problems develop, you can expect to grow old along with your friends." He seemed satisfied with this answer and went on to talk of other things. Direct straightforward answers are readily accepted by the school age child. Two boys with lymphoma who had become friendly while in the clinic were hospitalized simultaneously for problems with their disease. One 8-year-old boy in remission was quite ill with pneumonia, while the other, age 9, was terminally ill after multiple relapses. The 8-year-old, although sick himself, turned to his caretakers to express sadness and concern about his friend. He also asked how his disease compared with that of his friend. The caretaker's response was simple and truthful, "Medicines that have worked to keep your disease away did not work for him."

The boy accepted this answer. He had developed sufficient trust in his caretakers to confide his concerns in them and to discuss his feelings with them. Parents also should be encouraged to answer their child's questions in an honest and straightforward fashion.

Caretakers should listen carefully to the questions asked by the school age child and answer them without drawing unnecessary conclusions or projecting concerns or complexities that are not present. However, if the child does not ask about prognosis or details of the disease, the caretakers still have the responsibility to inform the child of the nature of the disease and the purpose and means of therapy.

School age children often manifest a greater acceptance of disease and therapy than do children of other age groups. They seem to carry on without allowing fears to overwhelm them or treatment schedules to disrupt their life-styles. They may even appear complacent about their disease. Caretakers, however, should not assume that the child is without worry or fear. The school age child is confronting self-frailty and isolation at a time when achievement and socialization are important developmental goals. Despite an apparent calm, caretakers should be alert for subtle expressions of anxiety in the school age child and be available to provide assurance and support.

Adolescent—years 12 to 18

Developmental needs. The child's progression from the quiet of the school age years to the turmoil of adolescence is as striking and yet familiar as winter changing to spring. Rapid growth, both physical and mental, causes the adolescent to take a new view of him or herself and the world in which he or she lives. Sexuality becomes a new and exciting dimension in the child's life. Erickson[7] and others point out that the major task of the adolescent is to establish a self-identity. The personality becomes honed through the resolution of various developmental issues: separation of self from parents, establishment of independence and self-determination, creation of an ego ideal, formulation of a healthy self-image, verification of authority, and acceptance of newly acquired sexuality. In other words, life for the adolescent is a complex of multiple forces that at the same time can be demanding, confusing, exhilarating, anxiety producing, satisfying, stressful, and joyous. It is a time when the child blossoms into an adult. During this period, the adolescent often develops specific behavioral problems. He or she may display a self-interest and concern that is almost to the exclusion of others. This narcissism is a natural concomitant of the struggle to establish self-identity. Depression, marked by withdrawal, abrupt mood swings, and anger, is another manifestation of the adolescent's struggle to establish self-identity. Excessive risk taking and other tests of environmental mastery are not uncommon at this turbulent time. Behavior fluctuates between maturity and childishness because the adolescent is ambivalent; he or she is astride two worlds, seeking the adventure of adulthood, yet clinging to the security of childhood.

Osteogenic sarcoma, one type of bone cancer, is a particularly devastating disease that occurs during adolescence. This disease is most frequent during the pubertal years when the child's bone growth is most rapid. This aggressively malignant tumor most often affects long bones, especially the proximal tibia, proximal humerus, or distal femur. Frequently, the child will report a history of trauma at the involved site, but this history is probably a sign of the early sensitivity of the site rather than a causal event. Early signs of disease include pain, swelling, and sometimes a limp if a leg bone is involved. Radiographic studies show a distinctive sunburst pattern of malignant bone formation with other areas of bone destruction. Definitive diagnosis of this disease always requires biopsy.

Osteogenic sarcoma is a highly malignant and aggressive disease. If untreated, the tumor will continue to grow and will cause increased pain, swelling, and loss of function in the affected limb. Surface erosion and ulceration may develop. Treatment frequently requires amputation for complete removal of the bone in which the tumor resides. While local control can usually be achieved through aggressive surgery, this tumor unfortunately has a high potential for pulmonary metastases. Before mutilating surgery is performed, the adolescent with osteogenic sarcoma is carefully evaluated for evidence of metastatic disease. If metastases are found, amputation may not be indicated. Despite a negative preoperative evaluation, lung metastases will frequently appear months after amputation has been performed. The overall survival rate, with surgery alone, is approximately 20%.[19] Because of this poor prognosis, various adjuvant chemotherapy programs have been initiated in an attempt to improve cure rates. These programs are generally administered for 18 months as long as the client remains free of disease. If metastases occur while on therapy, however, the adolescent is given more aggressive regimens. Because metastases most frequently occur in the lungs, single or multiple thoracotomies for tumor nodule removal may be performed. Often such procedures result in temporary palliation, even if cure cannot be achieved. Radiation therapy is not as effective as chemotherapy and surgery for treating osteogenic sarcoma but is sometimes used for local control of disease if surgery is inappropriate or unacceptable.

Problems related to cancer treatment. The adolescent with osteogenic sarcoma must face not only the grim diagnosis of cancer (with the threat of death) but also the overwhelming impact of the loss of a body part, often an entire leg. No less important is the strain imposed by long and arduous chemotherapy. After enduring all of this, the adolescent may still face spread of disease to the lungs, with resultant chest surgery and more intense chemotherapy.

Amputation is a shocking experience for anyone at any stage of life, but for the adolescent, with a fragile sense of identity and evolving body image, such a loss can be shattering. The adolescent is able to comprehend the reasons for a treatment as drastic as amputation to fight cancer, but this understanding will not eliminate the depression, sadness, and anger that results. It is an important responsibility of the caretakers to help the adolescent adjust to the loss.

In caring for the adolescent with osteogenic sarcoma, caretakers must first address their own response to amputation. Feelings of revulsion and remorse are natural and not uncommon, but, if not controlled, such feelings may interfere with the delivery of care. When intense, these feelings are likely to be communicated to the adolescent. The adolescent needs to know that his or her appearance after amputation is acceptable and that the caretakers will remain a source of support and encouragement. The fact of amputation should be dealt with openly, and caretakers should emphasize the adolescent's importance as a human being. Support of the adolescent amputee should be manifest in all aspects of postoperative care. Physical therapy, stump dressing changes, treatment of phantom pain, and surgical wound care should be performed in a relaxed manner so that the adolescent can express freely and openly feelings and frustrations about his or her adjustment to body disfigurement. The caretakers should encourage and support the acquisition and use of a prosthesis and can suggest appropriate clothing and activities.

The hair loss that results from chemotherapy also has great psychologic impact on the adolescent and represents yet another insult to the person who has undergone amputation. Both amputation and hair loss negatively affect the adolescent's self-image and how he or she will be perceived by others. Caretakers must not ignore the adolescent's intense concern about body image and strong reaction to any bodily damage. Feelings of anger, depression, and sadness are appropriate and must be acknowledged and managed. The caretakers, with a genuine belief in the personal strengths of the adolescent, can support his or her efforts to deal with this crisis.

One way to assess the adolescent's ability to adjust to a change in body image is by observing personal style and appearance. If the adolescent is poised and self-assured and takes care with personal appearance, adjustment is probably proceeding well. Caretakers should determine whether the adolescent has resumed usual social interactions with friends and at school. Compliments from caretakers to the adolescent about personal appearance and accomplishments are a good source of encouragement. The interest and concern of the caretakers can be quite important to the adolescent, even if at times he or she appears diffident and disinterested.

Caretakers should encourage the adolescent's emerging sense of humor as a way to release tension and anger. One 17-year-old girl, who lost her hair from chemotherapy approximately 2 months after amputation of her leg for osteogenic sarcoma, discussed the anger and sadness she felt about the loss of hair. She said that it was just too much to take after the loss of a leg, and she seriously questioned the need to continue therapy that caused her so much harm. The caretakers reassured her that hair loss was temporary and complimented her on the attractiveness of her wig. Several days later, at a clinic visit, she announced to her caretakers, "I know you guys try, but this is not one of my favorite health spas or beauty parlors." Such sarcasm provides a means of releasing some of the tension and depression surrounding loss. Often the adolescent will name the artificial leg, for example, Henrietta or Elmer and, when something goes wrong with the prosthesis, will say: "Henrietta is acting up again." This wit enables the foreign and strange object to be more easily incorporated into daily life.

Adolescents' perceptions. The school age child is able to understand details of his or her disease and will enjoy explaining these facts to others; however, the school age child does not experience the intense emotional impact of the disease. The adolescent, on the other hand, does suffer greatly from the emotional impact of the disease and, therefore, often uses study of the disease to distance himself or herself from its impact. The adolescent often approaches the facts of the disease with detachment, wishing to be included in academic pursuits such as viewing x-ray films, bone marrow aspirates, or blood slides. By focusing on the academic aspects of disease, the adolescent can avoid dealing with the emotional impact of personal jeopardy; however, intellectual involvement also can provide the adolescent with a mechanism for coping with the disease.

One 15-year-old girl, with recently diagnosed Hodgkin's disease, was fearful and resentful of the many painful studies and surgery that were necessary to properly stage her disease. Further insult was added when she was informed of the hair loss that would result from chemotherapy. She was sad and depressed throughout the hospitalization for diagnostic studies. During this period, the caretakers attempted to provide an atmosphere in which she could express feelings, ask questions, or simply cry. About 1 week after discharge, she had to be readmitted for further abdominal surgery to relieve a partial bowel obstruction. As a result, she became even more depressed and withdrawn. She stated that she did not know how much more she could take and questioned whether she would ever feel good again. While she was recovering from the bowel surgery, she was asked to discuss the diagnostic studies that she had undergone for Hodgkin's disease with a group of medical students. She agreed and was able to explain quite clearly and accurately the reasons the various studies had been performed. As her academic interest in the disease and the process of therapy grew, she involved herself in reading about her chemotherapy and looking at her tissue slides under the microscope. Her intellectual interest seemed to draw her out of her depression. She became quite enthusiastic and initiated much of her own postoperative surgical care, such as walking, deep breathing, and monitoring intravenous infusions. She also expressed concern that her chemotherapy had to be delayed because of her surgical complication. On discharge she borrowed hospital material and gave a detailed presentation in school to her classmates and teachers on the nature of Hodgkin's disease and her personal experiences with therapy. For this adolescent, talking to others about her disease proved therapeutic; her intellectual endeavors enabled her to overcome her fears and depression. Characteristically, the adolescent will seek out literature and information concerning cancer and will discuss with caretakers his or her ideas about the disease and treatment. This intellectualization can provide a way for the adolescent to tolerate the emotional strain of cancer therapy.

The intellectual ability of the adolescent enables comprehension of the potential consequence of cancer. The concept of death can be quite real and frightening. The adolescent is able to realize that personal survival may be at stake. Caretakers should recognize this awareness of death whenever they discuss the status of the disease with the adolescent. Honesty is essential for building the adolescent's trust in the caretakers. The adolescent should be given a clear and complete picture of the disease and therapy and should be involved in decisions concerning care. Also important is the style in which the adolescent is informed about the disease, its treatment, and prognosis. The caretaker must balance clear, accurate, and realistic information with a purpose and enthusiasm that encourages hope. The adolescent may have to face the reality of death, but he or she should not be denied the comfort of hope.

The relationship of caretakers with the adolescent is crucial to sustain him or her through the process of therapy. Caretakers cannot limit their involvement simply to the management of disease. They will become involved with the emotional, social, and personal life of the adolescent as well. At this time, the adolescent is forming the concept of who and what he or she would like to become; this concept is the ego ideal.[12,13] In working toward forming an ego ideal, the adolescent scrutinizes adults for admired values, traits, skills, and accomplishments so that he or she may emulate those values and qualities. Caretakers are closely observed by the adolescent and, in this way, often have a strong influence on the formation of the adolescent's ego ideal.

Individuation and separation, in conjunction with development of an ego ideal, are processes through which the adolescent strives to become an independent person.[16] The struggle is most obvious in the adolescent's relationship with his or her parents. The adolescent often demands rights and privileges from parents while criticizing their authority and values. The constraints and complications of therapy may well be viewed by the adolescent as another form of parental authority to which he or she must conform. As a result, he or she may feel that self-determination and independence are being threatened. Caretakers should make every effort to allow the adolescent as much control as possible by including him or her in the decision-making process and providing choice and flexibility whenever reasonable. By allowing the adolescent to bargain about certain aspects of care, he or she can be drawn into the process of therapy and become an interested, rather than an unwilling, participant. Adolescents may wish to determine the times of their clinic appointments and the order of events during the clinic visit, such as when they go to x-ray, have blood drawn, or have a bone marrow aspiration. Flexibility in various aspects of care can give the adolescent a needed sense of control and self-determination.

One 16-year-old girl with leukemia, early in her course of treatment, was passive when therapeutic procedures were performed. Also, she was often withdrawn and hostile with her caretakers. Her parents accepted this behavior but did attempt to dispel her sullen attitude and encourage her as much as possible. One day in the clinic, she suddenly and emphatically refused further intravenous chemotherapy. The caretakers and parents stressed the necessity for therapy and urged her to continue. She refused to change her mind, however, so the caretakers asked her to take time at home to reconsider her decision. She left, indicating that she would return to the clinic in a week. On the way home in the car with her parents, she announced that she was now ready to proceed with treatment. She returned to the clinic and the medicines were given. For this adolescent, it was important that she be able to assert some control over the process of therapy. Once she realized that she did have some control and could influence the intrusive events of therapy, she agreed to continue with treatment. Caretakers must understand what is happening and maintain flexibility so that they can handle such situations.

Although caretakers provide an important source of emotional support to the adolescent during therapy, they also represent adult authority at a time when the adolescent is questioning and challenging authority. The relationship between the caretakers and adolescent is unusual and ambivalent. On one hand, the adolescent will associate the caretakers with the impositions of the disease and therapy, and therefore direct his or her hostilities and frustrations toward the caretakers; yet the caretakers are those individuals who are there to help and support and who clearly best understand the difficulties that the adolescent with cancer must face.

Expected behavior manifestions of the adolescent's struggle for identity, such as narcissism, depression, and risk taking, can be accentuated by the stress of cancer. The psychologic and physiologic changes of this period are great and quite personal and cause the adolescent to focus on himself or herself. This self preoccupation has been called narcissism.[12,13] Adolescent depression often manifests itself by abrupt mood swings from deep despair to unbounded elation. Anger and hostility directed at others is often an expression of the adolescent's depression and dissatisfaction with self. The depth of depression depends on the level of self-esteem.[22] The adolescent often sets high standards for personal performance; if these expectations are not met, self-esteem will fall and depression will occur. Excessive depression in adolescents has been linked to learning difficulties, behavioral problems, and delinquency.[6,11,20] Hopelessness and despair in the adolescent with cancer can produce an immobility to the extent that he or she lacks the determination and energy necessary to tolerate the rigors of cancer therapy.

Risk taking and reckless behavior, such as the abuse of psychoactive drugs or the careless driving of an automobile or motorcycle, are ways in which the adolescent will test his or her environment. Restraints and rebuffs from the adult world cause the young person to fluctuate between feelings of omnipotence and helplessness. The adolescent is likely to feel angry and hostile about the constraints of therapy and may refuse treatment because of the pain and disruption. The adolescent may express omnipotence and denial by ignoring the disease and avoiding therapy. Caretakers should realize that such feelings are not unusual for the adolescent and should remind him or her of the disease's seriousness, without resorting to threats. Caretakers should also convey understanding and acceptance of the adolescent's conflicting feelings and assert their belief that he or she has the capacity to deal with these problems. The persistence of their commitment to the adolescent's care will demonstrate that the caretakers believe in the adolescent's inherent worth as a human being.

Parents must also affirm their belief in the unique value of their child as a human being and guide him or her through the difficulties of therapy. Without strong parental direction, the adolescent generally has a harder time coping with his or her disease. Cancer most likely will magnify whatever strain exists between parents and adolescents, but this strain should not be allowed to interfere with the adolescent's acceptance of therapy.

A 17-year-old girl with osteogenic sarcoma refused the adjuvant therapy program recommended after leg amputation. She expressed anger and helplessness about her disease and doubted that further treatment would be of any use. She also believed that her disease would not spread and stated that she was willing to take the risk rather than endure therapy. Her parents were ambivalent and would not advise her to take the recommended therapy. When the caretakers asked them to assist in trying to convince her to accept therapy, they simply stated that she should do whatever she thought was best. Although these parents said that they would want her to take therapy, they were afraid that she would blame them for any failures and for the illness and hair loss that she would suffer. These parents were overwhelmed by their child's disease and were too immersed in their own conflicts and needs to be a source of strength for their child. They were afraid and felt powerless to influence her. Because they were unable to assist her, she was alone with a decision of such major consequence.

This adolescent refused chemotherapy for several months; however, her relationship with the caretakers continued through occasional clinic checkups. The caretakers persisted in their efforts to convince her and her parents to proceed with therapy, and the repeated clinic visits served to remind her of the disease. Eventually, as a result of the strengthening relationship between her, the parents, and the caretakers, she was able to change from a passive victim to an active combatant against her disease. After much effort and persistence over the course of months, the caretakers finally were able to convince her and her parents of the need for therapy. Unfortunately, during this time, the tumor spread to her lungs. Although treatment had been significantly delayed, the renewed involvement of this girl and her parents in her therapy program enabled progress to be made in the treatment of her metastatic osteogenic sarcoma.

This example demonstrates the importance of both parents and caretakers in the crucial decisions that the adolescent with cancer must face. The respect and trust developed between the adolescent and the caretakers can be essential for proper implementation of therapy. Caretakers should not underestimate their influence on the adolescent. They should constantly be aware that the adolescent's various behaviors reflect not only the stress of the disease but also the turmoil of ongoing developmental struggles. The adolescent has the right to refuse therapy, but with strong support from parents and caretakers, the adolescent can be guided into appropriate decisions.

The adolescent is known for his or her embrace of and withdrawal from maturity. This progressive and regressive behavior is intensified in the adolescent with cancer. Once the adolescent understands and is familiar with such procedures as blood drawing, spinal taps, and bone marrow aspirations, he or she is able to tolerate them quite readily. Yet, these intrusive procedures can also be an arena in which the adolescent acts out fears and rage about the disease and therapy. How much the adolescent will act out and disrupt these procedures is often directly related to how well therapy is progressing. Behavioral problems frequently develop during times when the disease is not under control. It is not unusual for an adolescent, who tolerated painful procedures with no apparent concern in the past, to cry and call out for parents, refuse procedures, and in general be uncooperative when under stress of worsening disease. This developmental progression and regression is not unusual for the adolescent and should be understood as symptomatic of situational stress. When caretakers provide understanding and guidance, the adolescent will endure and continue to mature in the midst of the serious and threatening circumstance of cancer.

CONCLUSION

Cancer is a harsh intruder that not only threatens the life of the child but also disrupts development. Advances in pediatric oncology offer new hope of cure; however, cure is never certain. This uncertainty increases the stress for all concerned.

During the long, arduous, and trying period of therapy, caretakers must make a strong commitment to nurture the child's development. Building trust in the infant, acknowledging protest of the toddler, alleviating fears of the preschooler, answering questions for the school age child, and bargaining with the adolescent are all worthwhile efforts when the child actively makes developmental progress despite cancer therapy. Although the child's struggle to mature is complicated by the burden of cancer, the authors conclude that children are able to face the impact of cancer with surprising strength and resilience. If the child receives appropriate medical treatment and psychosocial care, developmental progress can continue and the child will be able to cope with the stress posed by the disease.

ACKNOWLEDGMENT

We wish to dedicate this chapter to the children, families, and staff of the Hematology-Oncology Clinic at Wyler Children's Hospital. This chapter was inspired by the strength and resilience of the Wyler pediatric cancer patients. We also wish to give special thanks to Amy Berk, Dianne Gallagher, Sarah Hathaway, and Don Voss, whose diligent assistance, perseverance, and constant encouragement enabled this chapter to be written. Special acknowledgment goes to Dr. John Moohr, whose personal style of medical care exemplifies the approach recommended in this chapter.

REFERENCES

1. Altman, A. J., and Schwartz, A. D.: Malignant diseases of infancy, childhood, and adolescence, New York, 1978, W. B. Saunders Co., p. 2.
2. Beckwith, J. B., and Palmer, N. F.: Histopathology and prognosis of Wilms' tumor—results from

the first National Wilms' Tumor Study, Cancer **41:**1937, 1978.

3. Bloom, H. J. G., et al.: Cancer in children—clinical management, New York, 1975, Springer-Verlag New York, Inc., p. 85.
4. Breslow, N. E., et al.: Wilms' tumor: prognostic factors for patients without metastases at diagnosis—results of the National Wilms' Tumor Study, Cancer **41:**1577, 1978.
5. Chilcote, R. R., et al.: Mediastinal mass and prognosis in acute lymphocytic leukemia (ALL) (abstract), Proceedings of the Twelfth Annual Meeting of the American Society of Clinical Oncology, May 4-7, 1976, **17:**292, 1976.
6. Chwast, J.: Depressive reactions manifested among adolescent delinquents, Am. J. Psychother. **12:**575, 1967.
7. Erickson, E. H.: Childhood and society, ed. 2, New York, 1963, W. W. Norton & Co., Inc., p. 247.
8. Fernbach, D. J.: Natural history of acute leukemia. In Sutow, W. W., Vietti, T. J., and Fernbach, D. J., editors: Clinical pediatric oncology, ed. 2, St. Louis, 1977, The C. V. Mosby Co.
9. Freud, S.: The basic writings of Sigmund Freud (translated and edited by A. A. Brill), New York, 1938, Modern Library, p. 580.
10. George, S., et al.: A reappraisal of the results of stopping therapy in childhood leukemia, N. Engl. J. Med. **300:**269, 1979.
11. Glaser, K.: Masked depression in children and adolescents, Am. J. Psychother. **21:**565, 1967.
12. Hendrick, I.: Narcissism and the prepuberty ego ideal, Am. J. Psychoanal. **12:**522, 1964.
13. Jacobson, E.: Adolescent moods and the remodeling of psychic structures in adolescents, Psychoanal. Study Child **16:**164, 1961.
14. Miller, R.: Etiology of childhood cancer. In Sutow, W. W., Vietti, T. J., and Fernbach, D. J., editors: Clinical pediatric oncology, ed. 2, St. Louis, 1977, The C. V. Mosby Co.
15. Paloyan, E., and Lawrence, A. M.: Thyroid neoplasms after radiation therapy for adolescent acne vulgaris, Arch. Dermatol. **114:**53, 1978.
16. Schaffer, R.: Concepts of self and identity and the experience of separation-individuation in adolescence, Psychoanal. Q. **42:**42, 1973.
17. Strong, L.: Genetic considerations in pediatric oncology. In Sutow, W. W., Vietti, T. J., and Fernbach, D. J., editors: Clinical pediatric oncology, ed. 2, St. Louis, 1977, The C. V. Mosby Co.
18. Sutow, W.: General aspects of childhood cancer. In Sutow, W. W., Vietti, T. J., and Fernbach, D. J., editors: Clinical pediatric oncology, ed. 2, St. Louis, 1977, The C. V. Mosby Co.
19. Taylor, W., et al.: Trends and variability in survival from osteosarcoma, Mayo Clin. Proc. **53:**695, 1978.
20. Toolan, J.: Depression in children and adolescence, Am. J. Orthopsychiatry **32:**404, 1962.
21. Vietti, T., Land, V., and Ragab, A.: Management of acute leukemia. In Sutow, W. W., Vietti, T. J., and Fernbach, D. J., editors: Clinical pediatric oncology, ed. 2, St. Louis, 1977, The C. V. Mosby Co.
22. Walters, P.: Depression, Int. Psychiatry Clin. **7:** 169, 1970.

24

Morbidity and the quality of life in clients with breast cancer

LISA BEGG MARINO

A diagnosis of breast cancer creates considerable psychologic and physiologic stress on the client—psychologic stress because of the value placed on the female breast in American society and physiologic stress because of the treatments commonly employed to arrest its progress. What exactly makes up these stresses and how they interact to cause morbidity that interferes with the quality of life for female clients is the focus of this chapter.

SCOPE OF BREAST CANCER PROBLEM

Incidence

In the United States in 1979, the incidence of breast cancer was estimated to be 108,000.[1] This number represents the most frequent cancer in women after nonmelanotic skin cancer.[17] The average age-specific incidence rate per 100,000 population for white females age 30 to 34 is 22.5; for those age 65 to 69, the rate is 234. The incidence for black females has a somewhat different pattern and a lower rate but also shows a large increase with advancing age.[14] In general, the United States incidence pattern shows two peaks, one about age 45 and the other much later. This pattern could suggest the existence of two different types of breast cancer—one primarily premenopausal, which is related to ovarian function, and the other postmenopausal, which accounts for two thirds of all cases.[17] International and migrant population studies are contributing clues about the etiology of breast cancer. Breast cancer can also occur in men, but the total annual incidence is less than 1,000 new cases and therefore will not be discussed other than to say that nurses can help identify cases by alerting male clients to the possibility of breast cancer occurring. Unfortunately, the same index of suspicion that many women have does not occur in men, with a more advanced stage being diagnosed. While the total cases may be few, many of these men die because of ignorance about breast cancer detection.

Risk factors for the development of breast cancer

Breast cancer in females is associated with a number of risk factors. The following is a list of factors that place a woman at high or low risk of developing breast cancer some time in her life:

Higher risk[17]
1. Direct family history, particularly if client's mother had bilateral breast cancer or cancer diagnosed while premenopausal
2. Nulliparous until after age 35
3. Previous diagnosis of breast cancer

Lower risk[17]
1. Certain ethnic groups such as Orientals
2. Risk decreases as age at first full-term birth occurred, that is, under age 15 lowest risk
3. Artificial menopause by bilateral oophorectomy

Less substantiated but currently associated with an increased risk
1. Early menarche and later menopause[19]
2. Excessive exposure to ionizing radiation[19]
3. Estrogen replacement therapy[19]
4. Large body size (particularly related to obesity and/or higher intake of animal fats)[19]
5. Nulliparity[19]
6. History of cancer of the endometrium, ovary, or colon[19]
7. Long-term use of reserpine[17]

Chief among these factors is the family history of breast cancer and having developed breast cancer previously. In cases where the mother has premenopausally had breast cancer, her daughter's risk can be *50 times* that of the general population at age 29.[17] Recognition of these risk factors can help nurses to identify women who are at higher risk and to help these women become more aware of how they can help themselves.

Likewise, women need to understand that most breast masses are benign so that avoidance in examining their breasts and delay in seeking medical evaluation will only harm them further. Fully *80% of all masses* found in the breast are benign. In fact, women can even be taught the most common areas in their breasts where a cancer is likely to appear. Fig. 24-1 demonstrates that nearly one half of all types of breast cancer appear in the upper outer quadrant. Nurses can teach women to examine their entire breast but pay special attention to this particular quadrant. Unfortunately, this concentration has one distinct disadvantage that can readily be seen in Fig. 24-2. The axilla contains many lymph nodes that facilitate the regional and distant spread of the primary breast cancer to other sites in the body, principally the contralateral breast, bone, liver, and brain. The recognition of the regional spread of breast cancer led Halstead to pioneer his standard radical mastectomy in 1894. The surgical procedure is still regarded by many surgeons as the procedure of choice for removing breast cancer. The importance of these regional lymph nodes is also the reason the surgeon will carefully disect them to determine the extent of the cancer's spread. The histologic presence or absence of cancer in the regional lymph nodes coupled with the histologic type of breast cancer are the most

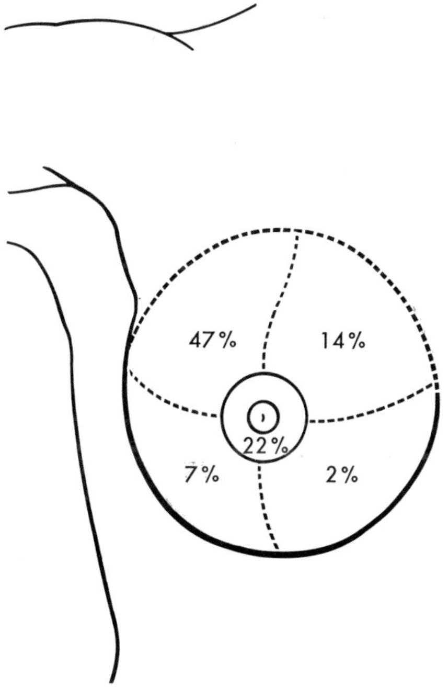

Fig. 24-1. Distribution of carcinomas within breast.

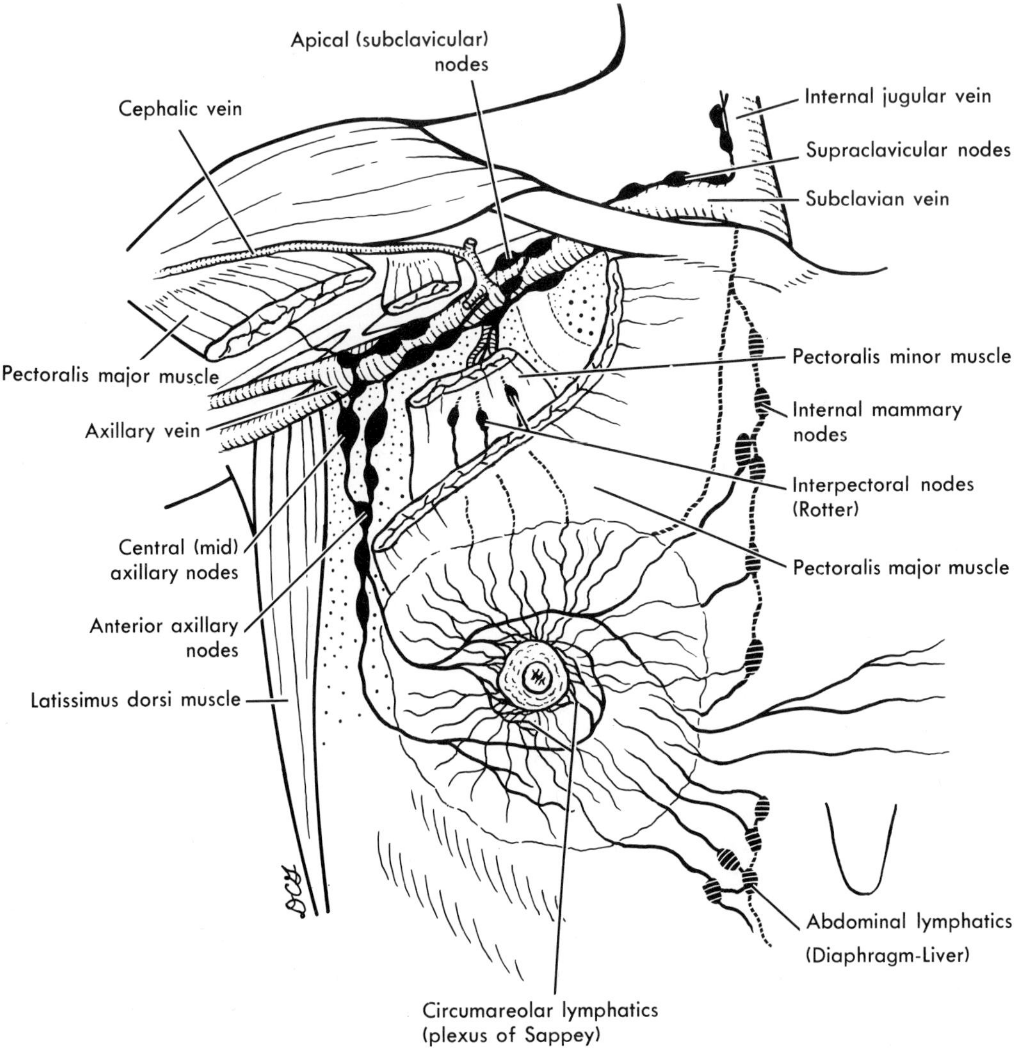

Fig. 24-2. Lymphatic drainage of the breast. (From Gallager, H. S., Leis, H. P., Jr., Snyderman, R. K., and Urban, J. A., editors: The breast, St. Louis, 1978, The C. V. Mosby Co.)

significant prognostic factors. The following is a list of the various types of breast cancer:[2]

A. Noninfiltrating
   1. Paget's disease with intraductal carcinoma
   2. In situ lobular carcinoma
   3. In situ intraductal carcinoma
B. Infiltrating
   1. Paget's disease with infiltrating carcinoma
   2. Ductal carcinoma
      a. Infiltrating, not otherwise specified
      b. Adenoid cystic
      c. Comedo
      d. Medullary
      e. Mucinous
      f. Papillary
      g. Lobular carcinoma, infiltrating

Infiltrating, also referred to as invasive carcinoma, specifically ductal carcinoma, encompasses about 60% to 70% of all breast cancers.[9] These cancers have 5- and 10-year survival rates from 54% and 32% (lobular infiltrating carcinoma) up to 83% and 56% (papillary).[16] Clients with negative axillary lymph nodes have only an 18% and 24% 5- and 10-year rate of treatment failure, respectively, compared to clients with more than four positive axillary lymph nodes who have 79% and 89% 5- and 10-year rates of treatment failure.[8]

Aside from prognostic significance, the lymph nodes and the histologic type of breast cancer largely determine what form of treatment needs to be employed. The form of treatment, in turn, largely determines the degree of morbidity the woman experiences. Further discussion relative to postmastectomy morbidity will be expanded on later in this chapter.

OVERALL CLIENT NEEDS

General needs

Just as with other forms of cancer, there are areas of general needs for each client and more specific needs based on their individual physical and psychologic state. The specific needs are largely dependent on the degree of disability resulting from the illness as well as the woman's perception of what is happening to her. For example, under general needs are such concerns as physical restoration and optimal functioning, cosmesis as it relates to the client's sexuality, comfort and coping measures, early detection of recurrent disease, and information gathering from diagnosis on as well as the general problem area of postmastectomy morbidity. These needs are important to virtually all women with breast cancer regardless of the disease extent and disability associated with their illness. Physical restoration is a major problem for these women because of the extensive loss of muscle as well as the shoulder dysfunction that results from the surgical procedure. Regardless of whether or not their cancer progresses, these women need to use their arms, hands, and upper torso in activities of daily living. Likewise, a woman's sexuality is important throughout her life, perhaps even more so if the cancer progression limits outside contacts and interests.

One research study that collected data through client interviews found that three basic changes occurred after mastectomy. First, mastectomy precipitated a period of shock; second, obvious changes in body appearance resulted; and third, the future became uncertain because of the fear of shortened life and the possibility of a slow, painful death.[15]

Specific needs

Specific needs are those needs that become more or less prominent depending on the client's state of wellness or illness. Examples of these needs are comfort needs immediately after mastectomy, if bony metastasis occurs, or at the end of life. Psychologic comfort specific to disclosure of diagnosis, immediately postmastectomy, during the return home when reintegration within the family is likely to occur.

Information gathering, important throughout the illness course, is especially important following confirmation that a breast cancer exists. It is during this period that the woman confronts the reality of the situation and forms a plan of action. Information as to available options is vital to any decision-making process. Because these options have lifelong implications, the woman needs to come to some agreement with herself as to what course of action to pursue.

CANCER MORBIDITY AND ITS IMPACT ON THE QUALITY OF LIFE

Morbidity is defined as a negative change in the physical or psychologic functioning of the client that is a direct result of the disease or its treatment. In the case of cancer morbidity, any impairment that is a result of the pathologic process or secondary to treatment would be included within this definition. Because of the debilitating aspects of cancer and the extensiveness and seriousness of many of its treatment regimens, morbidity in cancer is a major problem area. Chapter 22 discusses cancer morbidity from the perspective of a central need associated with numerous secondary needs such as loss of sexuality owing to disfigurement or a loss of mobility owing to a "frozen shoulder."

How cancer morbidity relates to, and impacts on, the quality of the woman's life is important for a number of reasons. First, 108,000 women were diagnosed with breast cancer in *1979*. Prior years produced significant numbers of cases with many more women to be afflicted in the future. Many of these women will suffer recurrence or death directly attributable to breast cancer. Second, the economic implications of breast cancer are even more staggering. In the United States, it is estimated that mere medical costs are *over $0.5 billion dollars each year.*[17]

Additionally, breast cancer incidence patterns demonstrate that one third of all new cases—35,000 of the 108,000 cases in 1979 alone—occur in women under the age of 50. There is never a good time to have cancer regardless of the woman's age, but it is particularly tragic for young women in the prime of life to be afflicted with a life-threatening illness.

How much morbidity associated with cancer in general and how it affects the quality of the client's life have not been documented to any great extent. Subjectively, most cancer clinicians can respond with their personal observations of the consequences they have observed in their clients, but few morbidity models exist. In one way, this fact is surprising in that the morbidity is readily observable to trained health personnel. Likewise, morbidity can be dealt with by most professional nurses. It is for this reason that the focus of this chapter will be on cancer morbidity specific to breast cancer and how the quality of the client's life is affected.

MORBIDITY ASSOCIATED WITH BREAST CANCER

Most of the morbidity that is associated with breast cancer can be attributed to its treatment. All major forms of cancer treatment can and are frequently employed in an attempt to control the breast cancer. Chief among these treatment forms is surgery; this form will be discussed next.

Morbidity resulting from breast cancer surgery

Surgery designed to eradicate breast cancer has been in existence since the late 1800's when William S. Halstead put forth the radical mastectomy procedure that bears his name. This procedure was the sole method of treating primary breast cancer for a number of years. Within the last 15 years, however, it has lost favor to less radical procedures. The following is a list of definitions[19] of each of these surgical procedures from the least to most extensive:

Limited procedures—Variety of names: local excision, partial mastectomy, extended tylectomy and lumpectomy, or segmental resection; excision consists of removing the mass plus varying amounts of surrounding normal breast tissue from 0 to 6 or 8 cm. The nipple and areola are not removed.

Subcutaneous mastectomy—Removal of the internal breast tissue, leaving the skin; if a cancer is confirmed, the breast and axillary lymph nodes are removed. After a period of time, an implant is inserted to restore the contour of the breast.

Total or simple mastectomy—Only the breast is removed, leaving the axillary nodes and pectoral muscles intact. This avoids the "sunken" chest that results from the more extensive procedures.

Modified radical mastectomy—Removal of entire breast combined with axillary node dissection; the underlying pectoralis major muscle is left in place, but the pectoralis minor muscle is usually removed along with the axillary nodes. All major lymphatic chains except the channel through the pectoralis major muscle are removed.

Halstead radical mastectomy—The entire breast including the pectoralis major and minor muscles and the lymph nodes of the axilla, fat, and skin overlying the involved area are removed.

Extended radical mastectomy—Excision of all tissue as in the Halstead radical mastectomy plus the internal mammary chain of lymph nodes; generally a section of the rib cage must be removed to reach these nodes.

Generally speaking, the more limited surgeries such as total mastectomy or limited procedures are employed for older women or for those women who are thought to have more extensive disease for which local tumor removal could not be curative. If the effects of age are discounted, there are generally fewer problems associated with the lesser procedures as opposed to the more extensive procedures such as the extended radical mastectomy. Fig. 24-3 illustrates part of the reason. The surgical procedure illustrated in these diagrams is the modified radi-

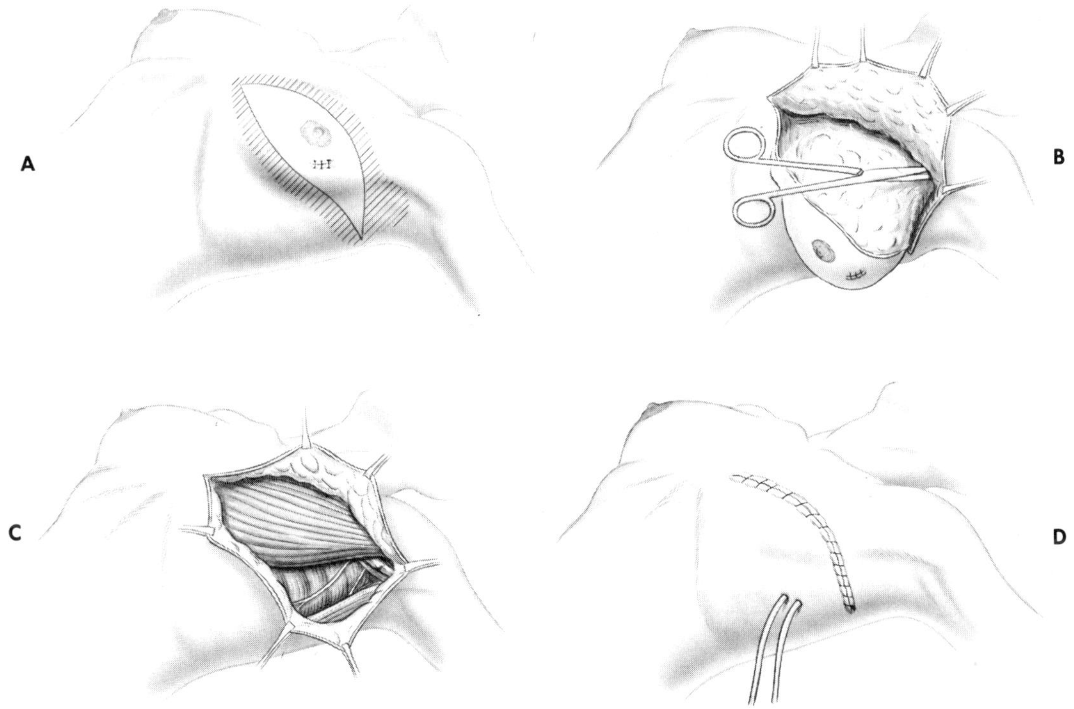

Fig. 24-3. A, Transverse incision marked on skin of left breast prior to total or modified radical mastectomy. **B,** Skin flaps above and below breast. Breast is being removed. **C,** Operative field after completion of modified radical mastectomy. **D,** Skin closure after total or modified radical mastectomy. (From Gallager, H. S., Leis, H. P., Jr., Snyderman, R. K., and Urban, J. A., editors: The breast, St. Louis, 1978, The C. V. Mosby Co.)

cal mastectomy. This procedure requires the surgeon to remove the entire breast, leaving only the pectoralis major muscle in place; the pectoralis minor muscle is generally removed along with axillary lymph nodes. The modified mastectomy is not as cosmetically disfiguring or functionally impairing as the Halstead radical mastectomy.

Physical dysfunction associated with breast cancer surgery. The three principal forms of physical dysfunction seen with mastectomy are lymphedema, arm and shoulder stiffness, and the loss of cosmesis.[18]

Lymphedema, or the collection of excess fluid within the arm, has been attributed to unusual trauma to the axillary blood vessels during surgery or a postoperative infection in the axillary areas. Regardless of the specific etiology, the mechanisms producing lymphedema are essentially the same: the lymph flow from the extremity is obstructed thereby causing an increase in the hydrostatic pressure. Measurement of the degree of arm dysfunction has been made by one researcher based on the following parameters: slight lymphedema, which caused the arm to enlarge 2.5 cm in circumference when compared with the arm on the side of the normal breast; moderate edema between 2.5 and 4.5 cm; and severe edema more than 4.5 cm. Client recordings were taken shortly after surgery and again at 18 months after mastectomy. Early in the postoperative period, 69% indicated some degree of lymphedema was present. Of these 193, however, 77% had slight edema, 14% had moderate lymphedema, and 9% had severe lymphedema. At 18 months after mastectomy, 77% had some evidence of lymphedema, with 70% of that total having slight enlargement and 15% each with moderate or severe lymphedema. Most of these women had undergone the Halstead radical mastectomy; the less extensive procedures produced a lesser chance of the development of lymphedema.[5]

Arm and shoulder stiffness causing arm dysfunction was commonly reported with lymphedema. Parameters of arm activity have been defined as: "good motor function if wide and free arm motion was present without limitation; moderate dysfunction was present if the client was unable to perform many tasks and to do others with restriction; severe dysfunction meant that the client could perform only the simplest tasks."[7] In at least one study, there was a relationship between arm dysfunction and the presence of lymphedema. Between the first and second interviews, the percentage of clients with good arm function rose from 42% to 76%, with the direct relationship between function and lymphedema present at both time points.[7]

Although arm dysfunction can be minimized by regular exercising, a woman who has lost her pectoralis major and minor muscles as a result of a Halstead radical mastectomy or extended radical mastectomy may never regain her full muscle strength in the afflicted arm; however, other muscles can compensate to a degree.[19]

Physical disability, in general, was evaluated in another study[4] utilizing cases and controls by asking the woman "Do you have any physical disability that prevents you from doing anything you should be able to do?" Those answering affirmatively were then asked to estimate the extent of disability from none to total disability. The results indicated the following: 19% of the 134 women reported significant disability and 16% of the 260 controls reported significant disability. The women were also asked to describe their current health status on a 5-point scale from excellent to very poor. Cases and controls were similar in the proportion estimating their health as good or excellent. However, cases did have a significantly larger proportion of responses in the poor to very poor category (10.4% versus 3.8%, respectively).

Psychologic dysfunction related to breast cancer surgery. Psychologic dysfunction related to mastectomy consists of the woman's attitude about herself, sexual activity, presence of depression, anxiety, and introversion. Studies in this area are limited because of the overall sample sizes as well as the methodologic problems in utilizing open-ended questions that can introduce well-known biases.[18]

In one study, women were asked to rate themselves with respect to happiness; all clients were 5 or more years after mastectomy. The great majority of cases and controls rated themselves as happy. However, a slightly higher proportion of cases than controls said they were unhappy, 6% and 2.7%, respectively.[4]

Another study measured attitude with "good" representing the client who had no complaints, "fair" when there were complaints about some aspect of the experience, and "poor" when the woman expressed her unhappiness with the entire illness. Comparing clients having undergone limited surgery versus those clients who have undergone a more radical form of mastectomy, a large difference between the two groups was indicated. For example, those clients who had undergone more limited surgery demonstrated an improvement in their attitude between the two interview periods, whereas the radical group's attitude worsened. The percentages in the radical group went from 56% to 38% for good, 41% to 58% said fair, and poor stayed at 4% each time.[7]

Postmastectomy depression and loss of self-esteem in a group of newly diagnosed breast cancer clients were compared with those of a control group of women with other forms of cancer. A clinical interview was conducted at 4 to 6 weeks postmastectomy and again at 6 to 8 months. A similar proportion (30%) of breast cancer clients and other cancer clients reported the syndrome of depression, lowered self-esteem, increased health concerns, and loss of energy. Peak emotional distress occurred in the breast cancer group about 2 to 3 months after mastectomy.[21]

Another study[4] compared women with breast cancer to a control group of cholecystectomy clients in a number of standard psychologic measures of depression and anxiety along with measures of self-esteem. The data were supplemented by additional data obtained through interviews. Significant differences relative to three of the measures employed (depression, anxiety, and introversion) were noted, with the mastectomy clients being more anxious, depressed, and introverted in their behavior. Since these client contacts were made 18 months to 5 years after mastectomy with the cases having undergone only total and modified mastectomies, the findings are highly significant.

Trained interviewers were employed in one study to ascertain the psychologic and social adjustment of women who presented with a breast lump that subsequently required that a mastectomy be performed. The women were interviewed in their homes before admission for biopsy, again at 4 months, and then at 1 year after mastectomy. Results at 4 months indicated that 27% of the mastectomized group were moderately to severely depressed compared to 12% of the controls. Additionally, a larger number of breast cancer clients were found to have suffered from sexual problems during the 1 year follow-up period. One third of the women who stated that they had a satisfactory sex life premastectomy stated they ceased all sexual activity or achieved no enjoyment from sex at 12 months postmastectomy. Only 8% of the control group made such statements.[12]

However, in another study of 34 married women[20] 4 years after mastectomy, no change in sexual frequency was noted in the majority of cases. In comparing those cases who did or did not acknowledge a decrease in their sexual frequency, the women with unchanged activity appeared to be better prepared for their surgeries, reported more interest in sex, were much more satisfied with their current sexual relationships, had fewer persisting complications and fewer symptoms of depression, were less likely to have had radical surgeries, were twice as likely to be under 46 years of age, and were more satisfied with their husband's companionship. Of all these characteristics, only sexual satisfaction and satisfaction with the husband's companionship differed significantly between the two groups.

Another study obtained data on the frequency of breast stimulation after mastectomy and found that of 41 married women,[20] 46% reported stimulation by touching the breast was common in comparison to 33% reporting it after mastectomy. In this group, frequency of intercourse also declined. An interesting observation was made that 63% of women in this group indicated a desire to discuss sexuality with a nurse but did not because of a perception that the nurse's attitude would prevent such discussion.

Clearly, undergoing a mastectomy, regardless of its extensiveness, creates additional stress to women. Unfortunately, the mastectomy may be only the beginning of a series of treatments aimed at eradicating the breast cancer. If this is in fact the case, a *series* of stresses may occur so that the woman is required to adjust to repeated situations in order to maintain psychic equilibrium.

Nursing interventions. The findings of physical and psychologic morbidity have numerous implications for all of the health care providers, but particularly so for the nurse. For example, while the nurse can do little about any intraoperative trauma, instruction on the importance of protecting the affected arm is very important and can do a great deal to prevent the worsening of any lymphedematous condition. Instruction to the woman to wear gloves while gardening or doing work that might irritate the skin of the affected arm is very important. Likewise, protection from injuries commonly sustained within the home, such as sewing accidents and use of abrasive compounds, is helpful. Many women do not realize the threat of injury that revolves around such seemingly innocuous procedures as vaccinations, blood pressure tests, or simple injections. Protecting the skin of the affected arm from sunburn and wearing loose clothing to cover the chest wall and arm are also important. Lastly, if lymphedema does occur, the woman should be made aware that resources are available to minimize the dysfunction through such measures as frequent and sustained arm elevation, customized sleeves to promote lymph drainage, exercise, and physical therapy.

The same situation is true for any shoulder or arm dysfunction. Prevention of deformity is always preferable to treatment so an exercise plan in consultation with the surgeon is important as is encouragement and explanation to family members so that the entire family can become involved. Identification of resources if problems do develop is an appropriate nursing function so that further problems can be avoided.

Most mastectomies do not result in a cosmetically attractive breast. While the nurse can do little about this fact, information and assistance in obtaining medical resources are important activities. For example, much controversy currently exists as to the most efficacious type of mastectomy to employ. Much research and pure rhetoric are being exchanged with no real resolution in sight. These disagreements place additional burdens on the woman and her family because there do not seem to be any clear-cut answers. The final decision is ultimately up to the woman and her family, but support during this trying period is helpful as well as providing the woman with information on alternative procedures. While the "partial" mastectomies such as segmented mastectomy and tylectomy have not shown to be efficacious, there are surgeons willing to perform such procedures. If the loss of the woman's breast is that significant, she may elect to undergo one of these procedures. Assisting the surgeon in explaining the advantages and disadvantages so that an informed decision can be made are appropriate nursing interventions.

Nursing interventions directed toward minimizing the psychologic dysfunction are more difficult because consultation and intervention on the part of a variety of health care providers is generally needed. Specifically, psychiatric consultation to minimize long-term depression and sexual counseling to promote successful adjustment appear to be worthwhile. The nurse, acting as a full team member, would be involved in assessing the woman and her family and intervening once the overall plans become known. To help identify women who may demonstrate this behavior a number of years after mastectomy, contacts with community agencies can be maintained as can general case finding among neighbors and acquaintances of nurses. Many women may suffer in silence because they are unaware that these feelings are quite common among clients with breast cancer or are unfamiliar with ways to seek help. This diminished productive life compounds the internal tragedy that the diagnosis creates.

Two important points from Woods' book *Human Sexuality in Health and Illness*[20] pertain to nursing interventions specific to clients' sexuality after mastectomy. One nursing function is to help the client explore her feelings about the consequences the mastectomy may have on her sexual life. It is important that the nurse retain a nonjudgmental attitude because the client may perceive that the nurse is unable or unwilling to discuss such a subject. Also, the nurse can reinforce the significance the Reach to Recovery volunteer can have to the client through behavioral modeling. Seeing a woman who has successfully adjusted to her mastectomy is important because it serves as a stimulus to the client to move on with life and reinforces the importance of the woman's total personality. The Reach to Recovery volunteer can counsel the client firsthand as to likely problems that must be dealt with as well as offering suggestions for successfully accomplishing these adjustments.

Morbidity associated with radiation therapy

There are eight reasons that radiotherapy for breast cancer has been administered: as an alternative to surgery, preoperative radiotherapy of operable or borderline inoperable tumors, systematic postoperative radiotherapy after radical surgery, as a therapy for known postoperative residual tumor, as postoperative surgical adjuvant therapy following purposefully limited surgery, as total radiotherapeutic management of inoperable carcinomas, for therapy of chest wall and postoperative regional recurrences, and as therapy for metastatic manifestations.[6] Many of these approaches are still regarded as controversial, but the reality is that women are being treated by such means with resulting morbidity. Part of the reason that morbidity results from radiotherapy is that multiple factors affect the therapeutic gain; for example, the dose and method of administering the irradiation can vary depending on the tumor cell type, the normal tissues to be irradiated, the time-dose relationship, the volume of irradiation, and the bulk of the tumor.[10] Specifically relating to tumor bulk, it has been shown that 4,500 to 5,000 rads are effective in eradicating microscopic amounts of breast cancer but that 6,000 rads are required for small but clinically apparent tumors and as high as 8,000 to 9,000 rads are required for very bulky tumors.[10] The higher the dose, the greater the risk of exceeding the soft tissue tolerance with the greater likelihood of complications such as necrosis, moist desquamation, rib fracture, and disabling fibrosis. It is not the purpose of this section to debate the efficacy of such treatments but to provide the reader with insights into what may happen to these women and what nursing care may be offered to assist them.

Morbidity associated with primary radiotherapy. Because of the documented morbidity associated with breast cancer surgery, many oncologists have researched the efficacy of using supervoltage radiotherapy as a primary treatment for stage I and stage II breast cancer. This type of therapy generally requires dosages in the range of 5,000 rads in 5 to 6 weeks followed by interstitial implantation of another 1,500 to 2,000 rads. This approach produces acute side-effects such as local skin changes of dry desquamation, hyperpigmentation, and areas of moist desquamation. Most incidents are transient so that side-effects disappear in 1 to 3 weeks after therapy. When recovery occurs, the interstitial implantation is done with a number of later complications possible. These untoward effects can range from self-limited problems such as an unproductive cough and mild shortness of breath to rib fractures.[10]

Morbidity associated with adjunctive radiotherapy. There are two reasons for which adjunctive radiotherapy is generally given in the management of primary breast cancer: first, when known postoperative residual tumor is present and, second, to accompany limited surgeries such as segmental mastectomy. In the former case, the surgeon may not have been able to completely remove all of the tumor in the woman's breast or axilla. Since numerous local problems can occur, radiotherapy is generally given in an attempt to eradicate the residual tumor bed. Because gross tumor is present, the dosage of radiotherapy must increase correspondingly. The underlying lung creates a problem in these types of cases, with pulmonary fibrosis being common. In fact, this particular problem most closely reflects the untoward effects seen in earlier years before it was completely understood that removing all gross tumor allowed a lesser dose of irradiation to be given with much less morbidity encountered. Radiotherapists now understand the importance of treating microscopic as opposed to gross tumors in terms of the frequency of complications.

When radiotherapy is given adjunctively after limited surgeries, it is done so as to eradicate any multicentric disease that may be present elsewhere in the breast. With supervoltage equipment and sufficient fractionalization, radiotherapy is well tolerated. Generally, there are no untoward effects other than minor dysplasia at about 3 weeks of therapy. Skin reactions are also limited to erythema and pigmentation with moist desquamation usually avoided. Physical therapy is generally ordered by the radiotherapist to avoid shoulder motion restrictions; these exercises need to be continued by the client on her own. There is generally no arm edema.[13]

Morbidity from palliative radiotherapy. Palliative radiotherapy can range from treating chest wall recurrences to pathologic bone fractures. In the case of chest wall recurrences, radiotherapy is so successful that many times the client is virtually cured of this recurrence. Esophagitis, nausea, and vomiting are usually the acute effects that are transient and disappear after treatment subsides. Pulmonary fibrosis is a more troublesome and later effect of this type of treatment.[3]

Radiotherapy can also be administered for stage III breast cancer where large tumors that are locally advanced cannot be treated by other means. As explained previously, when gross disease is present, higher dosages need to be given. Generally 6,000 rads by external beam therapy are needed. This treatment is justified despite the high incidence of subsequent distant spread because ulceration would eventually occur without such local treatment. In these cases, brisk erythema and, less frequently, moist desquamation can occur. Late effects can include mild telangiectasia and fibrosis.[3]

When radiotherapy is employed as palliation for metastatic bone lesions, benefits almost always outweigh any untoward effects because doses are much smaller and the client's discomfort mandates therapeutic intervention.

Nursing interventions. Nursing interventions relative to reducing the morbidity associated with radiation therapy center on two major approaches: client teaching to prevent or treat complications and working actively with the physician to monitor the client during and after treatment.

Client teaching is important to assure that the woman and her family understand how to care for the skin during and after treatment so that further irritation does not occur. Approaches generally vary from one radiation therapy department to another, so the nurse needs to become familiar with the rationale and procedures in use locally. Another area where client teaching is important is to minimize shoulder dysfunction through effective and repeated exercising. Many radiotherapists now order a physical therapy assessment so that proper assessment and personalized instruction can be given. It is important for the nurse to attend these sessions so that follow-up instruction can be given and reinforcement of the need to continue these exercises after treatment is completed to preserve shoulder function can be accomplished.

Detecting complications is also important to prevent major disability and here the nurse can be helpful to the entire health care provider team by careful periodic assessment of the client to determine if esophagitis, nausea, or vomiting has occurred. Moreover, reinforcing the need to consult with the physician in the future is important if shortness of breath, telangiectasia, and fibrosis are to be detected.

Morbidity secondary to cancer chemotherapy for breast cancer

Cancer chemotherapy is now routinely administered for high-risk clients as well as those clients with metastatic breast cancer. Adjuvant chemotherapy or the use of chemotherapy after mastectomy is still regarded as investigational, although it is widely employed. Chemotherapy for advanced breast cancer is now considered standard although certain single agents or combinations of agents may still be regarded as investigational or under continued study.

For those agents employed for some time in treating breast cancer, both early and recurrent disease, the side-effects are well known. For example, myelosuppression, cardiotoxicity, neurotoxicity, stomatitis, diarrhea, alopecia, nausea, and vomiting are toxicities associated with a variety of chemotherapeutic agents. The toxicities from these agents can range from life-threatening to nuisance level. Because of this wide range as well as the fact that most chemotherapy is administered on an outpatient basis, it is important that the client and family be actively involved in all aspects of care. Likewise, toxicity may vary depending on the client's stage of disease in that adequate renal and liver functioning can be significant in reducing problems as can a high nutritional level. Since chemotherapy is not specific to cancer cells, a delicate balance between therapeutic and toxic levels must be maintained.

Long-term morbidity associated with chemotherapy is only now being assessed as clients are surviving for longer periods. For example, most chemotherapeutic regimens are given over many months so that the long-term effect of repeated myelosuppression still needs to be evaluated. Unfortunately, reports of clients being diagnosed with second cancers are increasing. However, it remains to be shown whether these cancers are a natural consequence of breast cancer and are only now appearing because more clients are achieving long-term survival. The other side of this important issue is whether or not these second cancers are caused in some way by the chemotherapy itself. There is some evidence to support this in that renal transplant clients have a higher incidence of cancer. This discovery is particularly troublesome given the documented morbidity from the other forms of treatment and the lack of other alternatives, and it is hoped that this severe morbidity will be balanced by continued increases in client survival.

Other long-term effects include potential loss of reproductive capacity because of suppressed function. This consequence is particularly true for the alkylating agents in premenopausal women. Additionally, some chemotherapeutic agents have been shown to be mutagenic in animals or potentially teratogenic in humans. Problems in this area may not occur, but women should be so advised.

Methotrexate, an antimetabolite, can cause hepatotoxicity, nephrotoxicity, and pulmonary damage.

Hormonal therapy, although distinct from antitumor chemotherapy, is generally discussed with chemotherapy in terms of toxicities. Hormonal therapy has currently been revived because of the ability of hormonal receptor assays to better detect responders. There are two approaches to hormonal therapy, additive or ablative. Additive hormonal therapy involves the use of estrogens, androgens, progestins, glucocorticoids, or antiestrogens. Ablative procedures are designed to remove sources of estrogen and include oophorectomy, adrenalectomy, and hypophysectomy.

The additive side-effects include nausea, vomiting, fluid and salt retention, masculinization, anorexia, hypercalcemia, hot flashes, pruritis, and uterine bleeding. The ablative procedures permanently remove the source or sources of estrogen, thereby rendering the client sterile. Additionally, cortisone replacement therapy is required, which necessitates that the client assume self-responsibility so that cortisone can be maintained.

Nursing interventions. Many interventions relative to chemo- and hormonal therapies require a combination of diligent client-family teaching, observation, and supportive interventions. Client-family teaching is required because many of these types of treatments have life-threatening toxicities and are usually administered outside the hospital. Actively involving the client and family better assures an increased level of understanding so that toxicities can be detected as early as possible with the client helping herself as much as possible. Additionally, these treatments can extend over a prolonged period so that continuity and coordination can be beneficial. Nurses are in ideal positions to assume these responsibilities.

Observation through careful review of laboratory tests, maintenance of contact with the client and family over time, and periodic physical assessment can help the physician determine the therapeutic effects and possible toxicities of these agents and more closely monitor the client's physical and psychologic states.

Supporting the client to minimize toxicities is a very important nursing function so that interference with important life events can be minimized at the same time maximal therapeutic effect can be achieved. Monitoring adequate nutritional intake can provide the client with added strength as well as reduce such toxicities as hemorrhagic cystitis owing to cytoxan administration when adequate fluid intake is not maintained. Likewise, assisting clients to establish adequate rest periods and activity levels allows them to have control over their lives while permitting therapy to continue at maximal levels. A detailed discussion of nursing interventions relative to the specific agents employed in cancer management is included in Chapter 14 of this book.

Morbidity associated with immunotherapy for breast cancer

Immunotherapy in general is still considered investigational but has shown some promise in advanced stages of breast cancer. Agents such as bacillus Calmette Guérin (BCG) and *Corynebacterium parvum* (*C. parvum*) are examples of active, nonspecific immunotherapeutic agents commonly employed in breast cancer.

Side-effects from these agents vary depending on the route of administration. For example, BCG can be administered intradermally, intralesionally, intrapleurally, or via the scarification method. If BCG is given intradermally, generally only local effects will be seen. Mild irritation and malaise are the most common. However, when given via the scarification method, a flulike syndrome consisting of malaise, chills, fever, nausea, and vomiting lasting up to 1 week after treatment is very common. Additionally, scarification is an accurate term in that scars are visible in the treated areas.

Side-effects of *C. parvum* vary with subcutaneous or intravenous administration. Local reactions in the form of swelling and soreness are most common when *C. parvum* is administered subcutaneously. Occasionally, ulceration and abscess formation may also occur. Intravenous use produces much more severe toxicity such as rigor, severe nausea and vomiting, and hypotension.

Rarely is immunotherapy employed singularly in breast cancer management, so it is important that the nurse be familiar with all possible toxicities and any synergistic effects that may occur.

Nursing interventions. As with chemotherapy, nursing interventions combine client-family teaching, observation, and supportive measures. Specifically, clients and their families need to be taught what is a minor toxicity and what is severe enough to call in or appear for an evaluation. Additionally, dosages can be adjusted according to the level of toxicity experienced by the client so this information needs to be accurately and completely reported back to the physician. Supportive measures include working with the client to devise an acceptable activity schedule during periods of treatment and appropriate intervals to administer antiemetic and antipyretic medication to relieve toxicity. Immunotherapy is generally administered during the more advanced stages of breast cancer, so it is important for the nurse to develop an integrated plan to support the client and family.

MORBIDITY DIRECTLY RELATED TO DISEASE PROGRESSION

Thus far, morbidity secondary to cancer treatment has been discussed. Unfortunately, the pathologic process itself contributes to diminished psychologic and physical functioning of the client. McCorkle[11] has developed a list of common disease-related physical symptoms and has offered suggestions for their care. There are four main groups of symptoms: bone, chest and soft tissue, brain, and viscera. Since many women do develop metastatic breast cancer, it is imperative that nurses understand more fully the pathology and resulting nursing interventions that can ease the client's discomfort.

CASE STUDY

A client whose clinical situation parallels many of the problems discussed in this chapter was Judy, a 36-year-old Caucasian female. Judy's case is vividly recallable because of the circumstances of her illness and the fact that most of her health care providers were truly saddened by the problems she experienced that ultimately caused her death 2 years later.

Personal history

Judy, a bookkeeper by training, was the mother of two small children, Duncan, a 4-year-old girl, and Jason, a 7-year-old boy. She was married to Jim, who was 4 years her senior and a certified public accountant. They had been married 9 years and characterized their marriage as an essentially happy one. Jim made a good living that enabled them to have their own home, entertain at frequent intervals, and take annual "family-style" vacations. Judy had planned to return to a full-time bookkeeping position once Duncan started in school and was currently only accepting free-lance jobs with small companies. She was an attractive, dark-tanned woman who looked slightly younger than her stated age.

Background to illness

Judy knew how to do breast self-examination (BSE) but did so infrequently because of the "rush" she was always in with the children, her home, and Jim. She did happen to think of BSE one month while taking a shower. It was at that time she noticed a small hard lump in her left breast. She became very anxious, immediately left the shower, and standing before a mirror checked herself again. The lump was still there, and as she said many times, she thought it had gotten larger in those few minutes. Judy wanted to call her husband and blurt out her fears that she had cancer, but Jim was on a business trip and would not be home until later that evening. No immediate family was near her. That night Jim and Judy discussed what had happened and Jim confirmed that he felt a hard lump in her left breast. They decided the next day to call Judy's gyneocologist and ask him how best to proceed.

The gynecologist asked Judy to come in that afternoon so he could check the mass himself. Judy did so and was told that there was, in fact, a small mass in the upper outer quadrant of her breast. The gynecologist suggested that a surgeon be consulted. The call to the surgeon was made while Judy sat in the office; the appointment with the surgeon was set for the next afternoon. Jim had been unable to go with Judy but decided to go with her to the surgeon because neither one of them knew him and Judy was getting increasingly anxious.

The surgeon examined Judy and confirmed to the two of them that he, too, had felt a small mass and suggested a biopsy as soon as possible. He cautioned Judy that most breast lumps were benign particularly for women her age, but biopsy was the only way to determine for sure if a cancer did exist. He also mentioned that from his experience, if the biopsy proved positive, it was best for everyone to do a mastectomy immediately. Judy remembered phrases such as "you're a young woman; we should take care of this thing right away and not delay; lots of women have radical mastectomies and go on to live normal lives." Judy and Jim wanted to think things over that night and promised to get back to the surgeon the next day. That night, they discussed Judy's lump over and over again. They cried a lot and they called Judy's gynecologist and asked him what he thought. He had already heard from the surgeon and said it was really their decision, but he knew the surgeon and felt that Judy would be given good care. No options were presented to Judy, and since she did not know anyone with breast cancer, she assumed the radical mastectomy was the only procedure available to her. Reluctantly, they decided to call the surgeon and have him schedule the biopsy and possible mastectomy. This was done, and they were told later that day that she would be admitted to the hospital in 2 days with surgery scheduled the following morning.

Period of hospitalization

Judy spent 2 fretful days. Part of her anxiety was for herself, but she also recalled dwelling on her life with Jim and the children and how she did not want to die. She worried how her elderly parents would take the news, since she was an only child. She wanted to call them but decided it was best to wait to find out if she did have cancer. Judy spent the day before she was admitted looking around the house, looking at Duncan, and remembering all the happy family times they had. She tried to remember that both her gynecologist and surgeon had kept saying that most breast tumors were benign but had a bad feeling that hers would be malignant.

Jim took Judy to the hospital and it was at this time that I first met her. It was customary at this particular hospital for the admitting nurse to conduct an admission survey, which was done by Judy's primary nurse, Helen. This assessment revealed a very anxious client and husband who expected the worst to happen to them. Judy revealed her belief that a cancer would be found and that she would have to have the radical mastectomy, which she had signed for along with the excisional biopsy operative permit. The nurse, reaffirming the surgeon's comments, told Judy that most breast masses in women Judy's age were benign and that in all likelihood hers would be also. Not to mislead Judy, however, Helen explained what the plan would be if a radical mastectomy was necessary. Information about the pressure dressing, the arm exercises, and consultation with community health nurses to assess any home adjustments would be available, if desired.

Judy remained tearful most of the evening, particularly after Jim went home to the children. Aside from worry about herself, Judy had ambivalent feelings about not calling her parents, but she decided that her plan was best for them. She would ask Jim to call them if it was found that she did have breast cancer.

Judy was very open about discussing her feelings preoperatively. She was most worried about dying, but she also feared the deformities that were common to radical mastectomy procedures. She was frank in admitting that she liked to wear nice clothes and enjoyed her life very much. She did not want to lose what she and Jim had worked so hard for. She also worried about Jim's reaction, even though she was confident of their relationship. She knew that she could not possibly be as attractive to him if she lost her breast. She hoped for the best but admitted that she expected the worst.

Judy did not sleep well but decided to go ahead with the procedure and was prepared for the operation. She went to the operating room without seeing Jim because they had agreed that he should get Jason off to school and wait with Duncan for the caretaker to arrive. He arrived at Judy's room about 9 AM and was told by Helen that the unit had received word that Judy was undergoing the mastectomy. Helen stayed with Jim for awhile as he expressed his fears about how he would be able to deal with Judy's cancer.

He loved her so much that he did not want to let her down but admitted that he was overwhelmed himself. Helen cautioned Jim that these were perfectly normal feelings owing to the suddenness of the situation and the seriousness of Judy's illness. Interestingly, Jim expressed many of the same feelings that Judy had about how he hoped this operation would not damage their relationship, but he felt that it was such a distortion that it would almost have to. Helen said she could appreciate Jim's fears, as they were expressed by other thoughtful people, but that there were qualified resources available to him if he felt the need to pursue this further. It was about this time that Judy's surgeon arrived to tell Jim that Judy was now in the recovery room and would be back in her room in about 2 hours. He mentioned that it would take a few days to obtain all the information about Judy's cancer, but he was hopeful that she would do all right. If no complications developed, he expected Judy to be discharged in 8 days.

Judy's postoperative course was uneventful except to her. She recalled the first time that her dressing was changed and how shocked she was with the bruised, swollen appearance of the outer segment of her breast. She was particularly upset as she had expected a "flat chest." Her surgeon cautioned her that she was only a few days postoperative and that the edema was due to the surgical manipulation. Unfortunately, the surgeon had to inform Judy and Jim that the pathologic review revealed the cancer was present in three of the axillary lymph nodes; the type of breast cancer she had was infiltrating ductal carcinoma. He mentioned that he had asked the oncology team to evaluate her case for any additional therapy.

I was part of the oncology team that evaluated Judy in terms of the appropriateness of instituting adjuvant chemotherapy because of her high-risk status for tumor recurrence. We discussed with Judy and her husband that this treatment was part of a research effort to determine if tumor recurrence could be minimized by administering cancer chemotherapeutic agents. Detailed discussion took place as to the potential risks and benefits, the cost, the time requirements, and what they could expect from us. The discussion was open and friendly with Judy saying that she wanted to think about the options we had presented and asking us to return the next evening. We did so and found that Judy wanted to undergo chemotherapy treatments and understood that she could drop out if she wished and that changes in her condition as well as the concepts of treating breast cancer would be discussed with both of them. A consent form was signed and plans to begin the treatments in a few weeks were made. Judy was discharged by her surgeon as expected.

Posthospital course

It was our belief that many clients needed support and possible aid in adjusting to the home environment and so we routinely called all our clients a few days after their discharge. We did so in Judy's case and detected a great deal of tension in Judy's voice. From what she had told us it appeared that Judy was upset at her lack of strength and her perceptions of how fast she should be convalescing. A community referral had been made by Helen, but since it was marked as "routine," the nurse had not arranged to see Judy. We convinced the nurse to see Judy the next day and to call us with her impressions. This was done and we were saddened to hear that Judy's appearance did not seem the same. Her house was not neat and she seemed depressed. The community nurse, Helen, and the oncology nurses talked via the phone and decided to suggest that Judy's mother might be a reasonable resource to help out in this initial period. Judy and her mother thought this was a good temporary solution, with her mother scheduled to arrive in a few days. Judy said she felt much better having her mother there to help with the housework and play with the children. Judy was able to get more rest now and seemed in better spirits until she started to try on her old clothes to see how she could conceal her chest. Everyone tried to dissuade Judy, but she persisted and was very distraught to find that her fitted clothes did not look good. To add to her troubles, Judy's arm and hand started to swell and a diagnosis by her surgeon of lymphedema was made. Rest, elevation, a pressure sleeve, loose clothing, and protection of the affected arm were suggested. Plans continued for Judy to start on a combination chemotherapy regimen at 6-week intervals. Tests were completed and an orientation visit to the clinic was made. I was surprised at Judy's appearance, as it was obvious that she was not taking the same care with herself as when I saw her in the hospital. Judy admitted that she was surprised at how she was functioning but felt that her outlook would improve. Mention was made of resource people in addition to the team, but Judy elected to continue the relationship she had with us.

Over the next 9 months Judy received six courses of treatments, all but the first at reduced levels because of significant toxicity. This development surprised the team since Judy's laboratory parameters were all within the normal range, and her age and general good health were working for her. Many of us had a "gut" feeling that Judy's case would not end happily. Nothing could be shown to be wrong, but deep in our hearts we knew Judy would have problems. However, Judy's status remained the same. The surgeon had little success in reducing the lymphedema, which limited Judy functionally and cosmetically. No tumor recurrence could be found although she still received only partial doses of her chemotherapy. Then it happened. It was 13 months since Judy's mastectomy when she developed a cord compression. Her mother had been visiting her and ran to her bedroom to investigate her screams. Judy blurted out that she could not move her legs. Her mother called Jim immediately and he in turn called the ambulance. We met Judy in the emergency room and scheduled her for a myelogram and a possible decompression laminectomy. Judy was confirmed to have the cord compression, successfully underwent the laminectomy, and had her paralysis reversed. Her chemotherapy program was discontinued because of the tumor recurrence. This period was prior to the routine use of hormonal receptors, so Judy was offered a second program of chemotherapy. The other team members and myself continued to see and talk with Judy and were distressed at her deterioration. She was depressed and seemed to lack that "spark of life" that we had seen initially. Judy confirmed that she did not feel good about herself; she did not like her physical appearance, her diminished arm strength, her almost constant worrying that she was going to die, and her increasing isolation from her family. A meeting between Judy, Jim, a psychiatric nurse, and myself was arranged and possible plans for improving Judy's state of mind were discussed. We settled on a psychiatric consultation as the plan to pursue. Judy went weekly to the psychiatrist and Jim joined her at monthly intervals. They both felt they were being helped but continued to be depressed about Judy's physical limitations. Judy was tolerating her chemotherapy, so this was not producing a significant strain on her. All of us were becoming more hopeful until Jim called to discuss something that was troubling him. He mentioned that Judy seemed to be getting forgetful and that her moods would change abruptly. Sometimes Judy would get very angry at Jim, and this distressed him as this was not their usual pattern of communication. I reported this information to the oncologist and we asked

Judy to come in early for a checkup. She and Jim were quite anxious when they arrived at the office. A brain scan and neurologic consultation were arranged and the preliminary diagnosis of brain metastasis was made; this was confirmed afterward. The chemotherapy was discontinued and radiation therapy to the brain was scheduled. Judy was upset to hear that she would probably lose her hair from the treatments. Jim was assuming a greater burden in their relationship as Judy was less able to deal with these problems, her home, and basic decision making. The radiation therapy gave her temporary relief, but her physical condition and mental state continued to deteriorate so that major efforts on the part of the oncologist, the community nurse, Jim, and myself were needed to care for Judy. Eventually, she became so disoriented that she did not even recognize Jim or her mother. It was at this time that our support was transferred to them since they were the ones most in need of understanding. Judy was periodically readmitted to the hospital but died at home 22 months after her mastectomy. Jim, her parents, and the private duty nurse were able to care for her during the latter months.

Because of the distressing circumstances of Judy's condition and our own need to come to some resolution, the community nurse and I maintained periodic contact with Jim. He was so emotionally drained by the events that it took him many months to even begin to recover. Judy's mother remained with him until he could secure full-time childcare and then left. Jim had some ambivalent feelings about Judy but basically felt he had done well by her and cherished their time together. After about a year, he moved closer to his in-laws so that they could help him with the children since they were so young that he worried about providing a good environment for them.

All of the cancer team members, including myself, felt great frustration with this case. Judy's course had been rapidly downhill, and it had been difficult for us to deal with our limitations. In retrospect, we were frustrated because we could do so little for Judy. Her lymphedema could be lessened but not eliminated; the chest wall distortions were almost inevitable with a radical mastectomy; her body image was what it was and so all we could do was to reinforce our belief that she was still a worthy person and offer psychiatric support. Her disease progression was slowed by the radiation therapy, but her mental state continued to deteriorate and this placed great strain on her family and the staff as well. In situations such as Judy's, it is important for the clinician to acknowledge that there were some positive aspects. Judy and Jim did stay together. They were not always completely responsive to each other's needs, but it is almost impossible for people to always respond the way others want them to. Judy and her mother grew closer together as they worked to keep a busy household functioning. Most of us learned an important lesson from this—it is important not to abandon an ill person, even though the situation may be quite overwhelming, because it is possible to alleviate some of the suffering, thereby improving the quality of life. In Judy's case, we were able to do this.

CONCLUSION

This chapter has presented the morbidity that is commonly associated with breast cancer in women and the various treatments that are employed in an attempt to control the disease progression. Some of these untoward consequences are preventable or at least can be minimized by careful instruction of the client and family in ways to protect the woman's affected arm, to carry out a long-term exercise program, and to help them to identify and consult with resources should problems develop. In other situations in which morbidity is a predictable sequelae to the therapeutic intervention, the nurse can work actively with the other health care providers to assure that the client and family understand what may happen to them so that they can consider all possible options before making a decision. This latter professional role is becoming increasingly important as the controversies continue over the risks and benefits of breast cancer screening and therapeutic regimens. No one person has all the answers or can predict the future consequences of these interventions so that the final decision must remain with the client and her family. Because these situations, with all their unknowns, can be anxiety provoking, nurses can perform a valuable function by maintaining communication with these women so that support and information can be provided as needed to minimize or prevent any morbidity and its negative impact on the quality of these women's lives.

REFERENCES

1. American Cancer Society: 1979 facts and figures, New York, 1979, American Cancer Society, Inc.
2. American Joint Committee for Cancer Staging and End-Results Reporting: Manual for staging of cancer, 1977, Chicago, 1977, The Committee.
3. Chu, F.: Radiation therapy for locally advanced, recurrent or disseminated breast cancer. In Gallager, H. S., Leis, H. P., Jr., Snyderman, R. K., and Urban, J. A., editors: The breast, St. Louis, 1978, The C. V. Mosby Co.
4. Craig, T., Comstock, G. W., and Geiser, P. B.: The quality of survival in breast cancer: a case-control comparison, Cancer **33:**1451, 1974.
5. Daland, E. M.: Incidence of swollen arms after radical mastectomy and suggestions for prevention, N. Engl. J. Med. **242:**497, 1950.
6. del Regato, J. A., and Spjut, H. J., editors: Ackerman and del Regato's cancer diagnosis, treatment and prognosis, ed. 5, St. Louis, 1977, The C. V. Mosby Co.
7. Eisenberg, H. S., and Goldenberg, I. S.: Measurement of quality of survival of breast cancer patients. In Hayward, J. L., and Bulbrook, R. D., editors: Clinical evaluation of breast cancer, New York, 1966, Academic Press, Inc.
8. Fisher, B., and Gebhardt, M. C.: The evolution of breast cancer surgery: past, present and future, Semin. Oncol. **5**(4):385, 1978.
9. Gallager, H. S., Leis, H. P., Jr., Snyderman, R. K., and Urban, J. A., editors: The breast, St. Louis, 1978, The C. V. Mosby Co.
10. Harris, J. R., Levene, M. B., and Hellman, S.: The role of radiation therapy in the primary treatment of carcinoma of the breast, Semin. Oncol. **5**(4):403, 1978.
11. McCorkle, M. R.: Coping with physical symptoms in metastatic breast cancer, Am. J. Nurs. **73:**1034, 1973.
12. McGuire, P.: Psychiatric problems after mastectomy. In Brand, P. C., and Vankeep, P. A., editors: Breast cancer, psychosocial aspects of early detection and treatment, Baltimore, 1978, University Park Press.
13. Montague, E. D.: Radiotherapy as primary modality in treatment of curable breast cancer. In Gallager, H. S., Leis, H. P., Jr., Snyderman, R. K., and Urban, J. A., editors: The breast, St. Louis, 1978, The C. V. Mosby Co.
14. National Cancer Institute: Third National Cancer Survey, NCI Monograph No. 41, Washington, D.C., 1975, U.S. Government Printing Office.
15. Quint, J. C.: The impact of mastectomy, Am. J. Nurs. **63:**88, 1963.
16. Rilke, F., et al.: The importance of pathology in prognosis and management of breast cancer, Semin. Oncol. **5**(4):360, 1978.
17. Saracci, R., and Ripetto, F.: Epidemiology of breast cancer, Semin. Oncol. **5**(4):342, 1978.
18. Talbott, E. E., Marino, L. B., and Mueller, D. P.: The evaluation of post-mastectomy morbidity: a review of the literature, Prev. Med. **8:**429, 1979.
19. U.S. Department of Health, Education and Welfare: The breast cancer digest, Publication No. 79-1691, Bethesda, Md., 1979, Department of Health, Education and Welfare.
20. Woods, N. F.: Human sexuality in health and illness, ed. 2, St. Louis, 1979, The C. V. Mosby Co.
21. Worden, J. W., and Weisserman, A. D.: The fallacy in post mastectomy depression, Am. J. Med. Sci. **293:**169, 1977.

25

Nutritional problems in clients having gastrointestinal cancer

PHYLLIS PALKA CULLEN

SCOPE OF THE GASTROINTESTINAL CANCERS

Nurses in all settings working with cancer clients will have significant contact and involvement with individuals having cancers of the gastrointestinal system. It is well recognized that colorectal cancers remain among the highest in estimated new cases and annual deaths in the United States. The American Cancer Society in 1979 estimated 112,000 new cases with 51,900 estimated deaths. It is less well recognized that there were an additional 70,900 estimated new cases occurring elsewhere in the gastrointestinal system, making a total that year of 182,900 estimated new cases for all gastrointestinal cancers.[2] Therefore, this chapter will include discussion of the care of clients having cancer of the gastrointestinal tract, in general, not exclusively colorectal cancers.

Tumors invade several different organs of the gastrointestinal system. For most of these sites obstruction is the primary medical problem. This can be mechanical or it may be an interference in the secretory or absorptive functions of the system. Gastrointestinal cancer sites include the esophagus, stomach, small intestine, pancreas, liver, gallbladder, colon, and rectum. Table 25-1 provides an overview of these sites, including common signs and symptoms.

Incidence

The incidence of these gastrointestinal cancers has remained quite constant for several years with the 5-year survival generally being low. Most often nurses care for clients with advanced gastrointestinal cancers. Because of this fact, there is more widespread use of endoscopic procedures and more early detection screening programs that may lead to a larger proportion of clients being seen with primary and early gastrointestinal cancers.

Since there are still large numbers of individuals who have metastatic gastrointestinal cancers, it is this population that will now be discussed. These clients often provide a good example of the chronicity of cancer. Contrary to what is often believed, the diagnosis of advanced or metastatic gastrointestinal cancer does not mean the person is "terminal" or near death. Often, clients will live with metastatic gastrointestinal cancer for many months or even years, frequently without symptoms. Others may be in and out of the hospital with multiple acute and chronic problems. Still others will be in the end stage of their disease and near death. These differences within the same group require different care priorities.

PHASES OF CARE

To help the nurse establish guidelines of care for clients in these different stages, Table 25-2 represents these three *distinct* phases of metastatic gastrointestinal cancer.

Phase I

It is during phase I that the beginnings of a solid nurse-client relationship are established. Expectations are discussed. The clients usually will need help sorting out the facts of their diagnosis, the details of treatment and testing, and their feelings about having a serious chronic illness.

This is the best time for the nurse to learn about the client's preillness life-style and preferences. These facts may be helpful later, for example, in encouraging hobbies and suggesting recipes.

Also, during this early phase of metastatic illness, the client will probably have the time and energy to complete unfinished tasks. These might be taking a long dreamed of vacation, completing an unfinished building project, settling a legal or financial matter, or making a reconciliation. In a good nurse-client relationship it is possible to communicate that this may be an opportune time for such activities.

Phase II

It is often during phase II that clients and their families need the most support. With disease symptoms present, the diagnosis often becomes more real. Readjustments in employment status, living situations, and family structure may occur now. Home visits by a public health nurse should also begin. The nurse should make a thorough assessment of the client's support systems.

With physical changes occurring frequently and social readjustments being made, the nurse will need to revise the plan of care almost constantly during this phase. It is now that the benefits of the early relationship developed in phase I begin paying off. It is now that a stronger nurse-client relationship is developed to help with the ups and downs and the preparations for a possible death in the future.

Phase III

If ever there was a time for sensitivity, kindness, and putting aside personal fears, it is during the short phase III. As nurses, this is a time for control of the client's care. Medical treatment will generally be less aggressive and the priorities will now become those controlled by nurses. The provision of comfort measures, pain control, and psychosocial support should constitute most of the care to clients near death. Nurses need to be true client advocates at such times as when extra pain medication is needed or when hospital routines need to be altered. It should be remembered that hydration is necessary for comfort. Nurses need to consider that not all clients wish to die in the hospital. Alternate arrangements may take extra nursing effort. Finally, nurses need to work at helping clients maintain as much control as possible and die with dignity.

• • •

Hopefully, this concept of the three phases will help achieve awareness of the differences that occur within the population of individuals having metastatic gastrointestinal cancer.

One of the major functional problems that may occur in persons with gastrointestinal cancer is nutrition. Nutritional needs exist throughout the gamut of these diseases. In-

Table 25-1. Overview of gastrointestinal cancers

Site	Estimated U.S. incidence, 1979		Signs and symptoms	Metastases
	New cases	Deaths		
Esophagus[2,11]	8,400	7,500	Dysphagia in 90%, anorexia, weight loss, persistent cough, hematemesis, cervical adenopathy, left vocal cord paralysis, hemoptysis	Liver, lungs, pleura
Gastric[2,11]	23,000	14,100	Ulcer symptoms, vague epigastric discomfort with or without anorexia and weight loss, iron deficiency anemia	Liver, lungs, bone
Small intestine[2,11]	2,200	700	Obstruction, bleeding, abdominal mass; less common—perforation and malabsorption syndrome; symptoms of carcinoid syndrome—abdominal cramps, watery diarrhea, flushing, asthmatic type symptoms; valvular lesions of the right heart	Liver
Pancreas[1,2]	23,000	20,200	Muscle weakness, anorexia, weight loss, gaseousness, and nausea; pain in 70%-80% of clients in the region of epigastrium or back; pain is usually dull or boring; also jaundice, palpable gallbladder, and recent onset of diabetes	Liver
Liver[1,2]	11,600 (includes biliary passages) Less than 1% 5-year survival	9,200	Aching upper abdominal pain in 70% of clients; often becomes more severe and constant and radiates to the back; weakness, anorexia, bloating, hepatomegaly, ascites; mild jaundice occasionally	Distally
Gallbladder[1,2]	American Cancer Society does not provide this breakdown.		Anorexia, vague abdominal pains, and weight loss; history of gallbladder attacks with signs and symptoms indistinguishable from cholecystitis and cholelithiasis	Liver
Colorectal[1,2]	112,000	51,900	*Right colonic lesions*—unexplained anemia and gastrointestinal tract bleeding; *sigmoid*—obstruction; *rectum*—rectal pain, gross blood per rectum, pencil thin stools with feeling of incomplete evacuation	Liver, lungs

Table 25-2. Clients with metastatic gastrointestinal cancer*

Population	Characteristics	Needs, concerns
Phase I: clients having early recurrence, residual disease, controlled minimal disease	Largely asymptomatic; almost complete return to preillness life-style; few acute problems	Nutrition, psychosocial support, client teaching, assessment
Phase II: clients having progressive disease, disease controlled after a moderate amount of progression	Symptomatic; increased dependence on family members for assistance with day-to-day activities; acute problems often requiring hospitalization; possible sudden improvements and sudden decline over months and years	Nutrition; pain control/comfort; ambulation/transportation; psychosocial support for family and client; provision of additional resources; client teaching
Phase III: clients having end-stage, extensive disease	Near death; usual life expectancy of few hours or days; virtually complete dependence; manifestations of present or impending death	Nutrition/hydration; comfort/pain control; resources/homecare; psychosocial support for family and client

*Reprinted with permission from the September issue of *Nursing '76,* Copyright © 1976, Intermed Communications, Inc. All rights reserved.

deed, nutritional depletion is often an immediate cause of death with gastrointestinal cancers. Therefore, the topic of nutrition, especially with this group, has been selected for further discussion.

NUTRITION AS A FUNCTIONAL PROBLEM

Nutrition intervention, diet therapy, elemental, manipulate, pump, hyperalimentation, enteral, parenteral, supplemental—feed, eat, diet, gorge, starve, hunger, appetite, dinner party, stuffed, pot luck are all part of a huge vocabulary relating to nutrition.

The first group of terms is generally associated with nutrition in the ill; the latter group is generally associated with nutrition in the healthy. Some overlap does exist, but generally the vocabulary, and surely the tone, differs when discussing nutrition with the sick client as opposed to the healthy friend.

It is sometimes easy when using these scientific terms to forget that the discussion is focusing on a functional area of the client's life with which there has *always* been involvement. Eating is something everyone has done and has feelings about, whether conscious or unconscious. As with so many other areas of teaching, the nurse must begin by learning what the client knows, what misconceptions are present, and, finally, what emotional issues are involved.

Looking at a few of these issues will indicate the magnitude of emotional components involved, and why the nurse should be the primary health care provider intervening in this functional area of nutrition will be presented. Finally, a review of nutrition in the cancer problem will be included followed by specific guidelines for the nurse working with cancer clients requiring nutritional intervention.

Emotional aspects associated with nutrition

Why do people eat? A few reasons might include: to be sociable, to relieve hunger pangs, to satisfy our taste buds, to make someone we care about happy, to counteract boredom, and to celebrate.

Perhaps it is more insightful to ask, what if we don't eat? Others may judge us to be "sick" or "neglected"; infants may be labeled "failure to thrive." If the reason is dieting to lose weight and we are obviously obese, we will probably be applauded. If the reason is dieting to lose weight, but we are only a few pounds overweight, our hostess may tag us "unsociable" or "vain." Along these same lines nurses, as well as society in general, sometimes use how well a person eats as a measure of good or bad, happy or unhappy. Some examples are a family member calls the unit and asks, "How is my mother today?" and the nurse responds "Much better. She was up in a chair and ate most of her breakfast." or "Not much change. She wants to stay in bed; didn't touch her tray." When a friend or neighbor has suffered a loss, have we not heard remarks like, "He's so sad. He hardly talks, and he's eating like a bird." On the positive side, "How was your trip?" "Oh, we had a *great* time. We ate our way through San Francisco."

Obviously, these terms give an indication of the emotional connotations associated with eating. These phrases also indicate that the clients who are also part of the society at large bring their own biases relating to food and nutrition along with them when they become ill.

The nurse as the provider

Why should the nurse have a major role in the nutritional aspect of the cancer client's care and treatment? Of the members of the health care team, nurses most often have the best overall access and skills necessary for dealing with the whole gamut of nutritional problems.

Some necessary skills include: assessing, coordinating, teaching, planning, implementing, motivating, supporting, and evaluating. Physicians may help by prescribing hyperalimentation formulas, antiemetics, or by diagnosing deficiencies and imbalances. Nutritionists may be best able to teach a specific diet plan. Social workers can help to support and identify resources. When nutritional problems are severe, it may take a *whole team effort* to be successful. Regardless, the nurse should be present whenever possible during discussions to provide continuity.

So often, motivation and encouragement make the greatest difference to the success of the program. If the nurse has helped the client set and meet realistic goals elsewhere in the care plan, the prescribed plan for nutrition may also be successful because of the trust that has been established. Likewise, if the nurse feels this elemental diet is important and workable, the client may give it a try.[9]

Obviously, the client with a cancer of the gastrointestinal tract may have a very severe long-term nutritional problem relating to a variety of causes. Clients with malignancies of other sites may have severe problems or their problems may be only moderate and short term. The nurse needs to realize that nutritional problems with cancer occur for a *variety of reasons* in several different settings. Some of these are: *preoperative,* disease-induced problems such as a gastrointestinal obstruction or problems relating to the necessary preparations before surgery; *postoperative,* such as the effect of surgery, absorptive changes, fistulas, difficulty swallowing, gastric dumping, inadequate pancreatic enzymes; *treatment related,* such as nausea, vomiting, diarrhea, or anorexia with chemotherapy or radiation therapy; or *disease-induced nutritional problems with advanced malignancy,* such as severe anorexia, cachexia, mechanical obstructions in colorectal cancer, or taste changes. Other problem areas can probably be identified in each nurse's sphere of practice.

Review of the nutrition problem in cancer

Because nutrition is such a major problem, the past few years have seen a marked increase in the volume of literature relating to cancer and nutrition. Much concentration has been given to why cancer clients are often unable to take in adequate nutrition orally. Some of the most common causes cited are difficulty in swallowing, premature sensation of fullness, nausea and vomiting, digestive difficulties with pancreatic cancers, dumping syndrome, and anorexia. Of these, perhaps the most difficult to combat over long intervals is anorexia, or loss of appetite, with resulting cachexia and muscle wasting. Work and interest in this area is increasing, but definite answers as to why anorexia and cachexia exist with cancer are not currently available.

Cachexia. Several factors have been identified as contributing to cachexia especially in clients with advanced cancer. Some are mechanical obstruction, hemorrhage, nausea and vomiting, malabsorption, and general loss of appetite.

However, the factors contributing to weight loss as the earliest manifestation of cancer or in the presence of adequate nutritional intake are not so clearly identifiable. Complex biochemical and metabolic changes occurring with cancer are being researched. Two areas being studied are the phenomenon of increased energy expenditure in tumor-bearing hosts and the area of tumor production of disruptive metabolites.

Theologides[16] offers a summary of work done as well as new hypotheses for what he describes as a "profound systematic derangement of the host metabolism" in some individuals with cancer. The cancer, he believes, might be throwing the entire metabolism of the tumor-bearing host into a chaotic state by producing low molecular weight metabolites.

Anorexia. One of the most commonly recognized causative factors of anorexia is abnormalities in the client's taste sensation. Much work in this area has been done by De Wys[10] who, in testing a series of 50 cancer clients with a spectrum of malignancies of variable extent, noted 25 having a general reduction in the pleasureable aspect of taste. Cancer clients were tested for salty (NaCl), sour (HCl), sweet (sucrose), and bitter (urea) tastes. Recognition and detection thresholds for salty and sour were similar to those of the control group. However, cancer clients did have an *elevated* threshold for sweets and a *lower* threshold for bitter tastes; that is, a higher concentration of sucrose would be required to taste something sweet, but these same people were more sensitive to the bitter tastes than were the controls. The sucrose results could be correlated with the presence of the symptom of decreased taste sensation. The increased sensitivity to bitter taste may have some correlation to meat aversion, which is frequently seen in cancer clients. Also, abnormality of taste could be correlated with the client's body burden of tumor and the likelihood of weight loss. De Wys further noted that many physiologic reflexes were triggered by positive taste stimuli. Cancer clients who have elevated taste thresholds may not trigger these reflexes, perhaps explaining some symptoms of the anorexic client. Some reflexes not triggered might lead to inadequate salivation with difficulty in swallowing as a consequence, inadequate gastric secretions paired with a sense of early fullness, and inadequate pancreatic secretions leading to slow digestion of the first meal of the day. Obviously, this aspect of altered taste sensations in many cancer clients has clinical significance.

Assessment and identification of the nutritional problem

Before outlining guidelines of care, a discussion of assessment and identification of the problem must be included. Although not always possible, prevention of protein-calorie malnutrition should be the nurse's goal. Butler[5] has devised a nutritional assessment tool for nurses in which she includes identification of common procedures and treatments that often lead to nutritional deficiencies, such as the prolonged use of a minimal diet, intravenous fluids, or mechanical interference with self-feeding.

Defining malnutrition. When protein-calorie malnutrition is already suspected, the health care provider may need studies to validate and parameters to follow. Copeland uses the following parameters in defining malnutrition in the cancer client: a weight loss of 10 pounds or more from the ideal body weight, serum albumin below 3.4 gm, a peripheral lymphocyte count of less than 20%, and anergy to a battery of recall skin test antigens. He found that these parameters return to normal in the majority of clients treated with intravenous hyperalimentation.[7]

It has also been pointed out that a general failure to recognize protein-calorie malnutrition may lie in the widespread use of weight for height measurement alone. Sensitive measures for determining body protein stores, namely, arm muscle circumference and serum albumin levels, are either seldom used or not generally appreciated.

Clinical observations. The health care providers, particularly the nurse, need to use clinical observation to identify malnourished persons. The physical changes of extreme thinness, poor tissue turgor and color, and decreased strength and mobility are quite obvious. Butler[5] suggests considering personality changes as correlating with malnutrition. She saw clients who were originally outgoing and even tempered change following weight loss. They became apathetic, withdrawn, whiney, self-centered, and, in general, unwilling to participate in any activity. She cites physical complaints with starvation, including dizziness when rising, weakness and fatigue, an inability to laugh heartily, muscle soreness, and edema. Again, because nurses are the most constant observers of clients they are in the best position to note any changes. Of course, there are many possible variables for these personality changes such as depression owing to disease prognosis, changed body image, or discomfort. Butler suggests that the nurse consider how many of these behaviors might be *reversible* with improved nutrition. Fortunately, the client's nutritional state can be improved by mechanical interventions.

Nutritional routes. Nutrition can be provided by two main routes. The first is parenteral, through a central or peripheral intraveneous line. The second main route is enteral, which is from within the intestine. Enteral can further be divided into the oral and tube feeding routes. In addition to routes, the nurse should also consider the extent of nutritional intervention. Parenteral can be used for total nutrition or it can be supplemental. Also with enteral, an elemental diet such as a tube feeding might be chosen to provide total baseline nutritional support. Bury[4] explains that the elemental diet is an outgrowth of the early United States space program. This term, elemental diet, has come to mean a chemically formulated powdered food source that is used in a liquid form. When an amount supplying 1,800 calories or more daily is used, total baseline nutritional support is provided with the exception of cobalt and vitamin K. The enteral route, especially with oral feedings, is also used for supplemental nutrition.

The extent and mode of nutritional treatment necessary is determined by the health care providers. Questions that should be asked are: Does the client need a supplement or total nutritional support? Can this nutritional support be accomplished orally? Is tube feeding indicated or is the client a candidate for parenteral support? If oral or tube feedings are the possible choices, is an elemental diet indicated?

Evaluating the client. Before a decision can be reached, some physical baseline information on the client must be gathered to allow for evaluation: height and weight; mobility; strength; performance status; abdominal girth; presence of ascites; skin condition, color, turgor, and presence of areas of breakdown. Also, when possible, arm muscle circumference, serum albumin levels, and skin tests for common recall antigens including purified protein derivative of tuberculin (PPD), mumps, and candida are obtained.

Guidelines for nursing care

Guidelines for nursing care in the categories of oral feedings, tube feedings, and parenteral nutrition will be presented. Once these preliminary observations are completed, the nurse develops a guideline for care.

The client who is receiving oral feedings. As stated earlier, the precise causes of weight loss in individuals with cancer are not known, hence the dietary interventions can only be general. The primary goal is to prevent weight loss and provide an abundant supply of high-quality protein. To meet these goals, clients will often need an intake of 2,500 to 3,500 calories or more if weight gain is desired. A list of high-protein foods as well as recipes for using them should be provided.

Likewise, clients are often given elemental diets orally before surgery; postoperatively, most clients and those receiving chemotherapy or radiation therapy still primarily receive nutritional therapy orally. With postoperative or treatment clients having very high nutritional requirements that cannot be met orally, the health care providers have the option of using tube feedings or parenteral nutrition. When working with cancer clients having nutritional problems resulting from advanced disease, parenteral hyperalimentation is often not the treatment of choice. High cost, usually a long hospitalization period, and increased risk of sepsis are some factors making it less appropriate with the client having end-stage cancer. The appropriate population for receiving nutrition via tube feeding will be discussed later, but with many clients in phases II and III of advanced disease, tube feeding at home cannot be managed well. This is because clients lack family members willing or able to take on this additional responsibility. This leaves only the oral route to pursue.

Questions to ask the client. The nurse needs to determine what the exact nutritional problem is. Is the problem nausea and vomiting with therapy? Is the problem a result of surgery, as with gastrectomy or pancreatectomy? Is the problem a consequence of advanced disease or anorexia? If the client is suffering from nausea and vomiting that are treatment related, how long after treatment do the nausea and vomiting begin; how often does the client vomit; how long is it until the episode ends; and when are antiemetics taken during this period and how effective are they? If vomiting is inevitable and a 1-day problem, offer the client the alternatives of eating regular food before the episode begins so there will be bulk to expel or keeping the stomach relatively empty, therefore vomiting a small volume of gastric juices and bile primarily. Some clients report less muscle soreness if vomiting occurs with a full stomach. Another question to ask is if the nausea persists between vomiting episodes or whether lying quietly between episodes helps alleviate the nausea. Can the client retain small sips of fluid? The nurse needs to remind the client of the need to replace lost fluids, instructing the client and family to call if vomiting exceeds 12 to 18 hours and severe dehydration becomes a threat.

Problems commonly seen following gastrectomy. Sometimes clients who have a gastrectomy for stomach or pancreatic cancer experience the dumping syndrome. They need to be taught to recognize this syndrome, which may include possible sensations such as nausea, flushing, abdominal cramping, epigastric fullness, weakness, and perspiration; tachycardia, tachypnea, and pallor may occur less often. The client may find lying down provides relief. These symptoms may be one or many and will usually begin about 15 minutes after eating. The client should be told that dumping syndrome symptoms tend to improve with time. Understandably, persistent symptoms may lead to food aversion on the part of the client. If this does occur, the nurse may suggest a diet high in protein, moderate in fat, and relatively restricted in carbohydrates; small frequent feedings should also be taken. It has also been suggested that omitting liquids at meals may be beneficial.[14] This is a situation where the nurse should work closely with the nutritionist or dietitian.

Problems commonly seen following pancreatectomy. Nutritional intervention will be one of the major tasks of the nurse caring for a client who has had a pancreatectomy. First, the dumping syndrome just described may occur. Next, the surgery leads to loss of digestive enzymes; clients must be taught the necessity of taking enzymes orally with meals. An effective pattern is taking enzymes immediately *before* each meal and snack. The appropriate number will be determined by the physician, but the client should report episodes of moderate to severe "indigestion" as this may be due to too few enzymes. These oral enzymes are expensive so some attempt to determine the correct amount for each client should be made. Also, a few tablespoons of antacid immediately after eating is helpful. The client who has had a surgical resection of the pancreas develops diabetes mellitus, often of the "brittle" type. This, of course, requires instructing the client in the correct use of insulin, as well as instruction in urine testing, the signs of hypoglycemia, and a diet regimen. These efforts generally require the full participation of all the health care providers.

Anorexia. When clients suffer from anorexia or impaired taste sensations, the nursing care requires several different steps. First, the nurse needs to obtain a history of intake, including the time and number of meals and snacks, type of food eaten, amount taken at each sitting, most difficult foods to eat (meat aversion is a common problem), and best liked foods before this illness. Second, the nurse needs to explore possible reasons for the client's inability to eat, such as nausea, gas, pain, fullness, no taste or bad taste, or any combination of these. The nurse can share information with the client on the changes in taste sensation commonly observed with cancer. Outpatients sometimes whisper to the nurse that the whole problem with their inability to eat is "My wife's cooking has become horrible." Although humorous, this conclusion is understandable if the client has not been told that taste changes do occur.

The nurse also needs to meet with the client and the individual preparing the meals. The following suggestions may prove helpful in preparing meals: adding extra flavorings or spices to help combat blandness, experimenting, diminishing the bitter taste clients sometimes detect in meat by offering it cold, and serving only small portions at any one time. If the client is turned off by the smell of food, the client should be taken away from the kitchen while the food is being prepared. The nurse should explain that a high-protein diet is important and *may* improve the client's response to treatment. The nurse needs to provide the client and family with a list of high-protein foods, exploring protein alternatives to meat; offering recipes, if available; and discussing the usefulness of frequent snacks. A few mouthfuls every 2 hours can constitute an extra meal by the end of the day. Suggest menu planning and use of a food diary. As stated initially, nursing assessment of the client's current knowledge of nutrition, any possible misconceptions, and related emotional issues is imperative. These assessments should also be made with the person who prepares the meals.

An example of how to operationalize these assessments is as follows: Mr. and Mrs. D. and I sat together one afternoon in the outpatient clinic and discussed nutrition. Mr. D., our client with gastric cancer, was very depressed, stating that he couldn't eat but would listen. Mrs. D. was a very anxious and vocal wife. She was near panic over Mr. D.'s weight loss and thin appearance. As I presented material, she took notes, nodded, and thanked me for the suggestions. Mr. D. acknowledged that perhaps he could try the plan. I especially emphasized the areas of small frequent meals and high-protein foods. The following week we were all disappointed that Mr. D. continued to lose weight. What had he eaten? Mrs. D. smiled proudly and announced that she had worked especially hard in the kitchen and made homemade chicken soup. She started dinner on several days by presenting Mr. D. with a large bowl of the soup. He ate as much as he could but never had room left for the rest of the meal.

To Mrs. D. chicken soup was the ultimate in good nutrition—lots of vitamins and love. Unfortunately, Mr. D. needed protein, too. I had failed to initially assess Mrs. D.'s beliefs. Even over a period of time, I was not able to alter her misconceptions.

If applicable, the nurse can instruct the client and family in the use of food supplements. Commercial preparations are available for between meal use. Liquid glucose polymers are now available for use as a calorie supplement source. This liquid, which is derived solely from carbohydrates, can be added to traditional food to boost caloric intake. Some preparations contain as much as 32 calories per tablespoon. If lactose intolerance is not a problem, there are many blenderized high-calorie preparations that can be made at home; ice cream can be used extensively as a base for these preparations.

With anorexia, the setting and appearance of meals becomes very important. Some clients report that 4 ounces of wine or ½ can of beer before a meal perks their appetite. The number of possible suggestions is limitless. All the nurse needs to do is to make a good assessment of the client and be creative. If the nurse demonstrates a degree of sensitivity to how difficult eating may be, provides a lot of positive reinforcement and follow-up to the client and family, as well as provides a sound plan, a degree of success can be achieved with the anorexic client.[9]

The nurse should also realize that for many clients their weight gain or loss is seen as a parameter of disease control. Rapid weight loss on the scale, loss of appetite, and baggy slacks are understandable signs to the client that all is not well. The client recognizes these developments as probable signs of disease progression, so the nurse should be aware of any possible anxiety as the client steps on the office or clinic scale and be available to listen and offer support.

The phase III client. The nurse needs to also consider care guidelines for the hospitalized cancer client who may be near death or in phase III. Helping the client to retain the function of eating can be very beneficial for psychologic welfare. The nurse may provide a before mealtime wash-up so that the client will be more alert, provide mouth care and insert dentures if applicable, help the client into a comfortable sitting or semisitting position, and remove clutter such as tape and other equipment from the bedside table. The client may need to be fed or assisted promptly when the tray arrives. If extra foods are stored at the bedside, they should be of the right temperature. Perhaps, most important, the nurse can help make the client's mealtime a social experience by alloting a pocket of time for a relaxing, unhurried mealtime with the client.

The client using tube feeding. There has been a marked increase recently in the use of tube feedings with cancer clients. Improved methods of catheter insertion have emerged with more common usage of "long-tubes" of thin gauge that are placed into the duodenum or jejunum. However, despite great efforts by pharmaceutical firms, clients often still find elemental diet preparations unpalatable. This is largely due to the taste and odor of organic amino acids not being well masked by flavorings in use today.

However, tube feedings are appropriate for a wide spectrum of cancer clients. Elemental tube feedings are now often used preoperatively instead of oral clear liquid diets. For postoperative clients, the extra protein aids in healing. In some instances, "long-tubes" are inserted at the time of the operation itself. Hospitalized clients receiving chemotherapy and radiation therapy are sometimes spared weight loss by the use of tube feedings of elemental diets or supplemental formulas during such treatments.

Clients with advanced disease who suffer from anorexia are also appropriate candidates for tube feedings if they wish. Also tube feedings are often safely used in outpatient clinic settings if a good support person can arrange to provide monitoring.

These elemental diets are helpful because their main characteristic is ease of absorption. Elemental diets, as generally given, need a minimum of help from the gastrointestinal tract. They are liquid, bulk free, and usually lactose free. Elemental preparations are also nearly fat free, vary in osmolality, contain protein primarily in the forms of amino acids or protein hydrolypsate, are high in carbohydrate, are hypertonic as normally diluted, and have an acidic pH. There are also many elemental preparations available commercially. Bury[4] provides an in-depth discussion of these diets with much of her information applicable to cancer clients.

Gravity tube feeding with a standard size nasogastric tube placed in the stomach is an age-old practice. However, the standardized tubes usually cause a sore throat and difficulty in swallowing. Continuous feeding into the stomach often leads to distention or a bolus may lead to diarrhea. Therefore, planning and adhering to a tailored time schedule is very important. The use of small lumen tubes such as the pediatric size is becoming popular for both gastric and duodenal/jejunal feedings; client comfort is also greatly improved with their use. Detailed information on catheter insertion and placement is provided by Page and co-workers.[12]

Some care guidelines for nurses with clients receiving tube feedings are to always be aware of the danger of aspiration; raise the head of the bed 30 degrees as a good safety measure; provide good mouth care; maintain accurate intake and output; check the position of the tube regularly with fluoroscopy, as many of the tubes are radiopaque;

monitor fluid, electrolytes, and albumin; measure urine fractionals; determine if a pancreatic enzyme supplement is necessary if feedings are via a "long tube"; and keep a record of changes in the baseline data of the client.

Another consideration that the nurse needs to be aware of is that gastrointestinal disturbances including abdominal cramping, nausea, vomiting, and diarrhea can be a problem relating to osmolality. This problem is usually controlled by beginning with weak solutions at a slow rate and moving up one step at a time over 4 to 7 days. If the feedings are given intermittently, the tube can be flushed with a small amount of cranberry juice and clamped. The staff should familiarize themselves and the client with the safe and proper operation of the infusion pump.

If tube feedings are used with a cancer client at home, it is necessary to provide good written instructions and emergency phone numbers so contact can be made when problems arise. If a pump is used for continual infusion, the client and his family should consider the use of a portable battery-operated rechargeable model. The nurse needs to be sure the client receives the necessary laboratory tests for fluid and electrolyte evaluation. Referral to a home health agency should also be considered. When a decision is made to use long-term tube feeding, the nurse needs to spend time with the client answering questions and alleviating fears. Some clients with advanced disease, perhaps colorectal cancer, who begin tube feedings at home because of severe anorexia, show signs of depression or perhaps grief. These persons sometimes verbalize their fear of never eating again. This can sometimes be the case, but the nurse can point out that this avenue of nutrition can be reversible. For example, a mutual decision can be made to remove the tube; in fact, some clients do remove tubes themselves. Again, food and eating have strong emotional components and these should be recognized and acknowledged by the health care providers.

The client receiving parenteral nutrition. The second major nutritional route, *parenteral* nutrition, most often involves the use of intravenous hyperalimentation. Cancer clients, whether preoperative, pretreatment, or mid-treatment, are now sometimes considered excellent candidates for intravenous hyperalimentation. However, the client with advanced disease who has a poor performance status and is not receiving active treatment is rarely considered a good candidate and almost never a candidate for ambulatory parenteral nutrition.[15] Copeland and co-workers[8] make a strong case for the use of intravenous hyperalimentation as an adjunct to cancer treatments such as chemotherapy. In their study, they showed a positive correlation between the nutritional status of the client and the chemotherapeutic tumor response. They concluded that "intravenous hyperalimentation can be a valuable adjunct to cancer chemotherapy by improving the nutritional status, increasing the total deliverable dose of anticancer agent per unit of time, and reducing the incidence and severity of the toxic gastrointestinal side effects without adversely stimulating malignant cell growth or producing septic complications."[8]

The use, care, and management of cancer clients receiving total parenteral nutrition, commonly known as TPN, generally are the same as with other client populations. The TPN solutions generally contain amino acids, hypertonic dextrose, water, vitamins, electrolytes, and some trace element additives. Recently, a fat-emulsion preparation has become available that is being used as a supplement to the hypertonic dextrose therapy.

The client should have a good understanding of why a course of TPN has been chosen. The nurse needs to teach the client about the insertion procedure and work on practicing the Valsalva maneuver—taking a deep breath, holding it, and bearing down. During the insertion procedure, the nurse will assist with positioning the client, maintaining asepsis, and providing client support.

TPN preparations are tailored to the client's needs and are generally mixed in the pharmacy under a laminar hood. Also, since these hypertonic dextrose solutions are excellent sources for bacterial growth, solutions must not be left hanging longer than the procedure dictates, usually 12 hours. The nurse must be especially alert for early signs of infection with the cancer client receiving TPN. For example, clients receiving chemotherapy may become myelosuppressed, so diligent care of solutions, lines, and dressing sites is mandatory to prevent a life-threatening infection. An infusion pump is generally used with the TPN program to avoid the inadvertent infusion of large amounts of solution; close timing and monitoring the fluid with a slow increase in rate over several days is necessary. In addition to blood chemistry profiles, clients will need their urine checked for glycosuria and regular insulin may be ordered as an additive to the solution.

Mouth care of the client, including the use of rinses, lip balms, and hard candy, if allowed, should be done. Before engaging in the care of clients receiving TPN, the nurse should become thoroughly familiar with the excellent nursing resources in the literature. For detailed care of the client receiving TPN, see Phillips[13] or Colley.[6] In another excellent source, Borgen[3] emphasizes the need for skilled emotional support. She points out that some clients for whom eating was especially pleasurable may hallucinate about food when they cannot eat. She reminds us that food has many different meanings and levels of importance of which we should try to remain aware.

CONCLUSION

In conclusion, a note of caution is advised. Some clients and family members seem to grasp onto the situation of increasing their oral nutritional intake as one of the few opportunities to make a personal positive contribution toward control of their cancer. Diet planning, special shopping trips. long hours in the kitchen, and constant encouragement to the client to eat seem to fill some family members' days. Unfortunately, this concentration can lead to nagging. The nurse should counsel clients to attempt to follow the diet plans and eat those extra snacks while acknowledging that sometimes they may not be able to do so. Likewise, the family should be told that the client may ask for a certain food and when it is served refuse it. This reaction is quite common because the memory of food taste or odor may vary greatly from what is actually served. The client knows this preparation may take extra effort on the part of loved ones and this sometimes leads to unnecessary guilt.

The nurse needs to recognize that although nutritional intervention may be important, clients should not be pushed beyond their limits. If pain, fullness, or nausea are precipitated regularly by adherence to the nutritional plan or domestic conflicts result, the quality of life in our clients with advanced disease is not being promoted.

CASE HISTORY

Mrs. M., a 62-year-old woman, was referred to us following surgery for moderately differentiated adenocarcinoma of the head of the pancreas. Secondary lymphatic, muscular, and perineural invasion was also present. The surgical procedure employed was a Whipple resection, which is the removal of the head (and sometimes the neck) of the pancreas; removal of adjacent stomach, distal portion of common duct, and duodenum.

Prior to her illness, Mrs. M., a social worker, was very active with her job as well as with voluntary work on several boards and committees of urban service organizations. She lived with her husband and had a sister living nearby.

Mrs. M. appeared to us, when we first met her in our clinic, to be a sensitive, calm, and intelligent woman who recognized that this change in her health was going to require many changes in her daily living. We realized that there was much critical teaching and planning to be done.

First we discussed the changes occurring owing to surgery: diabetes and absence of pancreatic enzymes. Next we noted that Mrs. M.'s weight of 92 pounds was low even considering that she had always been petite. Prior to her illness she weighed 110 pounds. She expressed hope that she might again weigh at least 100 pounds.

Her immediate complaints included loss of appetite, feelings of indigestion, and fatigue. She told us she was depressed and felt very uncertain about what to expect of the future.

The immediate medical treatment for her cancer included a course of radiation therapy, 4,000 rads to the pancreas, over 7 weeks, with chemotherapy during the first 3 days of radiation therapy. Then, after appropriate evaluation, she would begin a series of chemotherapy treatments with combined agents.

It was clear that we needed a plan—the first of many. Mrs. M. needed to learn many things about diabetes. We taught her how to measure sugar and acetone in her urine and the procedure for administering insulin. We reviewed the signs of hypoglycemia owing to excessive insulin, ketoacidosis, and appropriate actions for dealing with each.

We explained the need for oral medication containing amylase, lipase, and trypsin to control the problems of pancreatic insufficiency. She learned about the need for, and use of, antacids.

Perhaps most importantly we worked out a diet plan. Mrs. M. needed a strict eating schedule not only for gaining weight and avoiding increased cachexia but also for anchoring the other medication and urine testing times. We aimed for 1,800 calories in six meals. As a starting point, we emphasized high protein, considering her postoperative state with radiation therapy and chemotherapy. Often individuals with pancreatic insufficiency are given a bland, low-fat diet. Diabetic individuals are usually instructed to avoid sugars, and often a lactose-free diet is necessary in adults, especially after radiation. We decided that if we included all these restrictions initially, there would be less chance of getting Mrs. M. eating again. Therefore, we proceeded with an 1,800 calorie, six-meal, high-protein diet and made modifications as problems occurred.

Mrs. M., despite her fatigue, anorexia, and depressed feelings, took the basic plan and set to work implementing it. Often we forget about the work involved in following a diet. She taught her husband and a sister all we had taught her. She knew she needed some backup support.

Her weight loss trend stopped immediately and it was not many weeks before she began a slow, steady gain in weight, strength, and activity. At 5 months postoperative, her weight was up to 96 pounds and at 8 months she reached her initial goal of 100 pounds. At 1½ years postoperatively she weighed 102 pounds and continued to a high of 108 pounds. She had no signs of fluid retention, so we accepted these weights as true body weight changes.

After those first few months we discussed in depth her eating pattern and how she managed it. She told us that each evening initially she and her sister would plan a menu for the next day for 1,800 calories in six meals. Mrs. M. often found this very difficult since she had severe anorexia. Her sister would then go out for the necessary groceries. During those early months, her sister helped with the meals.

Mrs. M. clearly took the responsibility of adhering to a plan very seriously. Her plan follows: meals at 7:15 AM, 10:30 AM, 1:30 PM, 4:00 PM, and 6:00 PM; juice at 9:00 PM; late night snack at 11:00 PM. Before each of the six meals two enzyme tablets equalling 12 per day were taken, and 30 minutes after each meal, at bedtime, and as needed 2 tablespoons antacid were taken. NPH insulin was taken each morning. Urine fractionals were measured before breakfast, before dinner, and before the late night snack.

In addition to sticking to the plan, Mrs. M. also was an excellent historian, which was important in aiding the continual reevaluation of her nutritional needs. Her insulin level began at 5 μ NPH and over time was increased to 32 μ NPH based on urine fractionals, blood glucose levels, and symptoms of hyperglycemia.

As her appetite improved, a total of 500 calories of a liquid, nutritionally balanced, elemental diet containing medium-chain triglycerides was added in two servings. This made her daily caloric intake 2,300 calories. Other changes included a gradual increase in oral enzymes when she experienced steatorrhea. At 12 enzyme tablets per day, her bowel movements were normal.

Over a 2-year period postoperatively, Mrs. M.'s pancreatic cancer was evaluated as stable. She received chemotherapy 5 days every 5 weeks over this period. Each week she came in for complete blood count, differential, and platelet blood studies. She was familiar with the normal levels.

At the start of Mrs. M.'s third year with us she developed progression of her pancreatic cancer based on scans and physical examination measurements of her liver span. Her chemotherapeutic agents were changed, but progression continued. Mrs. M. remained asymptomatic and physically active. She did not return to her job as a social worker but had resumed some volunteer work.

During this third year, Mrs. M. had a bout of herpes zoster, her chronic anemia worsened, and her diabetes became very difficult to control. Late in the year her appetite decreased markedly, but she lost only 5 pounds over several months.

We continued to modify the plan—the enzyme preparation was changed to one that would allow her to take fewer pills. Her insulin levels changed from 21 μ NPH to 32 μ NPH back down to 20 μ NPH over 15 months. Also, we changed the elemental diet preparations.

Mrs. M. died 3½ years after coming to us. During most of this time, she retained full activity status and remained asymptomatic. She always had a neat appearance and gracious manner. She dealt with problems, delays, and errors firmly, maturely, and effectively. It appeared that she had always taken responsibility for, and control of, her life, allowing her to continue this behavior in her time of illness.

Mrs. M. told us while stable that she credited the stability in part to a firm adherence to the nutritional plan—perhaps it helped. In any instance, Mrs. M. fully participated in her care.

She seemed never to have forgotten how low she felt postoperatively and was always willing to talk with other clients who were suffering from anorexia. Also, she had a special relationship with each team member, allowing us all to help. It is unusual for a person with pancreatic cancer of Mrs. M.'s stage to survive 3½ years, but the most heartening phenomenon was how well she lived.

SUMMARY

Nutrition is just one functional problem of clients having gastrointestinal cancer. Other functional problem areas include changes in body image, pain control-comfort, stoma care, and sleep-rest-activity balance. Several of these problems are common to many advanced cancer clients regardless of the cancer site. Discussion of these nursing care aspects, therefore, may be found throughout cancer nursing literature and should be reviewed.

Gastrointestinal cancers are treated with four modalities: surgery, chemotherapy, radiation therapy, and immunotherapy. Increased efforts are being made in the areas of prevention and early detection. Nurses are active in public health settings promoting screening for occult blood and instruction in the use of high-fiber diets.

With many functional problems, several modalities of treatment in varied settings, it is obvious that care of clients with gastrointestinal cancer is a complex task requiring an interdisciplinary health care provider team in care, treatment, and research. One of the most important team members in this area is the nurse.

REFERENCES

1. Adams, J.: Cancer of the major digestive glands. In Rubin, P., editor: Clinical oncology, New York, 1978, American Cancer Society, Inc.
2. American Cancer Society: 1979 cancer facts and figures, New York, 1979, American Cancer Society, Inc.
3. Borgen, L.: Total parenteral nutrition in adults, Am. J. Nurs. **78:**224, 1978.
4. Bury, K. D.: Elemental diets. In Fischer, J. E., editor: Total parenteral nutrition, Boston, 1976, Little Brown & Co.
5. Butler, J.: A tool for assessing the nutritional status of cancer patients, Oncol. Nurs. Forum **5:**11, 1978.
6. Colley, R., and Wilson, J.: Meeting patients' nutritional needs with hyperalimentation, Nursing '79 **9:**76, 1979.
7. Copeland, E. M.: Parenteral nutrition in cancer patients, Digestive Disease Week, Post Graduate Course: Gastrointestinal Cancer, San Antonio, Texas, May 17-18, 1975.
8. Copeland, E. M., et al.: Intravenous hyperalimentation as an adjunct to cancer chemotherapy, Am. J. Surg. **129:**167, 1975.
9. Cullen, P. P.: Patients with colo-rectal cancer: how to assess and meet their needs, Nursing '76 **6:**45, 1976.
10. De Wys, W.: Changes in taste sensation in cancer patients: correlation with calorie intake. In Kare, M., and Mallor, O., editors: The chemical senses and nutrition, New York, 1977, Academic Press, Inc.
11. Morton, J.: Alimentary tract cancer. In Rubin, P., editor: Clinical oncology, New York, 1978, American Cancer Society, Inc.
12. Page, C. P., et al.: Continual catheter administration of an elemental diet, Surg. Gynecol. Obstet. **142:**184, 1976.
13. Phillips, K.: Nursing care in parenteral nutrition. In Fischer, J. E., editor: Total parenteral nutrition, Boston, 1976, Little Brown & Co.
14. Shils, M.: Nutritional problems arising from the treatment of cancer. In Nutrition and cancer, New York, 1972, American Cancer Society, Inc.
15. Solassol, C., and Jayeux, H.: Ambulatory parenteral nutrition. In Fischer, J. E., editor: Total parenteral nutrition, Boston, 1976, Little Brown & Co.
16. Theologides, A.: Pathogenesis of cachexia in cancer: a review and a hypothesis, Cancer **29**(2):484, 1972.

26

Infection control in clients with acute leukemia

MARY D. BATES and MARY BETH ORTON

Less than a decade ago acute leukemia in adults was considered by many to be an untreatable and incurable disease. Active chemotherapeutic agents were unavailable, and the majority of clients died from complications of infection or hemorrhage. There have been several major advances in the management of adult acute leukemia; in the field of chemotherapy, supportive therapy such as antibiotics, platelets, and white blood cells and immunotherapy have resulted in increased complete remission rates and prolonged survivals. This chapter focuses on infections in acute leukemia. However, a review of the disease process including treatment modalities and usual complications is necessary to facilitate the understanding of infection control in the leukemia client.

INCIDENCE

The adult acute leukemia (AAL) population is comprised of approximately 75% acute myelogenous leukemia (AML), 15% to 20% acute lymphocytic leukemia (ALL), and 5% to 10% of the clients have acute undifferentiated leukemia (AUL). In general, clients with AML have a lower rate of complete remission than clients with ALL. However, once in complete remission, the remission duration for myelogenous leukemias is often longer than for lymphocytic and undifferentiated leukemias. In contrast, clients with ALL/AUL have a higher remission rate, but remissions are of a shorter duration.

PATHOPHYSIOLOGY OF ACUTE LEUKEMIA

The word "leukemia" literally is defined as "white blood." Clients with leukemia may have many white blood cells present in their blood—hence the term "leukemia." However, it is known that leukemia is not only a proliferation of white blood cells in the peripheral blood, but it is also a complex disease process that originates in the bone marrow.

The bone marrow is the organ primarily responsible for the production of blood components (that is, white blood cells, red blood cells, plasma cells, and platelets). There is a constant turnover of these components in the body, and the supply is replenished from a stem cell pool in the bone marrow. The stem cell is a highly specialized

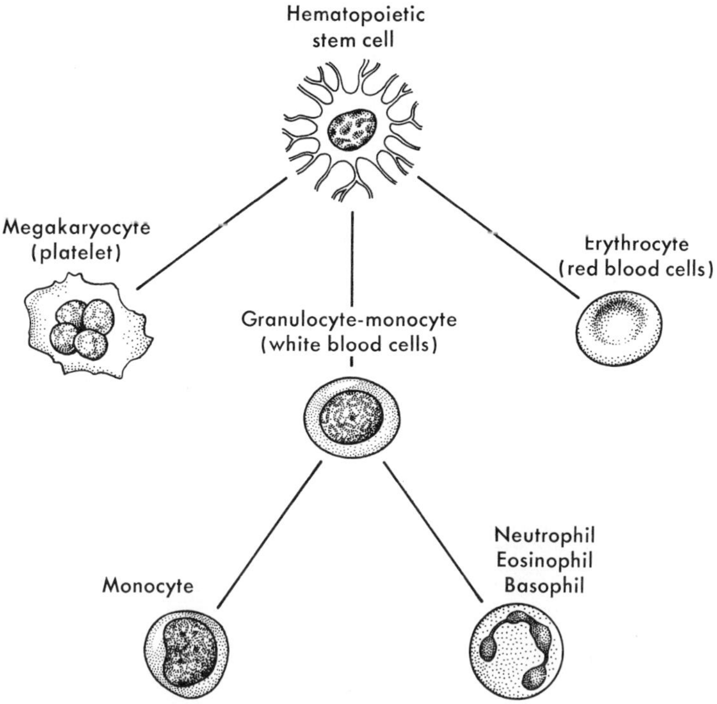

Fig. 26-1. Schematic illustration of stem cell differentiation.

cell in many ways. It has the ability to replicate itself by the process of mitosis, thereby maintaining an adequate stem cell pool in the bone marrow. In addition, the stem cell can become committed to one of the blood component cell lines and differentiate into either white blood cells, red blood cells, platelets, or plasma cells. Once the stem cell is committed to a particular cell line, it matures and results in a functioning cell of the peripheral blood. For example, the mature neutrophil found in the peripheral blood originates from the committed stem cell that has matured through the various cell stages in the bone marrow to the blood.

In the leukemia client, there is a functional abnormality in maintaining hemostasis in the bone marrow. This can occur in any cell line in the bone marrow as well as in any stage of the stem cell's development. The white cell series is most commonly involved in the leukemic process. The leukemic white cell loses its ability to mature, which results in an accumulation of immature nonfunctioning cells in the bone marrow. Eventually, immature blast cells are released into the bloodstream and can be determined by a differential white blood cell count. Normally blast cells are not present in the peripheral blood.

CLINICAL PRESENTATION

Clinical manifestations of acute leukemia found at the time of initial diagnosis are related to the major complications of the disease: anemia, neutropenia, thrombocytopenia, coagulopathies, and infiltration with leukemia cells. Presenting signs and symptoms of acute leukemia vary in each client because the presenting symptoms of leukemia are nonspecific and associated with many other illnesses. Leukemia often goes undiagnosed until further evaluation of the complete blood count, including differential counts, and examination of the bone marrow specimen are completed.

TREATMENT OF ACUTE LEUKEMIA

The purpose of chemotherapy is to destroy a sufficient number of leukemia cells in the bone marrow to permit regrowth of residual bone marrow elements. Usually a period of profound bone marrow hypoplasia is induced to achieve this goal. The initial effect of chemotherapy can be seen with a reduction or clearing in the number of circulating blasts in the peripheral blood. The most reliable indication of response to chemotherapy is through bone marrow analysis. Therefore, during remission induction, clients can expect frequent bone marrow aspirations to be performed.

Clients with high white blood cell counts (greater than 50,000/mm^3) require urgent medical management. With a high number of circulating leukemia cells, there is a risk of leukemia cell growth in the walls of cerebral blood vessels. Subsequent rupture of the vessels leads to catastrophic intracerebral hemorrhage. Leukapheresis (a technique designed to physically remove white blood cells from the client's circulation) and chemotherapy (such as intravenous hydroxyurea or cytosine arabinoside (Ara-C)) should be employed immediately.

Achievement of complete remission is the ultimate goal of chemotherapy. The criteria for complete remission is a normal cellular bone marrow with less than 5% blast cells. The bone marrow should show normal regeneration of all bone marrow elements, and the peripheral blood count should have returned to the normal range. At the time of diagnosis, there are approximately 100 billion leukemia cells in the body located in the bone marrow and extramedullary (or outside the bone marrow such as lymph nodes). Chemotherapy-induced complete remission reduces the leukemia tumor burden by approximately 90 billion cells. It is postulated that after successful remission-induction therapy there remains approximately 10 billion leukemia cells that are undetectable by present laboratory methods. Additional chemotherapy is necessary after complete remission to further reduce the amount of leukemia cells present. Some of the frequently used agents in acute leukemia are listed in Table 26-1 along with an indication of the degree of neutropenia caused by each agent.

Table 26-1. Chemotherapeutic agents commonly employed in the treatment of acute leukemia

Anthracycline antibiotics	
Doxorubicin (Adriamycin)	+++
Rubidazone	+++
Daunomycin	+++
Antimetabolites	
Cytosine arabinoside (ara-C)	+++
6-mercaptopurine	+++
Thioguanine	+++
Methotrexate	+++
Alkylating agent	
Cyclophosphamide (Cytoxan)	++
Vinca alkaloid	
Vincristine (Oncovin)	+
Steroid	
Prednisone	−
Antineoplastic enzyme	
L-asparaginase	−

+++ = Severe neutropenia; ++ = moderate neutropenia; + = possible mild neutropenia; − = no evidence of neutropenia.

Many different combinations of the drugs listed in Table 26-1 are used in the chemotherapy of acute leukemia. Some of the usual combinations are listed below:

AdOAP—*Ad*riamycin *O*ncovin *A*ra-C *P*rednisone

ROAP—*R*ubidizone *O*ncovin *A*ra-C *P*rednisone
OAP—*O*ncovin *A*ra-C *P*rednisone
POMP—6-Mercapto*p*urine *O*ncovin *M*ethotrexate *P*rednisone
TAD—*T*hioguanine *A*ra-C *D*aunorubicin
VP—*V*incristine *P*rednisone
ARA-C-TG—*A*ra-C *T*hio*g*uanine

A detailed review of chemotherapy and the side-effects encountered can be found in Chapter 14.

MANAGEMENT OF COMPLICATIONS OF ACUTE LEUKEMIA

The leukemic disease process gives rise to many serious complications. Without immediate treatment these complications may be fatal. The three major complications of leukemia are anemia, hemorrhage, and infection.

Anemia

Anemia is defined as a reduction in the circulating red blood cell mass. Anemia often accounts for the vague clinical picture of weakness, pallor, and fatigue. It is common for a client to have a hemoglobin of 6 to 10 gm% when initially diagnosed. Hemoglobin levels of less than 6 gm% are very serious and should be corrected immediately.

Anemia reduces the oxygen-carrying capacity of the blood. In the leukemic client, anemia is often insidious in onset, allowing for a physiologic adaptation. Clients are often able to tolerate hemoglobins as low as 6 gm% without being seriously handicapped. Tachycardia and an increased pulse pressure may be present. Clients will begin to see a decrease in exercise tolerance and may experience shortness of breath on exertion. In severe anemia, manifestations of headache, vertigo, muscular weakness, and drowsiness are seen. Clients may occasionally experience a variety of gastrointestinal complaints, such as nausea, diarrhea, anorexia, and abdominal discomfort. Symptoms of anemia in the leukemia client are alleviated only through the control of the leukemia and supportive therapy with blood transfusions.[1]

General nursing measures are aimed at minimizing the effects of anemia to promote client comfort. The nurse should assist the client in determining the activity tolerance and ways of conserving energy. When planning nursing care, it is important to organize daily activities, diagnostic tests, and therapeutic procedures to ensure sufficient rest time. This is particularly important for the new leukemia client who is undergoing multiple diagnostic and therapeutic procedures when first admitted to the hospital. At the other end of the spectrum, in some clients and families a tendency toward overprotection exists because of fear of their diagnosis. The nurse must intervene to encourage adequate exercise as well as rest for the client. Clients who have lived with leukemia for some time can usually sense when their "counts" are down and set activity limits accordingly.

Monitoring vital signs is important in assessing many different parameters in the leukemia client. A rise in the pulse and respiratory rate may be indicative of a further decrease in hemoglobin level. This should alert the nurse to further assess the client's condition and notify the physician of any changes. Anemia can be temporarily managed by transfusion of blood cells. However, the only method for long-term management is by control of the leukemic process. Clients are usually transfused to maintain the hemoglobin about 8 gm%. Packed red blood cells as opposed to whole blood are indicated. There are several advantages for utilizing packed cells: multiple units of blood may be transfused with minimal danger of circulatory overload and chances of transfusion reaction owing to plasma protein factors or antibodies in the donor plasma are reduced, especially if leukocyte-poor, washed, or frozen red blood cells are used.[18] "Leukocyte-poor" blood is the component remaining after removal of leukocytes and platelets from the whole blood; "washing" the cells removes any plasma, white blood cells, or platelets that may remain after the cells are packed. The purpose of giving washed, leukocyte-poor blood is therefore to prevent transfusion-associated fever reactions in cases where the presence of leukoagglutinins and antiplatelet antibodies have been demonstrated or are suspected and to prevent sensitization to leukocytes and platelets in potential candidates for long-term blood cells and platelet transfusions.[9]

Hemorrhage

The second major complication of leukemia and its treatment is hemorrhage. Bleeding tendencies develop as a result of thrombocytopenia (a decrease in circulating platelets). Platelets function to promote hemostasis by participating in clot formation and providing support for the endothelial lining of the blood vessels. Injury to tissue results in adherence of platelets to the site of the injury. There is also an increase in the local aggregation of platelets to the site of the injury, which results in the formation of a platelet plug to control hemorrhage. The platelet plug is one of the initial stages in the coagulation process to establish a more permanent platelet/fibrin clot.

Platelets also function to maintain the integrity of blood vessel endothelium. Platelets are attracted to the spaces that occur between endothelial cells. Platelets adhere to the blood vessel lining and become part of the extracellular structure. This prevents leakage of blood into the interstitial tissue.

Failure to maintain an intact endothelial lining of blood vessels results in small hemorrhages into the cutaneous tissue called petechiae. Petechiae may occur spontaneously and are most often found in the dependent parts of the body. Bruising, as a result of very mild trauma, is common in the thrombocytopenic client.

Bleeding as a result of thrombocytopenia is usually mild. Petechiae and ecchymosis, although cosmetically disturbing, present no physical danger to the client. However, even minimal leakage from intracranial blood vessels may be catastrophic owing to increased intracranial pressure resulting from the bleeding. Massive hemorrhage, particularly in the gastrointestinal tract and pulmonary system, usually do not result from thrombocytopenia alone. Coagulation disturbances such as disseminated intravascular coagulation and mucosal ulceration predispose the client to major hemorrhages.

Clot formation may also be affected by factors that cause abnormalities in platelet functions such as drugs (aspirin, high-dose penicillin, indomethacin, and phenylbutazone). In addition, disturbances in the leukemic stem cells may give rise to abnormal platelets that are unable to function effectively in maintaining hemostasis. The presence of an enlarged spleen usually results in an increased number of platelets being sequestered by the spleen and thus not functioning in the circulating pool of platelets. The presence of infection, sepsis, and fever further complicates the platelet deficiency by consuming the platelets in the process of disseminated intravascular coagulation.

Thrombocytopenic bleeding is best managed by prophylactic platelet transfusions to maintain a platelet count greater than $20{,}000/mm^3$. The incidence of severe hemorrhage is rare above this level. Platelets can be collected from either whole blood donated from multiple donors or 2 to 4 units of blood from individual donors. In the latter process, the donor's platelets are removed by a plateletpheresis technique, which allows the return of the donor's plasma and red cells, thus enabling more frequent donations from the same person.

The nursing interventions for the thrombocytopenic client are aimed at preventing and controlling hemorrhage. This can best be accomplished by early documentation of any signs or symptoms of bleeding. Bleeding can occur virtually anywhere in the body. The nurse must assess the client for any signs or symptoms of bleeding. Common sites for bleeding are in the skin, with the presence of petechiae, ecchymosis, and hematomas. Bleeding is also common in the urine and ranges from microscopic to gross hematuria. Epistaxis, scleral hemorrhages, and gingival bleeding may occur. Females may have extremely heavy menstrual bleeding that necessitates control with hormonal therapy.

Major complications of thrombycytopenia involve bleeding into the gastrointestinal tract, lungs, and central nervous system. These hemorrhages can occur spontaneously or as a result of trauma.

Symptoms of an intracranial hemorrhage may have an insidious onset, and the nurse must be alert to signs of impending danger. Depending on the location of hemorrhage in the brain, the client may experience visual disturbances, loss of motor function, differences in pupil accommodation to light, headaches, and changes in the level of consciousness. Treatment with platelet transfusion must be initiated immediately once the signs of intracranial hemorrhage are recognized.

Vague complaints of abdominal tenderness may be the first step of gastrointestinal hemorrhage. On assessment, melena or hematemesis as well as unexplained drop in hemoglobin and hematocrit may be found. Gastrointestinal hemorrhage is usually treated symptomatically. A nasogastric tube is inserted to prevent severe abdominal distention. Iced saline lavages also may be instituted to help control gastrointestinal bleeding. Estimated blood loss should be replaced with packed red blood cells and intravenous fluids to restore circulatory volume. Platelet transfusions and transfusions of fresh frozen plasma containing clotting factors may be beneficial. Prednisone, a common chemotherapeutic agent used in the treatment of acute leukemia, is known to cause gastric disturbances and should be used with caution in clients where gastrointestinal bleeding is suspected.

Intrapulmonic hemorrhage presents an emergency situation. The client will experience increasing respiratory difficulty. Respirations become very labored and shallow. Rales can be heard on auscultation. Coughing is productive of copious amounts of blood-streaked sputum and blood clots. Excessive endotracheal suctioning may cause further hemorrhage from trauma by the suction catheter. Intrapulmonic hemorrhage can be controlled only by platelet, fresh frozen plasma, and red blood cell transfusions to replace blood lost. The client often requires intubation and mechanical ventilatory assistance.

Bleeding in the leukemia client can be associated with other problems in addition to thrombocytopenia. Clients with progranulocytic leukemia have a higher tendency to develop disseminated intravascular coagulation (DIC), which is a complex coagulation disturbance that further complicates the bleeding tendency; DIC is also associated with septicemia. Liver failure or liver involvement in the leukemic process may result in a decreased production of clotting factors and vitamin K, which are vital to the coagulation system. Assessment and treatment of all deficiencies in the clotting process are necessary to restore adequate functioning of the coagulation system.

Infection

Interest in the role of infections in cancer clients has steadily increased over the past decade. Major advances in chemotherapy have brought about stabilization of malignant diseases to the point where investi-

Table 26-2. Fatal infections related to type of malignancy

Malignancy	No. of clients	Disseminated	% clients with pneumonia	Peritonitis	% dying of infection
Acute leukemia	366	65	28	0.1	70
Lymphoma	206	53	40	3	51
Genitourinary	208	48	34	10	58
Gastrointestinal	142	45	39	13	49
Lung	104	20	78	2	44
Head and neck	94	19	74	2	46
Melanoma	78	35	59	3	37

Reproduced with permission from Bodey, G. P., Sr., et al.: Supportive care in the management of the cancer patient. In Clark, R. L., and Howe, C. D., editors: Cancer patient care at M. D. Anderson Hospital and Tumor Institute. Copyright © 1976 by Year Book Medical Publishers, Inc., Chicago.

gators are now able to turn their attention to secondary problems. However, infection continues to be a major factor in mortality in cancer clients (Table 26-2).

There are several factors that predispose the cancer client to infection. Neutropenia as a result of the disease process and/or myelosuppressive treatment modalities is a major contributing factor in the incidence of infection. Immunosuppression, malnutrition, and long periods of hospitalization result in increased risks of infection in the client with cancer. The principles and treatment modalities used in the management of infection discussed in the remainder of this chapter, although specifically related to acute leukemia, can be readily applied to all cancer clients.

Infection as a functional problem. Infection is the major cause of morbidity and mortality in acute leukemia. The incidence of infection is particularly high during the remission induction phase of treatment. High doses of myelosuppressive chemotherapeutic agents that are given in attempts to control leukemia also cause neutropenia, which increases the risk of infection. Chemotherapeutic regimens used in the management of other cancers also cause neutropenia, thus predisposing the client to infection. Therefore, principles and guidelines detailed in the following section should be applied to *any* neutropenic client.

Of 366 clients with acute leukemia studied at M. D. Anderson Hospital and Tumor Institute, 70% ultimately died of infection and not their leukemia. Severe infection is unlikely in clients with an absolute granulocyte count greater than $1{,}000/mm^3$:

$$\text{Absolute granulocyte count} = \frac{\%\ \text{Granulocytes} \times \text{Total WBC}}{100}$$

There is a reciprocal relationship between the incidence and severity of infection and the number of circulating granulocytes. A direct relationship exists between the duration of neutropenia and the risk of infection.[5]

Recent advances in infection control, isolation and culture of pathogenic organisms, antibiotic therapy, and granulocyte transfusions have helped to decrease the number of fatal infections in the leukemic population. The use of the protected environment (laminar airflow room or life island) has further reduced the number of infectious episodes experienced with the use of intensive high-dose chemotherapy.[3]

The management of infections in leukemia

clients is a complex process that requires constant surveillance by the health care team. Several considerations in the management of infection in the leukemia client are summarized in the list below:

1. The classic signs and symptoms of infection are absent because of neutropenia.
2. Untreated infection may disseminate rapidly and lead to death.
3. Most infections are caused by gram-negative bacilli.
4. Infections may be caused by nonpathogenic and unusual organisms.
5. Some antibiotics are less efficacious in neutropenic clients.
6. Neutropenic clients are subject to repeated infections caused by the same organism.
7. Multiple organisms may cause infections in the same or separate sites simultaneously.
8. Superinfection is a frequent occurrence.

The infectious process in the acute leukemia client presents a most confusing paradoxical picture. The usual signs and symptoms of infection and inflammation are not always present in the leukemia population. The client may have an open lesion without purulent drainage, a pneumonia without sputum production, or an abscess without pus formation.

Because leukemic white cells are very immature, they are not able to fight infection. Also the myelosuppressive effects of chemotherapy reduce the number of white blood cells, leukemic and normal, and further reduce the body's ability to fight infection. Without functioning granulocytes, the defenses of the body are compromised. The white count itself is nondiagnostic of infection and often misleading. In a normal individual, an increased white count may signal infection. In the leukemic client, it may signify that the leukemia is still uncontrolled. The most important parameter in assessing white blood cell count is the evidence of functioning neutrophils determined by the differential white blood cell count.

Common symptoms. Temperature must be analyzed very carefully as an indication of infection. In many studies, a temperature of 101° F or greater in neutropenic clients (absolute granulocyte count less than 1,000/mm^3) is used as an indicator of probable or potential infection. The cause of the elevated temperature other than infection must be considered. Has the client received any packed red blood cells, platelets, or white blood cell transfusions? Was any chemotherapy or immunotherapy such as Rubidazone, Neocarzinostatin, 5-Azacytidine, *C. parvum,* MER, or BCG given? Did the client receive any antifungal therapy with amphotericin B? All of these agents are known to cause fever and may confuse the nurse in attempting to assess a possible infection.

When a client's temperature spikes greater than 101° F, routine cultures are taken from blood, urine, throat, sputum, stool, and any other clinical foci. If no other cause of fever such as administration of blood products can be determined, antibiotics are administered immediately. A chest x-ray film should be taken at this time because subclinical pneumonia is a common cause of fever. When possible, cultures should be completed prior to initiating antibiotics because antibiotic therapy may interfere with proper identification of the causative organism.

Clients with leukemia who do have infection may not exhibit any signs of elevated temperature. Prednisone, as well as other corticosteroids, may suppress temperature and mask other inflammatory responses to infection. Tylenol and aspirin, commonly used as mild analgesics, also cause a reduction in elevated temperatures. These agents, as well as other products containing aspirin and acetaminophen, should be used only when the infectious process is clearly understood and controlled.

Fevers of unknown origin (FUO) are common in leukemia clients. An FUO can be defined as a condition in which a temperature elevation exists unrelated to transfusion of blood products or other pyrogenic agents and no causative organisms can be cultured. Nearly 50% of the febrile leukemia clients have no documented source of infection. However, initial treatment of fevers in the neutropenic client with broad-spectrum antibiotics is necessary to prevent rapid dissemination of a potentially fatal infection. In many instances, a thorough workup for infection yields no causative organism, and multiple antibiotic regimens fail to control the elevated temperature. It is hypothesized that the leukemic disease process may be responsible for some of the fevers for which no other cause can be found. Supportive care with antibiotics during the febrile period is integral to client survival, but only through the control of the leukemia can the client hope to remain free of serious infection.

In the neutropenic client, infections can be caused by organisms normally found in the body's microbial flora (endogenous) as well as by foreign organisms (exogenous). Infections that are caused by normally nonpathogenic organisms are called "opportunistic" infections. Opportunistic infections occur in clients with compromised defenses (that is, granulocytopenia) and clients receiving antibiotic therapy. Antibiotics may disrupt the natural balance of microbial flora and predispose the client to infections by drug-resistant organisms. Therefore, clients may become infected with multiple organisms that further complicate the clinical picture. It is not uncommon for clients to have repeated infections with the same organism. A detailed account of the client's infectious history gives important clues to possible etiologies of the infection.[6]

Common causative organisms. The majority of infections in leukemia clients are caused by gram-negative aerobic bacilli, namely *Pseudomonas aeruginosa, Klebsiella,* and *Escherichia coli.*[24] These organisms are a part of the normal gastrointestinal tract flora but may become pathogenic in the neutropenic client. *Staphylococcus aureus* is the most common pathogen among gram-positive bacteria. Fungi, specifically of the *Candida* genus, are routinely cultured from various body orifices in the neutropenic client. Disseminated fungal infections account for 15% of the fatal infections in the leukemia population.[21] Viral infections caused by rhinoviruses, adenoviruses, and enteroviruses have essentially the same frequency and clinical course in leukemia clients as in the normal population. However, infections caused by herpes zoster, herpes simplex, and cytomegalovirus (CMV) pose a serious threat to the compromised host.

Infection can occur anywhere in the body. Skin and mucous membranes provide natural protective barriers against invasion by pathogenic organisms. Any invasion of the integument creates a source of potential infection. Warm, moist skin provides an excellent medium for bacterial and fungal growth; hence, infections are commonly found in the groin, axilla, perineum, and perirectal areas, between folds of fatty tissue in obese patients, and under the breasts. Stomatitis and mucositis are frequent complications of chemotherapy and predispose the client to infections of the oral cavity. These infections may be classified as mild; however, careful management is warranted to prevent spread of the infection.

Infectious complications occur frequently in the upper respiratory tract and lungs. Dissemination of a preexisting pulmonary infection may result in septicemia. However, septicemia has also been found to be the primary infection in the leukemia client subsequent to direct invasion of a pathogenic organism.

Treatment of infection. As previously stated, infections in leukemia clients are best managed when the leukemic process is under control. Fortunately, the availability of efficacious antibiotic therapy and granulocyte transfusions decreases the incidence of fatal infections, thereby allowing adequate trial for remission induction with chemotherapeutic agents.

Leukemia clients are generally treated with broad-spectrum antibiotics initially when infection is first suspected. Because of the increased incidence of gram-negative bacterial infections, treatment with aminoglycosides (that is, tobramycin, gentamicin) and/or cephalosporins (cephalothin, cephamandole) is recommended.[21] A penicillin derivative such as carbenicillin or ticarcillin is recommended as treatment for *Pseudomonas* infections.[20] Sulfamethoxazole-trimethorprim may be effective in bacterial infections that do not respond to the above agents, and also as front-line therapy for protozoal infections.

Every attempt must be made to identify the causative organism as well as antibiotic sensitivity to ensure effective antibiotic therapy. Changes in antibiotics may be necessary if the causative organism proves resistant to the antibiotics or the clinical picture does not improve. Antibiotics may be added to the original antibiotic schema if an additional resistant organism is discovered. Antifungal agents, such as amphotericin B, may be prescribed for documented fungal infections or highly suspected cases of fungus.

In leukemia clients, antibiotics are usually administered intravenously. Thrombocytopenia prohibits the intramuscular administration of drugs, and oral administration is usually less effective because of impaired gastrointestinal absorption. Antibiotics are prescribed at intervals designed to maintain therapeutic blood levels. Continuous administration of aminoglycosides and cephalosporins yields the most constant, therapeutic blood levels of these antibiotics. Continuous infusions can be safely administered via infusion pumps. The availability of battery-operated pumps further enhances the safety and convenience of continuous infusions by allowing client mobility without interruption of continuous therapy.

Administration of antibiotic therapy is not without serious complications. Nephrotoxicity and ototoxicity are side-effects of aminoglycoside therapy and are related to dosage and blood levels. Routine determinations of serum creatinine and BUN should be monitored as indicators of renal function. Tinnitus is an indicator of possible ototoxicity and should be reported to the physician as soon as it is recognized. Electrolyte imbalance is frequently associated with penicillin derivatives. Hypokalemia can be controlled by concomitant administration of IV or oral potassium supplements. Hypocalcemia and hypomagnesemia may occur after prolonged administration of combination antibiotic therapy. Parenteral replacement of calcium and magnesium may be indicated.

Antifungal therapy with amphotericin B may produce severe nephrotoxicity with prolonged administration in addition to hypokalemia. Severe chills and fever are also common with the administration of amphotericin B. Premedication with antihistamines and/or hydrocortisone may decrease these side-effects. Meperidine sulfate given as a premedication or when fever and chills begin has been empirically found to be effective in reducing these symptoms.

Chemical phlebitis from the intravenous administration of antibiotics is not uncommon, particularly when infusion is via scalp vein needle. The use of central venous catheters has significantly reduced the incidence of phlebitis.

Gastrointestinal side-effects from antibiotic therapy are usually mild but cause client discomfort. Nausea, vomiting, and diarrhea may be controlled with antiemetics and antidiarrheals. The sensation of "tasting" intravenous antibiotics further increases nausea and vomiting and may lead to anorexia. These side-effects are temporary and subside with discontinuance of the drug(s). Because nutrition plays an important role in maintaining the metabolic state of the client, careful assessment of the client's nutritional status and calorie intake is necessary. Fever results in an increased metabolic rate and may also increase nutritional requirements. When nutritional needs cannot be met orally, parenteral nutritional support with intravenous hyperalimentation may be indicated.

There are several reasons for antibiotic failure in the leukemia population. One of the most important reasons is delay in initiating antibiotic therapy in the febrile, neutropenic client. It is imperative that febrile episodes be immediately reported to the physician and that prescribed antibiotics be administered promptly. Delay in initiating antibiotic therapy may lead to rapid dissemination of the infection and possible death.

It is known that some antibiotics are less effective in neutropenic clients. Control of infection requires appropriate antibiotic therapy as well as functioning neutrophils. When neutrophil function is suboptimal, owing to neutropenia and impaired phagocytic action, otherwise appropriate antibiotic therapy may not be successful. Cephalothin, gentamicin, and tobramycin have been found to be less effective in neutropenic clients.[21]

Any factors that interfere with tissue penetration of antibiotics may decrease effectiveness of therapy. Tumor infiltration or decreased blood supply to the infection site may result in inadequate antibiotic therapy. Deficiencies in host defense mechanisms as a result of the disease process and immunosuppressive chemotherapy are major deterrents to the control of infection.

Prophylactic antibiotic therapy. Studies have been conducted to determine the benefits of prophylactic antibiotic therapy in neutropenic clients prior to heralding signs and symptoms of infection. Conflicting results have been reported on the effectiveness of prophylactic antibiotics when used in a general hospital setting. However, when prophylactic intravenous antibiotics are used in combination with a protective environment (including oral nonabsorbable antibiotics, topical antibiotic preparations, sterile diet, and special bathing procedures), the incidence and severity of infection is significantly reduced.[22]

Granulocyte transfusions. Granulocyte transfusions play an important role in the management of infections in the neutropenic client. Granulocytes are collected via a blood cell separator, which selectively removes white blood cells from the peripheral blood and returns red blood cells, plasma, and platelets to the donor. Historically, granulocytes have been collected from CML donors and related HLA-matched donors to control infection. In non-CML donors, agents such as steroid hormones are used to induce a temporary leukocytosis, enabling a greater number of white blood cells to be pheresed. The use of granulocyte transfusions has significantly improved the neutropenic client's response to infection.[19] Prophylactic granulocyte transfusions are currently being investigated to determine their effectiveness in preventing infections in the neutropenic client. In these studies, neutropenic clients are started on granulocyte transfusions prior to developing fever and/or other signs and symptoms of infection.

Granulocyte transfusions are mainly available at comprehensive cancer centers and require the efforts of trained staff as well as volunteer donors. Most often, blood relatives are utilized for granulocyte donations, but in some instances, successful transfusions have been collected from unrelated donors. The collection of white blood cells by leukapheresis involves minimal risk to the donor. Because of more refined leukapheresis techniques and development of less expensive equipment, granulocyte collection and transfusions are becoming more prevalent particularly in major cancer treatment facilities.[17]

The nursing considerations for a client receiving white blood cell transfusions are similar to a client receiving other blood products. The nurse should be alert for signs and symptoms of blood reaction: chills, flushing, rash, hives, hyper/hypotension, and tachycardia. There is a minimal risk of an anaphylactic reaction to granulocyte transfusions, but this is unlikely when using non-CML donors. When anaphylactic symptoms occur, the granulocytes should be discontinued, the physician notified, and appropriate emergency treatment administered. Common agents used for white blood cell reactions are antihistamines, such as diphenylhydramine, and steroids, such as hydrocortisone. Epinephrine should be available for treatment of anaphylactic reactions.

Transfused white blood cells have a tendency to migrate to the area of infection. Therefore, a client with a cellulitis or perianal lesion may complain of pain at the site of infection secondary to the migration of transfused granulocytes. Clients with documented pneumonias, particularly bilateral pneumonias, must be carefully monitored for possible respiratory complications during or following granulocyte transfusions. Symptoms of shortness of breath, increased respiratory rate and effort, tachycardia, and restlessness may be indicators of pulmonary consolidation with white blood cells. In extreme bilateral pulmonary consolidation with white blood cells, ventilation may be severely compromised to the point of requiring mechanical ventilatory assistance. Although these reactions are rare, the nurse must be aware of the risks associated with white blood cell transfusions and provide nursing intervention accordingly.

NURSING INTERVENTIONS

Some of the general nursing considerations and interventions are depicted in the standard nursing care plan (Table 26-3) for infections in the leukemia client. The goal of nursing care is to prevent infections from occurring. However, in the leukemia population, infections continue to occur despite meticulous nursing and medical attention. A secondary goal then is early detection and appropriate treatment of infections.

Preventive nursing aspects

Prevention of infection in acute leukemia is virtually impossible despite scrupulous nursing and medical care. Neutropenia is so profound in acute leukemia that infections or fevers of unknown origin are an expected result of the myelosuppressive therapy. However, meticulous nursing care will help to limit the morbidity and mortality associated with infection.

One of the most important and, unfortunately, often neglected infection control measures is handwashing. It is imperative that hands be thoroughly scrubbed prior to, as well as between, client contact. Many infections are transmitted via direct contact

Table 26-3. Nursing care plan

Date	Initials	Client needs and problems	Nursing action
2/1/79	R. N.	Potential infection owing to granulocytopenia and lymphocytopenia Goals: Prevention/early detection/treatment of infection	Maintain adequate handwashing techniques (particularly between client contacts). Utilize aseptic and sterile technique as indicated. Assess for any signs/symptoms of infection. Check skin, mouth, rectal/vaginal areas, lungs, site of indwelling catheters, or tubes. Maintain integrity of skin and mucous membranes as a protective barrier. Be aware of drugs that mask fever and other signs and symptoms of infection (aspirin, acetaminophen, steroids, or products containing any of these drugs). Promote optimum personal hygiene. Assist as necessary. Maintain a clean and safe environment. Empty and clean drainage receptacles (suction apparatus) at end of each shift. Screen personnel and visitors with contagious infection. Monitor white blood cell counts, particularly differential count of granulocytes. Monitor vital signs at least every 4 hours, and report temperature above 101° F and significant drop in systolic blood pressure immediately to the physician. Promptly obtain all cultures as ordered and monitor results. Administer antibiotics as ordered. Initiate and maintain appropriate isolation techniques for documented infection according to hospital policy. Implement client and family instructions regarding above measures.

from employees to clients. Another common mode of transmission is fecal contamination. Clients and staff must be careful to employ thorough handwashing after bowel movements and attending to personal hygiene.

It is also important to maintain a clean, uncluttered environment. Any drainage receptacles must be emptied and cleaned at least once each shift. The fluid in these containers provides an excellent media for microbial growth. A clean environment is essential to decreasing the incidence of nosocomial infections.

Any break in the body's protective barriers (skin and mucous membranes) provides a port of entry for microorganisms. Proper aseptic and sterile technique should be followed for invasive procedures.

In the leukemia client, an intravenous access line is necessary for administration of antibiotics, chemotherapy, and blood products. However, this creates a constant potential source of infection. Urinary catheterization, arterial cannulation, and invasive procedures (such as bone marrow aspiration, spinal tap punctures, and biopsies) are common causes of infections, particularly in the neutropenic, immunosuppressed leukemic client.

Meticulous care of intravenous and/or intra-arterial sites is most important. Many antibiotics and chemotherapeutic agents the client receives cause phlebitis, which further increases the chance of infection. The use of an antiseptic germicidal ointment, such as povidone-iodine (Betadine), is recommended at the puncture site. Sterile dressing changes at central venous catheter sites are recommended three times a week. Many hospitals recommend that intravenous sites be changed every 48 hours. However, in the leukemic client, this may not be feasible. Venous access in clients is usually obtained by insertion of scalp vein needles. Scalp vein needles often result in subcutaneous infiltration, necessitating frequent changes of sites. Also, redness and tenderness at insertion site or phlebitis often result in 3 to 5 days, and intravenous sites are changed at that time. Peripheral venous access becomes almost impossible in some leukemia clients and central venous access by subclavian or jugular catheter is required.

Recently studies have been completed on peripherally inserted silicone central venous catheters—Intrasil. These catheters are inserted by specially trained nurses through the basilic or cephalic vein. The catheter sites are cleaned and dressed with alcohol and povidone-iodine, and sterile dressings are applied three times a week and as needed. Dressing changes are performed by the infusion therapy team. These catheters have been kept in place from 2 to 180 days. The infection rate with these catheters is minimal, even in the leukemia client. However, the infection rate is directly proportional to the number of times the infusion system is opened for blood drawing, changing piggyback lines, and so forth.[16]

Prevention of infectious complications in the bedridden, neutropenic client creates one of the most challenging exercises in nursing. Frequent position changes, the use of Zimfoam mattresses, and active and passive motion exercises help to reduce the incidence of skin breakdown and subsequent infection. Severe thrombocytopenia is considered by some to be a limiting factor for activity. However, clients are able to safely tolerate mild forms of exercise (that is, range of motion and activities of daily living) even with platelet counts below 10,000/mm^3. The benefits of preventing infectious complications must be weighed against the risk of thrombocytopenic bleeding.

Because pulmonary infections are common in neutropenic clients, it is important to promote optimum ventilation. Clients mostly confined to bed must be encouraged to cough and deep breathe at frequent intervals as well as to change positions. Incentive spirometry and blow bottles are utilized to promote maximum expansion of the lungs and prevent infection and atelectasis.

Early detection of infectious complications is one of the primary responsibilities of the nurse. Vital signs must be taken at least every 4 hours, and significant deviations should be reported to the physician. The role of temperature as a heralding sign of infection has already been discussed. When fever is present, a careful scrutiny of the client is necessary to determine any clinical focus of infection. Physical examination is important to identify potential sources of infection. It is important to emphasize the nurse's responsibility in thoroughly investigating the many possible "hidden" sites of infections.

SPECIFIC TREATMENT MEASURES

Any open skin lesion is a potential site of infection and should be treated prophylactically. Lesions may be cleansed with povidone-iodine, followed with an application of topical povidone-iodine ointment. Sterile dressings may be needed. Without adequate neutrophils, drainage from an open lesion may not be present. Therefore, the absence of drainage is not indicative of a clean wound: cultures should be obtained from all open lesions, especially when the client is febrile.

Often the client will have specific complaints that alert the nurse to possible infection. Pain, burning, or frequency of urination are suggestive of a urinary tract infection. Proper collection of clean, voided midstream urine is vital for the isolation and identification of the infecting organism. Antibiotics should be initiated if the client is febrile but may be changed once the culture reports and sensitivity analysis are completed. The nurse should encourage the client to drink plenty of fluids to help prevent stasis of the urine in the bladder, which may further complicate the infection.

If a pulmonary infection is suspected, the physician may order a sputum culture. This culture may be difficult to obtain in the neutropenic client. Treatment with IPPB (intermittent positive pressure breathing) may be necessary to obtain a sputum specimen. Nasotracheal and transtracheal aspirations are other methods of obtaining material for culture and sensitivity tests. There are cases when extensive workup of pneumonia, including open lung biopsy, fails to yield the etiologic organism.

A sore mouth or throat is a common complaint among leukemia clients. Examination of the oral cavity may yield conclusive evidence about a possible infection. Oral candidiasis produces "white patchy areas" on the roof of the mouth, tongue, and throat. Chemotherapy-induced stomatitis may precede infection. Nursing intervention is aimed at prevention and early treatment of oral cavity infections.[7]

Time is a necessary ingredient in healing stomatitis and mucositis; any physical measures that promote comfort and keep the oral cavity clean are of the utmost importance. Specific treatment of oral candidiasis may incorporate a variety of agents. Nystatin (Mycostatin) in solution may be used to swish, gargle, and swallow; antifungal lozenges are helpful in treating candida. The dissolving lozenges have a more prolonged direct contact with the oral candidiasis and therefore are more therapeutic than liquid preparations. Vaginal troches or suppositories, such as nystatin or clotrimazole, are usually well tolerated orally when dissolved.

Toothbrushing with a soft toothbrush after meals continues to be important. Toothettes (sponge toothbrushes) are utilized if the client experiences gingival bleeding. Waterpiks are encouraged as an additional hygiene measure. In instances in which there is an increased amount of saliva production and oral secretions, clients may utilize tonsil-tip suction catheters to aspirate their own secretions. When possible, a dental consultation should be initiated prior to chemotherapy to assess the condition of the teeth and facilitate any needed dental work. Dentures may be temporarily removed if the client experiences complications of stomatitis.

There are many mouth rinses available. Frequent oral hygiene should be encouraged. Often the client may try a variety of oral rinse preparations before finding a satisfactory agent. Commonly used oral hygiene agents include Cēpacol, Listerine, and other commercially prepared rinses. These preparations may be beneficial initially but not well tolerated when inflammation begins and mucous membranes become denuded. Mouth rinses with salt and soda solutions (normal saline and bicarbonate) and hydrogen peroxide and water are often soothing. Xylocaine viscous used as a gargle and benzocaine (Cetacaine) topical spray are beneficial when stomatitis extends to the oral cavity and the client has difficulty swallowing. These agents have a temporary effect and should be used just prior to meals to promote dietary intake. At times, parenteral nutrition may be indicated when adequate nutritional support cannot be maintained because of severe stomatitis and dysphagia.

A mixture of diphenylhydramine and kaolin-pectin solution has been helpful for many clients in reducing discomfort and promoting healing. The kaolin-pectin acts as a protective coating on the oral mucosa, and the antihistamine effects of diphenylhydramine reduce the "sting" of the inflammation.

Lip lesions from herpes simplex are not uncommon in the neutropenic client. The lips should be kept well lubricated, and in some instances antiviral agents, such as adenine-arabinoside, will be applied. Gentian violet may also be useful when topically applied to the lesions.

Infections in the perirectal, vaginal, and groin areas are occasionally seen in neutropenic clients. It is essential that the nurse examine these areas for any sign or symptom of infection or inflammation. Careful perineal cleansing after bowel movements is necessary to prevent infection, particularly in the bedridden client. Hemorrhoids are a source of potential infection and must be observed for signs of inflammation or ulceration.[8]

Perirectal pain or discomfort may be the first signal the client has an abscess or fistula formation. Sitz baths, whirlpools, and tub baths are encouraged for clients with rectal lesions to promote comfort and healing. Open lesions may be cleansed with povidone-iodine (Betadine), followed by irrigations with normal saline. In severe cases of fecal-draining rectal fistulas, all oral intake may be prohibited and intravenous hyperalimentation administered until the rectal fistula heals. Surgical interventions and radiation therapy are sometimes beneficial.

Rectal temperature taking is often avoided to reduce the chance of infection in the neutropenic client. However, rectal temperatures may be necessary to obtain an accurate febrile picture. Proper lubrication and careful insertion of the thermometer should minimize complications. Stool softeners and mild laxatives are indicated to prevent straining from a hard bowel movement and to avoid fecal impaction. If an impaction occurs, the physician should be notified and extreme caution used in manual removal of feces.

Sepsis/septic shock

There is risk, particularly during remission-induction therapy, of a client developing septicemia and subsequently septic shock. The effective management of septic shock requires aggressive medical and nursing treatment. Antibiotics must be carefully administered and monitored. White blood cells and corticosteroids may be indicated. Vasopressors, such as dopamine, may be necessary to maintain systolic blood pressure and adequate renal perfusion. Mechanical ventilatory assistance and intubation are utilized when tissue oxygenation is not effectively maintained. Usually, intubation is elective and can be organized before an emergency situation exists. At times, the justification of such an aggressive therapeutic approach in leukemia clients is difficult. However, it must be remembered that if the client can be successfully managed during this crisis situation and the leukemia process controlled, there is a chance for a prolonged remission.

Isolation techniques

Isolation procedures may vary in different institutions. However, the principles remain the same. Reverse isolation is sometimes utilized in neutropenic clients as a measure to protect the client from potential sources of infection. Reverse isolation alone (gown, mask, and gloves) is not effective in significantly reducing the incidence and severity of infection. Most infections in the neutropenic client are endogenous; therefore, reverse isolation does not protect the client.

Studies have shown that masks alone are of minimal benefit in infection control for the neutropenic client. The only form of reverse isolation that significantly reduces the incidence and severity of infection is the protected environment program utilizing laminar airflow facilities or life island units in combination with other sterile procedures.

Isolation should be instituted for clients with documented infections known to be contagious to the general population. In addition, isolation guidelines must take into consideration the additional susceptibilities of the compromised immunosuppressed neutropenic client.

Complete (maximum, strict) isolation is utilized to prevent the transmission of communicable diseases that are spread by direct contact or airborne routes of transmission. Complete isolation incorporates the use of a single-client room with private bath facilities. All persons coming in contact with the client must don gown, mask, and gloves before entering the client's room.

Infections that require strict isolation in the leukemia population include:

- Active pulmonary tuberculosis (until adequate INH therapy is given)
- *Staphylococcus aureus* (septicemia, pneumonias, and extensively draining wounds)
- Group A beta hemolytic streptococcus (pneumonias, pharyngitis, and wound infections)
- Exanthematous infections (herpes zoster, measles, varicella, rubeola, rubella)

Protected environment

The *protected environment* (PE) program has proved to be effective in reducing the incidence and severity of infections during the remission-induction phase in the acute leukemia population. The original PE or "life island" units, designed in 1965, consist of an airtight plastic bubble that encloses a hospital bed. Air is pumped through high-efficiency particulate air (HEPA) filters that are capable of filtering microorganisms greater than 0.3 μ in diameter. The airflow is turbulent and exchanges at a rate of 10 to 15 times per hour. The plastic bubble or canopy provides a protective physical barrier from staff and visitors.[4]

There are disadvantages in the "life island" system in that client activity is limited because of the size of the bubble. The plastic material has a tendency to tear or rip with excessive movement or tension and presents a risk of environmental contamination. There is no plumbing facility with the life island system and bathwater must be heated and supplied by alternate methods.

The PE was further refined and improved in 1966 when a laminar airflow room (LAFR) was designed. This unit is built around a wall of HEPA filters. Air flows in a constant linear direction through the filters and is exchanged at a rate of 380 times per hour. This provides for more efficient filtration of particles from the air. The LAFR is better tolerated by the client because activity is not as limited as in the life island bubble. Sterile water can be made available through the use of special water filters, thus eliminating the need for outside water supply. The convenience of hot and cold running water is an obvious advantage to the client as well as the nursing staff. The LAFR also affords greater client accessibility. If necessary, personnel may don sterile attire and enter the room with minimal risk of contamination to the client.

The primary use of the PE is protection from infection during periods of profound myelosuppression from high-dose chemotherapy. Chemotherapy may be safely administered at higher (more effective) dosages when the client is in a protected environment unit.

Studies done at M. D. Anderson Hospital and Tumor Institute have demonstrated that clients treated in a PE have fewer infectious episodes than those in the general ward. The rate of remission is slightly, although not significantly, higher in clients in the PE. However, remission duration and survival rates were found to be significantly higher in clients treated in the PE. This difference has been attributed to the increased doses of chemotherapy that can be given in the PE because of reduced risk of infection.

Success of the PE unit is dependent on many interrelated factors. All clients in the unit should receive prophylactic or therapeutic antibiotics. Suppression of the normal flora of the skin, mucosa, and bowel is necessary to reduce contamination. The use of oral, nonabsorbable antibiotics and topical applications of antibiotic creams has proved to be efficacious in reducing the normal microbial flora.[2]

All food items must be sterilized before they are eaten. Any equipment entering the room must be sterilized and placed in the room by aseptic techniques. Client and room contamination must be monitored by air sampling and culture analysis. Particular items in the client's room (such as overbed tray, nurse call light, and television) should be cultured. Weekly cultures of the skin, nose, throat, ears, vagina, and stool should be obtained and monitored by the nursing staff and physician. Often contamination may be decreased by reinforcement from the nursing staff as to the purpose and application of the topical antibiotic and the importance of scrupulous personal hygiene.

Clients are encouraged to be as independent as possible in the LAFR. They are taught to apply all topical antibiotics and instructed to bathe from head to toe including daily shampoo with bacteriostatic soap. Clients who are not feeling well or are unable to care for themselves must be assisted by the nursing team to assure continuity of all procedures and to minimize bodily contamination.

Caring for the client in a PE presents a challenge to the nursing team. The needs of the client are sometimes magnified by the profound sense of isolation the client experiences. The average client's stay in the PE is 10 weeks. During that time, the client must be reassured that although physically isolated, every effort will be made to minimize the negative effect of isolation. The nursing team along with the physician, social worker, dietitian, and chaplain play an active role in meeting the needs of the isolated client, whether they be mental, physical, psychosocial, or spiritual. Continued positive reinforcement is important in maintaining client participation and cooperation during the isolation period.

INFECTIONS IN THE OUTPATIENT LEUKEMIA POPULATION

One of the basic philosophies in cancer nursing is to provide nursing interventions that improve not only the quantity but also the quality of life. With this in mind, plans for discharge are always considered when client management is feasible and safe in an outpatient setting. Studies have shown that many infections are hospital acquired; therefore, outpatient management of a leukemia client may indeed be safer from an infection-control standpoint. Generally, initial remission-induction therapy requires hospitalization because of the continuous administration of intense chemotherapeutic regimens.

Soon after remission-induction therapy, the client may be discharged and additional chemotherapy courses administered in an outpatient setting. There are some infection control guidelines the client must follow as an outpatient because subsequent courses of chemotherapy may still provide a risk of infection when the client is myelosuppressed. However, the trend and duration of myelosuppression are usually more predictable and manageable during maintenance chemotherapy.

Client and family instruction begins when the client is first diagnosed with leukemia. The client and family usually play an active role in the management of leukemia. Much time and effort is spent on client/family education. The guidelines for infection control may be familiar to the client because of previous hospitalization experience. However, on discharge the client assumes much more responsibility in managing self-care. Infection is the major cause for readmission in the leukemia client, therefore, the signs and symptoms to look for and general guidelines to follow must be understood.

The purpose of discharge teaching is to promote client independence and involvement in care and to ensure the safest outpatient course possible. The client and family are instructed on the danger of infection in leukemia clients and the importance and necessity of treatment. The schema of chemotherapy is reviewed, along with the client's usual response to therapy.

It is not necessary for clients to take their temperature every 4 hours when discharged unless there is a particular problem. Usually, clients are able to tell if their temperature is rising and should check it at that time. A temperature elevation greater than 101° F for 4 hours should be reported to the physician. Any other sign or symptom of infection, as previously discussed, should also be reported. The client is instructed not to take drugs containing aspirin or acetaminophen that may mask temperatures unless prescribed by the physician. No other medications (especially antibiotics) should be taken unless ordered by the physician. When antibiotics are ordered, the clients are instructed to continue taking the medication for the prescribed number of days even if they become symptomatically better.

It is usual for client/family to have many questions regarding infection control when the client is discharged. They have become accustomed to the protective nurturing aspect of hospitalization and may actually be fearful of discharge. Instructions are given to promote as much independence as possible and to reduce any unnecessary limitations. Often the client needlessly refrains from activities because of fear of infection when this is unnecessary from a medical standpoint.

Clients are instructed to avoid obviously contagious individuals. With that exception, it is safe to resume normal group activities and be exposed to crowds. Clients commonly ask about the risk of catching "colds or flu" from crowds. In general, this need not concern clients when they are in complete remission because the clinical course for viruses and colds is essentially the same as in the overall population.

Virtually all physical activities can be resumed when the client is in complete remission. It is usually necessary to build up some physical tolerance after discharge, and the time it takes to "get back to normal" varies with each client. Most clients in complete remission are able to return to their usual activities.

Questions may arise regarding sexual and physical contact. Sexual practices usually may be resumed without danger of infection when discharged; however, the importance of cleanliness and personal hygiene should be discussed. It is not unusual for clients to have a fear of resuming sexual intercourse after hospitalization, particularly if there has been a prolonged period of abstinence. It is important to allay any unnecessary fears of anxiety and promote open communications regarding sexual activity.

CASE STUDY

Mr. J. O. is a 24-year-old white male who sought medical attention from his local physician because of a 2-day history of blurred vision. The physical examination revealed bilateral retinal hemorrhages, and further workup revealed a platelet count of 20,000/mm³, hemoglobin of 8 gm%, and a white count of 75,000/mm³ with many circulating blast cells. Bone marrow analysis was performed, and a diagnosis of AML was made the same day. After discussion of alternative methods of therapy, J. O. elected to be referred to M. D. Anderson Hospital and Tumor Institute, a major comprehensive cancer research center, for treatment.

Nursing admission assessment elicited a complex list of client needs and problems as well as potential problems that could arise as a result of treatment. The following lists the major client needs and problems on admission.

Active problems

1. Newly diagnosed, untreated acute leukemia
2. Blurred vision
3. High circulating WBC's
4. Low platelet count
5. Scattered petechiae
6. Anemia
7. Wife 4 months pregnant
8. Relocation of wife to Houston
9. Interruption of medical school
10. Minimal knowledge of leukemia and treatment
11. Admission to protected environment 2 days prior to Christmas holidays

Potential problems

1. Infection
2. Hemorrhage
3. Anemia
4. Physical isolation from wife (with protected environment)
5. Limited control of environment and usual activities
6. Failure to respond to treatment
7. Inability to cope with stress of initial diagnosis, treatment, and long-term management of disease

Nursing interventions were directed at minimizing the actual client problems, preventing potential problems from occurring, and initiating appropriate interventions for complications that arose.

J. O. was treated in the protected environment with AdOAP (Adriamycin, Oncovin, Ara-C, and prednisone), prophylactic systemic antibiotics, and topical prophylactic ointment and gels. The first week in the protected environment was uneventful, except for the holiday fanfare with sterile turkey and dressing and Santa's visit. A bone marrow analysis on day 8 of course 1 revealed no reduction in leukemic infiltrate. The client's peripheral white blood count decreased from 169,000/mm³ to 1,300 on day 9 with an AGC less than 1,000. He became febrile and his systemic prophylactic antibiotics were discontinued and he was started on carbenicillin and netilmicin intravenously. A central venous line was inserted for optimum venous access.

Subsequent bone marrow aspirations continued to show no improvement in leukemia status and an additional 5 days of Ara-C and weekly VCR were given. On day 23 of the initial AdOAP course, his leukemia infiltrate was still unchanged and a second course of AdOAP was begun. This course was altered to provide 10 days of prednisone therapy and weekly administrations of vincristine because his morphologic diagnosis changed from AML to ALL. J. O.'s fever pattern continued, although masked by prednisone therapy. No source of infection was identified. Platelet counts hovered at 10,000 to 20,000/mm^3 with no incidence of hemorrhage.

Bone marrow analysis on day 11 of the second course revealed a hypocellular bone marrow and hopes for possible response to chemotherapy. Course 3 was begun on day 16 with a hemoglobin of 10.2 gm%, platelets of 21,000/mm^3, and a white blood count of 900/mm^3.

The problems began about 1 week after the initiation of course 3. J. O.'s white cell count ranged from 400 to 800 and his platelet count from 8,000 to 20,000/mm^3. On day 11, J. O. developed a fever of 103° F. Routine cultures were taken and a chest x-ray film was within normal limits. His antibiotics were again changed. On day 12, J. O. showed no response to the new antibiotics and the decision to start white cell transfusions was made. J. O. also noted the onset of dizziness. A check of his hemoglobin revealed a decrease in a matter of hours without any obvious signs of hemorrhage.

During this time J. O. became very weak and lethargic. He had to depend on the nursing staff for all his needs. He was bathed twice daily with pHisoHex and sterile water, his antibiotic creams and gels were applied, and he was fed sterile food by the nursing staff. His wife, now 6 months pregnant, slept nightly beside the life island bubble and never left her husband's side.

On days 14 and 17, bone marrow analysis again revealed a hypocellular marrow, a report that carried both joy and deepening concern for the client with it. The hypocellular marrow meant that the leukemic cells had been destroyed but that the normal marrow elements had not yet begun to regenerate. The fear of a regeneration of leukemic cells also loomed in the air.

On day 17 of the third course, J. O. developed melena. The next day, with a platelet count of 9,000/mm^3, J. O. had two episodes of rectal bleeding in which he lost approximately 250 ml of blood. After the gastrointestinal bleeding, his hemoglobin had dropped from 9.8 gm% to 7.8 gm%. He was immediately transfused with 2 units of packed red blood cells and 4 units of platelets. After the platelet transfusion, no further indications of hemorrhage were found.

White cell transfusions continued on a daily basis as J. O. remained febrile. Five hours after J. O. received a white blood cell transfusion, he developed tachypnea with very shallow respirations at 50 per minute. A chest x-ray film at that time showed increased pulmonary infiltrates. *Pseudomonas aeruginosa* was identified on an earlier blood culture. Arterial blood gas analysis showed $Pa{O_2}$, 58%; $P{CO_2}$, 18, and pH, 7.55. His temperature spiked at 105° F. The clinical picture was consistent with a pneumonia and consolidation of white blood cells in the lungs. J. O. was started on hydrocortisone, 500 mg every 6 hours. The wide strip of adhesive tape used to prevent air leakage from around the zipper on the life island bubble was removed in order to facilitate emergency entry into the bubble should that become necessary.

As a result of the steroid therapy, J. O. became less tachypneic and his temperature defervesced to 100° F. However, J. O.'s problems were not over yet. He began to complain of muffled hearing. This was thought to be due to the use of aminoglycoside antibiotics that J. O. was receiving. However, the antibiotics could not be discontinued as they were needed to control his very serious infection.

On day 20 of the third course, just 2 days after the episode of rectal bleeding and 1 day after the episode of tachypnea and high fever, he was started on antifungal therapy with amphotericin B. A superinfection of candida was suspected because of his high fever (105° F despite antibiotics and white cell transfusions) and its rapid response to steroid therapy.

As J. O.'s condition seemed to stabilize, he again had an episode of rectal hemorrhage. His hemoglobin dropped by 2 gm%. He was transfused with packed red blood cells and platelets. Once again his condition stabilized.

Throughout the next 2 weeks J. O.'s condition gradually improved. His strength increased and he was able to bathe himself and sit up in bed for his meals. Bone marrow analysis on days 17, 20, 25, 28, 32, and 35 continued to be hypocellular without enough cells to be counted. His peripheral white cell count and platelet counts began to increase steadily from day 35. A bone marrow analysis on day 39 was done. Although still hypocellular, there were no leukemic cells. This fact, together with his increasingly normal peripheral blood counts, led the physicians to believe that J. O. had achieved a very early complete remission.

J. O.'s future now looked very encouraging. The physical therapy department was consulted to help start an active exercise program in the bubble for J. O. He had lost much strength and muscle mass when he became so critically ill. He worked at his exercises faithfully. J. O. even began to read through his medical textbooks, which had been sterilized for him at the beginning of his hospitalization. His wife, now 7 months pregnant, finally got the rest she so richly deserved. She had spent many sleepless days and nights standing next to the bubble, holding onto her husband through the plastic gloves and hoping and praying he would survive.

Finally on day 47 of the third course, 85 days after J. O. entered the hospital, their prayers were answered. Bone marrow analysis revealed a blast cell count of 2%. Hemoglobin was now 10.9 gm%, platelets were 153,000/mm^3, and white cells were 1,800 with an absolute granulocyte count of greater than 1,000. J. O. had achieved a complete remission. He was released from the bubble amid cheers from the medical and nursing team. His wife, who had not even touched her husband in almost 3 months, just put her arms around him and cried.

After a routine lumbar puncture with prophylactic intrathecal cytosine arabinoside, J. O. was discharged from the hospital to begin his maintenance chemotherapy as an outpatient.

Discussion

J. O.'s case included several of the complications associated with leukemia and its treatment. The most significant principle to highlight is that high doses of chemotherapy were administered, rendering the bone marrow hypoplastic for several weeks, and measures of protective isolation, antibiotics, granulocyte, platelet, and red blood transfusions were utilized to support him until his bone marrow regenerated with normal cells.

J. O. required constant nursing attention during the critical phases of his illness. He suffered physical complications as well as severe psychologic and emotional stress. Therefore, nursing interventions were aimed at meeting both his physical and emotional needs.

He was hospitalized for 86 days to undergo chemotherapy for complete remission. Eighty-three days were spent in a sterile life island bubble. His success story is a result of the efforts of many individuals, years of intensive research, and the availability of unconventional methods to treat a life-threatening disease. J. O. is currently off all chemotherapy, active in medical school, and enjoying his wife and 2-year-old son.

CONCLUSION

Remission induction therapy for acute leukemia is best managed in major treatment centers that have supportive therapy available as well as highly trained individuals monitoring client care. Many advances have been made in the chemotherapy of leukemia. The major cause of morbidity and mortality is infection. The utilization of protected environments, antibiotic therapy, and granulocyte transfusions have significantly reduced the mortality from infections.

Historically, leukemia has been considered a fatal disease; however, with appropriate treatment, many clients can expect complete remission from the disease with hope for long-term survival. Nurses can be valuable members of the team treating these clients by stressing the importance of infection control procedures as well as providing instruction to the client and family.

REFERENCES

1. Beland, I.: Clinical nursing: pathophysiological and psychological approaches, New York, 1970, Macmillan, Inc.
2. Bodey, G. P.: Isolation for the compromised host, J.A.M.A. **233:**543, 1975.
3. Bodey, G. P., and Rodriquez, V.: Protected environment-prophylactic antibiotic programmes; microbiological studies, Clin. Haematol. **5**(2):395, 1976.
4. Bodey, G. P., Watson, P., Cooper, C., and Freireich, E. J.: Protected environment units for cancer patients, CA **21:**214, 1971.
5. Bodey, G. P., et al.: Supportive care in the management of the cancer patient. In Clark, R. L., and Howell, C. D., editors: Cancer patient care, Chicago, 1976, Year Book Medical Publishers, Inc., p. 581.
6. Bouchard, R., and Owens, N.: Nursing care of the cancer patient, ed. 3, St. Louis, 1976, The C. V. Mosby Co.
7. Bruya, M., and Maderia, N.: Stomatitis after chemotherapy, Am. J. Nurs. **75**(8):1349, 1975.
8. Burkhalter, P. K., and Donley, D. L.: Dynamics of oncology nursing, New York, 1978, McGraw-Hill Book Co.
9. Clark, R. L., and Howe, C. D.: Cancer patient care, Chicago, 1976, Year Book Medical Publishers, Inc.
10. Donley, D.: Nursing the patient who is immunosuppressed, Am. J. Nurs. **76**(10):1619, 1976.
11. Donovan, M. I., and Pierce, S. G.: Cancer care nursing, New York, 1976, Appleton-Century-Crofts.
12. Freireich, E. J., et al.: Therapy of acute myelogenous leukemia, Cancer **42**(2):874, 1978.
13. Gunz, F., and Baekie, A.: Leukemia, New York, 1974, Grune & Stratton, Inc.
14. Keating, M. J., et al.: Acute leukemia in adults, 1977, CA **27**(1):2, 1977.
15. Keating, M. K.: Personal communication, 1979.
16. Lawson, M., Bottino, J., and McCredie, K.: Long term infusion therapy, Am. J. Nurs. **6:**1100, 1979.
17. Levine, A. S., and Deisseroth, A. B.: Recent developments in the supportive therapy of acute myelogenous leukemia, Cancer **42**(2):883, 1978.
18. Lister, T. A., and Yankee, R. A.: Blood component therapy, Clin. Haematol. **7**(2):407, 1978.
19. McCredie, K., et al.: Blood components in the care of the cancer patient, Curr. Probl. Cancer **III**(1):4, 1978.
20. Madhaven, T., and Van Slyck, E.: Using drugs for the compromised patient: infections in acute leukemia, Drug Ther. **7:**56, 1977.
21. Rodriquez, V., and Bodey, G. P.: Antibacterial therapy—special considerations in neutropenic patients, Clin. Haematol. **5**(2):347, 1976.
22. Rodriquez, V., et al.: Randomized trial of protected environment-prophylactic antibiotics in 145 adults with acute leukemia, Medicine **57**(3):253, 1978.
23. Schumann, D., and Coindreau, P.: The adult with acute leukemia, Nurs. Clin. North Am. **7:**743, 1972.
24. Valdivieso, M.: Bacterial infections in haematological diseases, Clin. Haematol. **5**(2):229, 1976.
25. Weirnick, P. H.: Treatment of acute leukemia in adults, Clin. Haematol. **7**(2):259, 1978.

27

Female sexuality and gynecologic cancer

SAUNDRA ELAINE SAUNDERS

RECOGNITION OF A NEED

In the treatment of clients for gynecologic cancer today, it might seem obvious that whatever treatment is done to or for the client can be interpreted as an assault on the individual's sexuality. Yet only a few years ago it was not routine to discuss sexual changes with the individual. Emphasis was placed on the expected effectiveness of the treatment and the anatomic changes. Very little, if any, emphasis was placed on sexual consequences nor was the individual or anyone significant to the individual given much opportunity to ask questions concerning sexuality or to explore alternatives that would be acceptable for both parties.

The reluctance of the caregiver to discuss sexual matters may have been due to several factors. Among these are embarrassment in discussing the topic of sex and sexual function, a lack of basic knowledge in regard to alternate forms and methods of sexual expression, not knowing what resources are available to the individual for sexual counseling, and a tendency to totally interchange the terms sexuality and sexual activity when sexuality is indeed a far broader concept.

In response to the so-called sexual revolution, some members of the health care system have begun to look at how concepts used in sexual counseling for the "healthy" populace might be applied to the care of those individuals who, through an illness, find themselves in the acute care setting. A knowledge of body image development and how the concept of sexuality relates to that development and its importance should be a starting point in helping the health caregiver learn how to intervene more effectively when there is a potential for sexual dysfunction. Included in this learning of concepts should be time for self-awareness concerning attitudes toward sexuality, as well as possible dysfunctions and alternatives or options.

THE CONCEPT OF SEXUALITY

Body image

Body image is a combination of individuals' perceptions and the cues that people receive from the environment and those around them; it has been identified by Kolb[3] as having four major components. First, the *body perception* consists of the accumulated reactions of the individual to sensory experiencing of the body. It begins with tactile stimuli through early self-exploration and is later expanded with visual cues as the individual grows and observes through sight the changes that occur within and of the body. Second, the individual *body concept* relates to those thoughts, feelings, attitudes, and memories that evolve as the individual views his or her body in relation to others. Third, the *body ego* is an idealized body image brought about by the perceptions and viewing aspects of the individual's personality. The ego functions to integrate any change or disparity within the body image that may lead to an arousal of either painful or pleasurable effects. Fourth, the *body ideal* is the concept the individual holds as being desirable and against which the individual measures his or her perceptions and concepts held in regard to his or her own body.

Therefore, it can be seen that body image encompasses both the physical and emotional aspects of an individual's self-concepts. Body image is ever-changing and calls for adjustment throughout the individual's life in the normal maturing and aging process. It can include such perceptions as the size, shape, and posture of the body; the attitudes held toward the function, use, and necessary care of the body; as well as the personality type and emotional changes and responses of the individual in relation to his or her own body and to others.

Finally, the self-concept perceptions of the body image are further tempered by input from the environment as well as the response of others toward the individual.

Definition and components of sexuality

Sexuality in its entirety becomes a major part of the individual's body image as he or she matures and begins to explore the meanings of his or her own maleness or femaleness. It is that part of the body image that deals with the individual's instincts, drives, and behaviors, in relation to being sexual and to sexual activity. The individual's sexual identity is composed of attributes that are either predominantly male or female with neither grouping of attributes existing without a portion of the other.

Sexuality is usually seen as that force that encourages us toward seeking a mate and developing a relationship of sharing both passive and aggressive aspects of ourselves. Sharing not only through our thoughts and actions of caring but also through our bodies as we nurture and give pleasure to ourselves and others.

Sexuality includes a range of relationships among females and males. The term "sexuality" encompasses such concepts as attractiveness versus repulsiveness, openness in relationships versus guardedness or isolation, and warmth and nurturing versus coldness and fear of giving or an inability to receive. None of these concepts is an all-or-nothing idea, rather they can be found on a continuum. The messages individuals give themselves as well as those they receive from others will determine how fully they will grow and function as sexual beings. The way individuals view themselves as sexual beings, both giving and receiving, will determine how they will relate to others of their own or the opposite sex.

When feminine sexuality is considered alone, some of the concepts initially brought to mind are attractiveness, shapeliness, seductiveness, softness, warmth, nurturing, and mothering. All of the above can be greatly altered when a woman finds herself confronted with a dread disease that can not only threaten her life but also her reproductivity and desirability as well.

When a woman has a gynecologic cancer, her life-style may be threatened more profoundly than can be perceived on the surface initially, owing to the fact that a major portion of her self-concepts, rooted in her being, will need to undergo alteration and reassimilation. Her ability to effectively assimilate changes in her sexual self caused by the disease and/or treatment will depend on how well she relates to herself and her relationships with others. A healthy assimilation depends on the responsiveness of those around her and the help she receives.

ASSAULT TO SEXUALITY

The stigma of cancer

Cancer in general carries with it a stigma not seen with most other life-threatening or chronic illnesses outside of perhaps leprosy, venereal disease, and mental illness. The word "cancer" conjures up ideas of lack of control, dirtiness, foulness, contagion, pain, despair, punishment, and death. With all these negatives how does one begin to help the victims of cancer salvage reasonable lives for themselves?

Time and again my clients refer to their inability to discuss their illness with friends because of a fear of being repulsed or repulsive. The messages they receive are that cancer happens to those who are unclean or have little control over their lives and therefore they are feared as much as the disease itself.

Jean was a young divorced woman with cervical cancer who had been in the hospital for some time undergoing a workup and external radiation therapy. She had been isolated from her family because of the great distance, and she looked forward with longing to a weekend pass when she would see her family. When she returned on Monday, I found her in tears and was told by the staff that she had been crying continuously since her return. We initially thought she was homesick but later found that she was "heartsick" and felt worthless. She stated that she would never return home and undergo that humiliation again. It seemed that her family and friends appeared to fear her and considered her disease to be contagious. They had not allowed her to eat with the family but forced her to eat elsewhere on disposable dishes. She was only allowed in certain rooms that were sprayed heavily with disinfectant. She was not allowed to use the usual family bathroom, and worse yet, she had not received one *touch* from those she had previously missed so much. Jean was isolated, apparently untouchable, and therefore unlovable and worthless.

One of the first things the staff gave to Jean was our "touch" whenever the opportunity arose to begin to instill the concept that we saw her as a worthy human being, capable of being loved and cared about. We allowed her to vent her anger at her isolation and gave her feedback on what might be causing the isolation (mainly fear on the part of the family and friends stemming from ignorance of what caused the illness, the potential dangers, and what could be expected). We tried to reach the family in hopes of determining their concerns and giving them information, but we were unable to overcome a fear so great that it prevented even Jean's mother, to whom she had formerly felt close, from visiting her.

The family physician was advised of the problem and was willing to meet with the family and try to be a support person for Jean as she returned to her former life-style. In the meantime, for the remainder of her hospitalization we encouraged Jean in activities that could reinforce her self-worth including assisting the volunteers and doing odd jobs with and for the staff. We wanted to help her acquire a self-concept strong enough to weather any negative feedback she might receive.

As she was reinforced with concepts of her ability to be productive and assured that those who understood what was happening to her still found her acceptable and not repulsive, she was able to better determine how to use resources to work out her own fears. She learned that some people would always be fearful and therefore unable to be close and helpful, but that there were others who could overcome fears with knowledge and therefore could be receptive to her. To the former she became more tolerant and toward the latter she became more able to be vulnerable and therefore to give and receive. None of this was done overnight but spanned many months with a lot of sincere help until she was able to emerge as a stronger person.

The preceding success is not always the case, however, and I wonder what would have happened to Jean had we not been able to perceive her needs and openly share our concerns and caring before she had a chance to become completely isolated.

It is imperative that we open up avenues to the loved ones of the cancer client for information seeking and exploring of feelings and needs. Recently two clients discussed with me what had happened to their marriages since the occurrence of cancer. Mary was now 5 years from her original bout with cancer and on the verge of getting a divorce. Her husband had not touched Mary since her original diagnosis, and when she had encouraged him to speak with the physician, he had refused saying he could not discuss such topics with someone else. The two of them had therefore lived in cohabitation with essentially no communication. Mary became so demoralized over this that she gained over 150 pounds, which succeeded in giving her another self-inflicted reason for being undesirable.

Recently she had undergone a local excision of a small lesion on the vulva to rule out recurrence of her cervical cancer. The lesion was benign, and most of the vulva remained intact. In discussing the effects, if any, on her ability to be sexually active, she shared her fears of the last 5 years and her feelings of being repulsive—so why not be? At this time she felt she had tried to reach her husband and felt it was time to give up the marriage and realize that he simply had no desire to be helped.

As we talked, we discussed her feelings about herself. She did wish to be sexually active. The cancer had not frightened her away; inconsistency in her lover had. As we reviewed her assets, she was able to agree that she was a pretty, warm, outgoing, and intelligent person, all positives in developing a new image of herself as able to withstand trauma and to be an attractive and lovable individual. On discharge she had enrolled in Weight Watcher's, hopefully on her way to a better self-image.

Her roommate, however, felt differently. Ruth's husband was being very close and loving. He was not afraid of her cancer, either catching it or spreading it. He was fearful for his wife. Having lost his mother to uterine cancer, this only pushed him to remain even closer to his wife. He was angry at the threat to her life and wished to be as strong for her as he possibly could be. He wanted to hold her close to him for as much time as possible.

Ruth, however, was frightened, felt fragile, and had some feelings that sexual activity was related to her disease. After talking with Ruth and her husband they were both able to share their concerns with me and with one another during several discussions. Throughout this time, Ruth began feeling freer and less fearful, and her husband found ways to express his love with consideration to the timing of her feelings and fears, giving her room to explore and grow.

A colleague in psychiatry once stated that no one was known to have died from a hug, but an individual sure could die from the lack of one. Being lovable and hugable is very important to our survival as sexual beings and individuals. Disseminating information and attitudes designed to dispel the stigma of cancer would certainly have a great deal of impact on the approachability of the person with cancer and therefore be a constantly worthwhile goal.

Cancer as a chronic illness

The chronicity of cancer can and often does have a great impact on the individual's sexuality and sexual responsiveness. There are constant interruptions and alterations in the life-style of the individual made necessary by prolonged treatment and follow-up. The constant reminder of the illness caused by frequent return appointments has been pointed to by several clients as causing them periodic episodes of anxiety that affects their relationship with their loved ones. Several have felt a "burden" when a loved one needs to make special effort to provide transportation to and from the appointments or treatment. Roles often change or are reversed during the illness, requiring understanding and assistance as the individual attempts to adjust to a new life-style.

Perhaps the gains and losses of the illness, with remissions and exacerbation or treatment for palliation, is what affects the individual's sense of herself and her sexuality the most. Chronic weakness, fatigue, loss or thinning of hair, and loss of muscle and fatty masses that affect body contour can in differing degrees lead to a sense of fragility, self-abhorrence, inadequacy, and defeatism. At such times, the individual often has little interest in "sexual activity," and yet to prevent isolation she definitely needs the touch, closeness, and strength of those she loves and wants so to be loved by.

Recently, a student in my class had read a small book written by a woman who had suffered breast cancer and had subsequently undergone several remissions and exacerbations of the disease. In the book she described how she felt about riding the waves of gains and losses that sometimes seemed pleasantly rolling, giving her time to adjust to the change, and at other times overwhelmingly tumultuous, leaving her little sense of control. The student, her husband, and friends developed a 15-minute film portraying the feelings the woman expressed. Looking in mirrors and finally being afraid to look for the changes wrought in one's own face can have a frightening and wearing quality of its own. When the individual feels her worst, what is helpful are times for rest and renewal along with the added care that allows any of us to look our best. Encouraging and helping the chronically ill woman to continue her usual routine to enhance her attractiveness allows her to present her best image to herself and those she loves. Planning for that time is just as important as the treatment and medications necessary to her care.

As health professionals, we need to be cognizant of just how disruptive chronic illness is and how little "normal" sharing time couples have for their hopes, fears, and love. Once we recognize this concept, facilitating closeness can be a worthwhile and rewarding goal. Allowing extended visiting privileges and privacy not only when someone is dying of cancer but when they are living and fighting with it can be a warm and rewarding experience.

Susan spent much of the last 1½ years of her life in the hospital with recurrent ovarian cancer and small bowel obstruction. Her husband was captain of a freighter that traveled from our shores to Europe and back. They had been married 5 years after having been separated by the iron curtain for 12 years before their marriage. Their love for each other was apparent and there was so little time to be at home and alone.

Susan was a striking woman with thick auburn hair she kept immaculate even when weakened with her illness. We talked about the unfairness of the disease coming at this point in their lives and the changes it had wrought in her life. As she spoke through her tears and her concerns about the vomiting and her chemotherapy became apparent, Charles suddenly came to her side and caressed her hair. She asked if something were wrong and he said only that he wished to touch her. The beauty they shared was shared with me for a moment and yet every day I find health professionals living by rules that do not allow for such moments.

Somehow when we bring individuals into our institutions we expect them to harness their sexual needs and expressions or assume that their needs center on treatment for the disease and have nothing to do with the sexual beings they are. I wonder what effect our response has on the expression of those same needs once they return to their own homes. It would seem so simple to pull curtains, close doors, plan for private time, encourage closeness and touch, and yet we have to seemingly walk out on a limb to do just that. In so doing, the people we serve and we ourselves miss out on one of the greatest gifts, particularly at times of stress and vulnerability, that of human sharing and loving.

Cancer treatment

Surgical procedures. Treatment for cancer, necessary to survival, can assault the individual's sexuality as intensely if not more so than the illness itself. Surgery is the one treatment modality in which time and energy needs to be allowed for the necessary changes in body image. Whether the individual experiences a change in body function such as a colostomy or ileal conduit, suffers a visible loss such as a breast, or "only" has a scar that designates the loss of the ability to reproduce with loss of the uterus, an adjustment time is necessary. Time needs to be given to these women to allow them to share their feelings and fears about their survival and about themselves as functioning women.

Too often in the past we have assumed that to be rid of such a threatening disease was the ultimate answer and goal. However, when considering quality of life, it would seem that the individual would need to be able to perceive herself as continuing with living with some aspect of normalcy for any treatment to be an effective and reasonable addition to the individual's life.

With this in mind, encouraging the practice of giving the individual time to assimilate information concerning the recommended surgery and its outcomes, sharing concerns with loved ones regarding the changes, and looking at any possible options can have impact on the eventual rehabilitation of the individual. Whenever possible, effort should be made to include sexual partners or significant others in discussing outcomes of treatment. This gives the professional an opportunity to assess the needs of both individuals as well as to facilitate more open communication between the partners in a hopefully nonthreatening atmosphere.

If there is not a sexual partner, it should not be assumed that the interest in sexual matters may not be just as important when considering the future. The more involved the partners can become and the more they have an outlet to verbalize fears and frustrations, the better able they will be to adapt and be supportive and close following surgery. If they cannot do this, it can be a time to work through the loss and find other means of support for the person with cancer.

Ann was 33 years old when told she needed a vulvectomy and abdominoperineal resection for cancer of the vulva. Her husband was 29 years old, and they had two children. She knew she could remain sexually active following the vulvectomy with reconstructive surgery, but her feelings about the impending colostomy truly threatened her integrity as a desirable and functional woman. She had worked in a nursing home where ostomy appliances were old, malodorous, and ineffective. In a discussion with her husband, she cried and said she could not be an embarrassment to him and their children.

We explored the literature on ostomies and new appliances together with an emphasis on the normalcy of life that many ostomates have acquired for themselves. Ann became more positive, and her husband, shy of expressing his needs and now knowing hers, willingly accepted help from the husband of an ostomate from the Ostomy Association. Of course there were adjustments, but Ann and her husband have weathered them and are supportive to each other and sexually active at this time. Her husband felt that had someone not given them the time to share concerns and ongoing support that allowed him to be an active part of his wife's care, he might not have handled the necessary changes so well. Both could be proud of their sharing.

Audrey underwent a vulvectomy 36 years into a rewarding marriage. The surgery and its results were carefully explained to both her and her husband, including the morbidity of wound breakdown. Audrey's husband felt that as long as Audrey would be alright, they would work through the change. Audrey, however, was afraid that her husband would be repulsed by her. Time was given to both individuals to express their concerns individually and together.

When it was time for Audrey to be discharged, she still needed wound care which her husband said he would willingly do. We discussed with him thoroughly what he would see before he watched the dressing procedure. Audrey anxiously watched his face as he observed the procedure. He could not look at his wife and later talked with the nurse about how large the scar seemed and how painful he had imagined it would be. Although he had held her hand, his inability to look at Audrey had convinced her that he could not love her tattered self and she wept quietly much of the evening and night, unable to be consoled.

The next day Audrey's husband arrived at the time of the dressing change, strode over to the sink to wash his hands, turned to smile at his wife and the nurse, and said, "Now, what is it that I need to do?" Audrey beamed, and as her husband proceeded with his lesson, he openly shared his concern of hurting her and finished off with a hug and a kiss. He had spent a sleepless night because he wanted so to rise to the occasion and was frightened he might not and, therefore, hurt the woman he loved. They both needed time to work through their own fears before they could again be the loving team they had always been.

Many others are not so fortunate. Some relationships will not last through such an assault. Emphasizing positive aspects of the individuals and their sexuality as well as allowing them grieving time can be the most beneficial interventions we can use. We have not extended ourselves enough if an individual leaves our care permanently convinced she is less than feminine.

Radiation therapy. Radiation therapy can assault sexuality through remote means, owing to weakness, fatigue, and malaise as side-effects from therapy over extensive areas of the body, or directly, when treatment calls for pelvic irradiation. For the former the same concepts apply as for chronic illness. When considering pelvic irradiation, the effects can include sterilization for the premenopausal woman; cessation of menses, which is an outward evidence of feminity to some; and the formation of pelvic fibrosis with subsequent painful or interrupted coitus.

The young woman needs to be fully informed of the effects of radiation on ovarian function and what options are available should she suffer symptoms of menopause. These symptoms occur gradually as the dosage increases and may not even be noticed by many individuals, whereas surgical removal of the ovaries usually can be expected to present dramatic symptoms within a few days after surgery. Again, it is helpful to assist the woman to identify the clues she uses to recognize herself as a feminine being and to allow her time to explore her feelings regarding the proposed change.

We know that pelvic fibrosis will occur, and without proper intervention the pelvic tissues will lose all of their flexibility and resiliency. The vagina becomes a narrow and hardened tube that either prevents coitus secondary to vaginal inadequacy or coitus may become so painful that the individual elects to cease having sexual relations.

To prevent the formation of extensive fibrosis, we ask our clients to use a vaginal dilator on a daily basis during and up to 6 months following therapy. The use of the dilator breaks down forming adhesions and allows for distensibility of the vagina. The dilator is made from clear Lucite and has a curved handle for comfort in its use.

Asking someone to use a vaginal dilator can have many ramifications. Some individuals will relate the use of the dilator to a form of masturbation. Their attitude in this regard will determine how readily they will accept its use as part of their therapy. Therefore, those attitudes need to be carefully explored in a nonthreatening manner. Time is given to the individuals to discuss the pros and cons and their feelings regarding the device.

Many individuals have coined sometimes comical names for their dilators or the activity itself. They are encouraged to remain sexually active if they have been previously and are told that on the days they have vaginal intercourse they need not use the dilator. This is another way to give them permission to be sexually active. Comparison studies of our client population have shown that those individuals using a dilator have less pelvic fibrosis, easier and more well-defined pelvic examinations, and have remained sexually active, while the reverse has been found for those individuals who have not used the dilator.

Some physicians feel that if a client understands that it is permissible to have sexual intercourse, she can maintain patency of the vagina in this way. However, this does not take into account what would seem a fairly common fear of individuals that intercourse might cause injury, spread the disease, or allow for contagion to the partner. These fears often prevent sexual activity for some at least until treatment is over.

For those who do have fibrosis preventing intercourse, counseling should be available to explore needs of sexual expression and different approaches to fulfilling those needs. Showing tolerance and giving permission to explore such concerns is an important aspect of these individuals' care if we are to help them maintain a sense of wholeness and feminine worth. It is suggested that including private time for the assessment of sexual concerns should be a part of any interview with an individual who is about to undergo a treatment that will assault her sexuality.

Cancer chemotherapy. Probably the most obvious assaults to sexuality when the individual is undergoing chemotherapy have to do with such things as hair loss and weight loss when experiencing the side-effects of nausea and vomiting. The American Cancer Society in many institutions provides a free supply of wigs to be given to individuals using drugs that are likely to cause hair loss. It is recommended that the time to discuss and select wigs is before the therapy is instituted. Armed with the immediate ability to disguise hair loss, if and when it occurs, gives a feeling of security. Most women dread being bald and an object of ridicule or awe. Hair is seen as a part of the individual's total image. For a woman who considers herself plain, having beautiful full-bodied hair that is kept immaculate may be viewed as a feminine extension of herself. Many view hair as seductive. To be threatened by a loss of this cherished body part is overwhelming in itself but can be dealt with more easily if props are readily available to disguise the loss of a beautifying attribute.

It takes time to adjust to a smaller frame, and certain clothing styles are more becoming to the individual who has suffered weight loss. Taking time to give feedback, encouragement, and suggestions can be most helpful. We should be sure to give compliments when a woman looks nice, but it is not helpful if she perceives the compliment as a kindness rather than a true evaluation.

Betty illustrated this concept when she reacted negatively to her physician telling her she looked like a rose only 5 days after starting her on hyperalimentation for severe cachexia. She stated that she could look in the mirror and realize that he was giving her a well-intentioned lie. Because of such white lies, she was having trouble with her feelings and needs for a "trust" relationship with her physician and the staff. She did, however, appreciate suggestions for enhancing her coloring and appearance with makeup and clothing as well as an honest discussion that optimum results from hyperalimentation would be a long time coming until body stores could be replenished.

Once this was shared with her physician, a more open and honest relationship developed with the giving and receiving of truthful feedback. Betty had been a pretty young woman before her illness, and as months passed her prettiness returned and she was able to recognize it.

So often in wanting to be helpful we miss our chance to really be so by glazing over the facts of the individual's situation and therefore closing the door to an opportunity for the individual to honestly explore the change in herself. This interferes with her ability to integrate the change into her body image and allow her more comfort with that change.

Fatigue is another problem frequently faced by the individual on chemotherapy. Considering all the activities we may demand daily of their depleted energy level, oftentimes there is little time left to do favorite activities that enhance the individual personality or time to attend to self-care, such as makeup and hair styling, that enhances the view that the world has of us. For some reason this aspect of care becomes less important to those of us who are busy giving treatment care. Yet, sexuality and femininity being such important components of the individual's self-concept would seem to demand that we make time for its enhancement. Working out schedules to allow adequate rest in order to partake in favorite activities could become a reasonable must. Paying attention to hygiene needs and feminine toilet routines when the individual is too weak or declining to request them are parts of nursing intervention that are important to the maintenance of the individual's feelings of self-worth.

Sexuality and terminal cancer

Too often during the terminal stages of life it is assumed that the individual has no interest in her sexuality. The need for loving and closeness and the comfort they bring never cease. *Hope* is an important factor in involvement with loving and living. Interest in sexuality returns as hope revives with remission, feelings of increased strength, and the minimization of side-effects of treatment.

As the disease takes its toll, the individual may feel repugnant to herself and her loved ones and friends. Helpful interventions to remember are that the best appearance possible is a must, as well as involvement in favorite activities and sharing. Closeness and gentleness are needed at all times, but particularly when sexual activity is interrupted. We should see that that closeness is not interrupted.

Giving permission to be sexually active is important to maintain a sense of normalcy even when fatigue interferes. Society in the past has separated touching, embracing, and loving from the individual with terminal illness. There are many acts besides sexual intercourse that allow the individual enjoyment and a sense of being lovable that should be permitted and encouraged. Privacy is important, although many times it seems difficult to obtain. The individual needs time to herself and time with her loved ones.

CONSIDERATIONS FOR REHABILITATION

Wholeness

Wholeness is a concept that can be seen throughout nursing literature. The importance of dealing with both the body and mind of the client is repeated innumerable times. Yet, until recently, sexuality, which is perceived by some as physical instinct and by others as emotional response, has often been left out of consideration for the individual's health care needs. Murray, when discussing body image, states that "sexual identification is a central personal characteristic, and any circumstances that alter or endanger this identification can have a marked effect on the person's self-concept."[6] Fisher,[1] when he talks about individuals endowing their bodies with special properties that form an elaborate concept of selfhood, goes on to state that sexuality for women takes on an even larger context of being able to produce life.

Treatment for gynecologic cancer directly alters and endangers the woman's sexual identification, at least temporarily. It not only effects a change in bodily contour and/or function, but it also effects a change in the individual's sense of herself as a giving and nurturing human being.

Initial responses may involve feelings of fear, not only caused by loss of control over her body and its functioning but also caused by feelings of loss and inadequacy in continuing relationships with loved ones and an expectation of rejection by them. Weakness and fatigue in response to illness and treatment as well as depression and mourning over any disfigurement or functional loss lead to a sense of being fragile and incapable of dealing with life in a productive manner. Feelings of fragility can lead to the separation of the woman from her usual activities, including sexual activity. Thus, this effectively separates her from the love and reassurance she may need to rebuild her self-concept and get on with her life.

Occasionally a woman may welcome this feeling of fragility in order to interrupt sexual activity that has been less than desirable to her. This, however, may lead her into the interruption of other relationships as well if she continues to view herself in a semi-invalid state.

In order to avoid this crippling self-concept, it is important to open up conversations regarding impending changes in the life-style of the individual as soon as she begins to deal with the knowledge of her disease and the treatment to be used. Careful assessment of the woman's self-concept, her feelings as a sexual being, and how she relates her sexuality to her life-style gives a base from which the nurse can guide exploration of feelings, concerns, and response to her change in body image. The final self-concept will be defined by the woman, but to assist her to affect a healthy change in that concept, the nurse should know the strengths, weaknesses, hopes, dreams, and coping behavior of the client.

In assessing the individual's ability to

adapt to a change in her body image after an assault to her sexuality, asking several questions will help guide the nurse as she intervenes to help the individual return to a sense of wholeness. What was the woman's previous view of herself in relation to her general life situations including the physical, social, and emotional aspects? How has this view of herself been influenced by the diagnosis of cancer? What is her understanding of what is happening to her and what can be expected or planned for in the future? Who are her significant others, and what are their concerns? What sense does she have of her own femininity, and how does this relate to other aspects of her life? And lastly, but exceedingly important, how effective is she in expressing her needs to others?

Having the information gleaned by this assessment and sharing initial concerns opens avenues for rehabilitation efforts. Having a sense that someone cares, understands, and perceives her needs can benefit the woman in lessening her isolation and therefore possible depression as she deals with the changes in herself.

Desirability

Kolb[3] reminds us that the general attitude of society toward physical disfigurement is that of disapproval, repulsion, and rejection. All human beings have, somewhere within them, the need to be desired, approachable, cared for, and loved. A woman who has recently suffered, or is about to suffer, an assault to her sexuality through cancer and/or treatment can often have feelings of shame, embarrassment, repulsion, and fear of not being approachable and lovable. This can occur even without outward signs of disfigurement. Understanding that women of all ages from teens to old age have an interest in sexual activity and being desirable, should lead nurses to explore ways that they might helpfully intervene. Being aware of certain influences is also necessary to be helpful.

Cultural and social class attitudes affect the development of a concept of sexuality and desirability. For the young woman whose culture dictates that desirability is linked to the ability to reproduce, a change in that ability presents a more exacting crisis for her than it might for someone who does not have that pressure. For the older woman who enjoys sexual activity against the dictates of her culture, an assault could lead to feelings of shame and guilt. If a woman can no longer take care of her family, but needs their care, she may have the added burden of feeling worthless for their caring and, therefore, undesirable.

Religious background can determine underlying values that affect a woman's response to changes in sexual activity or her sense of being a valued person. Certain religious beliefs might dictate to her how she should respond to the change in herself. If there is any guilt attached to her sexuality, she will need to have additional time and feedback. Clergy can be quite helpful to religious individuals as they return to relationships after such trauma. However, we probably do not use their assistance as often as we might in helping couples overcome concerns and fears.

It is important for the nurse working with the woman with gynecologic cancer to know what her usual sexual practices have been. This knowledge gives a baseline from which to work when exploring the changes that will occur with therapy and what alternatives are available. It is important that the nurse not use her own concept of "adequate sexuality" when looking to alternatives. The "normal sexuality" for that individual and her sexual activity will form the basis for intervention. By giving permission to discuss specific concerns openly, the nurse is most helpful in dealing with sexual changes and concepts. Proceeding from the usual expressions of sexuality for the individual client, the discussion continues to alternatives in a comfortable and tolerant atmosphere. The woman will need time to herself. However, time must also be given to her consort. Discussion alone and together can help to facilitate open communication.

Reality-type issues need to be confronted. These include such issues as anatomic changes that will require different positions and forms of stimulation, the interruption and/or cessation of vaginal intercourse, the exploration of alternate means of sexual expression, impotency in an older partner after an extended absence from his wife during treatment, as well as feelings of fragility or repugnance of some care needs. When discussing sexual activity, an emphasis on the mechanics of love making is more appropriate, necessary, and helpful than generalities with little guidance.

The earlier assessment of what is "normal" for the individual and her concept of herself as a sexual being guides the nurse as to what kinds of information are acceptable and appropriate for sharing. It also helps in the timing of information, with the need for constant reassessment of where the individual is in relation to her changing image. Throughout this exploration and adjustment, using love, patience, imagination, and a sense of humor that allows both the nurse and client to be naturally human can be immeasurably helpful.

Individuality

Murray[5] states that the ability to cope with a body image crisis is influenced by the degree and number of changes that will affect the individual's life-style with her family, occupation, and social group. Time needs to be given to investigating what changes will be necessitated in how she relates to her family, whether or not she will be able to continue a career, and whether she will be able to relate to friends and the community with warm feelings of security.

Efforts to maintain the individual's integrity in other aspects of her life, such as returning to usual activities and responsibilities as soon as possible, are important to the care of the individual. When she can feel physically stronger and confident in successes in dealing with an altered life-style, she will be started toward the development of a healthy and productive self-concept. Kaplan expresses the thought that "self-esteem, self-respect, and even self-love are necessary for the development of healthy human sexual relationships with other or both sexes."[2] When the nurse can encourage the return of these essentials to her client's self-image, much has been done to enhance recovery. As a woman begins again to take risks and return to former activities that gave her feelings of self-worth, she will be able to reach out to those she loves and develop new relationships while strengthening old ones.

Finally, certain concepts in dealing with the woman who has undergone a body image crisis that can affect her sense of herself as a sexual being should be reiterated. Labrum[4] has said that the greatest help we can give is by attending, responding, initiating, and communicating with the individual we wish to serve.

With that in mind, the nurse must never assume the client's level of knowledge but should be able to anticipate needs for information and education. The nurse initiating the opening of pathways for the client to express needs and take an active role in decisions for her care is a facilitator indeed for recovery. Hygiene and appearance are of utmost importance. The nurse can assist the client in measures to help her feel good about herself and be as active and productive as her condition allows.

Being honest, realistic, and creative in helping the client feel better about herself are some of the more helpful attitudes of the nurse caring for the person with cancer. The nurse can give time to significant others to express their needs as well and allow them to explore how they might take an active role in maintaining a sense of importance and independence in their loved one. We are sexual beings and need time for privacy to share with loved ones, which can be one of the best avenues of support available.

CONCLUSION

The nurse needs to be ever attentive in assessing the client's self-concept. The nurse will need to listen carefully to what the person is saying about herself, particularly in regard to changes in attitudes concerning herself and her life-style. That is the key to more fully facilitating the recovery and rehabilitation of clients.

REFERENCES

1. Fisher, S.: Body consciousness, New York, 1974, Jason Aronsen, Inc.
2. Kaplan, R.: Aspects of human sexuality, Dubuque, Ia., 1973, Wm. C. Brown Co., Publishers.
3. Kolb, L. C.: Disturbance of the body image. In Arieti, S., editor: American handbook of psychiatry, ed. 2, New York, 1975, Basic Books, Inc., vol. IV.
4. Labrum, A. H.: Psychological factors in gynecologic cancer, Primary Care **3**(4):811, 1976.
5. Murray, R. L. E.: Principles in nursing intervention for the adult patient with body image change, Nurs. Clin. North Am. **7**(4):697, 1972.
6. Murray, R. L. E.: Body image development in adulthood, Nurs. Clin. North Am. **7**(4):617, 1972.

ADDITIONAL READING

Donahue, V. C., and Knapp, R. C.: Sexual rehabilitation of gynecologic cancer patients, Obstet. Gynecol. **49**(1):118, 1977.

Knapp, R. C., and Donahue, V. C.: Gynecologic surgery: its threat to sexuality, Consultant **12:**55, 1972.

McCloskey, J. C.: How to make the most of body image theory in nursing practice, Nursing '76 **76:**68, 1976.

Severyn, B. R.: Nursing implications with a loss of body function, ANA Clinical Sessions p. 233, 1969.

Sutherland, A. M., and Orback, C. E.: Psychological impact of cancer and cancer surgery, Cancer **6**(5): 958, 1953.

Tiedt, E.: Psychodynamic process of the oncology experience, Nurs. Forum **14**(3):264, 1975.

28

Changes in body image associated with head and neck cancer

MARY JO DROPKIN

The term "head and neck cancer" refers to a malignancy in the area that lies above the clavicle but excludes the brain, spinal cord, axial skeleton, and vertebrae. The exact etiology of head and neck cancer is unknown, but excluding skin lesions, the tumors are frequently found in conjunction with a history of heavy smoking and excessive alcohol intake. It is estimated that 72,600 cases of head and neck cancer occur each year in the United States, accounting for 22,550 deaths annually (Table 28-1). The incidence is higher in males than in females. The lesion usually is first seen in the fifth or sixth decade of life. While head and neck cancers comprise only 5% to 6% of all cancers, special attention is warranted by them owing to the drastic structural, functional, and psychosocial disturbances that can result from the disease as well as its treatment.

CHARACTERISTICS OF HEAD AND NECK CANCER

Ninety percent of all head and neck tumors are classified histologically as epidermoid or squamous cell and can occur anywhere along the surface epithelium of the upper respiratory or digestive systems. Other cell types that are less frequently observed include adenocarcinomas, sarcomas, and lymphomas. The course of head and neck cancer and the success of treatment depend on the location of the primary site. Although many lesions that arise in the area are amenable to detection and treatment in the early stages of disease, the anatomic complexity of this region frequently predisposes to aggressive tumor growth and subtle clinical manifestations.

The head and neck are highly vascular with an extensive lymphatic network and contain a number of vital structures in close proximity. Several factors, therefore, must be considered prior to treatment of cancer in this area. Each individual must be evaluated with regard to the size and location of the primary site, invasion of surrounding structures, presence of metastatic disease, histopathology of the lesion, and possible severity of functional compromise. Current treatment modalities primarily include surgery, radiation, or a combination of the two. The position of many of the tumors may prevent complete surgical removal giving rise to a high recurrence rate in this population. Additionally, the diversification of anatomic structures frequently presents difficulties with regard to radiotherapy. Despite a radical therapeutic approach as well as recent improvement in control of local disease, 5-year survival rates for moderately advanced disease remain poor. This is attributed to a noted increase in the occurrence of distant metastases.[38] Chemotherapy in conjunction with surgery or radiation is presently being more widely used in an attempt to improve survival rates.

Head and neck cancer as well as its treatment can present drastic physiologic alterations with major psychologic and social implications. Such changes are incompatible with a person's predisease or pretreatment body image. Alterations in appearance and modes of communication, respiration, or deglutition can be not only emotionally devastating but can also result in disorders that are considered socially unacceptable, such as continuous drooling. A unique approach to nursing care is essential to accommodate the complex needs of this population. It is the primary purpose of this chapter to demonstrate that a plan of care based on the framework of adaptation to illness through alteration in body image provides the most comprehensive support system to these people for their physiologic, psychologic, and social adjustment. The case history of a person who underwent extensive treatment for cancer of the larynx follows the discussion of body image and is presented to illustrate utilization of body image as the central theme in nursing management of the head and neck cancer patient.

BODY IMAGE: DEFINING THE CONCEPT THROUGH RESEARCH

The concept of body image was initiated by neurologists and psychiatrists in an attempt to determine the nature of distorted body perception observed in many of their clients. Further interest in body image has been generated, particularly over the past 20 years, as its significance to pathologic as well as normal behavior is increasingly recognized. Research reports have often been conflicting and inconclusive because of the difficulty in quantifying subjective feelings about the body. Although no single study to

Table 28-1. Head and neck cancer: estimated new cancer cases and deaths, 1980*

Site	Estimated new cases			Estimated deaths		
	Male	**Female**	**Total**	**Male**	**Female**	**Total**
Buccal cavity and pharynx	17,900	7,600	25,500	6,100	2,700	8,800
Lip	4,000	400	4,400	150	25	175
Tongue	3,200	1,600	4,800	1,400	600	2,000
Salivary gland				400	250	650
Floor of mouth	5,600	3,700	9,300	400	125	525
Other and unspecified mouth				950	500	1,450
Pharynx	5,100	1,900	7,000	2,800	1,200	4,000
Larynx	9,000	1,700	10,700	2,900	600	3,500
Eye	900	900	1,800	200	200	400
Thyroid	2,600	6,500	9,100	350	700	1,050
TOTAL	48,300	24,300	72,600	15,650	6,900	22,550

*From American Cancer Society: 1980 cancer facts and figures, New York, 1979, American Cancer Society, Inc., p. 9.

date has illustrated the total manner in which the individual experiences his body, a comprehensive review of the literature reveals a more composite picture of this highly complex phenomenon.

The body, as the core of man's existence, is the structure within which all life events are experienced. The body becomes the medium or agency through which life acquires significance. Life experiences must be dynamically assimilated, therefore, in a manner that makes them meaningful to the body. This process is accomplished with the development of a comprehensive mental "picture" of the body or body image. Ultimately, body image is dependent on the individual's perceptual capacity as well as his ability to interpret and organize life events. Essentially, however, body image is the unique perception each person has of his or her own body as a physiologic, psychologic, and sociocultural entity.

The body is perceived as a physiologic object through awareness of its spatial dimensions. This awareness consists of comprehension of an external boundary and sensitivity to internal sensations.[18] The external boundary is comprised of the anatomic features and superficial sensations that occur on the body surface. The anatomic features can be visualized, are recognized as self from an early age,[12] and distinguish the individual from other objects in the environment. External sensations are received and interpreted by the central nervous system. Acknowledgment of this boundary occurs at a conscious as well as unconscious level. Although one's exterior would seem self-evident, people vary a great deal in their perception of their own boundary. Despite the fact that cause and effect remain unclear, individuals who are acutely aware of their body boundary are more reactive to stimulation at exterior sites such as the skin and muscles. They tend to contract superficial ailments such as arthritis or skin rashes but at the same time perceive this boundary as a protection from injury. The reverse is true for those with a less clearly defined body boundary. These people are less physiologically reactive at exterior sites and tend to channel energy inward. They are inclined to contract internal disorders such as gastric ulcers and feel more vulnerable to external injury.[18] Such differences in body boundary awareness may be exemplified by the varying reactions of clients to invasive procedures such as injections. While it is not known whether one perception of boundary is more normal than another, the person who lacks a clear definition of body boundary is likely to experience more discomfort or anxiety with these procedures than one with a clearly demarcated boundary.

The occurrence of internal sensations such as neurologic, metabolic, hormonal, or endocrine can also provide perception of the body as a physiologic entity. The amount of attention directed to these sensations may range from minimal to maximal and varies among individuals. The hypochondriac is an extreme example of hypersensitivity to internal bodily sensations. The reasons why some people are more aware of internal sensations than others remain uncertain. Possibly the frequency of activity and/or the significance of the bodily region in which it occurs might account for the noted variation in acknowledgment. Ultimately, realization of physiologic activity can provide conception of visceral space and form the basis for cognitive decision as well as selected behavior.[18] For instance, when a rumbling is heard or felt in the abdominal region, one becomes aware that "my stomach is growling." Based on an association with hunger, a decision is made whether or not to eat, and the appropriate behavioral response is initiated.

Many internal and external physiologic

responses are associated with "feelings." Increased heart rate and respirations, as well as muscular tension and sweating, are experienced as fear. Yet these same sensations can be modified with learned relaxation techniques or conscious body perception.[19] The body thus achieves significance as a psychologic object through its animation of emotion and intellect. As "self," bodily structures, functions, and sensations assume additional importance, and the body can only be experienced as the self is experienced. There is a definite relationship, in other words, between the way one evaluates oneself as a person and how that individual feels about his or her body.[18] Satisfaction with bodily parts, for example, has been repeatedly linked with a positive self-concept.[42,48] Dissatisfaction, on the other hand, is usually associated with anxiety in the form of somatic complaints.[23]

As the body is integrated into self, selected meanings or values are assigned to specific body regions. Certain structures and functions become more important than others. This selected attention probably occurs at an unconscious level and varies from one person to another. Concern with the particular function(s) in the area might account for such emphasis or possibly the individual wishes to personify qualities that have been ascribed to the area. One may perceive the heart, for example, as more vital to life than any other organ. Or as commonly used phrases such as "heart of gold" imply, the heart may represent qualities of generosity or kindness to the individual who considers himself a giving person. The same organ or structure, in other words, may have different connotations to different people. Some interesting variations in body focus have been noted between men and women's perception of the same structure. Legs, for example, are primarily perceived by men as a source of strength or locomotion. Women primarily view their legs as a source of attractiveness.[47]

Many studies that have illustrated similar differences in body perception between the sexes attribute it to sociocultural overlap. It has been speculated that women tend to perceive their bodies more within the context of social interaction than men do.[18] Generally, however, an inherent relationship exists between sociocultural experience and body perception.[37,43] One's role in society may designate meaning and significance to a body part. The hands, for instance, may be considered highly valuable to a surgeon, artist, or carpenter but have different meaning for each based on professional implications such as dexterity, creativity, or strength. Sociocultural factors also affect the individual's most basic care of the body as well as relationships with others. In this society, special emphasis is placed on bodily appearance. Conclusions about one's self are made by others based on physical attributes.[29] The individual also develops a variety of behaviors such as grooming and dietary habits and the use of clothing or cosmetics that are ultimately designed to facilitate acceptance of the body to others as well as the individual. The need for social acceptance is not equally strong, however, in all people. The individual with a well-defined body boundary and positive self-concept is likely to assume that others react to him in a similarly positive manner. Social interaction is thus facilitated, and the need for others' approval reduced.

In summary, body image might be described as a perceptual homeostasis. It is an adaptive mechanism that maintains equilibrium among the physiologic, psychologic, and sociocultural components of the body. It is a cognitive system developed by the individual to determine the nature and purpose of the structure in which he exists and through which he conducts himself in his environment. Many aspects of body image have defied measurement to date owing to its highly subjective nature and the fact that this type of self-assessment can be idealistic, unrealistic, or otherwise inaccurate. Through persistent research, however, the complexity of body image not only continues to be appreciated, but provides endless possibilities for further investigation.

DEVELOPMENT OF BODY IMAGE

Although many aspects of body image such as boundary perception are not significantly altered over time,[17] the body's meaning to the individual changes in the process of growth and development. The obese person, for example, may have felt quite stigmatized during adolescence but may feel content with the same boundary perception later in life. Emphasis shifts, in other words, according to the physiologic, psychologic, and sociocultural events experienced with age.

In infancy and early childhood, the body is primarily experienced on the physiologic level. The newborn experiences bodily sensations such as hunger or pain but is unable to understand or interpret them. The developing child is increasingly exposed to environmental experiences and with sensorimotor development learns to assume mastery over the environment. Body boundary is initially formulated during this period and is accompanied by recognition of self as separate from mother and others.[18,32] In adolescence and young adulthood, sociocultural awareness seems to dominate body image development. The physiologic and emotional changes that occur are frequently considered in relation to the peer group. Attitudes concerning bodily appearance and function are strongly influenced by those with whom the individual has established meaningful relationships. Finally during the later adult years through senescence, self-concept becomes the dominant influence on body image. Introspection occurs with regard to past experiences, and previous misconceptions of body image are resolved. The body is more fully accepted, and ongoing physiologic and sociocultural changes are more easily integrated into self. Physical appearance and peer approval assume less importance as the development of a positive self-concept becomes more meaningful in preparation for aging.

Head and neck cancer most frequently is seen during this latter period of body image development. The individual with a mature and realistic concept of his body has ideally attained acceptance of his body in spite of the fact that structural and functional changes that are occurring indicate physical decline. The hair is graying and/or thinning, loss of elastic fibers and subcutaneous tissue causes wrinkles to become more apparent—particularly those that have been formed from habitual facial expressions. Energy requirements diminish and weight now gained more easily is distributed toward the hips and abdomen. Visual and auditory acuity decrease, and hormonal changes give rise to the male and female climacteric.[21] Although the aging process occurs at varying rates in different individuals, those who have been unable to achieve inner gratification or who have remained intensely concerned about bodily appearance or function through this period have a more difficult time integrating such changes into their body image. Additional sociocultural changes may necessitate role modification or redefinition such as the "empty nest" syndrome of the housewife and mother or acknowledgment of previously unfulfilled ambitions by the career person. The typical evolution of body image to this stage in life entails development of a secure and positive sense of self. This sense of self, in turn, provides the individual a means to cope with additional changes of old age including acceptance of death.

Thus, physiologic, psychologic, and sociocultural experiences simultaneously affect body image development and designate the dimensions of its components. One type of influence seems to dominate as the individual ages, however, and in this manner may alter the significance of the body in various stages of life. Generally, sensorimotor development is the primary influence on body image in childhood; the appearance of the body to others dominates adolescence and young adulthood; and finally, achievement of inner gratification becomes the most significant aspect of body image development in middle age and senescence.

SIGNIFICANCE OF THE HEAD AND NECK TO BODY IMAGE

The head and neck area is consistently regarded as a highly valued region of the body.[18] It is the location of the brain, upper respiratory tract, and upper digestive system. The anatomic characteristics of its external boundary have dual significance as facial features and the major sense organs. Several external sensations are experienced here. Energy from the visible spectrum is converted to action potential in the optic nerve providing visual impressions. Sound waves are converted to action potential in the auditory nerve furnishing the sensation of hearing. The presence of olfactory receptors in the nasal mucosa account for odor distinction, and the taste buds and gustatory receptors located in the mucosa of the epiglottis, pharynx, and surface of the tongue determine taste sensations. Internal sensations in this area include the sense of equilibrium originating in the inner ear, which provides orientation in space, and the vibratory sensation of voice production.

The head and neck region is also considered the center for thought processes and logic, learning, memory, and perception. Neuromuscular action in this area accounts for multiple facial expressions that can convey emotion or modify speech. The face, as the most basic representation of self, provides identity.[1] Each facial feature assumes additional importance in terms of self-identification as well as its functional capacity. Sensory ability to perceive the environment and obtain information as well as the ingestion of food and inhalation of air designate the general theme of incorporation or "taking in" to this region of the body.[18]

Communication with others is accomplished with voice production. Perception of others occurs through visual stimulation primarily provided by the face.[30] The intensity of social interaction also depends in large part on such mutual visual impressions,[35] and in this manner, feedback for "self" is acquired. Anthropologists exhibit interest in the sociocultural significance of the face, particularly in a fully clothed society. As such, one's worth as a person is frequently assessed according to facial characteristics.[30] Deviance from society's aesthetic expectations is often judged harshly or deemed socially unacceptable.

The head and neck, therefore, might be regarded as the essence of body image. Its action as a medium for physiologic, psychologic, and sociocultural existence provides an optimal illustration of the multidimensional experience of the body.

SIGNIFICANCE OF BODY IMAGE TO NURSING CARE OF THE HEAD AND NECK CANCER PATIENT

Physical alteration dictates alteration in body image, constituting adaptation to bodily changes. These alterations can prove quite disrupting or anxiety provoking to the individual,[23] particularly when representation of self is at stake. Diagnosis of head and neck cancer, therefore, can have a devastating impact on body image. Diagnosis itself provokes but one of a series of body image conflicts the individual will ultimately undergo.

The person who has developed head and

neck cancer may have experienced some degree of body image alteration even prior to diagnosis. A sizable intraoral lesion might be visualized or felt with the tongue, or an "invisible" defect in the area could present as hoarseness or dysphagia. The anxiety that accompanies these changes may either prompt or deter the individual from seeking medical attention in the early stages of the disease.[8] Once diagnosis is fairly well established, a grief process is initiated as a part of self is "lost" to malignancy.[36] The experience of grief may be heightened as the part is further lost to treatment or extended disease. Associated fears of visible disfigurement or functional loss cause additional disruption. Generally, the individual who has maintained a mature and secure body image before illness can resolve these conflicts somewhat more readily.[22]

In many cases, however, the individual who develops head and neck cancer has been an alcoholic, thereby sustaining a distorted body perception prior to illness. Body image studies that have been conducted specifically with alcoholics indicate that they tend toward either a very negative body perception accompanied by difficulty communicating with others or maintain an artificially favorable body image secondary to drinking.[7,46] It is feasible that this latter group as a patient population might not comprehend the impact of cancer or its treatment for up to 1 year after sobriety.[46] Alcoholism thus compounds or delays the adaptive process.

Major head and neck surgery probably constitutes the most rapid and aggressive assault on body image from which all individuals will need time to recover. The term "time lag" has been used to describe this period during which these patients must reintegrate drastic physical changes into self.[5] Depending on the extent of disease or treatment as well as the person's preexisting body image, such reintegration can be facilitated by nursing care specifically directed toward body image reorganization. Following such surgery, the reaction of the nurse becomes highly meaningful as this is usually the first person to view the client's altered appearance. Evidence of compassion as well as technical competence can serve to reassure the patient that he will not be rejected or abandoned because of the way he looks and can promote the first step in the reestablishment of self-esteem. The quality of nursing interaction can indicate to these people that they have indeed maintained an identity that has not been irreparably altered. Anxiety about the bodily alteration can gradually be reduced and attention redirected to self as the substance of continued life.[13]

Untreated or surgically resected head and neck cancer can, however, prove to be a very disconcerting sight. With this particular population the nurse is not able to utilize the defense of depersonalization or detachment of disease or operative site from the client. This region represents identification to the patient as well as to the nurse. The nurse, therefore, might experience some degree of anxiety during direct encounters. Research indicates that the intensity of one's reaction to another's visible disfigurement depends on the integrity of the viewer's body image.[16] One with a well-defined body perception is likely to view such disablement more favorably, and the threat of experiencing a similar occurrence is not as great.[31] The nurse, then, must also adapt to the patient's physical alterations in order to deliver comprehensive care. In addition to value change, or emphasizing self over physical characteristics, nurse and client also adapt through confining the defect and viewing physical limitations as assets rather than liabilities.[13] A defect, particularly in the head and neck, may initially represent a defect in self. Through administration of nursing care as well as the encouragement of self-care, each of which necessitate viewing and touching the site, the defect becomes anatomically confined and finally perceptually limited. When considered in relation to the norm, such defects in function or appearance may seem quite detrimental. When considered in relation to the reality of disease and treatment, however, a more optimistic view can be attained by nurse and patient.

Unfortunately, the literature presently indicates that physiologic adaptation in terms of mastication, deglutition, and phonation may never be fully achieved by many of these people in spite of multidisciplinary rehabilitative efforts.[34] Psychologic and sociocultural compensation is, therefore, essential to body image adaptation. A large percentage of these clients are able to cope with their physical defects. Difficulty arises, however, in situations that involve others' reactions.[45] Thus, any evidence of inner strength or self-acceptance must be acknowledged and supported by others as early into the treatment period as possible.

In summary, adaptation through alteration in body image with head and neck cancer can not only aid the patient in maintaining an optimal quality to his life but can ultimately prevent social reclusiveness or isolation[44] and promote compliance with self-care activities that may be necessary for continued survival.[4,14]

PHYSIOLOGIC ALTERATION: CANCER OF THE LARYNX

A brief discussion of the anatomy of the larynx is warranted at this point to facilitate understanding the pathophysiologic processes described in the following case history.

The larynx measures approximately 4.5 cm in length in the adult male and 3.5 cm in the adult female. Patency of the organ is maintained by its bony and cartilaginous framework. Skeletal structures include the hyoid bone, thyroid and cricoid cartilages, epiglottis, and arytenoid cartilages as shown in Fig. 28-1. Attachment of the hyoid bone to prelaryngeal muscles, the mandible, and the skull helps to maintain the position of the larynx within the neck as well as to raise it during phonation and deglutition. The thyroid and cricoid cartilages shield the larynx externally. The thyroid is the largest cartilaginous structure in the larynx. In males, the angle of its alae is more narrow than that of females, thus forming a subcutaneous projection referred to as the Adam's apple. The cricoid cartilage lies just below the vocal cords and is the only complete ring in the respiratory tract. Its lower border indicates the inferior margin of the larynx, which is located at the level of the sixth cervical vertebra. At this point, the larynx becomes continuous with the trachea. The arytenoid cartilages are paired, pyramid-shaped, and lie side-by-side in the posterior aspect of the cricoid cartilage. Muscular processes attached to these structures account for the abduction or adduction of the vocal cords. Finally, the epiglottis is a thin leaf-shaped fibroelastic cartilage. Its base is attached by a ligament to the thyroid cartilage. From that point, it arches diagonally upward and backward. Its anterior surface is attached to the hyoid bone. Thus, movement by the thyroid cartilage and hyoid bone largely determines the position of the epiglottis and may contribute to laryngeal constriction during swallowing. The free edge of the epiglottis constitutes the superior margin of the larynx and lies just behind the base of the tongue.

Generally, ligamentous attachments connect and stabilize the position of the separate but adjacent cartilaginous structures. Fig. 28-2 illustrates the relationship of ligaments to the skeletal structures of the larynx.

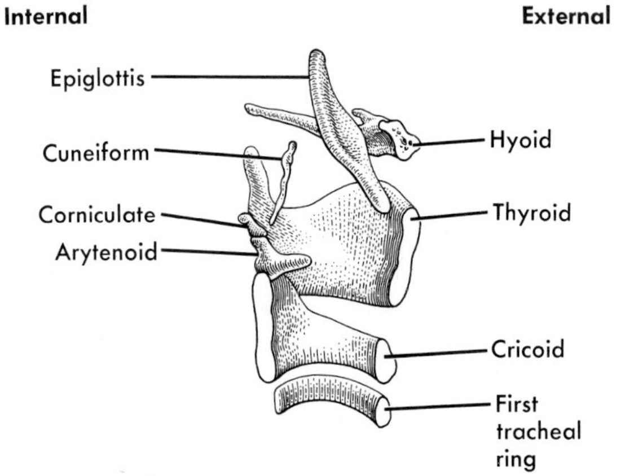

Fig. 28-1. Skeletal framework.

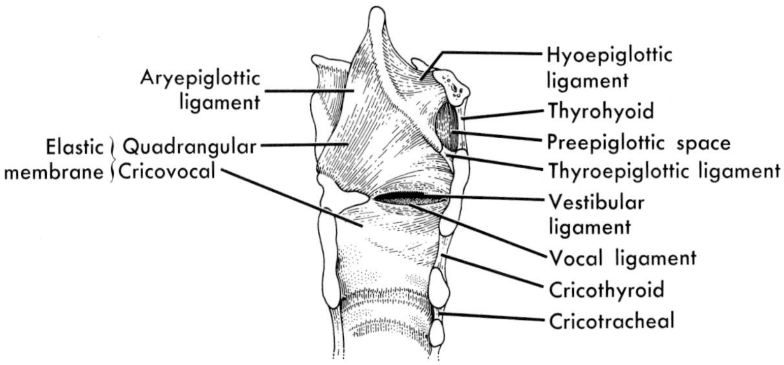

Fig. 28-2. Ligaments of larynx.

Muscular action on the larynx is primarily derived from two sources—the extrinsic and the intrinsix musculature (Fig. 28-3). The extrinsic musculature consists of pharyngeal and strap muscles and control fixation as well as movement of the whole organ. Upward movement is regulated by the elevator group: anterior and posterior digastric, stylohyoid, geniohyoid, and mylohyoid muscles from cranial nerves V and VII. Downward movement is accomplished by the depressor group: thyrohyoid, sternohyoid, and omohyoid muscles. These muscles also affect the laryngeal functions of deglutition and phonation. The intrinsic musculature is paired, with the exception of the interarytenoid muscle, and serves to modify the size of the superior laryngeal orifice as well as the length, tension, abduction, and adduction of the cords (Fig. 28-4).

The cavity of the larynx is lined with mucous membrane, which is continuous with that of the pharynx above and the trachea below. Stratified squamous epithelium lines the epiglottis and the vocal cords. The remainder of the larynx is lined by pseudo-

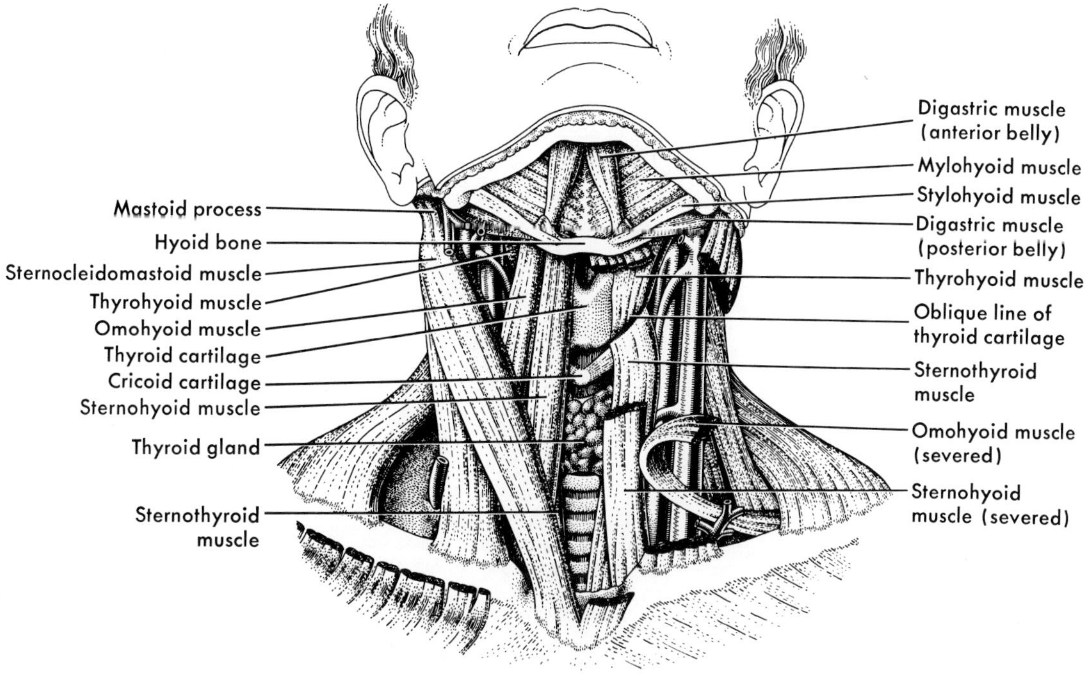

Fig. 28-3. Extrinsic muscles of larynx.

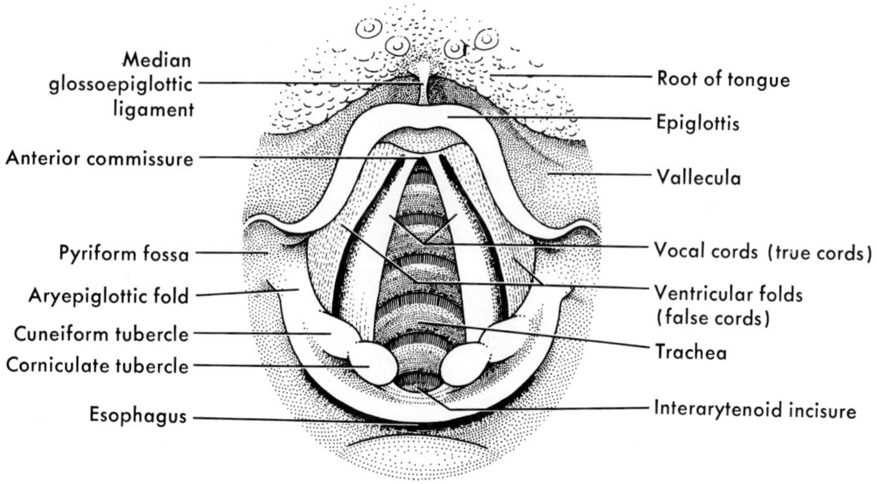

Fig. 28-4. Normal larynx, inspiration.

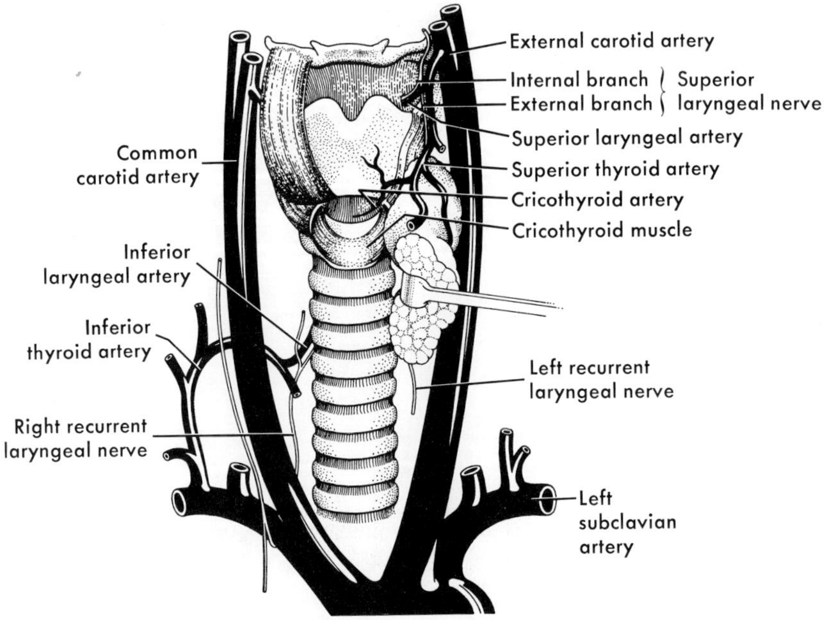

Fig. 28-5. Arterial supply.

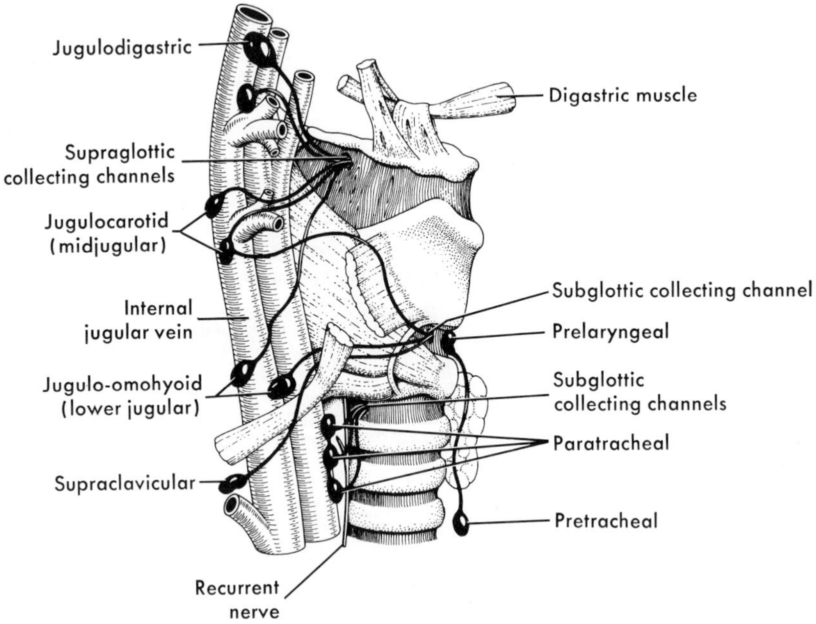

Fig. 28-6. Lymphatic drainage.

stratified ciliated columnar epithelium. For surgical as well as anatomically descriptive purposes, the larynx is divided into three parts: supraglottic, glottic, and subglottic. The supraglottic region of the larynx extends from the superior tip of the epiglottis to the bilateral mucosal folds immediately above the vocal cords, or the false cords. The glottic region extends from the inferior margin of the false cords to just below the inferior margin of the true cords. Each of the true vocal cords is a prominent white fold of mucous membrane overlying the vocalis muscle (a part of the thyroarytenoid muscle) and extends from the interior angle of the thyroid cartilage to the base of each arytenoid cartilage. Finally, the subglottic larynx extends from just below the inferior margin of the true vocal cords to the inferior margin of the cricoid cartilage.

The arterial blood supply of the larynx is primarily derived from two sources: the superior and inferior laryngeal branches of the superior and inferior thyroid arteries. Venous return from the larynx is accomplished by the superior laryngeal vein and the superior and middle thyroid veins into the internal jugular vein (Fig. 28-5). Basically, two branches of the vagus nerve supply the larynx. They include the external and internal branches of the superior laryngeal nerve and the terminal branches of the recurrent laryngeal nerve. The lymphatic network of the larynx is well developed in all regions except that of the true vocal cords, where there is a paucity of subepithelial tissue. The laryngeal lymphatic system is divided into two parts by this area, one draining superiorly, the other inferiorly (Fig. 28-6). The lymphatic network of the supraglottic region is extensive and more developed than that of the subglottic region. Ninety-eight percent of all supraglottic lymphatic drainage ends in the deep cervical nodes, with the remainder passing to the lower cervical or spinal accessory chains.[3]

CASE HISTORY

Diagnosis

Owing to the anatomic complexity of this region, proximity of structures, and aggressive tumor action, definitive diagnosis of the primary site may be difficult and is ultimately contingent on pathologic examination—in the following case, the base of the epiglottis. The extensive lymphatic network to the supraglottic larynx would seem to account for the rapid invasion of surrounding structures as well as early metastases to regional lymph nodes noted in this type of neoplasm.[28] People frequently remain asymptomatic in the early stages of the disease. The first clinical sign may, in fact, be enlarged cervical nodes.[11] Survival rate, however, is decreased significantly by the time cervical metastases are evident and decreased further in the presence of bilateral nodes.[33]

Mr. W. was a 55-year-old man whose initial complaint of sore throat was treated unsuccessfully by several physicians with antibiotics and other local treatments. On referral to an otolaryngologist, his chief complaints included sore throat, dysphagia, and hoarseness for a period of 6 months to 1 year. In addition, at this time Mr. W. had reported a 25 pound weight loss and progressive easy fatigue. Past medical history was unremarkable. This man had smoked heavily in the past, but had not smoked for 3 years prior to examination except for an occasional cigar. The client also had a history of alcohol abuse but had not consumed any alcohol for 1 year prior to examination.

Physical examination of the head and neck was within normal limits except for abnormalities in the larynx and in the neck. Indirect laryngoscopy revealed a large mass in the supraglottic region. The vocal cords were not well visualized at this time secondary to the presence of the mass. Examination of the neck revealed bilateral palpable

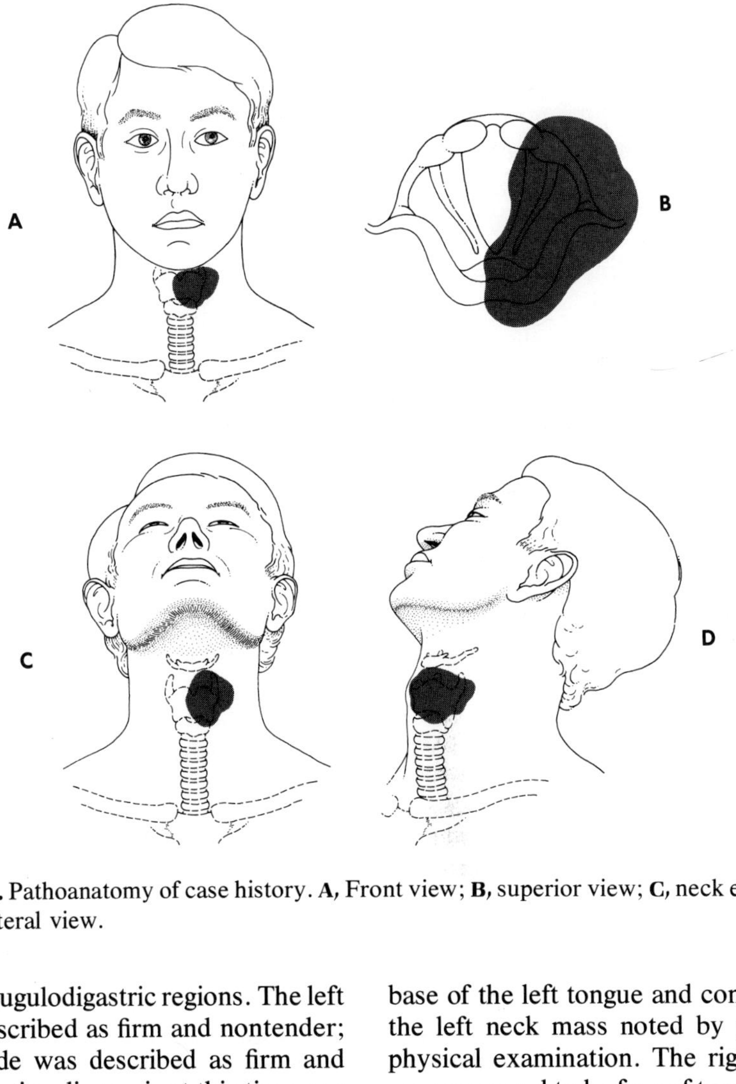

Fig. 28-7. Pathoanatomy of case history. **A,** Front view; **B,** superior view; **C,** neck extended; **D,** left lateral view.

nodes in the jugulodigastric regions. The left node was described as firm and nontender; the right node was described as firm and mobile. Tentative diagnosis at this time was carcinoma of the supraglottic larynx.

Tomograms of the larynx and laryngo-esophogram confirmed the presence of a left supraglottic mass that impaired the patient's swallowing when in an upright position. Metastatic workup included chest films and liver and spleen scans. Chest films revealed emphysematous changes; liver and spleen scans revealed hepatomegaly of unknown origin. Panendoscopy revealed a large left hypopharyngeal tumor extending from the base of the left tongue and contiguous with the left neck mass noted by palpation on physical examination. The right subglottic area appeared to be free of tumor, but gross involvement was noted in the left subglottic region. Multiple biopsies were obtained. Pathologic examination indicated all specimens to be negative with the exception of the right base of the epiglottis, which exhibited keratinizing squamous cell carcinoma (Fig. 28-7).

Treatment

Although small supraglottic lesions would ordinarily be treated by radiation or conservative surgery alone, combination therapy or radiation plus surgery is generally agreed on to be the treatment of choice for extensive lesions. The larynx poses a particular challenge to the radiotherapist, however, because of the heterogenicity of its normal structures. Techniques that avoid damage, such as perichondritis or necrosis of the bony/cartilaginous structures, but that effect tumoricidal action on soft tissue are necessary to facilitate later surgical excision.[15]

Total laryngectomy is the surgical treatment of choice for extensive supraglottic tumors.[28] Radical neck dissection is indicated for metastases.

Briefly, wide-field or total laryngectomy includes removal of the hyoid bone, preepiglottic space, strap muscles, and one or more tracheal rings. Radical neck dissection, in continuity with the laryngectomy, entails removal of the contents of one side of the neck including the sternocleidomastoid muscle, the internal jugular vein with its associated lymph nodes and the glandular contents of the submaxillary triangle. The carotid artery, vagus, sympathetic, and phrenic nerves are spared, as well as the scalene and prevertebral muscle groups.

As a result of the findings on panendoscopy and histologic examination in Mr. W.'s case, consultation with the Department of Radiology was sought. It was recommended that the client be treated with 5,500 rads of cobalt prior to surgical excision of the tumor. The total dose of radiation was delivered over a 5½-week period. The course of treatment was uneventful, and the patient was discharged for 5½ weeks. On return, physical examination of the throat revealed a supraglottic mass on the left that obstructed the view of the left true cord. The right cord was visualized at this time and appeared normal. Diffuse erythema was noted secondary to radiation therapy. Bilateral cervical adenopathy remained unchanged. Total laryngectomy and staged bilateral radical neck dissection were planned. Mr. W. underwent total laryngectomy, left radical neck dissection, creation of pharyngostome, and application of a dermis graft taken from the left thigh over the carotid artery. Pathologic examination of the specimen revealed squamous cell carcinoma and indicated that clear surgical margins had been obtained.

Complications

Advances in radiotherapy have helped to minimize but not to eliminate the complications of combined treatment. Variations in types of incisions, suture materials, and the use of dermis grafts have helped to reduce complications from a surgical point of view. Heavily irradiated skin in the head and neck area, however, never regains its original thickness, but remains fragile and vulnerable to healing difficulty following subsequent surgical trauma.[2] Although secondary skin reactions are not the primary deterrent to postoperative wound healing, they compound existent problems presented by the surgery itself. Surgery of the head and neck poses unique problems to postoperative wound healing. Salivary contamination, removal of large amounts of tissue, elevation of large skin flaps, and postoperative dead space all contribute to healing difficulty.[25]

On Mr. W.'s fourth postoperative day, suture line dehiscence was noted on the left lateral neck immediately adjacent to his pharyngostome. Following a period of observation to determine the extent of dehiscence, additional sutures were placed but failed to close the area. At this time, carotid exposure was noted in spite of placement of the dermis graft. Multiple wound care regimens were initiated such as dressing changes, zinc sulfate (via feeding tube), and high-caloric/high-protein diet. Gradually, over several weeks, granulation tissue was observed in the region. Mr. W. was discharged for 1 week. On return to the hospital, primary closure of the pharyngostome was attempted with a left deltopectoral flap. On the second postoperative day, cyanosis was noted on the medial edge of the tube pedicle, which ultimately became necrotic. A second attempt at débridement and closure of the fistula was tried under local anesthesia but failed within 5 days. The patient was continued on multiple wound care regimens including pressure dressings to the area. Finally, the remainder of the flap was implanted and he was discharged for a second time pending further reconstructive surgery. While at home, the client experienced a sudden and profuse bleeding episode from the neck and expired.

BODY IMAGE ALTERATION: NURSING CARE

To most aptly apply body image theory to care of the patient who has undergone extensive treatment for head and neck cancer, the following discussion will be based on Roy's adaptation model for nursing practice. Utilization of this model entails conceptualization of man as having four basic modes of adaptation: (1) physiologic needs, (2) self-concept, (3) role function, and (4) interdependence relations.[39] Nursing management, established according to this perception, will be examined in each of the four adaptive modes.

Physiologic needs

Following surgery, three major physiologic adaptations on the part of Mr. W. were identified as necessitating support through nursing management. These included: (1) deglutition, (2) respiration, and (3) phonation.

Deglutition. Mr. W. received nutrition and appropriate medication via nasogastric tube. He was taught to do the feedings himself and did so without difficulty. He received approximately 2,000 calories per day. Commercially prepared tube feeding was used and supplemented with liquids of the client's choice following complaints of hunger. Zinc sulfate as well as a high-protein/high-caloric diet were integral aspects of the intensive wound healing regimen. At this time, however, Mr. W. frequently complained of nausea and reduced his intake accordingly. Small, slowly administered, frequent feedings of the diet were recommended as well as the use of antacid medication when needed. These recommendations proved effective since ultimately his nausea diminished, granulation of the neck wound was observed, and progressive weight gain was noted.

Normally, the process of deglutition requires a closed system immediately following entrance of the bolus of food into the oropharynx. At this time, the mouth is closed and the passage between the nasopharynx and oropharynx is occluded by the soft palate. Muscular action causing the larynx and pharynx to elevate and then descend also assists propulsion of the bolus into the esophagus. Although the act of deglutition is too rapid to be primarily peristaltic in nature, pressure differences within the cavity are also fundamental to the act of swallowing.[9] Thus, the presence of a pharyngostome precluded the closed system as well as the pressure necessary for the act of deglutition.

Body image research has determined that the mouth is attributed psychologic significance primarily in terms of its nutritive and incorporative functions as well as oral gratification.[18] Much of the physical and emotional satisfaction of oral intake is thus inhibited with the use of a feeding tube. Additionally, presentation of supplemental liquids on a tray was likely more aesthetically pleasing and more socially familiar to the client than implements used for tube feeding alone. Sitting with the patient while he took his feedings also helped to maintain some degree of a social atmosphere to his meals as well as to supervise his tube feeding technique.

Complaints of nausea that occurred simultaneous to the initiation of intensive wound healing regimen were likely caused by rapid administration of the feedings, the high fat content of high-caloric beverages, or were a side-effect of zinc administration.[20] Subsequent difficulty in wound healing was primarily attributed to salivary erosion of radiated tissue as described previously.

Control over the environment through self-administration of tube feeding and choice of supplemental content thus seemed to compensate for alteration in deglutition and consequent denial of oral intake.

Respiration. Postoperatively, Mr. W. experienced continuous salivary drainage from the pharyngostome—situated immediately above the laryngostome. Presence of the laryngectomy tube prevented some of this drainage from entering the chest in the early postoperative period. Eventually, however, the tube was removed to avoid excessive irritation to the tracheal wall. Neck dressings were initially inadequate to prevent large amounts of saliva from entering the lower respiratory tract. Ultimately, dressing technique was improved with regard to materials used and mode of application. Additionally, the dressing was changed more frequently. Mr. W. was suctioned as needed and taught to suction himself, but preferred to cough up his secretions when able. Humidity was directly provided at the bedside and indirectly with a moistened gauze bib when he was away from the bedside.

Normally, air delivered to the alveoli has been tempered, humidified, and cleansed as a result of its passage from the upper respiratory tract. These functions may be provided by the mouth or the nose. Surgical removal of the larynx precludes these essential functions by altering the route of inspired air from the nose and mouth to the laryngeal stoma alone. Exogenous measures must be taken, therefore, to provide optimal temperance, humidity, and cleansing via the stoma.

Because adequate exchange of alveolar gases requires moisture,[3] humidity was essential for this laryngectomized patient. This was accomplished by direct administration and by indirect means. Indirectly, the use of a moist 4 inch × 4 inch unfilled gauze tied around the neck and over the stoma as a bib was a major supportive measure. It did, in fact, serve to replace the functions once accomplished by the nose, although not as efficiently. Moisture was provided on inspiration of air through the gauze. Loss of moisture as well as heat during inspiration would be replaced during expiration through the gauze. Additionally, the gauze served to filter out foreign material that might, otherwise, enter the chest directly through the laryngeal stoma. Laryngectomees are, in fact, encouraged to wear a similar bib at all times after discharge from the hospital.[27] The pharyngostome dressing served to absorb copious amounts of saliva, thus reducing the amount entering the trachea as well as minimizing the erosive effect of continuous salivary drainage on the lateral neck wound.

Mr. W. assumed maximal control over the environment with self-suctioning and ultimately changing his own neck dressing. Complete physiologic adaptation was not possible in this case, since the patient expired prior to closure of the pharyngostome. Adaptation had been noted, however, in his active collaboration with the staff to diminish salivary flow into the stoma. Such participation in his care also indicated integration of altered respiration into self as the "taking in" significance of the nose and mouth was redirected to the laryngeal stoma.

Phonation. Mr. W. was provided with writing materials at all times. Additional measures were taken to provide for the client's safety as well as to maximize his communication—that is, call bell within reach and limitation of intravenous therapy to areas that would not interfere with writing. It was explained to the patient that he would not be able to effectively utilize esophageal speech until the pharyngostome was closed. In the interim, he did attempt to use the Cooper-Rand Electronic Speech Aid but was unable to do so productively because of copious amounts of saliva that would accumulate in his mouth. His handwriting was legible, and he was able to communicate his needs to the staff in this manner and without difficulty.

Mr. W. was able to write fairly rapidly and participated easily in one-to-one conversation. He was able to demonstrate his emotions through underlining, large print, and accompanying facial expressions. Although at times he had difficulty communicating anger and depression, with reassurance and encouragement he was able to directly relate these feelings to his loss of voice and discouraging postoperative course. Recognition of his dependence on writing materials was observed from his conscientious possession of pad and pencil at all times.

Normal phonation is accomplished through delicate synchronization of the intrinsic and extrinsic muscles of the larynx with the musculature of the pharynx, soft palate, tongue, and lips. Sound is produced by vibration of the vocal cords that, by lateral movement, produce oscillations of pressure in expired air. Changes in these vibrations occur with alterations in the resonating cavities above; that is, the hypopharynx, pharynx, nasopharynx, and mouth. The size of the structures and, therefore, the resonance of the sound can be altered by changing the position of the tongue, and lips. Changes in the position of the soft palate, tongue, teeth, and lips can further modify the vibration of sound. It is this ability of structures in the oral cavity to modify sound that makes it possible for the person whose larynx has been removed to eventually speak intelligibly by other means.[41]

Again, complete physiologic adaptation in this case was dependent on pharyngostome closure. The sound of one's own voice, however, is an important characteristic of body image. Its unique, recognizable sound is normally "taken in" by the ears. The voice is also associated with assertiveness and projection of behavior.[18] Loss of one's voice, therefore, can create feelings of anxiety and insecurity. By utilization of alternative means of expressing himself, Mr. W. was not only acknowledging his disability but confining it to lack of voice production as opposed to lack of communication. Supplemental actions by the client while writing further emphasized this confinement by nonverbally indicating behavior patterns that would otherwise be verbally disclosed through inflection or tone of voice. In this manner, assertive and independent behavior was frequently derived from his written self-expression. Also, his optimal participation in dialogue manifested self-assurance within a social situation. Nursing behavior, supportive to such self-expression, was likely an additional indication that the means of communication to which the patient had adapted was equally worthwhile to that which he had previously utilized. Thus, written communication was viewed as an asset in itself rather than a liability in comparison to normal speech.

Self-concept

A major self-concept adaptation in this case was necessitated by the visible alteration in physical appearance.

Initially, Mr. W. seemed to adapt without difficulty to the presence of laryngeal and pharyngeal stomas in addition to the left neck defect. Maximal self-care of the neck wound and laryngeal stoma was performed from the early postoperative period throughout hospitalization. At the time the deltopectoral flap was raised into a tube pedicle to his neck, however, the patient withdrew noticeably from the society of the ward. On encouragement, he was able to express negative feelings about his appearance as well as fear of others' reactions to it. Additionally, he was reassured that others' reactions to him, particularly within hospital society, would be based on the assumption that he had undergone surgical treatment for disease. Ultimately, with continued encouragement and support, his self-concept conflict seemed resolved as he returned to his former patterns of behavior and socialization on the ward.

Prior to surgery, Mr. W. had several weeks during which to maximally integrate the impending alterations. This, in turn, may have facilitated his early postoperative adaptation. The tube pedicle extending from the chest to the neck (required for closure of the pharyngostome), however, was an unexpected outcome. Although he was aware that the tube pedicle would only temporarily alter his appearance, he likely needed additional time to integrate its presence into self. Furthermore, Mr. W. had been successfully utilizing self-care as an adaptive mechanism. At this point, however, he was advised against touching or examining the pedicle because of the delicacy of this skin graft in already friable neck tissue. Thus, the anxiety he was experiencing as a result of this additional body image conflict probably accounted for his withdrawal from others.[40] He may also have been projecting his own initial negative response to others' reactions to him.[37] As Mr. W. was able to progressively ventilate his feelings over time and within a one-to-one interaction, his anxiety gradually diminished. Once again, supportive intervention primarily included encouragement of self-expression or emphasis on self as opposed to physical characteristics.

Role function

Mr. W. had been hospitalized for preoperative radiotherapy. Following surgery, however, he needed to develop different patterns of behavior. Adaptation of role function, therefore, required supportive intervention.

Prior to hospitalization, he had been actively employed and was sole provider for his ailing wife and teenaged daughter. While in the hospital, the client was frequently described as cooperative and uncomplaining by the nursing staff. He had assumed a major role in his care and performed self-care tasks independently and competently. His progress, however, was frequently described as discouraging by the medical staff. The initial reconstructive effort and its subsequent failure seemed to evoke the patient's first overt signs of anxiety, anger, and depression. These feelings seemed to be somewhat dissipated, however, following long periods of time spent with Mr. W. during which expression of his feelings and continued reassessment of his situation were encouraged. On return to the hospital, following a brief visit home, his spirits had improved remarkably. Although he did experience intermittent anxiety and depression during the remainder of his hospitalization, his attitude generally seemed more persevering. A marked elevation in his spirits was also noted in the days prior to his second visit home.

The individual cast into the role of patient with little or no preparation may experience increased anxiety or fear of social rejection if he feels unable to meet the demand placed on him during hospitalization.[6] Mr. W. initially adapted well to the demanding role of postoperative head and neck patient. He assumed maximal control over the environment through performance of self-care early in the course of hospitalization. The nursing staff, in turn, provided ongoing patient education by supervising self-care techniques, introducing new tasks as necessary, and explaining the rationale for all procedures.

In addition to alteration in physical appearance, Mr. W.'s anxiety, depression, anger, and expressed fear of social rejection may have also been generated by the postoperative complications he encountered. To him, his inability to heal properly may have represented failure to meet the demands placed on him in the patient role, thereby indicating failure to meet obligations within the society of the hospital. Reduction of situational stress was accomplished by repeated explanations of the physiologic bases for his healing difficulties, acknowledgment of his competent self-care, and suggestions for alternative measures as needed. During the early postoperative period, for example, Mr. W. and a staff member discussed the need for increasing caloric intake with a dietitian.

Additional social fortification seemed to be obtained from the client's home visits, at which times he was able to resume, at least in part, the role of caretaker with which he had been familiar prior to hospitalization. The results of a recent investigation would seem to support this assumption. It was concluded that the home environment of the laryngectomee is a critical factor in determination of successful rehabilitation.[26] Thus, acceptance of physiologic alterations as self ultimately eased interaction with others and, in turn, facilitated adaptation within the patient's concept of his own role function.

Interdependent relations

The average person who becomes hoarse as a result of laryngeal carcinoma sees three physicians and waits an average of 8 months before his larynx is examined and definitive diagnosis is made.[11] Supraglottic laryngeal carcinoma is usually advanced by this time and the client's prognosis is poor. Trust in others, particularly medical or nursing personnel, may therefore be weakened, and successful adaptation in the interdependence relations mode may be impeded.

It was evident from Mr. W.'s history that he had been dependent on habit-forming substances in the past. Although in this context he had made occasional references to not having been a "good husband," his current relationship with his family seemed stable. He frequently mentioned his wife and daughter fondly and remained in close contact with them by mail while in the hospital and away from home. Mr. W., with the exception of rare expressions of anger and frustration toward the staff, maintained a sound relationship with medical and nursing personnel. He developed a particularly close relationship with one nurse, however, and seemed to depend primarily on her for emotional support and reassurance. Evidence of this was in the form of feedback from the patient as well as from the staff. Additionally, his elevated spirits on return from his first home visit and enthusiastic preparation for the second seemed to manifest the continued support he derived from his family.

Manifestations of feelings that might indicate distrust for medical and nursing personnel were not overtly observed in this instance. The occasional expressions of anger and frustration directed toward the staff would seem more a reflection of the truly discouraging situation in which Mr. W. found himself. The expression of these feelings may have actually indicated a good deal of trust in the staff. That is, "negative" feelings could be openly expressed without fear of rejection or abandonment. Possibly mistrust of staff is precluded in the client who previously exhibited dependent behavior patterns. In this case, dependence seemed to have been transferred in an appropriately situational pattern. This assumption is supported by the conclusions of Dediarian and Clough,[10] who suggest that one's usual patterns of dependence and independence may vary under the stress of hospitalization. Mr. W.'s dependence patterns were likely exacerbated while in the hospital. The competence and independence he exhibited in self-care activities were indicative of a sound body image.[14] A good deal of his positive self-concept, however, seemed to be derived from his relationships with others. Thus, encouragement of independent behavior as well as allowance for dependent behavior, particularly during periods of increased stress, facilitated adaptation within the patient's normal interdependence relations patterns.

CONCLUSION

Nursing care of the head and neck cancer patient is examining and touching an extensive facial wound without being horrified, struggling to maintain pressure on a ruptured carotid artery, and shaving around a facial defect. It is being there for the first look in the mirror after surgery, appreciating laughter without sound, and encouraging expression of feelings that may be difficult and time consuming to write down. It is walking arm-in-arm around the hall with one so severely disfigured he was afraid to venture out alone, knowing that a prosthesis will be truly beneficial only after the defect is accepted, and engaging in face-to-face interaction.

Nursing care of the head and neck cancer patient is a direct encounter with each dimension of body image. As such, it is also a powerful support for its reintegration. Finally, it is frequently feeling awed by man's capacity for adaptation. Johnson's[24] observation seems to most aptly describe the respect that so many of these individuals command:

These patients are the ones who wanted, who fought, so desperately to live; and then, in failing that, manifested a courage that leaves us hushed and maybe even a little humbled. These are the real heroes . . . not us, the doctors and nurses.

REFERENCES

1. Allport, G. W.: Personality: a psychological interpretation, New York, 1937, Henry Holt & Co.
2. Aron, B.: Principles of radiation therapy. In Paparella, M., and Shumrick, D., editors: Otolaryngology, vol. 1, Basic sciences and related principles, Philadelphia, 1973, W. B. Saunders Co.
3. Ballenger, J. J.: Diseases of the nose, throat, and ear, Philadelphia, 1971, Lea & Febiger.
4. Bille, D. A.: The role of body image in patient compliance and education, Heart Lung **6:**143, 1977.
5. Blues, K.: A framework for nurses providing care to laryngectomy patients, Cancer Nurs. **1:**441, 1978.
6. Cleland, V.: The effect of stress on performance, Nurs. Res. **14:**292, 1965.
7. Cleveland, S. E., and Sikes, M. P.: Body image in chronic alcoholics and non-alcoholic psychiatric patients, J. Projective Techniques and Personality Assessment **30:**265, 1966.
8. Cobb, B., et al.: Patient-responsible delay of treatment in cancer, Cancer **7:**920, 1954.
9. Davies, J.: Embryology and anatomy of the face, palate, nose, and paranasal sinuses. In Paparella, M., and Shumrick, D., editors: Otolaryngology, Philadelphia, 1973, W. B. Saunders Co.
10. Dedarian, A., and Clough, D.: Patients' dependence and independence on the prehospitalization—post discharge continuum, Nurs. Res. **25:**27, 1976.
11. De Weese, D., and Saunders, W.: Textbook of otolaryngology, ed. 5, St. Louis, 1977, The C. V. Mosby Co.
12. Dixon, J. C.: Development of self recognition, J. Genet. Psychol. **91:**251, 1957.
13. Donovan, M., and Pierce, S.: Cancer care nursing, New York, 1976, Appleton-Century-Crofts.
14. Dropkin, M. J.: Influence of social approval upon postoperative compliance in patients undergoing radical head and neck surgery: a pilot exploration, Omaha, University of Nebraska, Unpublished master's thesis, 1978.
15. Ellis, F.: The present status of the N.S.D. concept as related to the larynx, Laryngoscope **85:**1531, 1975.
16. Epstein, S., and Shonz, F. C.: Attitudes toward persons with physical disabilities as a function of

attitude toward one's own body. Paper presented at annual meeting of American Psychological Association, St. Louis, Mo., 1962.
17. Fisher, S.: Body image boundaries in the aged, J. Psychol. **48:**315, 1959.
18. Fisher, S.: Body experience in fantasy and behavior, New York, 1970, Appleton-Century-Crofts.
19. Forgione, A. G., et al.: Fear, learning to cope, New York, 1979, Van Nostrand Reinhold Co.
20. Goodman, L., and Gillman, A.: The pharmacological basis of therapeutics, New York, 1965, Macmillan Inc.
21. Guyton, A. C.: Basic human physiology, Philadelphia, 1971, W. B. Saunders Co.
22. Haber, R. N.: Nature of the effects of set on perception, Psychol. Rev. **73:**335, 1966.
23. Johnson, L.: Body cathexis as a factor in somatic complaints, J. Consult. Clin. Psychol. **20:**145, 1956.
24. Johnson, P.: The gray areas—who decides? Am. J. Nurs. **77:**856, 1977.
25. Joseph, D., and Shumrick, D.: Risks of head and neck surgery in previously irradiated patients, Arch. Otolaryngol. **97:**381, 1973.
26. Kommers, M. S., et al.: Practical suggestions on counseling—how I do it: counseling the laryngectomized patient, Laryngoscope **87:**1961, 1977.
27. Levin, N., et al.: Sound the way for laryngectomies, Patient Care **5:**2, 1972.
28. MacComb, W., and Fletcher, G.: Cancer of the head and neck, Baltimore, 1971, The Williams & Wilkins Co.
29. MacGregor, F. C.: Psychosocial approach to patients with facial disfigurement. In Wood-Smith, D., and Porowski, P., editors: Nursing care for plastic surgery patients, St. Louis, 1967, The C. V. Mosby Co.
30. MacGregor, F. C.: Transformation and identity (the face and plastic surgery), New York, 1974, The New York Times Book Co.
31. Masson, R. L.: An investigation of the relationship between body image and attitudes expressed toward visibly disabled persons. Unpublished doctoral dissertation, New York, University of Buffalo, 1963.
32. Norris, C.: The professional nurse and body image. In Carlson, C., editor: Behavioral concepts and nursing intervention, Philadelphia, 1970, J. B. Lippincott Co.
33. Ogura, J., et al.: Conservative surgery for epidermoid carcinoma of the marginal area (aryepiglottic fold extension), Laryngoscope **85:**1801, 1975.
34. Olson, M. L., and Shedd, D. P.: Disability and rehabilitation in head and neck cancer patients after treatment, Head Neck Surg. **1:**52, 1978.
35. Park, R. E., and Burgess, E. W.: Introduction to the science of sociology, Chicago, 1969, University of Chicago Press.
36. Peck, A.: Emotional reactions to having cancer, Am. Roentgenol. Radium Ther. Nucl. Med. **114:**591, 1972.
37. Phillips, E.: Attitudes toward self and others: a brief questionnaire report, J. Consult. Clin. Psychol. **15:**79, 1951.
38. Probert, J. C., et al.: Patterns of spread of distant metastases in head and neck cancer, Cancer **33:**127, 1974.
39. Roy, S. C., and Riehl, J.: Conceptual models for nursing practice, New York, 1974, Appleton-Century-Crofts.
40. Sarnoff, I., and Zimbardo, P.: Anxiety, fear, and social affiliation, J. Abnorm. Soc. Psychol. **62:**356, 1961.
41. Saunders, W. H.: The larynx, Clin. Symp. **16:**67, 1964.
42. Secord, P. F., and Jourard, S. L.: The appraisal of body cathexis: body cathexis and the self, J. Consult. Clin. Psychol. **17:**343, 1957.
43. Stock, D.: An investigation into the interrelations between the self concept and feelings directed toward other persons and groups, J. Consult. Clin. Psychol. **13:**176, 1949.
44. Sutherland, A., et al.: The psychological impact of cancer and cancer surgery, Cancer **5:**857, 1952.
45. West, D. W.: Social adaptation patterns among cancer patients with facial disfigurements resulting from surgery, Arch. Phys. Med. Rehabil. **58:**473, 1977.
46. White, W. F., and Gaier, E. L.: Assessment of body image and self-concept among alcoholics with different intervals of sobriety, J. Clin. Psychol. **21:**374, 1965.
47. Wittreich, W., and Grace, M.: Body image and development. Technical report, Princeton University, Office of the Naval Reserves, March 29, 1955.
48. Zion, L. C.: Body concept as it relates to self-concept, Res. Q. **36:**490, 1965.

ADDITIONAL READING

Behnke, H., editor: Nursing management of patients with head and neck tumors. In Memorial Sloan Kettering Cancer Center: Guidelines for comprehensive nursing care in cancer, New York, 1973, Springer-Verlag Publishing Co., Inc.

Bower, F. L., editor: Normal development of body image, New York, 1977, John Wiley & Sons, Inc.

Catlin, D.: Surgery for head and neck lymphomas, Surgery **60:**1160, 1966.

Cobb, B.: Cancer: psychosocial factors. In Garrett, J., and Levin, E., editors: Rehabilitation practices with the physically disabled, New York, 1973, Columbia University Press.

Corbeil, M. E.: Nursing process for a patient with a body image disturbance, Nurs. Clin. North Am. **6:**155, 1971.

Costello, A. M.: Supporting the patient with problems related to body image. In Kruse, L. C., et al., editors: Cancer: pathophysiology, etiology, and management, St. Louis, 1979, The C. V. Mosby Co.

Creech, R. H.: The psychologic support of the cancer patient: a medical oncologist's viewpoint, Semin. Oncol. **2:**285, 1975.

Dropkin, L., et al.: Leiomyosarcoma of the nasal cavity and paranasal sinuses, Ann. Otol. Rhinol. Laryngol. **85:**399, 1976.

Francis, G. M.: Cancer: the emotional component, Am. J. Nurs. **69:**1677, 1969.

Frazell, E., et al.: The head and neck. In Nealon, T., editor: Management of the patient with cancer, Philadelphia, 1965, W. B. Saunders Co.

Horton, J., and Hill, G.: Clinical oncology, Philadelphia, 1977, W. B. Saunders Co.

Lee, L., and Lee, K. J.: A study of facial proportions and sketching of facial contours, Ear Nose Throat J. **58:**150, 1979.

McCloskey, J. C.: How to make the most of body image theory in nursing practice, Nursing '76 **6:**68, 1976.

Miller, R. N.: Psychological problems of patients with head and neck cancer. In Rehabilitation of the cancer patient, Chicago, 1972, Year Book Medical Publishers, Inc.

Murray, R. L. E.: Body image development in adulthood, Nurs. Clin. North Am. **7:**617, 1972.

Rossman, I., editor: Clinical geriatrics, Philadelphia, 1971, J. B. Lippincott Co.

Summers, G. W.: Physiologic problems following ablative surgery of the head and neck, Otolaryngol. Clin. North Am. **7:**217, 1974.

29

Safety problems encountered by clients with brain tumors

PEARL MOORE

Malignant brain tumors are of special interest to the nurse because the effects of this tumor are so devastating. This chapter presents a brief overview of current concepts about malignant brain tumors, including incidence, signs and symptoms, diagnostic methods, and treatment. A description of the numerous problems threatening the physical and psychologic safety of the client will also be considered along with the role of nursing intervention.

MALIGNANT BRAIN TUMORS

Clients with primary malignant brain tumors represent a small percentage of persons diagnosed with cancer. Of the estimated 765,000 new cancer cases for 1979, it was projected that 11,600 would be those of the central nervous system.[2] However, primary central nervous system cancer is the second most common cause of cancer death in children under age 15.[2] The reported actual incidence figures for brain metastases are variable. One author states that in 1977, of the 385,000 cancer deaths, 50,000 were directly attributable to central nervous system metastases.[6]

Malignant brain tumors may involve any of the brain structures or tissues. The most frequently occurring primary brain tumors of adulthood are in the malignant glioma group (Table 29-1). These tumors are usually located above the tentorium and involve the cerebral hemispheres. The gliomas, highly anaplastic and invasive tumors, are the most lethal brain cancer. The postoperative median survival time of 4.5 months substantiates this statement.[10] Although primary brain tumors often cross the cerebral hemisphere and sometimes seed into the spinal cord, distant metastasis has been rare.

Metastatic brain tumors may occur as a single lesion, but it is not uncommon for multiple brain metastases to be present. Kidney, lung, and breast tumors as well as melanomas commonly metastasize to the brain. Metastatic brain tumors are highly destructive growths, and, if untreated, the median survival is approximately 1 month.[5]

Signs and symptoms

The signs and symptoms of brain tumors occur as a result of increased intracranial pressure and interference with the function of the involved area of the brain. The most common presenting symptoms are headache, seizure, and a personality change.[11] Other symptoms include motor, speech, and sensory deficits, as well as visual disturbances and mental status changes (Table 29-2). The interested reader may wish to refer to neurology textbooks for information on clinicoanatomic correlations.

It is not unusual for symptoms of a brain tumor to be the first indication of cancer elsewhere in the body. In these instances, a search for the primary site is then undertaken. Conversely, evidence of brain metastases is often found at autopsy when, in fact, no clinical evidence was present.

Table 29-1. Incidence of brain tumors*

Classification	% incidence
Malignant glioma	
Glioblastoma multiforme	23.0
Astrocytoma	13.0
Ependymoma	1.8
Oligodendroglioma	1.6
Mixed and other gliomas	1.9
Medulloblastoma	1.5
Meningioma	16.0
Pituitary adenoma	8.2
Neurilemoma	5.7
Craniopharyngioma	2.8
Sarcoma	2.5
Hemangioblastoma	2.7
Pineal tumor	1.1
Metastatic	13.0
Other	6.0

*From Walker, M. D.: Brain and peripheral nervous system tumors. In Holland, J. F., and Frei, E., III, editors: Cancer medicine, Philadelphia, 1973, Lea & Febiger, p. 1388.

Diagnostic methods

Early diagnosis, a goal of cancer control, is very difficult in the client with a brain tumor. For example, headache, the most common presenting symptom, is often ignored or confused with a benign condition. In addition, the tumor may be small and thus cause no compressive symptoms, or the tumor may be located in a "silent" area of the brain. Finally, an economically feasible mass screening test is not available for this type of tumor.

Diagnosis of a client's tumor usually occurs when the symptoms become pronounced and disabling. The diagnosis is based on the history, visual examination, neurologic examination, and various neurodiagnostic techniques. These techniques include skull films, electroencephalograms,

Table 29-2. Major signs and symptoms of a brain tumor

General signs and symptoms resulting from increased intracranial pressure	Focal signs and symptoms resulting from interference in the function of a specific area of the brain
Cardinal signs	Mental status changes
Headache	Motor paresis or paralysis
Vomiting	Sensory deficits
Papilledema	Focal and psychic seizures
Mental disturbance	Speech disturbances
Decreased level of consciousness	Visual loss
Generalized seizures	Cranial nerve palsies
Vital sign changes	Ataxia
Vertigo	Diabetes insipidus
	Abnormal growth

cerebral angiograms, and brain scans. However, it is the sensitive and specific computerized axial tomography brain scan that has become the most valuable tool in diagnosing and localizing brain involvement.[4] The final diagnosis is not determined, however, until histopathologic confirmation is obtained.

Treatment

The first treatment administered to a client with a brain tumor is designed to reduce the increased intracranial pressure caused by the tumor and the associated edema. These treatments may include surgical decompression, the glucocorticoids, or the hyperosmolar agents.

All of the cancer treatment modalities are employed in treating the person with a primary malignant brain tumor. Each modality, however, is laden with problems when applied to the brain. For example, the surgical principle of decreasing the tumor burden is often impossible if the mass is a deep cerebral lesion or if it is located in a critical brain stem site. In administering radiation therapy, the relative radioresistance of the hypoxic brain tumor and the potential danger of radiation necrosis are ever present considerations. Other treatment problems may evolve from the brain tissue–capillary interface commonly known as the blood-brain barrier. The blood-brain barrier and the need for lipid solubility have severely limited the chemotherapeutic agents available to treat this tumor.

However, progress has been made in the management of these tumors, increasing survival time and improving the quality of life. Refined techniques have reduced surgical morbidity and mortality and have provided clients the time necessary to proceed with radiation and chemotherapy. Whole brain radiation therapy, as opposed to more restricted portal size therapy, has decreased tumor extension to other areas of the brain. In addition, increased dosage levels of radiation have increased survival times.[9] However, higher dose levels of radiation may approach the tolerance limits of normal tissue reparative processes. As brain tumors are hypoxic, the use of hypoxic cell radiosensitizing agents is also being evaluated in clients with brain tumors.[8]

Because the lipid-soluble nitrosourea compounds cross the blood-brain barrier with ease, better chemotherapeutic agents are now available. Agents employed in clinical chemotherapy of brain tumors include carmustine (BiCNU), lomustine (CeeNU), semustine (MeCCNU), procarbazine, and vincristine.[5] In a National Cancer Institute Brain Tumor Study Group controlled clinical trial, carmustine added to radiation therapy and surgery has increased the median survival time to 51 weeks.[9] Many other drugs, local or total body hyperthermia, and immunotherapy are being evaluated in other controlled clinical trials.

Although radiation therapy is the accepted treatment modality for the client with a metastatic brain tumor, surgical resection also offers immediate palliation and a specific tissue diagnosis. Surgery is indicated if the person has a solitary and accessible metastatic brain lesion secondary to a slow-growing systemic primary tumor and no evidence of other life-threatening metastatic involvement.[10] Both surgery and radiation therapy have demonstrated only a 3- to 6-month increase in the median survival time of clients with metastatic brain tumors, but the relief from the disabling intracranial symptoms has justified these measures.[5] To date, chemotherapy has not proved effective in the management of metastatic brain tumors.

Prevention or cure of brain tumors still has not been achieved. However, aggressive treatment does offer longer life. The nurse is instrumental in making this a better quality life. Helping clients cope with resultant problems is the most important contribution the nurse can make. Therefore, the remainder of this chapter is directed to that topic.

PROBLEMS ENCOUNTERED BY CLIENTS WITH BRAIN TUMORS

The problems encountered by clients with brain tumors result from a disturbed neurologic state, the treatment employed, and the crisis that follows. These problems may be further affected by the premorbid family dynamics that influence the client and by the coping techniques the client has acquired. Because most of these problems pose a significant threat to the client's physical or psychologic safety, they deserve serious consideration when planning the nursing intervention (Fig. 29-1).

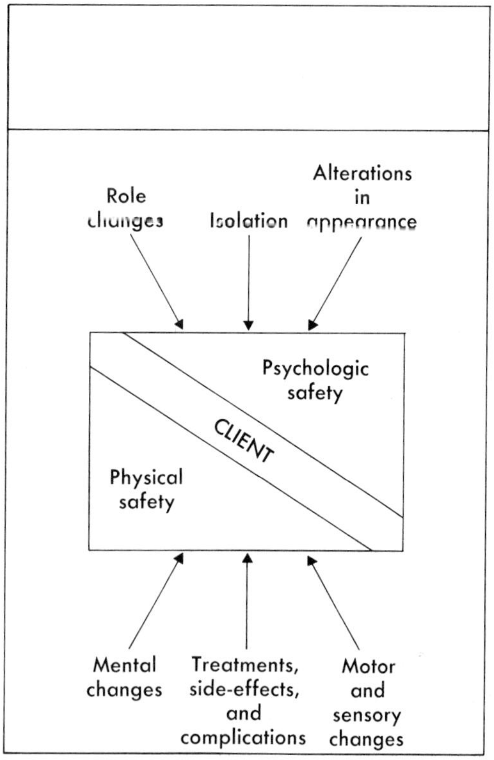

Fig. 29-1. Problems threatening clients' physical and psychologic safety.

Mental status changes

Clients with brain tumors frequently demonstrate changes in their mental status. These may include personality changes such as irritability, mood swings, or inappropriate behavior. Intellectual impairments such as memory deficits, impaired judgment, or disorientation may also be present. Communication disorders and a decreased level of consciousness are additional problems.

Such changes create a very hazardous situation. Accidents frequently happen to persons with even a slightly decreased level of consciousness. Persons with impaired judgment or inappropriate behavior take risks that often result in injuries. Because the manifestations of these problems are often quite subtle, the nurse must be certain that the client's family knows that these problems exist. An aware family is more likely to anticipate and eliminate possibly dangerous situations.

Although persons with any disease may fail to follow health teaching instructions, clients with mental status changes are especially prone to disregard instructions. Confused or memory-impaired persons may take their medications improperly. Depressed clients may fail to report symptoms indicative of disease progression, complications, or drug toxicity. Finally, persons with receptive speech problems may fail to understand instructions.

Since it is important to ensure that instructions are followed, family members are always included when teaching the client. Because of cognitive deficits, it will often be necessary to give the client instructions at a level different from those given the family. Teaching is adapted according to the client's particular learning deficiency. Examples include repetition for a memory-impaired person or visual aids for a person unable to interpret verbal speech. Effective teaching requires extreme patience on the part of the nurse, but protection of the client makes the effort worthwhile.

Motor and sensory function changes

Cerebral hemisphere and cerebellar tumors often result in motor function changes. Common symptoms include muscle weakness (paresis) or muscle paralysis (plegia), decreased muscle tone, involuntary or uncoordinated movements, and ataxia. Apraxia, the loss of ability to perform a previously learned act such as dressing or eating, is an additional symptom.

Clients with impaired motor function frequently sustain injuries from falls. Teaching clients and families proper ambulation and transfer techniques may reduce falls. The proper use of various aids such as rails, quad canes, walkers, and braces must also be stressed. In addition, a safe environment is essential in preventing accidents.

The major dangers threatening the person with impaired motor function, however, are the complications of immobility. These include (1) dependent edema, (2) pneumonia, (3) thrombophlebitis and pulmonary embolism, (4) renal calculi, and (5) skin breakdown. The nurse must teach the client what needs to be known to reduce these complications.

Prevention of the complications of immobility depends in large measure on vigilant nursing care. The incidence of thrombophlebitis and a resultant pulmonary embolus may be reduced by increased activity or by routine range of motion exercises when ambulation is impossible. The proper use of support hose may also be of benefit. Of course, leg pain, redness, or an edematous extremity must be reported immediately.

Other complications can also be prevented. For example, frequent position changes, coughing, and deep breathing may prevent pneumonia. Frequent position changes, keeping the skin well lubricated, and keeping the bed dry will aid in preventing a break in the skin integrity. The incidence of renal calculi can be reduced by an increased fluid intake, and if calcium stones are present, urine acidification with cranberry juice is helpful. Finally, dependent edema can be reduced by elevation of the extremities and support hose.

A word of caution is needed. All families are not physically or psychologically capable of taking care of the immobile client. In these instances, alternatives such as paid home helpers or extended care facilities must be explored.

The person with a brain tumor may also experience changes in sensory function. Symptoms include crude tactile sensory deficits, corticosensory perceptive losses, or disturbances of the special sense organs. The careful assessment of these losses is essential if the client is to be protected from injury and additional problems.

The type of intervention required for each person with sensory loss is contingent on the precautions that must be taken to avoid injuries. For example, a person with a tactile loss may have to be supervised closely when handling hot, cold, or sharp objects. Persons with visual field deficits need to have materials they require placed within their visual boundaries. Persons with more severe visual losses are, of course, not permitted to drive.

Side-effects and complications of treatment

Persons receiving chemotherapy for brain tumors are subject to the same problems as others receiving chemotherapy. The reader is referred to Chapter 14 for a discussion of these problems. In addition, neurosurgical postoperative nursing care is beyond the scope of this chapter.

Radiation therapy. Clients receiving whole brain radiation therapy will experience side-effects such as alopecia, cerebral edema, and fatigue. Severe cerebral edema will cause increased intracranial pressure and focal deficits similar to those caused by the tumor. If the nurse prepares clients for this occurrence and reassures them that the edema is manageable, clients and families can be spared much anxiety.

Glucocorticoids. The glucocorticoids, which play such a large role in the management of brain tumors, have been used in the treatment of cancer for both their antineoplastic and palliative effects. Persons wtih brain tumors often rely on substantial doses of the glucocorticoids for decreasing tumor-associated and radiation-associated cerebral edema. In addition, the subjective palliative effects of an increased sense of well-being and an improved appetite are of benefit.

Cortisol, also known as hydrocortisone, is the major glucocorticoid. There are many synthetic cortisol compounds on the market, varying in their therapeutic potency as well as in their potential for side-effects. Table 29-3 illustrates the relative anti-inflammatory and sodium-retaining potencies of five synthetic compounds compared to hydrocortisone.

Many side-effects are associated with the prolonged use of the glucocorticoids as follows:

Clinical problems related to prolonged glucocorticoid therapy

- Infection and delayed wound healing
- Electrolyte and fluid imbalance
- Gastric disturbances
- Steroid diabetes
- Musculoskeletal changes
  - Steroid myopathy
  - Osteoporosis
- Acute adrenal insufficiency
- Cushingoid changes
- Behavioral disturbances
- Other problems
  - Subcapsular cataracts
  - Renal calculi
  - Blood element alterations
  - Cardiac abnormalities
  - Menstrual irregularities
  - Inhibition of linear growth in children

The nurse has a responsibility to constantly assess for these side-effects and to teach clients how to cope with them. Problems associated with the major side-effects are considered here.

Clients receiving long-term glucocorticoids are very susceptible to infection owing to suppression of their normal immunologic, inflammatory, and healing responses. In

Table 29-3. Relative potencies of selected corticosteroids*

Compound	Relative anti-inflammatory potency	Relative sodium-retaining potency
Hydrocortisone (cortisol)	1.0	1.0
Cortisone	0.8	0.8
Prednisone	4.0	0.8
Prednisolone	4.0	0.8
Methylprednisolone	5.0	0.5
Dexamethasone	25.0	0

*Modified from Haynes, R. C., and Larner, J.: Adrenocorticotrophic hormones; adrenocortical steroids and their synthetic analogs; inhibitors of adrenocortical steroid biosynthesis. In Goodman, L. S., and Gillman, A., editors: The pharmacological basis of therapeutics, ed. 5, New York, 1975, Macmillan Inc., p. 1491.

addition, if the person is already generally debilitated, immobile, or myelosuppressed from chemotherapy, the chances of infection are further increased. To make the danger even greater, the normal responses to infection, inflammation and fever, are masked by the use of the glucocorticoids.

The nurse must constantly assess clients for evidence of infection and take all the steps necessary to prevent infection. Cultures should be taken for even the slightest symptom. Since a dormant tubercular process can be reactivated, frequent chest x-ray examinations and sputum cultures should be done and prophylactic isoniazid may be indicated. As glucocorticoids diminish the cellular immune response, tubercular skin tests are falsely negative. If the person on a glucocorticoid does contract an infection, large doses of antibiotics will be needed. In addition, because of the stress of the infection, the glucocorticoids may have to be increased to prevent adrenal crisis.

Fluid and electrolyte imbalance may occur as many glucocorticoids, particularly hydrocortisone, have some mineralocorticoid action.[3] The results are sodium and water retention and potassium loss. Thus, the person on glucocorticoids needs to be assessed frequently for edema, hypertension, weight gain, and hypokalemia. A low-sodium, high-potassium diet will need to be taught. In addition, scrupulous skin care is required by the edematous client to prevent skin breakdown.

Whether the glucocorticoids predispose persons to the development of peptic ulcers is a debated subject.[3] Many persons receiving glucocorticoids, however, do complain of gastric distress. The danger to these clients is that the early inflammatory symptoms are masked and, thus, the ulcer may perforate without any warning. Clients, particularly those with positive ulcer history, must be observed closely for the signs and symptoms of peptic ulcer. Health teaching for these clients includes encouragement of (1) a bland diet, (2) avoidance of caffeine, alcohol, and ulcerogenic drugs, (3) low-sodium antacids, (4) stool guaic testing, and (5) reporting even slight abdominal discomfort.

Because the glucocorticoids stimulate gluconeogenesis, diabetes may also occur. Steroid-induced diabetes is characterized by hyperglycemia and glycosuria with rare ketosis. Periodic blood glucose and frequent urine glucose monitoring is indicated, particularly in the client with a family history of diabetes mellitus. Clients should be instructed to report polydypsia and polyuria. A carbohydrate-restricted diet may be all that is necessary for controlling steroid-induced diabetes, although occasionally oral hypoglycemic agents or insulin is indicated. Known previous diabetics will require careful monitoring when receiving glucocorticoids.

The musculoskeletal side-effects of the glucocorticoids, steroid myopathy and osteoporosis, are very serious problems. Steroid myopathy is characterized by a weakness of the proximal muscles, particularly in the legs. This may be severe enough to prevent ambulation. Osteoporosis, a reduction in bone mass, often leads to pathologic fractures, particularly vertebral body compression fractures. Clients must be taught measures to prevent pathologic fractures. This would include (1) care in turning, (2) a firm mattress, and (3) prevention of falls. Clients who do sustain vertebral fractures often require back braces, bed boards, and various analgesics. Measures to decrease these musculoskeletal side-effects such as increased activity and increased protein and calcium intake may be helpful.

To prevent acute adrenal insufficiency, the nurse has a responsibility to see to it that clients always take their medications properly. Clients need reminders never to skip doses or to run out of medication. In addition, clients need to be cautioned that they require medication even when they feel well. Families need to know that if the client is unable to take oral medications, they must seek immediate medical help for parenteral glucocorticoid substitutes.

During abnormal periods of stress, clients are in further danger of developing acute adrenal insufficiency. At these times, they require increased dosages of the glucocorticoids. In addition, clients receiving concurrent phenytoin or phenobarbital may require increased dosages of the glucocorticoids owing to an increased cortisol hepatic metabolic rate.[12] Since most clients with brain tumors are also receiving anticonvulsants, this is important.

The use of alternate-day therapy administration, by diminishing hypothalamic-pituitary-adrenal suppression time, may do much to minimize these undesired side-effects. Only those glucocorticoids with a short hypothalamic-pituitary-adrenal axis suppression time and with low sodium-retaining properties are used in alternate-day therapy. Prednisone, prednisolone, and methylprednisolone meet this requirement.[7] Alternate-day therapy is instituted by doubling the maintenance dose and administering it as a single dose every other morning. This procedure mimics the natural circadian production of cortisol. In our experience, clients with brain tumors on alternate-day therapy have often required a tripling of the dose to control their neurologic symptoms.

Appearance changes

Persons with brain tumors experience many alterations in their appearance that may have an effect on their body image. Alterations engendered by the disease may include facial asymmetry or uncoordinated movements. Alterations induced by treatment include alopecia from radiation therapy and may include the cushingoid symptoms that result from the long-term use of the glucocorticoids. Cushingoid symptoms, caused by edema and a redistribution of body fat, include truncal obesity, "buffalo hump," thin arms and legs, "moon face," transparent skin, and striae. Less understood cushingoid symptoms include hirsutism and acne.

Such pronounced visible alterations cause all clients and families anxiety, particularly in a society that places so much value on physical beauty. The degree of anxiety depends, of course, on the value clients place on physical appearance. To many clients an altered appearance means the loss of earning power or sexual desirability. It may also mean vulnerability and isolation.

There is no blueprint to make nursing intervention easy and comfortable. The nurse must do the best that is possible to help the client cope. An atmosphere of caring and acceptance must be structured for clients who must be encouraged to express their feelings. The nurse and family need to realize that angry or withdrawn behavior is not an attack on them. To possibly ease the impact of the alterations, explanations of their physical bases can be helpful. Stressing the reversibility of temporary changes is important.

Since acceptance by others is essential in increasing the client's self-esteem, the nurse must prepare others for the client's appearance. If others respond in horror or revulsion, the effect on the client can be cataclysmic. The nurse must help others to understand how much the client needs support and acceptance.

Returning to work or school is very difficult for clients experiencing appearance alterations. Consider persons who made their living in a field with heavy public contact. Even if employers are willing to permit them to return to work, will the public be willing to accept them? Consider already image-conscious adolescents. Will they be willing to face their peers and will their peers be willing to accept them? Now nursing intervention is more important than ever. Frank and open discussions are required to prevent further deterioration of self-image. Referral to such resources as self-help groups or mental health therapists can be beneficial. In addition, many people have found great comfort and strength from literature that describes how others have coped.

Finally, clients should be encouraged to use whatever adornments will help them maintain or improve a positive self-image, for example, wigs, scarves, or pretty clothes.

Role change

Role change is a source of great stress to any person. Because of the general debilitating aspects of disease or treatment, many ill persons experience role changes. The neurologic impairments of clients with brain tumors, however, will more often prevent return to usual roles. Clients forced to watch as others assume their job or home responsibilities suffer a threat to their self-concept. In addition the economic burden of lost income or hiring others to perform home responsibilities creates further stress.

These clients often experience feelings of worthlessness and guilt because they no longer see themselves as productive or contributory. They may cry and rage against their helplessness. They may be angry and express their anger by being highly critical of others. Some turn their anger inward and become depressed or withdrawn, avoiding interaction with others. Or they may become infantile and superdependent on others.

Intervention should begin with an assessment of the client's fears and concerns regarding a role change. The venting of angry feelings should be encouraged. Unrealistic guilt needs to be explored. Steps should be taken to help clients achieve self-esteem. One way is to be certain that whenever possible clients participate in their own care.

Families need constant support. They need help in understanding the client's behavior, particularly in understanding that anger is not directed at them. The nurse must encourage the family to underscore the client's value as a useful and contributing family member regardless of role change. One suggestion that can be made is that the family should always include the client in family decisions.

Isolation

Another problem affecting a client and family is isolation. The fear of seizure, one of the most terrifying and anxiety-producing events, often causes a family to isolate themselves. The nurse can do much to reassure clients and families regarding seizure control. Inform them that increased dosages or different anticonvulsants will often stop seizure activity. Clients need to be cautioned, however, that because alcohol speeds up removal of anticonvulsants from the body, the possibility of a seizure is increased if they drink alcoholic beverages.[1]

Embarrassment, resulting from the client's appearance or behavioral changes, causes further isolation. This is difficult to cope with. However, explaining the bases of these changes may help to decrease their impact.

Some clients and families isolate themselves in another way. They turn their backs on the health care team, seeking unorthodox treatment methods. Given the poor prognosis, clients with brain tumors are particularly susceptible to cancer quackery. Steps can be taken to dissuade the client from seeking unorthodox treatment. The nurse must provide current information regarding both accepted and unaccepted methods of treatment. After all avenues have been discussed, it is less likely that the client will turn to unorthodox methods. In addition, since it is fear that often drives people to unorthodox treatments, we need to address that fear. We must assure clients that we will not desert them and hope must always be underscored.

Frequently the major cause of isolation is exhaustion. Families are often required to give constant, demanding care. In addition, there is strain caused by the numerous trips to the hospital for treatment. Families may feel trapped by their overburdening responsibility. To help the family, the nurse must serve as a sounding board for their exhaustion and frustration. The nurse must encourage family members to take a break in their routine without feeling guilty. Often the nurse has to provide reassurance that their feelings are normal. In addition, relief can be suggested in the form of volunteer or paid part-time home assistants.

CASE STUDY

A client whose problems illustrate many of the points made in this chapter was Carol, a 27-year-old wife and mother of two young children. Two years before I met her, Carol suddenly had a generalized seizure while working as a radiology technician. At that time, neurologic evaluation, including an angiogram, proved negative. During the next 2 years, Carol developed a personality change characterized as depression with "no interest in living." This change created a strain on the marriage, and her husband subsequently obtained a divorce and received custody of the children. Following their separation, she was admitted to a psychiatric facility for severe depression. On examination, the psychiatrist discovered that Carol had symptoms of a brain tumor and transferred her to a medical-surgical hospital for a CAT scan. A glioblastoma multiforme of the right parietal and occipital lobes was found and subtotally resected. I met Carol when she was transferred to our hospital for initiation of radiation therapy and chemotherapy.

Carol's treatment during our time together included 6,000 rads of whole brain radiation therapy divided into 32 daily fractions and 12 courses of oral chemotherapy (procarbazine). Treatment to control her severe cerebral edema required large doses of daily glucocorticoids and resulted in her becoming steroid dependent. In addition, she needed increasing dosages of anticonvulsants for seizure control.

Observations of Carol included serial CAT scans and monthly neurologic examinations. After 5 months of chemotherapy, her scan indicated a tumor recurrence. Subsequent scans showed no further increase in tumor size. Her major neurologic deficits included a left central facial weakness, left hemiparesis, an ataxic gait, and an expressive speech deficit.

During the time I cared for Carol, she was plagued by numerous treatment side-effects and complications, including (1) total alopecia; (2) severe bone marrow depression and abnormal liver enzyme studies necessitating treatment delays and dosage modifications; (3) severe nausea and vomiting requiring hospitalization for fluid and parenteral glucocorticoid replacement; (4) numerous urinary tract infections, oral candida mouth infections, and herpes zoster of the second and third division of the trigeminal nerve; (5) dependent edema of her left hand and both feet; (6) left leg thrombophlebitis requiring anticoagulation therapy; and (7) a generalized deossification of the vertebral bones with compression fractures of T_{12}, L_1, and L_4. With all these complications, Carol eventually became totally immobile, unable to leave her home.

Initial and subsequent assessments revealed that Carol, along with her physical problems, faced many psychosocial problems. First, Carol faced a multitude of losses. She lost her husband in a painful divorce. She lost custody of her children. Even the weekly visits with her children lost all joy, since they were fearful of her appearance. She lost her job. She had to give up her own apartment. After 10 years of being independent, it was difficult to move back to her mother's small home. Saddest of all, she lost her own positive self-image. The reflection in the mirror showed alopecia, a "moon facies," a left-sided facial droop, a leg brace, and a quad cane. Her assessment was, "I look like a freak."

Second, Carol felt alone. She had no close friends and did not belong to any clubs or organizations. She said that her job had been her social life. Her only support was her family. Yet, she was unable to discuss her illness with them because they became frightened when she cried. She felt she was a burden and useless. Attempts to be independent were stifled by the family's protectiveness. Both she and her mother felt they agitated one another but knew that they needed each other. As time went on, Carol became more frightened, unable to make decisions, and even contemplated suicide.

Prompt nursing intervention was necessary to help Carol cope with her numerous problems. Thorough health teaching was an important component of her care. At our initial meeting, I explained the cause of her various neurologic impairments, the purpose of all the treatments, and the possible side-effects she might encounter. We also discussed preventive measures that might protect her from complications. As Carol had a history of gastric ulcer and she was receiving high doses of steroid, measures to prevent ulcer reactivation were particularly stressed from the start. She did occasionally report positive stool guaics to us, and since she frequently had thrombocytopenia, this was serious. Although she never developed a serious bleeding problem or other evidence of ulcer, through her constant observations and prompt reporting, we would have been able to act quickly.

From the first course of chemotherapy, Carol had periods of severe leukopenia owing to bone marrow depression. She began to contract numerous infections and their control became a priority. As the steroids mask fever, Carol was instructed again to observe for and report any other evidence of infection. One nursing intervention that proved effective in decreasing one type of infection, stomatitis, and secondary candida infections was an oral hygiene routine and systematic mouth assessment. Despite preventive measures, Carol contracted another type of infection, facial herpes zoster. This added assault on her body image, her pain, and the danger of ocular complications was almost more than she or I could handle. However, with constant support, analgesics, and appropriate therapy, the herpes subsided and we were both relieved of this added stress.

Since Carol had a hemiparetic gait and would invert her left foot during ambulation, she was in constant danger of falling. I knew from my initial assessment how important independent ambulation was to her self-confidence. The physical therapist taught Carol how to do muscle strengthening exercises. With constant reinforcement of these exercises, a leg brace, and a quad cane, she ambulated independently for almost 2 years.

Seizure control was another important intervention for Carol's safety. I stressed the importance of taking her anticonvulsants regularly, and Carol's family understood how to protect her from injury during a seizure. With frequent monitoring of anticonvulsant blood levels and appropriate dosage regulations, her seizures were eventually well controlled.

Carol required some specific dietary instructions. When she developed dependent edema, she was again encouraged to limit her salt intake. Because procarbazine is a monoamine oxidase inhibitor, Carol was instructed to avoid foods high in tyramine. Because of her decreased activity and the analgesics, she developed severe constipation. My suggestion of adding bran to her diet proved effective.

Measures to prevent osteoporosis and pathologic vertebral fractures failed. As a result, Carol was faced with severe pain and further impeded mobility. A back brace and a bed board were prescribed, but her pain persisted. A major challenge in Carol's care had become pain control. Various analgesics were used, but prescribed dosages were ineffective. As a result of my suggestion, Carol was given control of their use and then experienced relief from her pain.

Providing Carol and her family emotional support was the second large component of her care. Carol and her family needed the opportunity to ventilate their fears, frustrations, and what they perceived as their inadequacies. I explored Carol's feelings of being a burden with her family and discussed her need for some control and independence. A satisfactory compromise was worked out that allowed Carol to do some small chores at home. While in the hospital, we had the recreational therapist meet Carol and she began to make artificial flowers. Her gifts of flowers began to appear in several departments throughout the hospital. This creative activity gave her much pleasure. After our discussions, Carol's sister and sister-in-law began alternating their weekly trips to the hospital with her. These trips eventually were followed by enjoyable luncheons and shopping excursions.

Attempts at normalcy were encouraged. Carol took delight in our compliments regarding her beautiful wigs and attractive clothes. I encouraged Carol's sister to speak with her children and explain why their mother appeared different. It was also important that she stress that their mother was the same person, only ill. Shortly after, Carol told me her visits with the children were much better. This time when she cried, it was with joy. In addition, as Carol told me she wasn't fearful of her appearance or speech when she was with people who understood her problems, we encouraged her to share her experiences with other clients. They appreciated and benefited from her efforts. The pride Carol felt from this was therapeutic.

As Carol's illness and depression increased, many other resource people and agencies were called on to offer help. The hospital chaplain developed a good rapport with Carol and arrangements were made for him to visit during her outpatient appointments. The psychiatrist from the health center's psychiatric liaison service met with Carol regularly to help her cope with her fears. Since financial concerns were also upsetting Carol, I contacted the state medical assistance department so that she could get needed financial aid.

When Carol became homebound, the American Cancer Society provided Carol with needed equipment to facilitate her home nursing. The people that she had the most contact with during her last few months of life were her local visiting nurses. They provided Carol and her family with constant emotional support and in Carol's own words were "angels." They taught her family how to provide the constant physical nursing that Carol required.

I spoke with Carol and her mother regularly on the phone during her last few months of life, but because she lived so far from the hospital, I never saw her again. Carol died of pneumonia at home 2½ years after we first met.

SUMMARY

This chapter has sought to provide nurses with the information they need to give high-level care to clients with malignant brain tumors. Many of the problems encountered by clients were explored. The intervention stressed was that of providing information and support as well as the prevention of complications. Caring for clients with brain tumors is both challenging and rewarding.

REFERENCES

1. Alcohol-Drug Interactions, FDA Drug Bulletin, Food and Drug Administration, Rockville, Md., **9:**11, 1978.
2. American Cancer Society: 1979 cancer facts and figures, New York, 1978, American Cancer Society, Inc., pp. 10, 14.
3. Goodman, L. S., and Gillman, A., editors: The pharmacological basis of therapeutics, ed. 5, New York, 1975, Macmillan Inc., p. 1480, 1496.
4. Olendorf, W. H.: The quest for an image of brain, Neurology **28:**517, 1978.
5. Posner, J. B., and Shapero, W. R.: Brain tumor, Arch. Neurol. **32:**781, 1975.
6. Shapero, W. R.: Management of primary malignant brain tumors, weekly update: neurology and neurosurgery, Princeton, N.J., 1978, Biomedia Inc., p. 2.
7. Thorn, G. W., editor: Steroid therapy: a clinical update for the 1970's, Kalamazoo, Mich., 1974, Upjohn Co., p. 35.
8. Urtasun, R., et al.: Radiation and high dose metronidazole (Flagyl) in supertentorial glioblastoma, N. Engl. J. Med. **294:**1364, 1976.
9. Walker, M.: Brain tumor study group: a survey of current activities. Modern concepts in brain tumor therapy: laboratory and clinical investigations, National Cancer Institute Monograph 46, Publication No. 77-1236, Bethesda, Md., 1977, U.S. Department of Health, Education and Welfare, p. 211.
10. Walker, M. D.: Brain and peripheral nervous system tumors. In Holland, J. F., and Frei, E., III, editors: Cancer medicine, Philadelphia, 1973, Lea & Febiger, p. 1396, 1398.
11. Walker, M. D.: Malignant brain tumors—a synopsis, CA **25:**115, 1975.
12. Werk, E. E., et al.: Interference in the effect of dexamethasone and diphenylhydantoin, N. Engl. J. Med. **281:**32, 1969.

ADDITIONAL READING

Barlogre, B., et al.: Total-body hyperthermia with and without chemotherapy of advanced human neoplasms, Cancer Res. **39:**1481, 1979.

Blount, M., and Kinney, A. B.: Chronic steroid therapy, Am. J. Nurs. **74:**1626, 1974.

Bouchard, R., and Owens, N. F.: Nursing care of the cancer patient, ed. 3, St. Louis, 1976, The C. V. Mosby Co., p. 140.

Conway, B. L.: Carini and Owens neurological and neurosurgical nursing, ed. 7, St. Louis, 1978, The C. V. Mosby Co., p. 369.

Erlich, S. S., and Davis, R.: Spinal subarachnoid metastasis from primary intracranial glioblastoma multiforme, Cancer **42:**2854, 1978.

Fager, C. A.: Indications for neurosurgical intervention in metastatic lesions of the central nervous system, Med. Clin. North Am. **59:**487, 1975.

Fewer, D., Wilson, C. B., and Levin, V. A.: Brain tumor chemotherapy, Springfield, Ill., 1976, Charles C Thomas, Publisher.

Heat plus drugs add up to better glioma treatment, Med. World News, p. 26, July 9, 1979.

Mahaley, M. S.: A current prospective for immunotherapy of brain tumors, Surg. Rounds **2:**50, 1979.

Rubenstein, L. J.: Tumors of the central nervous system. 2nd Series: Fascicle 6 of Atlas of tumor pathology, Washington, D.C., 1972, Armed Forces Institute of Pathology.

Simpson, J. F., and Magee, K. R.: Clinical evaluation of the nervous system, Boston, 1973, Little, Brown & Co.

Wilson, C. B.: Current concepts in cancer: brain tumors, N. Engl. J. Med. **300**(26):1469, 1979.

30

Male sexuality and genitourinary cancer

GARY R. HOUSTON and DOROTHY RODRIGUEZ

Clients with genitourinary cancer encompass the principles of nursing care for clients undergoing surgery, radiotherapy, and chemotherapy. Client and family education and goals of rehabilitation are also incorporated in their care.

This chapter will focus on nursing care of clients with cancer of the genitourinary system, including the kidney, bladder, testes, prostate, and penis. Effective nursing assessments and care plans can only be designed and implemented after a thorough understanding of the pathophysiology of the disease and related treatment modalities.

OVERVIEW OF INCIDENCE

This area is important to nursing because the estimated cases of the genitourinary cancers listed above result in a total of 120,000 or fully one sixth of the total new cancer cases projected for 1979. The total of 120,000 is broken down in Table 30-1.

In the male client, the estimated 1979 incidence of cancer by subsets indicates that just two of these cancers, cancer of the prostate with 17% and cancer of the urinary bladder with 10%, total 27% of all subsets.[10] Although estimated figures only, these point to the relative numbers and frequency of genitourinary cancers. The specific areas of each cancer will be discussed individually along with the themes of male sexuality and rehabilitation, which are important concepts for the nurse to consider throughout the disease process.

CANCER OF THE PROSTATE

Reportedly, carcinoma of the prostate ranks as the second most common malignant disease found in men.[23] The most frequently occurring cancer of the prostate is adenocarcinoma; transitional cell carcinoma and sarcoma have also been identified.

Symptomatology

Symptoms of prostate cancer include decreased urinary force and stream, nocturia, pain, bleeding, and, in some clients, acute urinary obstruction. To ascertain the size and firmness of the prostate, the physician or nurse examiner will perform a digital rectal examination. This procedure should be a routine component of the physical examination in all men past the age of 40.

As in most neoplasms, etiology of prostate cancer is uncertain. It has been suggested

Table 30-1. Subsets of genitourinary cancers*

Type of cancer	Estimated new cases for 1979
Prostate	64,000
Urinary bladder	35,000
Kidney and other	16,200
TOTAL	115,200

*From Silverberg, E.: Cancer statistics, 1979, CA **29**(1):14, 1979.

Table 30-2. Staging of prostate cancer*

Stage A	Unsuspected carcinoma found in one or two microscopic areas of the prostate obtained at operation for benign disease
Stage B	Tumor confined within the prostatic capsule without an elevation of the acid phosphatase level
Stage C	Tumor extending into extracapsular structure but confined to the local area
Stage D	Distant metastatic disease

*Reproduced with permission from Johnson, D. E., et al.: Urologic cancer. In Clark, R. L., and Howe, C. D., editors: Cancer patient care at M. D. Anderson Hospital and Tumor Institute. Copyright © 1976 by Year Book Medical Publishers, Inc., Chicago.

that incidence may increase with age, indicating continued exposure to carcinogens.[6] In addition, Johnson proposes that exposure to chemical and viral agents may have some bearing on the carcinogenesis of prostate cancer.

Staging of prostate cancer

Staging relative to this diagnosis is via the modified del Regato system presented in Table 30-2. Staging of the client suspected of having prostate cancer also includes analysis of the results of several diagnostic tests, including a complete blood count, liver profile studies, alkaline phosphatase, fractionated prostatic acid phosphatase, skeletal survey, bone scan, and excretory urogram. Serum acid phosphatase should not be done immediately following digital rectal examination because it can cause a false serum evaluation. Lymphangiogram is also helpful in determining if lymph node metastasis has occurred.

Treatment

Treatment of prostatic cancer parallels the identified state of the disease. Stage A is usually treated with transurethral resection and biopsy alone. Stage B disease is treated by total prostatectomy, and suspicious lymph nodes are removed for frozen section review by the pathology department. External radiotherapy is recommended for stage C, with a general dose of 6,500 to 7,000 rads delivered in about 7 weeks. Stage D recommendations include orchiectomy and subsequent estrogen therapy.

Radiotherapy plus surgical intervention for this type of tumor may pose problems and be of concern to the client. Treatment is relatively long term in that it includes radiotherapy treatment 5 days a week until the course of radiotherapy is completed. The therapy can take up to 7 weeks to complete, followed by several weeks of rest before the client undergoes a prostatectomy, if indicated. Frequently, the client will ask "How can I afford all this?" and "Will I have to stay off from work?" Generally, clients can continue their usual life-style during radiotherapy. Additionally, many employers will allow clients to continue working during their therapy. However, some clients must travel long distances to the city where treatments are offered so that an additional financial burden is required of the client. Suggestions of affordable and convenient housing where the client and family may prepare their own meals are very valuable. In addition, temporary work arrangements can sometimes be made for the duration of their therapy.

Nursing care

Minor complications during radiotherapy such as diarrhea and cystitis are sometimes encountered. The nurse can suggest that a low-residue diet be instituted, and antidiarrheal medication can be prescribed by the physician to help control the diarrhea. Analgesics and urinary antispasmodics have proven beneficial for the cystitis.[23]

If the client is admitted to the hospital for a prostatectomy, an accurate and thorough assessment of the client is extremely valuable. Identification of his needs and concerns should be of major importance and will influence his nursing care plan. Again, establishing the extent of the client's knowledge about his disease will alert the nurse to areas that need to be emphasized.

A postoperative urinary catheter allows urinary drainage and also helps maintain the urethrovesical anastomosis.[20] In the immediate postoperative period, urinary drainage is almost always bloody. The sight of this bloody drainage may exacerbate the client's fears and anxieties. He should be reassured that this is common, and that the condition should resolve within 3 to 4 days following surgery. During this time, it is vitally important that the client's fluid levels be monitored closely.

Urinary dribbling after the catheter is removed is not uncommon. Encouragement for the client that he will gradually regain complete urinary control is indicated. If the urinary incontinence presents a physical or psychologic problem, an external condom catheter or penile clamp may be utilized until continence is reestablished.

The topic of sexual activity may or may not be raised by the client and his partner; however, the nurse should spend time with the client to answer questions and explain sexual responses relative to the various treatment modalities that will be employed.

For example, radiotherapy may manifest adverse effects on sexual function. The treatments may cause external skin reactions including redness, tenderness, and sloughing. The tenderness may cause the client to abstain from activities such as caressing or intercourse, which would cause friction to the pelvic area. Radiotherapy reportedly may also result in neuropathy that can have an effect on sexual function.[8]

Those clients being treated by bilateral orchiectomy and estrogen therapy may notice a decrease in libido and potency. The estrogen therapy can result in feminization and gynecomastia, which may be an additional insult to the body image of the client.[8] Castration will result in the client being sterile but not necessarily impotent.The psychologic impact following castration relative to body image, the missing testicles, and obvious feminine qualities may have dramatic effects on the male's potency.

Transurethral resection of the prostate and partial prostatectomy may result in retrograde ejaculation, which has been referred to as "dry climax." Clients should be made aware that this situation may develop and is not an uncommon phenomenon. Total prostatectomy involving radical pelvic surgery may result in impotence secondary to interruption of the parasympathetic nerves.[21,23] Penile prosthesis, through implant, has recently emerged as an acceptable and successful prosthetic device for impotent clients. Available prostheses include semirigid silicone rods and an inflatable cylinder device.[23] If the prosthesis is pursued for implant, thorough explanation of the device is a necessity. Involving the client's sexual partner in the discussion is also beneficial.

CANCER OF THE BLADDER

Cancer of the bladder, like neoplasms in general, has multiple factors that contribute to its etiology and clinical course.[1] Unfortunately, the symptoms, prevention, and treatment of bladder cancer have received very little public attention. However, the incidence of bladder cancer is significantly high to demand attention. Incidence-wise, there is a male-to-female ratio of approximately 3:1 with 26,000 new cases of bladder cancer in men and 9,000 new cases in women annually being documented. The mortality rates exceed that of carcinoma of the uterine cervix.[7,10,12,16] Bladder cancer is primarily a disease occurring after the fifth decade of life. A recent review of Johnson and Lamy[11] of 214 clients with carcinoma of the bladder who underwent radical cystectomies and ileal conduit urinary diversion covered the range of 37 to 80 years of age with an average age of 63 years.

Certain environmental factors have been associated with an increased incidence of bladder cancer, such as exposure to dyes, smoking, coffee, certain industrial aromatic amines, and schistosomiasis.[6,18] Schistosomiasis is a parasitic disease rare in the United States but common in many other countries. Considerable data have been accumulated on saccharin as a bladder carcinogenic agent, but no definite association in humans has been offered. The full impact of carcinogens and other risk factors of bladder cancer remains unknown.

Symptoms

The most common presenting problem of bladder cancer is hematuria. The hematuria is usually grossly visible and may persist throughout the client's entire voiding process. Bladder irritability with urinary frequency is the second most common complaint. Unfortunately, the client's presenting symptoms may originate from metastatic sites such as the lungs, bones, or liver.

The four basic cell types of bladder carcinomas are transitional cell carcinoma, squamous cell carcinoma, adenocarcinoma, and undifferentiated cell type. The transitional cell type is the most common and accounts for 90% of all reported cases; squamous cell carcinomas account for 6% to 7% of the remainder of cancers.[12]

The stage and grade of the tumor must be determined prior to any treatment planning. The grade refers to the degree of cell differentiation, with grade I being well differentiated, grade II being papillary in type and less well differentiated, and grade III being poorly differentiated. The poorly differentiated cells are the most radiosensitive.[18]

The stage depends on the depth of pene-

Table 30-3. Jewett and Strong clinical staging for bladder carcinoma*

Stage O	Papillary tumor or carcinoma in situ (tumor confined to mucosa)
Stage A	Tumor invading the lamina propria but not the muscle of the bladder wall
Stage B_1	Tumor extending into the superficial half of the muscle layer
Stage B_2	Tumor showing deep muscle invasion
Stage C	Tumor penetrating through bladder wall into perivesical connective tissue
Stage D_1	Tumor fixed, invading lymph nodes below bifurcation of the aorta
Stage D_2	Metastasis to periaortic nodes and distant organs

*Reproduced with permission from Johnson, D. E., et al.: Urologic cancer. In Clark, R. L., and Howe, C. D., editors: Cancer patient care at M. D. Anderson Hospital and Tumor Institute. Copyright © 1976 by Year Book Medical Publishers, Inc., Chicago.

tration of the tumor into the bladder wall and the presence or absence of distant metastases. Two staging classifications are commonly used. The International Union Against Cancer (IUCC) proposes the TNM classification for bladder cancer.[6] A second widely used method proposed by Jewett and Strong and revised by Marshall is presented in Table 30-3.

To verify the cell type and clinical stage of bladder tumors, a physical examination, history, and series of diagnostic tests are necessary. It is important that an interdisciplinary team approach to comprehensive therapy be planned for the client from the onset. Previously, treatment was sequential in that the surgeon resected the tumor, on recurrence the radiation oncologist was consulted, and lastly when the cancer was far advanced, the chemotherapist was asked to consult. Currently, appropriate comprehensive treatment must be planned at the time of diagnosis.

The diagnostic tests indicated are as follows: cystourethroscopy and bimanual examination with the client under anesthesia, adequate biopsies, chest x-ray films, skeletal survey, excretory urogram, and serum liver profile studies.[12] Lymphangiography studies have been demonstrated by some urologists as being very valuable for the staging of bladder tumors.[12]

Treatment

Treatment of cancer of the bladder varies with the clinical stage and can range from transurethral resection and intravesical drug instillation for O/A stage disease with few tumors to preoperative radiotherapy, total cystectomy, and ileal conduit urinary diversion for B_2 and C disease. Stage D_1 disease is treated with radiotherapy and stage D_2 with systemic chemotherapy.[12] Postoperatively, adjuvant chemotherapy with high-risk stage B_2 and C disease is also being utilized. The interdisciplinary approach of radiotherapy, surgery, and chemotherapy has markedly improved the cure rates for bladder carcinoma, but coordination of the complex care remains a challenge to the nurse.

Nursing care

The impact of the therapies for bladder cancer on sexual function has many variables, since the causative factors have not been explicitly identified and isolated. Male clients who have undergone a radical cystectomy have historically been thought to be impotent because of surgical disruption of the vascular and nerve supplies to the penis. However, some clients are anecdotally relating the ability to have complete or partial penile erections and a still larger number of clients are reporting the experience of orgasm. The degree of the problem related to physiologic disruption or psychologic impact is difficult to determine. The client's anecdotes and different responses point to the need for more thorough investigations of what actually accounts for penile potency and what the therapies for cancer actually do to affect sexual performance. The same thought is true for the clients receiving radiation therapy. There is a question of what degree of sexual function is due to the long-term scarring and fibrotic effects of radiotherapy and what degree is due to the psychologic effects of genital cancer, the impact of a life-threatening disease, or the implications of a genitourinary disease that is so directly related to sexual function. All of the sexual myths of a person's background regarding masturbation, sexual promiscuity, or ego image can emerge as guilt or shame emotions at this time. More questions than answers can be raised by the client, so the documentation of needs is fertile ground for nurse investigation.

Cystectomy with subsequent urinary diversion and a history of immediate and

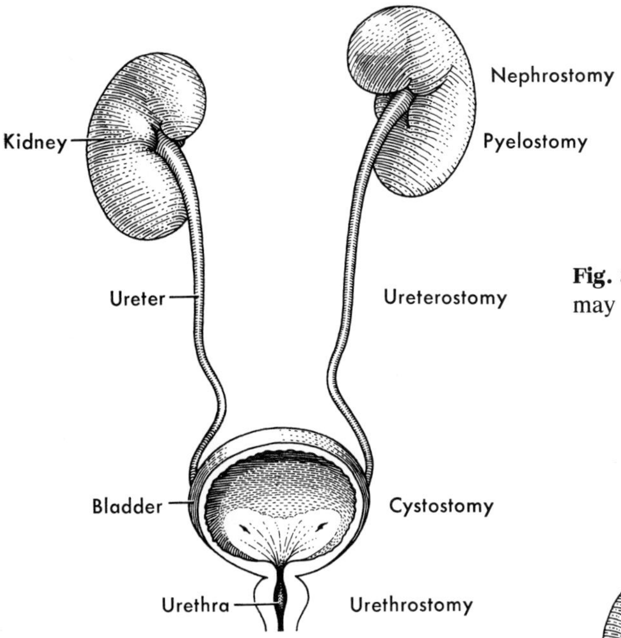

Fig. 30-1. Urinary diversion procedures that may be performed in urinary system.

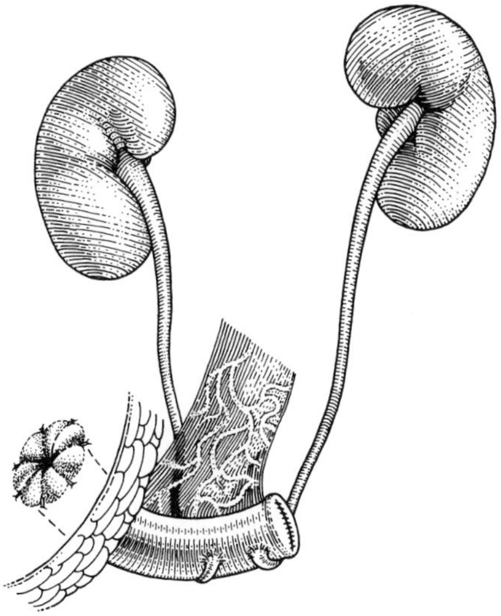

Fig. 30-2. Schematic drawing of ileal conduit urinary diversion.

long-term complications is a formidable operation. Today with improved surgical techniques, aggressive postoperative care, and enterostomal therapy support, more urologists are willing to embark on this extensive surgical approach.

There are several types of urinary diversions. Essentially any opening into the urinary system can be considered a urinary diversion. There are various types of urinary diversions presented in Fig. 30-1. The most common type of urinary diversion is the ileal or colon conduit as demonstrated in Fig. 30-2. The nursing care discussed later in this chapter will be related to that type of diversion.

CANCER OF THE KIDNEY

The most frequently reported malignancies of the kidney are renal cell carcinoma, transitional cell carcinoma, and Wilms' tumor, with Wilms' tumor generally seen in childhood.[9] Clients who develop these cancers often have symptoms of hematuria or flank pain as well as the occasional client who has an abdominal or flank mass present at the time of diagnosis.

Cancer of the kidney is a disease generally occurring in the fourth to seventh decade of life, wtih the disease being predominant in men by a ratio of 3:1. As in all other neoplasms, certain predisposing factors have been identified as potential contributors to cancer of the kidney. Heavy cigarette smoking and phenacetin abuse have been associated with renal disease. Wynder and Whitmore[23] suggested that fat/cholesterol may contribute to evolving renal adenocarcinoma in that a "lipid rich" saturation level may increase susceptibility to other carcinogens.

Staging

Staging is indicated prior to initiation of treatment. Table 30-4 demonstrates the clinical staging system for renal carcinoma as originally projected by Flecks and Tadesky, modified by Rolson, Churchill, and Anderson and cited by Johnson.[12]

In addition to physical examination and history, arteriographic studies, chest x-ray films, skeletal surveys, and serum liver profile studies are indicated for accurate diagnosis.

Treatment

In general, the indicated treatment for clients with renal carcinoma who do not have demonstrated metastasis is radical nephrectomy. Renal infarction or renal artery occlusion has been utilized 48 to 72 hours preoperatively in renal disease as an adjunct to surgical removal of the kidney.[9] The technique of renal infarction involves injecting an embolitic material into the renal artery to occlude the vessel. Reportedly, the blood supply to the kidney is reduced and there is less surgical bleeding.[5] This technique results in edema of the renal unit, which also facilitates surgical dissection.

Table 30-4. Clinical staging system for renal carcinoma

Stage I	Tumor within capsule
Stage II	Tumor invasion of perinephric fat (confined to Gerota's fascia)
Stage III	Tumor involvement of regional lymph nodes and/or renal vein and cava
Stage IV	Adjacent organs or distant metastases

Nursing care

Following the infarction, pain, fever, gastrointestinal upset, including nausea and vomiting, are fairly common. The amount of pain following infarction varies, but generally requires an intramuscular pain medication for control. In 1977, Bergreen[2] indicated that most clients will experience moderate pain for up to 36 hours postinfarction. Additionally, the client's temperature may remain elevated for several days following the renal infarction. Reassurance during this period when there is discomfort is important to the client and his family. Answering their questions honestly and thoroughly can help build and strengthen trust and confidence.

Nausea and vomiting may vary with each client. Antiemetics offer some relief and help decrease the client's anxiety. Accurate monitoring of fluid intake and output is essential. Gastrointestinal upset may result in decreased oral intake, thus requiring intravenous fluid replacement.

During the period between renal infarction and nephrectomy, the client usually has many questions. This is a time to listen and allow the client and family to talk about their feelings. A common question asked is, "Will I be able to live with only one kidney?" Reassurance from the nurse is valuable at this time. Preoperative teaching stresses that fluid intake following nephrectomy must be maintained. Clients should force fluids of choice to 2,500 ml per day. Water has been called the "white wine of health" and it should be actively included in the fluid regimen. Likewise, potential hazards such as fad diets should be avoided, and the clients should be advised to consult with their physician before beginning any dietary program that may result in excessive protein catabolism and subsequent ketosis. Preoperative teaching should continue with an explanation as well as demonstrations of proper techniques for turning, coughing and deep breathing, administration of IV fluids, function of the nasogastric tube, and care of the incision. Having assessed the client's level of knowledge, the nurse should strive to augment this knowledge so the client knows what to expect during the impending procedure.

Once the nephrectomy is performed, careful attention must be given to the client's fluid and electrolyte balance. Clients should be involved early in their own care and independence should be stressed. This allows clients to have some control over their own rehabilitative program.

For precautionary measures, clients should be encouraged to have frequent blood pressure checks if they are prone to hypertension. With only the one renal unit remaining, nephrotic pressure gradient changes relative to high blood pressure are of major concern.

The most common sites of metastases from the kidney are the lung, liver, and bone. Unfortunately, the response to adjuvant radiotherapy and chemotherapy, relative to long-term survival and cure, has not improved significantly in the last 10 years so that most of the clients the nurse will come in contact with will be in some stage of advanced disease.

CANCER OF THE TESTES

Testicular cancers make up approximately 2% of all malignancies in men. However, this disease ranks *second* as the cause of death from *all* neoplasms in men between 20 to 34 years of age.[12] Tumors of this type are extremely rare in blacks, comprising less than 2% of all reported cancer cases.

Symptoms

Presenting symptoms often include testicular edema or mass, testicular pain, and, in some cases, gynecomastia. Frequently, a testicular lesion is discovered on examination following an accident or injury to the scrotum. Often there is a delay between awareness of existing symptoms and the seeking of medical interpretation. Self-testicular examination should be taught to the general public and its use encouraged by nurses. This teaching, as described in Chapter 10, should encompass techniques for examination, signs, symptoms, and the need for medical consultation without delay.

Cancer of the testes includes the following histologic types: seminoma, embryonal carcinoma, teratoma, teratocarcinoma, and choriocarcinoma. It has been projected that a diagnosis of seminoma yields the best prognosis, and a diagnosis of choriocarcinoma yields the poorest.[12] Johnson[12] has indicated that 3.6% to 11.6% of testicular tumors arise in cryptorchid testes. Suspicious masses or edema in the testes or scrotum should be aggressively managed, since they are often considered malignant until proven otherwise.

Staging

Diagnostic tests often ordered to help determine the diagnosis include serum liver profile studies, HCG titer, alpha-fetoprotein determination, and lymphangiogram. In addition, a complete history should be taken and a physical examination should be performed. The staging classifications for testicular cancer are currently being revised, but generally the earlier stages have a better prognosis.

Treatment

Treatment following orchiectomy differs somewhat with each stage. Stages I and II A will generally receive radiotherapy to the involved areas. Stage II B receives, in addition, prophylactic radiotherapy to the mediastinal area. Stage III will receive a combination of radiotherapy and chemotherapy. These progressive modalities have offered marked improvement in the survival of clients.

Because of a significant percentage of clients presenting with periaortic lymph node metastases, clients are generally offered the additional surgery of retroperitoneal lymphadenectomy.[23] During embryonic development, the testes develop in the retroperitoneal cavity and descend past the inguinal ligament into the scrotal sac in about the eighth month. The usual metastatic spread is generally via these retroperitoneal tracts.[15] If the lymph node specimens are negative, no further treatment is usually indicated. However, with a positive lymph node specimen, the aforementioned radiotherapy treatments or chemotherapy is initiated.

Chemotherapeutic agents, as discussed in Chapter 14, that have been utilized for these clients include individualized combinations of bleomycin, cyclophosphamide (Cytoxan), vincristine (Oncovin), methotrexate, and 5-fluorouracil. Common side-effects of these agents are stomatitis, alopecia, nausea, and vomiting. These uncomfortable manifestations are seen during and after treatment.

Nursing care

Mineral oil combined with Milk of Magnesia and applied to the gums and lips with a lemon and glycerin swab may offer some soothing relief for stomatitis. Often, as a result of the stomatitis, the client's oral intake decreases dramatically. Fluids should be encouraged and Popsicles are usually popular with the clients during this time. Analgesics and antiemetics should also be a major component of symptom relief. These can be included in the individualized care plan for the client.

The client may be concerned about his loss of hair. Volunteers and social service workers can be active in providing wigs if the client so desires. Some men are not concerned with their alopecia and may even wear buttons stating "Bald is Beautiful"; however, it is important to listen to your client. Frequently, the client speaks, but the nurse does not listen. The purpose of a care plan is to reflect concerns and solutions that the client has identified for himself, not what the nurse identifies for him. Discuss aspects of his care with the client as well as the care team. In this way, the nurse will be better able to identify realistic and achievable goals with the client.

Body image may be threatened by any of these treatment techniques. It is of paramount importance to assess the client relative to his view of himself. Each person has a right to his own feelings and attitudes, and the nursing team should not impose its values on the client.

Orchiectomy may constitute an extremely threatening situation to a man. Although a unilateral orchiectomy will not alter the man's sterility or potency, it may have a bearing on his perception of his wholeness and masculinity. Bilateral removal of the testicles can result in depression, as well as the feeling and belief that he is less of a man. Sterility as a result of castration may devastate the young couple who are planning a family.

Studies are currently under way to determine and identify effects of chemotherapeutic agents on male sexuality.[8] Management of cancer clients with chemotherapy can also produce weight loss and alopecia that tend to exacerbate their uncertainties about self-esteem.

Many of the chemotherapeutic agents used for clients with cancer are toxic to cells. This toxicity, as a result of the action of some of the alkylating agents and antimetabolites, may manifest itself with an alteration in spermatogenesis.[19] Stohs[19] indicated that functional sperm production will probably return following the chemotherapy; however, it may not do so for several years or more following the therapy with antineoplastic drugs.

Statements have been made that chemotherapy has an adverse effect on libido and may result in impotence; however, definitive research relative to this point is difficult to document in the literature. Impotence, secondary to antineoplastic agents, is most probably a result of neurotoxicity.[8,19] In addition, other drugs that the client may be taking concomitantly can influence potency problems. It has been identified that some sedatives and hypnotics interfere with sexual function.[19,22] Further investigation into the effects of chemotherapeutic agents as well as other therapeutic drugs would reveal valuable and desirable information.

CANCER OF THE PENIS

Squamous cell carcinoma of the penis is fairly uncommon. It makes up about 2% of all genitourinary tumors.[11] Penile cancer occurs more frequently in men with poor personal and sexual hygiene.

Symptoms

Presenting symptoms commonly involve a penile lesion that may be mistaken for a venereal disease. Failure to seek early medical attention may center around the fear of embarrassment of discovering or confirming a venereal disease.

Johnson[12] and Wynder and Whitmore[23] stated that more than half of the clients have inguinal lymphadenopathy at the time of medical examination and diagnosis. Frequently, this lymphadenopathy is an inflammatory response rather than metastatic disease.

Treatment

The generally indicated treatment is penile resection. Partial amputation is considered only if there will be sufficient penile shaft left to enable the client to stand and direct his urinary stream.[23] If this is not possible, the penile shaft is removed and a perineal urethrostomy is surgically created. This urethral diversion does not alter urinary continence.

Nursing care

Amputation of the penis can have a dramatic psychosocial impact on the client and his spouse. Although the client will still be able to achieve orgasm from touch and friction, penile-vaginal stimulation will no longer be possible and so may be a major threat to his masculinity and body image.

Concomitant with these feelings may also be the fact that he will now have to sit on the toilet to urinate. This can cause severe psychosocial problems and has even resulted in some men avoiding social activities where they would have to urinate in public restrooms.

All of these cancers require major adjustment on the part of the client and family. One of the most important adjustments is in the area of sexuality, particularly male sexuality.

MALE SEXUALITY

The client's sexuality can be such a source of concern, anxiety, and frustration for nurses that it becomes a neglected area. In fact, it is such an area of neglect that it can be speculated that sexuality is perhpas the least comfortable social aspect for nurses to deal with. Unfortunately, the need is a great one since sexuality is not only a means of procreation but also a means of exhibiting love, concern, and affection.

Sexuality is a unique method of communication between people, both tangibly and intangibly. Sexuality involves the entire body, not just the sex organs or the erogenous zones. A person's sexual self-concept involves a synthesis of biologic, psychologic, and social forces.

Awareness of the client's body image is well developed by young adulthood and has a definite effect on the individual's ability to relate to other people. Society has encouraged the male to be aggressive and strong so there can be serious problems if sexual dysfunction does occur. Keuhnelian[14] indicated that males have internalized a number of liabilities, one of which is probably the interchangeability of self-esteem and self-competence. Thus, it can be deduced that if self-competence or virility is threatened or destroyed, self-esteem will be affected if not diminished. The importance of sex in self-esteem varies among cultures, but men in the American society tend to place great importance on virility as a major factor in the development and maintenance of their self-esteem.

Problems specific to genitourinary cancers

Unfortunately, sexual problems are commonly seen in clients with a diagnosis of cancer. Often sexual relations are abstained from during adjustment to the diagnosis and the subsequent management. Cancers of the bladder, with subsequent surgical intervention and urinary diversion, not only alter the physiologic process of the client but also his body image. The treatments commonly employed may be viewed as mutilating, disfiguring, and distasteful to the client. As a major thrust toward rehabilitation, reassurance and caring should be stressed by nurses so that couples can attempt to decrease their negative feelings as they strive to return to their former life-styles. The nurse can advise the couple that caring may be expressed through touching, caressing, or an affectionate manner appropriate to the individual couple.

Dr. Mary Calderone has indicated that sexual problems can be separated into primary and secondary aspects. The primary aspects are those problems that are relative to the sexual apparatus or the functioning of the client's sexual system. The secondary aspects are those problems that develop as a result of other conditions within the body.[17] These concepts are directly applicable to cancer clients who have undergone various surgical procedures to their sexual system as well as those clients whose treatment modalities may have altered other body systems.

The word "cancer" carries with it a devastating emotional impact for most people. Undue suffering and pain is often thought of in relation to the cancer client. Understanding the client's needs for sexual expression during the course of treatment should enable the nurse to discuss these subjects without inflicting personal values or moral judgments into the discussion. It is vitally important that the nurse remain nonjudgmental about a client's sexual preference or behavior.

As stated previously, cancer may have a devastating effect on a person, physically as well as psychologically and socially. Psychologic integrity may be further attacked if the cancer involves the sex organs or genitalia. The sudden realization that a malignancy involves the sex organs may threaten the client's confidence of sexual expression. The client may withdraw and become immobilized at any mention of sexuality. Conversely, he may "act out" sexually in an attempt to stabilize his masculinity. It has been speculated that sexual response is 90% above the shoulders, and the suggestion of impotence may be internalized to the point of *actual* impotence. Before discussing sexuality with the client, the nurse must recognize and acknowledge that there are varied feelings and attitudes toward sexuality in general as well as male sexuality. By discussing sexuality confidently and openly with sensitivity and concern, the nurse is better able to create an effective atmosphere for counseling.

Nursing approaches

The nursing process is germane to any discussion of male sexuality. Nursing assessment relative to a discussion on male sexuality should include a section on sexual history. This can be done without offense if the client is assured of the nurse's concern for him as a person and a beginning relationship has been established.

Following the data-gathering phrase, the nurse must plan for the appropriate intervention. It is of paramount importance that nurses realize their own limitations and make referrals if further or additional counseling is indicated. Various brochures and pamphlets are available through the United Ostomy Association and the American Cancer Society that are helpful in explaining words, feelings, and techniques relative to male sexuality. Many clients may prefer to read the information and then ask questions. Thus, the nurse is individualizing the client's care. The establishment of an individualized care plan provides an excellent time to correct any misinformation that couples may have. Often the nurse must sanction the client to discuss his sexuality.

The nurse's assessment should also include the knowledge base of the staff, as well as their feelings and attitudes about male sexuality. By exposing myths and fallacies, the staff will be able to provide continuity and support in professional encounters. Having established this open communication, nurses are better able to provide realistic and appropriate intervention for this particular population of clients.

Outcome criteria and appropriateness of clients' goals must be evaluated as ongoing components of the nursing process. Evaluation might include the establishment of rapport, realistic therapeutic intervention, and concern over what could have been done to further develop the client-nurse relationship.

Nurses, physicians, and other health care providers touch the client as they deliver care. Touch is a valuable therapeutic tool because it can relay feelings of support and caring as well as decrease anxiety and fear in the client. Because the spouse is not at the bedside throughout the entire 24-hour period, the client may be seen projecting his sexual expressions to the attendant staff. In some cases, the spouse is uncertain about touching the client, yet the nurse touches freely. This may be viewed as rejection by the spouse and acceptance of the nurse.

Sex education should be directed not just to the client and his sexual partner but to the staff as well. Collaborating and consulting with other members of the health team may evolve into an instrumental approach to supporting male clients with sexual concerns.

The nurse can become involved in research in the area of formalizing new educational approaches of support for the client, his sexual partner, and the staff. In addition, evaluating current progress to determine the effects of sexual health intervention may be beneficial. Acknowledging that man is a sexual being and that sexuality is an integral part of the individual's personality and totalness is important. Sexuality only ends with the termination of life, so it can be readily observed that including sexuality in the components of care extended to the client is a vital part of his plan of care.

As a result of the professional's anxiety, as well as the anxiety and fears of the client and his partner, the sexual needs of the client are often ignored by the nurse. Therefore, it is of paramount importance to realize that male sexuality and sexual expression are intertwined with all facets of the client, whether biologically, psychologically, or socially. Because male sexuality is a part of the total being, the art of acknowledging, caring, and supporting the client within his realm of sexual quality as his life continues can be the ultimate in rehabilitation.

Along with male sexuality, rehabilitation of the client with a genitourinary cancer must consider stomal care.

STOMAL CARE

Nursing care of a client with a cystectomy and/or ileal conduit diversion involves preoperative teaching and support, intense postoperative care, client and family teaching, and continuous concern toward rehabilitation.

Case study

A typical client was a 58-year-old white man with stage C transitional cell carcinoma of the bladder. His presenting symptom was hematuria. His initial examination with staging and planning of his therapy was done by the urologist and radiotherapist. His planned treatment was 5,000 rads external beam radiotherapy in 25 fractions over a 5-week period followed by 6 weeks at home for convalescence. A single stage radical cystectomy and ileal conduit urinary diversion would then be performed.

Once the planned treatment is explained to the client and his family, systems of support are necessary. Consider the weighty factors in this situation:

Cancer: A life-threatening diagnosis

Radical surgery: Involving a personal and private function of elimination

Resulting ostomy: Necessitating continuous use of a stomal appliance

Long-term treatment: Approximately 4 months; 5 weeks of radiotherapy plus 6 weeks of rest, 4 weeks of hospitalization plus convalescence; expense and time away from the job; a significant change in the client's body image along with interference or impairment of sexual function

What overwhelming questions will occur to the client?

1. Will my spouse still love and desire me?
2. Can I return to work? To social life?
3. Will I live?
4. How can I care for a urinary diversion?
5. Where will I stay during my treatments?
6. Am I too old for this surgery?
7. Can I financially afford this?

Underlying all these is a doubt, or maybe even a hope, that this treatment really is necessary. The client may or may not feel sick. Consequently, the commitment to this decision is not made easily.

To ensure benefit immediately following the client's diagnostic tests, the enterostomal therapist, or ET, can meet the client and his family to begin what will become a long-term relationship. The enterostomal therapist should take this initial interview only as far as the client is prepared to go. The enterostomal therapist should closely observe the client's response and not expose him to too much at one time. Frequently, it is a time when the client asks questions that have no answers: "What have I done? I am not sick; is this really necessary?" Ambivalence and confusion may be noted here. Clients are frequently seeking reassurance that they have not done anything to cause the cancer. Confidence in the cancer care team and the institution during this life-threatening period is important. Recognition by the enterostomal therapist that this is a serious operation and a big decision for the client is important. The client's real fears should not be belittled with the general comment, "You will do fine." The client will recognize the superficiality of this and begin to sense that the enterostomal therapist is not interested in serious problems.

Explanations regarding the surgery and postoperative care should be initiated at this time because it helps to clarify the client's understanding and begins removing any misconceptions that exist about the planned treatment. Staff nurses working with the client should follow through with adequate and individualized support and teaching. Frequently, social workers are involved with the care team. They can be very beneficial to the client and family. The social worker can offer support and assistance as the client and family activate plans for the longevity of the treatment, living accommodations, and the social supports they will need.

During this initial assessment, there may be very little teacher-learner activity aside from the beginning establishment of a trusting relationship. The client and his family are frequently stunned, angered, confused, and very emotionally vulnerable. Their greatest need is time for assimilation and adjustment. Preoperatively, the nurse should continue with client teaching regarding surgery, recovery room procedures, and the immediate recovery period. It is beneficial for the client to see an appliance and discuss postoperative care. The enterostomal therapist should explain that in the immediate postoperative period the *nurses* will care for the ostomy. This serves to relieve the clients of any responsibility for their own care when they are in the immediate recovery period and still acutely ill. When they become stronger, however, they should be advised to learn their own care. It is important to reinforce this idea that *they* will be able to care for their own ostomy *before* discharge from the hospital.

Careful preoperative attention is given to the placement of the stoma. The client is examined, preferably by the urologist and enterostomal therapist together. The client should be examined in the lying, sitting, and standing positions. The site that is selected should be readily accessible to the client and should have adequate surface area to support a faceplate. Consequently, care is taken to avoid placing the stoma near a bony prominence, in the beltline, close to the umbilicus, close to scars where valleys exist, on the undersurface of the panniculus in obese patients, or on an incision. If there is some question as to whether the selected site will support a faceplate, the client should wear a urinary appliance a few days before surgery to determine the most suitable area. The appliance should contain 100 to 150 ml of water or saline solution so that possible leaks can be evaluated.

Clients with a history of allergies should be skin tested before surgery with several of the ostomy adhesives. Patch tests of adhesives are done on the side of the abdomen *opposite* the ostomy site. Each adhesive is left in place and evaluated after 48 hours. Fortunately, most of the modern appliances and adhesives are hypoallergenic and cause very little skin reaction.

Relative to the surgery, the client may undergo a single-stage or multiple-stage radical cystectomy and ileal conduit urinary diversion. A nasogastric tube or gastrostomy tube will be inserted into the stomach to protect the ileal anastomosis. Because of the proximity of the bladder and prostate to the rectum in the male, it is very important that no rectal procedure, such as taking rectal temperatures or administering an enema, be undertaken because of the risk of perforation through the rectum.

Early ambulation is a must along with postoperative breathing exercises; coughing and leg exercises are begun as soon as the client wakes up from the anesthetic.

In surgery, the urologist or the operating room nurses may apply a skin barrier and a clear temporary urinary bag to the ileal conduit. The skin barrier will serve to protect the peristomal dermis already abraded by the preparation for surgery. It is important to continuously protect the peristomal area and keep the urinary drainage from prolonged contact with the skin. Ureteral stents may be present to support the ureteroileal anastomosis as shown in Fig. 30-3. The urinary bag should be connected to straight drainage with a urometer for measuring hourly outputs in the immediate postoperative period.

Ideally, the enterostomal therapist should see the clients as soon as they are admitted to the recovery room because it is important to note the color and characteristics of the stoma so there will be guidelines to detect any changes later. Any separation from the mucosoepithelial junction or uncontrollable bleeding should be immediately corrected by the surgeon. Likewise, the stoma should be observed daily to detect any signs of insufficient blood supply. If the conduit segment is not viable, emergency reconstruction of a conduit becomes necessary.

The enterostomal therapist begins the plan of care for the client's ileal conduit in the recovery room. This helps coordinate information regarding the client's care for the staff nurse involved. Immediate care, short- and long-term client goals, needed instructions, and discharge planning notes are included.

It is very important that the client's plan of care include the client. Aside from the client's immediate physiologic and emotional needs, a large part of the plan of care relates to client and family learning.

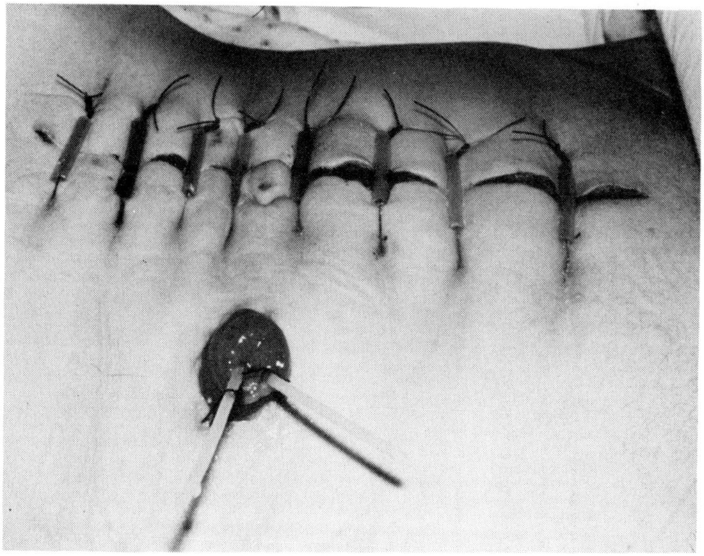

Fig. 30-3. Ileal conduit urinary diversion—new stoma with ureteral stents in place postoperatively.

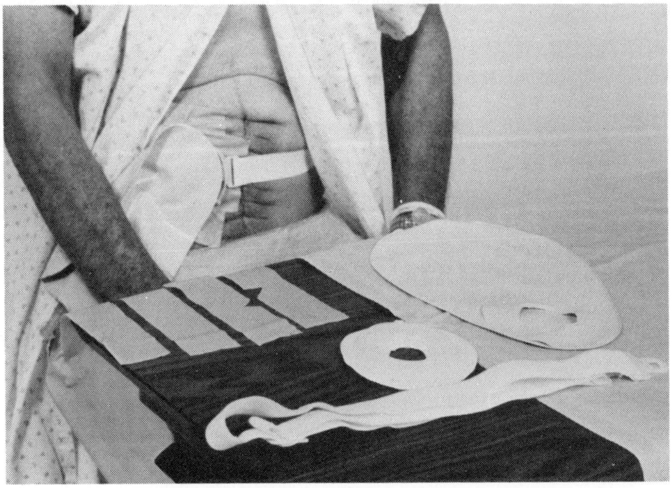

Fig. 30-4. Client with urinary diversion practicing application of his appliance.

There are two very important points to be considered in client teaching. First, teaching cannot be left to chance. Everyone may share in the teaching role, but it is vital that one person be designated to be ultimately responsible for the outcome. Second, learning does not take place unless there is some activity whether it be mental, physical, or both on the part of the learner. The client must be an active, rather than passive, learner to successfully demonstrate that care can be satisfactorily given. For clients to accept their ostomy, they must be able to *care* for it. It is important they they not be dependent on others for the care shown in Fig. 30-4.

Protection and care of the conduit and peristomal skin is very important. The use of a skin barrier immediately after surgery will preserve the skin. When selecting the proper appliance for the client to wear, the following aspects should be considered:

- Availability of the appliance
- Characteristics of the client's abdomen, be it flabby, firm, or low waisted
- Location of stoma relative to proximity to bony prominences, near wrinkle, skin fold, or incision, in beltline or horizontal to another stoma
- Characteristics of the stoma such as flush or skin level, protrusion, retraction to one side, or in a valley
- Personal variables of the client as to dexterity, vision, type of work, and body size

There is a large variety of urinary appliances, both temporary and reusable. A flush or protruding stoma well located on the abdomen may be fitted with a disposable faceplate. If there is a retraction or valley near the stoma, a convex faceplate will be needed to provide an adhesive seal. A skin barrier is not necessary if the appliance has a proper fit. The faceplate of the appliance should be $^{1}/_{16}$ to $^{1}/_{8}$ inch larger than the stoma.

Clients should be taught how to care for their skin. When removing the appliance, they should be instructed to gently push the skin away from the adhesive using a warm, moist guaze sponge or washcloth to aid in the removal. The use of soaps and solvents is not necessary. Any adhesive remaining on

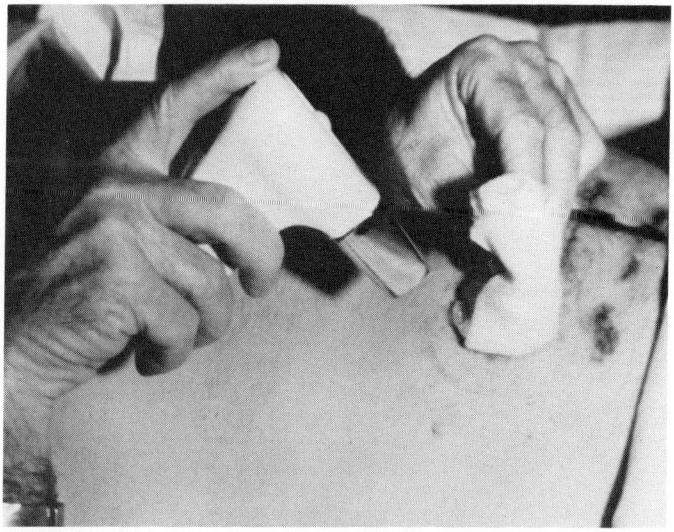

Fig. 30-5. Client drying skin around urinary stoma, using gauze wick to absorb urine.

the skin can be rolled off gently with a dry gauze sponge or washcloth. Excessive rubbing will damage the epithelium. The skin should be washed well with warm water and dried thoroughly. The appliance should be changed every 5 to 7 days or as much as needed. The client can shower or bathe with the appliance on or off. Water will not run into or hurt the stoma.

If skin problems do occur, it is important to assess the potential causes and treat them as well as the symptoms. Acute skin problems might arise from urinary leakage, monilia infection, or contact dermatitis. Hyperplasia of the epithelium can become a chronic skin problem.

Nursing care of acute skin problems (Fig. 30-5) includes:

1. Rinsing the skin with warm water
2. Drying the skin thoroughly with a hair dryer set on cool
3. Applying Karaya gum powder to reddened areas
4. Applying nystatin (Mycostatin) or other antifungal powder, if a monilia infection is present
5. Covering the powder with a plasticized dressing, such as skin prep, and allowing it to dry
6. Applying a skin barrier
7. Applying a properly fitting urinary appliance

Hyperplasia of the epithelium is a term used to describe epithelium that extends on the mucosa of the stoma. The nursing care for this problem involves softening the hyperplasia with acetic acid applied directly to the skin when the appliance is changed. A close-fitting appliance exposing only normal mucosa should then be applied (Fig. 30-6).

Clients who have undergone a urinary diversion procedure should be instructed to drink *at least* 2 to 3 quarts of fluids daily. The physician may prescribe ascorbic acid tablets, which help keep the urine acidic. This reduces the possibility of infection and keeps down the odor of urine. Cleanliness is a must for the client's ostomy and equip-

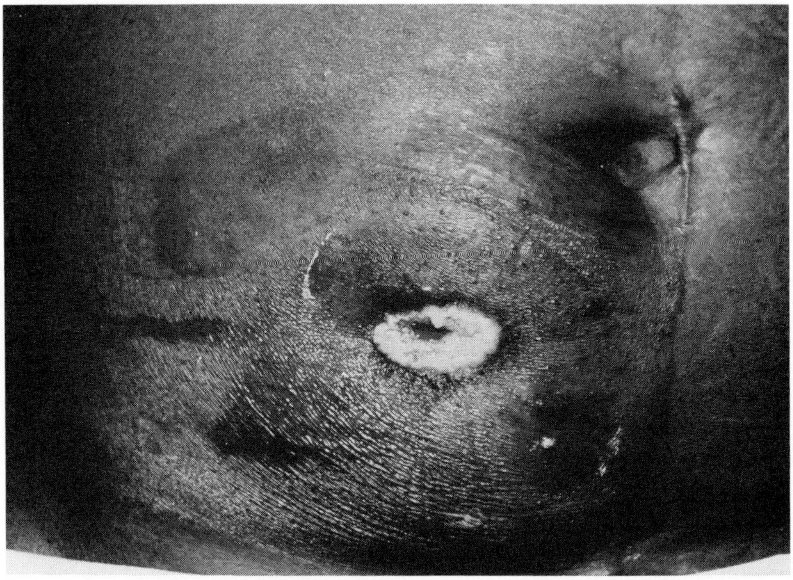

Fig. 30-6. Hyperplasia changes around urinary stoma.

ment. Clients should be taught how to care properly for their conduit, peristomal skin, and appliances to reduce the possibility of skin and stomal complications.

The entire process of preoperative care, intense postoperative care, and client teaching efforts is focused on rehabilitation of these clients, that is, helping them return to living their lives the way they were before their illness. Attitude can be a powerful influence on this process as the client responds to the staff's attitude as well as the family's attitude. A positive, confident, and sincere attitude will be sensed by the client. A false attitude or faked expression can be picked up just as easily and turned into doubt. Nurses may spend half of their visits molding attitudes and preparing clients and their families to receive what they need to share in terms of teaching and acceptance.

Sometimes an optimum attitude can be found in one visit; sometimes it is a 3-week struggle, and to be realistic, sometimes there will be failures. The nurse may not be able to change the character of a lifetime. For example, the cancer and the surgery may be superimposed on a lifetime of anger. Generally, however, the nurse's efforts will be successfully realized. Most clients are eager to learn and are motivated to be independent.

The enterostomal therapist should be available to the clients periodically to reassess their methods of care, their readiness for further learning, fitting of their appliance, and other social, economic, and family adjustments. This *test of teaching* is realized when clients have returned to their customary way of life.

REFERENCES

1. Ambrose, E. G., and Roe, J. J. C., editors: Biology of cancer, ed. 2, New York, 1975, Halsted Press, p. 2.
2. Bergreen, P., et al.: Therapeutic renal infarction, J. Urol. **118**:372, 1977.
3. Blandy, J. P.: Transurethral resection, Baltimore, 1971, University Park Press.
4. Calderone, M. J.: Sexual problems in medical practice, J.A.M.A. **23**(pt.2), 1968.

5. Cancer Bulletin vol. 31 (pt. 1), January-February, 1979.
6. deKernion, J. B., and Skinner, D. G.: Epidemiology, diagnosis and staging of bladder cancer. In Skinner, D. G., and deKernion, J. B.: Genitourinary cancer, Philadelphia, 1978, W. B. Saunders Co.
7. del Regato, J. A.: Radiotherapy for carcinoma of the prostate: a report from the Committee for the Cooperative Study of Radiotherapy for Carcinoma of the Prostate, Colorado Springs, Penrose Cancer Hospital, 1968, p. 10.
8. Donovan, M. I., and Pierce, S. G.: Cancer care nursing, New York, 1976, Appleton-Century-Crofts.
9. Harrison, J. H., et al.: Campbell's urology, ed. 4, vol. 1, Philadelphia, 1978, W. B. Saunders Co.
10. Holleb, A. I.: Cancer statistics, CA **29**(1):14, 1979.
11. Johnson, D. E., and Lamy, S. M.: Complications of a single stage radical cystectomy and ileal conduit diversion: review of 214 cases, J. Urol. **117**:171 (pt. 2), 1900.
12. Johnson, D. E., et al.: Urologic cancer. In Clark, R. L., and Howe, C. D., editors: Cancer patient care at M. D. Anderson Hospital and Tumor Institute, Chicago, 1976, Year Book Medical Publishers, Inc., p. 367.
13. Johnson, D. E.: Personal communication, 1979.
14. Kenhnelian, J. G., and Sanders, V. E.: Urologic nursing, New York, 1970, Macmillan Inc.
15. Patten, B. M.: Human embryology, ed. 3, New York, 1968, McGraw-Hill Book Co.
16. Silverberg, E.: Cancer statistics—1977, CA **27**:26 (pt. 1), 1977.
17. Skinner, D. G., and deKernion, J. B.: Genitourinary cancer, Philadelphia, 1978, W. B. Saunders Co.
18. Smith, S. L.: Nursing care, ed. 9, Los Altos, Calif., 1978, Lange Medical Publications.
19. Stohs, S. J.: Drugs and sexual function, U.S. Pharmacist, November-December, 1975.
20. Whitehead, S. L.: Nursing care of the adult urology patient, New York, 1970, Appleton-Century-Crofts.
21. Wood, R. Y., and Rose, K.: Penile implants for impotence, Am. J. Nurs. Feb., 1968.
22. Woods, N. F.: Human sexuality in health and illness, ed. 2, St. Louis, 1979, The C. V. Mosby Co.
23. Wynder, E., and Whitmore, W.: Epidemiology of adenocarcinoma of the kidney, J. Natl. Cancer Inst. **53**(6):1619, 1974.

VII

CONCLUSION

31

Cancer nursing: current progress and future trends

LISA BEGG MARINO

This chapter will synthesize the material presented in this book into two major areas: current progress and future trends.

The section on current progress represents nursing achievements that have already taken place and have impacted on some aspect of cancer health care. The section on future trends has been included so that the reader can see how the progress that has been obtained to date can serve as a starting point for even potentially greater future achievements. This chapter will demonstrate the substantial progress nurses have achieved currently and provide strong evidence to show that continued successes are well under way. Reading this chapter should also reinforce to the reader the interrelatedness of general and specialized (cancer) nursing practice as well as the value of working cooperatively with other health care providers to enhance the level of care being given.

Chapter 1 presented a conceptual framework for cancer nursing that began by discussing such major points as the health-disease continuum, the health care system, all health care providers, and the nurse as provider before focusing on cancer nursing as a specialty. This is because the specialty of cancer nursing does not exist in a vacuum, rather it is related to, and subject to, changes in all the other health areas. Nurses need to remain cognizant of this point so that future endeavors can reflect overall health care trends.

Each of the two sections will be presented within the nursing practice, education, and research framework so the reader can see the breadth of the current achievements as well as the elements common to all professional nursing regardless of specialty.

CURRENT PROGRESS

Current progress in cancer nursing has centered primarily on practice endeavors, but achievements have also been registered in cancer nursing education and research.

Cancer nursing practice

Within practice, cancer nurses have developed outcome standards for cancer nursing practice, articulated a nursing role in information gathering as it pertains to an ethical basis for practice, created a functioning network of nurses willing to consult with one another, begun to identify specific client and family needs or high-incidence problem areas, while demonstrating the benefit of nurses' coordinating care between and within care settings.

Outcome standards. The *Outcome Standards For Cancer Nursing Practice* were developed in 1979 by joint effort between the Oncology Nursing Society (ONS) and the American Nurses' Association (ANA).[1] These ten standards cover major areas of need or high-incidence problem areas and were developed by cancer specialist nurses from across the United States with input from ANA representatives. They are intended to serve as guidelines to nurses who care for clients at risk for, or actually diagnosed with, cancer. In addition to assisting individual nurses, these standards represent the first effort to identify a nursing model of care for this population of clients. Before the standards were developed, no such model existed. Additionally, these standards serve as a beginning scope of cancer nursing practice because they are written in outcome format, so that evaluation of nursing interventions is possible. Moreover, these standards are designed to include all types of clients, all types of care based in various settings, and all forms of cancer. Contrary to much of the material that has been developed previously, these standards go beyond the medical model to base care on the nursing process. Therefore, it is possible to articulate required nursing skills and knowledge, nursing interventions, and client outcomes so that evaluation can be accomplished. These standards also are flexible enough that regional and local settings can adapt them to meet their particular client needs. This approach allows for individuality while reinforcing the commonality of cancer nursing practice regardless of the variety of subspecialty areas.

Ethical basis for cancer nursing practice. Traditionally, ethics as a framework for health care has been the province of medicine and law. It has been the province of medicine because judgment was needed to determine the efficacy of various treatments, to confirm a diagnosis, and to offer a prognosis. Attorneys interpreted the intent of our laws to protect the rights of clients and contributed to an assessment of whether any wrongdoing had taken place. Situations were rarely "black or white" but neither were they all that ambiguous either.

However, now with therapy successes salvaging more lives, coupled with the complex diagnostic and therapeutic procedures that could be undertaken, philosophies and cultural mores have undergone substantial changes. The consumer's perception of the amount of information needed and the right to make decisions that impact on the quality and duration of life have increased. Expectations increased as to the degree of participation in decision making about therapeutic options, initiation and cessation of treatment, and when to end attempts at control of the disease process. All these changes have blurred the decisions that have to be made and blurred the roles of physicians, nurses, and the other health care providers. During this transition phase, some nurses decided that their professional colleagues were capable of assuming greater responsibility to serve as key resources in the area of health ethics and set up guidelines for these interventions. These professional actions have been labeled differently, such as information gathering or an ethical basis for cancer nursing practice (in this book) to information (*Outcome Standards For Cancer Nursing Practice*). Regardless of the differences in labeling, these interventions require the nurse to work actively with the physician and the other health care providers to supply sufficient information on diagnosis, treatment, prognosis, potential risks, potential benefits, and methods the client and family can utilize to help their cause. This approach enhances client and family participation in decision making, thereby increasing the probability that an informed decision will be made. The changing roles of nursing have also influenced nurses' perceptions of how physicians function. For example, in prior years, many nurses were critical of physicians for their apparent indifference to clients by not disclosing the diagnosis or, subsequently, a poor prognosis. Exploration by nurses of the dynamics of decision making in these areas has helped them better appreciate the inherent stress and anguish the physician sometimes experiences in carrying out professional obligations to clients. This growing sensitivity to the dilemmas the physician encounters has enabled nurses to revise their actions so that more support is given the physician as well as assuming a greater role for themselves, specifically in terms of validating the client and family perceptions as to what is happening to them, the psychologic state they are in, and what they need from the health care provider to cope with this crisis. Many nurses now undertake such activities, making them key resources in health ethics. Generally, decisions and strategies on how best to convey this negative information to client and family reflect input from many of the providers and no longer the physician alone. This relieves the physician of some of the burden of disclosure as well as providing more comprehensive care to the client and family.

Nurse consultant roles. Until 1975, there was no formal mechanism for nurses working with cancer clients to communicate and learn from one another. That year I led the effort to found the Oncology Nursing Society to promote colleagueship among nurses interested in working with cancer clients, to generate new knowledge about cancer nursing along with promoting cancer research in general, and to enhance the level of care being given to the client and family. From a small group of nurses, this organization has grown now to a few thousand members from the United States, Canada, and parts of Europe and the British Isles. Activities include major standing committees dealing with clinical practice, education and research, an annual congress to provide a forum for nurses to present and exchange information, and a professional journal to further disseminate information.

Aside from the formal organizational activities that promote the nurse consultant roles, there are numerous informal member channels such as the exchange of speakers for regional or national conferences, written or phone consultations for specific professional situations, and directories of nurses who hold professional positions in the various practice settings, education, and research programs. Communication has also increased on a local level among nurses interested in or actually working with cancer clients.

Formal and informal communication has also permitted nurses to offer their expertise for major cancer research and demonstration projects, to begin to offer input on the creation of policies that impact on care, and to serve as official nurse representatives to national cancer organizations.

All of these activities have enhanced the perceptions that nurses have for each other as well as more correctly identifying to others that nurses have both the initiative and knowledge to impact on cancer health care.

Nurse coordinator roles. Nurse coordinator roles vary with the clinical setting and the educational background of the nurse, but there are some commonalities to each role. For example, most nurse coordinators care for a discrete population of clients, possibly based on a hospital unit, outpatient clinic, or community agency. This concentration has permitted these nurses to identify needs or problems for a specific population of clients. Many of the chapters in this book exemplify the knowledge base of cancer nurses by their articulation of needs of clients with childhood cancers; cancers of the breast, gastrointestinal tract, head and neck, brain, genitourinary tract; gynecologic cancers; and adult leukemia. This information had not been available in prior years to any great extent. Also, information is available as to phases of wellness and illness, general and specific needs, and important transitions or higher risk periods.

Along with having a discrete population of clients that enables nurses to identify common needs, nurse coordinators provide for continuity of care between settings. With the exception of the community nurse, maintaining liaison with client and family members over time was not commonly done by nurses. True, nurse-to-nurse referrals were and still are very common, but the referring nurse usually did not continue to oversee care as the nurse coordinator continues to do. Providing liaison and ensuring that care is coordinated thus allow clients to minimize lost time caused by laboratory and radiologic studies, more time to pursue valued activities, greater support to the family so that they can participate in the client's care, and increased compliance with treatment.

The notable fact about the evolution of the nurse coordinator roles is the innovation that has been brought to them. No longer do nurses feel constrained to only practice in traditional settings but are now responding to expressed client and family needs. Such examples are nurses who have independent practices, those who function as community-based coordinators, those who run detection-counseling-client teaching centers or rehabilitation clinics, and those who are in joint practice arrangements with physician colleagues.

The nurse as a coordinator complements the physician's goal of curing or controlling the client's cancer and fulfills a need that would not be met by most of the other health care providers.

Cancer nursing education

Cancer nursing education, like practice, has undergone many changes in the past 10 years, principally in the areas of graduate and continuing education as well as curriculum guidelines.

Graduate nursing education. There are currently more than eleven programs throughout the United States that offer a clinical specialization in cancer nursing. Most of them have articulated different educational models so that the final products, the new clinical nurse specialists, are capable of functioning in widely varying roles from community detection settings to sophisticated territory care settings. Since many of these programs were developed within the last 5 years, it will take a few more years before adequate time for evaluation of their worth is possible. However, as the care for this population of clients becomes more complex, it seems likely that cancer clinical nurse specialists will continue to be needed to contribute to the team efforts.

Continuing education (CE) in cancer nursing. Like graduate nurse education, most CE programs directed toward cancer nursing were begun only in the last few years. Since the majority of nurses cannot or do not want to obtain master degrees, CE is a voluntary mechanism to upgrade nurses' skills and knowledge about cancer clients. Some programs have a number of offerings while others may only have one annual program. Moreover, the level of training to which these programs are geared can vary substantially from the generalist nurse to those nurses who already have a substantial background in cancer. Programs need to be evaluated for their individual merits, but generally, CE programs fulfill a valuable service to update nursing knowledge about a rapidly changing specialty.

Curriculum guidelines. These guidelines are in the final stages of preparation by the Education Committee of the Oncology Nursing Society. The aim of developing generalized guidelines in cancer nursing education is to provide direction in an overall way for nursing educators throughout the United States. Just as with the standards developed by this organization, substantial input has been received so that the curriculum guidelines reflect current practices and client needs.

The guidelines are divided into two major areas: fundamental and advanced cancer nursing education. Fundamental is defined as baccalaureate level education and advanced is graduate nursing education and certificate programs in the continuing education areas. Both levels have short-term continuing education programs within them to acknowledge the needs of many nurses who do not yet have baccalaureate degrees or who wish to pursue limited continuing education courses.

These guidelines are intended to be adjusted to meet the regional and local needs, to acknowledge the heterogeneity of nurses and also of client-family needs and problems. On the national level, there is no way to accurately predict the local needs so it seems both appropriate and feasible to provide direction in a general sense and leave the actual implementation to the local center. However, consistency within the nursing profession is vitally important so that program coordinators are encouraged to follow the National League for Nursing or American Nurses' Association guidelines.

Cancer nursing research

Research relating to cancer nursing has been ongoing for some time, but it has only been recently that the number of research efforts has increased substantially. For example, in 1979 there was the First National Conference on Cancer Nursing Research, which attracted some 250 nurses to a program of research reports ranging from small-scale clinical research projects to sophisticated larger scale efforts. There is an enlarging core of nurses prepared to conduct research, particularly those with doctoral degrees, so that information on comfort, symptom management, client education, adaptation models, home care, and supportive care as well as other areas is being generated.

These efforts are being supported by the Research Committee of the Oncology Nursing Society. This committee, recently established, will aid nurses in methodologic problems that are common to clinical research.

Methodologic problems in clinical research are not unique to the nursing profession. Most other disciplines have similar problems because of the inherent difficulties of undertaking research in a clinical setting, the ethical dilemmas relative to when, if, and how interventions should be made during the conduct of the research, the small sample sizes common to this type of research, and the complexity of the problems being studied. Nurses should feel heartened that significant progress is being made but not be deluded into a false sense of security. For research conducted by nurses to be considered important it will have to consider major problem areas and have a detailed and rigorous research design along with meticulous data procedures. Nurses have made a great deal of progress to date and should be encouraged by the support and recognition they are receiving.

Along with conducting individual research, nurses are beginning to impact on the evaluation of the worthiness of research projects for funding. The fact that nurses now sit on these review committees is a major achievement.

FUTURE TRENDS

As with the section on current progress, this section will discuss the trends in nursing practice, education, and research.

Cancer nursing practice

There are numerous activities that have impact for the future. Among the major items are the evaluation of the standards that have been developed, joint physician-nurse standards development, which could lead to the establishment of standards for an entire population of cancer clients, and a certification program.

All the potential future activities evolve from the development of the *Outcome Standards For Cancer Nursing Practice*.[1]

Evaluation of nursing interventions based on the outcome criteria described in each standard would prove very helpful to the nursing profession by documenting if hospital stays were shortened, complications were lessened, client and family understanding was increased, or adjustment was promoted. There have been very few examples of the effectiveness of nursing interventions in the various care settings, nor has there been any documentation of diminished cost.

Joint standards to reflect medical practice as well as nursing practice are under way in a few select centers. This accomplishment had been envisioned at the time the nursing standards were developed because the standards could not be complete without both professional groups. In fact, it is preferable to include other health care providers such as social workers, dietitians, clergy, and community representatives. Starting with physician-nurse standards is logical, however, since physicians and nurses are the major providers and they must reach overall agreement.

Identifying a discrete population of cancer clients to articulate complete standards may also be accomplished in the future. By complete standards of care is meant the statement of guidelines for physical structure, number of care providers who are needed, along with the statement of client outcomes. Much success and enhanced care have occurred for the client needing a coronary care unit, which complies with the accredited standards in that area. The same success would be hoped for with cancer clients.

A certification program for cancer nurses may also be developed in future years to meet a need to protect the public. Certification is defined as a "process by which a non-governmental agency or association certifies that an individual licensed to practice a profession has met certain pre-determined standards specified by that profession for specialty practice. Its purpose is to assure various publics that an individual has mastered a body of knowledge and acquired skills in a particular specialty."[2] Certification indicates a minimum competence to practice in a specialty area, so clearly defined criteria need to be developed. The outcome standards form a core of the criteria by delineating a beginning scope of practice. Much more work needs to be done in this area to have a functioning certification program, but a beginning framework is there to build on.

Cancer nursing education

The numerous graduate and continuing education programs that have been under way for some time are identifying educational strategies to better prepare nurses to care for cancer clients as well as train greater numbers of skilled and knowledgeable nurses. Refinements are continuing to take place so that nurses trained in future years will have more integrated opportunities to learn about clients with these disorders. No longer should cancer nursing education be fragmented and limited in its scope. Future plans call for implementing curriculum guidelines for undergraduate nursing programs so that initial training can also reflect the major changes in cancer health care. This integration will undoubtedly improve nurses' perception of the potential impact they can have on care. This movement into cancer nursing can only serve to enhance the knowledge base being developed currently and promote a more sophisticated level of care from nurses functioning in a wide range of care facilities.

Additionally, the current proliferation of various types of cancer nursing education programs may necessitate the development of an independent accreditation process. Like certification, accreditation is a major professional undertaking that has many economic and social ramifications. A move toward accreditation should be taken only after very careful consideration as to its purpose, value to society, cost, and administration. Duplication of accrediting that is currently in place can never be supported, but a rational plan to promote the updating of educational programs to better prepare nurses in cancer care can benefit society in general as well as the nursing profession.

Cancer nursing research

This area of cancer nursing will be greatly expanded within the near future as the core of trained cancer nurses increases and skilled nurse researchers become more aware of opportunities in cancer research. Therapeutic research will continue in full force, but as the public and policymakers become more concerned with the impact these treatments have on the quality of life, nurses will have more visibility and become involved in information gathering, public-client education, and morbidity associated with treatment. The only serious constraint to preventing nursing from making large gains in research would be the shortage of funds. The fact of a limited economic outlook comes at a bad time for nurses who are finally getting into the research area, but concentration on reducing costs associated with care would help their proposals. For example, if it can be shown that cancer client education developed by nurses does reduce complications, shorten hospital stays, and promote compliance with diagnostic or treatment procedures, nurses will have shown the value of their work. Likewise, if supportive and preventive nursing interventions can reduce the morbidity associated with certain cancer treatments so that the quality of life and adjustment are greater, the value of nursing interventions will be demonstrated. If a nurse-coordinated clinic for detection or "end-of-life" care can be shown to be successful and cost-effective, nurses will have demonstrated their value in a very important way. These examples are not meant to minimize the many other appropriate and successful models of cancer nursing research, rather they are discussed to point up ways that nurses can successfully compete for research support in the public and private sectors.

CONCLUSION

This chapter specifically, as well as the book in its entirety, has discussed the many ways that nurses can and should intervene with people who have cancer. Cancer remains a major health care problem nationally and a very fearsome, isolating illness for the client and family to individually confront. Medicine has shown the significant contributions that can be made in the diagnosis and treatment of the numerous forms of cancer. Because of these achievements, numerous other important needs or problem areas have surfaced that are ideally suited to the professional nurse. Knowledge is being generated in practice, education, and research areas within nursing so that it is more likely that nurses will possess the ability to contribute significantly to the care of these clients. The basic abilities of nurses to be client educators and coordinators of care allow them to make significant contributions to cancer health care so that nursing's influence is being felt on local levels. National policymaking roles are still to be defined, but I am confident that the changing individual perceptions that nurses have of one another will eventually alter the public and political perceptions as well. Once this occurs, nurses will finally have the opportunity for impacting on cancer health care at the national level. Right now, nurses can rightly feel a sense of pride and accomplishment with the level of care they are providing to cancer clients and their families.

REFERENCES

1. Oncology Nursing Society and American Nurses' Association: Outcome standards for cancer nursing practice, Kansas City, Mo., 1979, American Nurses' Association.
2. The study of credentialing in nursing: a new approach, vol. I. The report of the committee, Kansas City, Mo., 1979, American Nurses' Association.

Index

A

Abdominal involvement, diet for patients receiving radiation therapy for, 280
Ablative surgery, 257
Absolute granulocyte count, 530
ABVD, as chemotherapeutic agent, 249
Acetaminophen, 354, 398
Acting out behavior, 412-413
Actinomycin-D, 247, 303, 312, 314-315
Active immunotherapy, 344-345
Acupuncture, 393
Adaptation, 7
Adjuvant therapy, 63-64
Adolescent, care needs of, 480-486
Adrenocortical steroids, 319
Advocacy, 368
Advocate, client-family, 110-111
Affected population, characteristics of, 26-28
Age
  and incidence of cancer, 26-28
  and survival rate, 30-31
Aging of population, 79
Alcohol, and oral cancer, 183-184, 185
Alkylating agents, 295, 297-299, 306-308
Alopecia, 282, 335, 377
American Cancer Society, 43-45
American College of Surgeons, Hospital Cancer Program of, 48
Aminoglutethimide, 320
Amphotericin B, 533
Analgesics, 394-400
Analysis, in epidemiologic studies, 151-153, 156-157
Androgens, 318, 320
Anemia, 335, 527-528
Anger, client, 60-61
Angles of recovery, 102, 103
Anorexia, 274-275, 334, 513-514, 516-518
Antibiotic therapy, prophylactic, in clients with acute leukemia, 534
Antiestrogens, 319, 320-321
Antimetabolites, 299-301, 308-311
Antitumor antibiotics, 303-304, 312-315
Anxiety, client, reducing, 82
Appearance changes, in client with brain tumor, 589-590
Artifact, 147-148
Asbestos, and relation to incidence of lung cancer, 194
L-Asparaginase, 304, 315-316, 458, 526
Aspirin, 398
Assertiveness, 130-131
Assessment information, potential sources of, 85
Attitudes, shift of, as sign of burnout, 119-121
5-Azacytidine, 301, 311

B

Bacillus Calmette-Guérin, 239, 346-348, 501
Bamfolin, 359
Biopsy, 252
Bladder cancer
  multimodality treatment for, 240
  nursing care for client with, 599-600
  nursing interventions, 205-206
  risk factors, 204
  staging for, 598
  symptoms, 598-599
  treatment, 599
Bleomycin, 304, 313-314, 457
Body image
  changes in, 451-452
    associated with head and neck cancer, 560-579
  of clients with gynecologic cancer, 547-548
  concepts of, defining, through research, 561-564

Body image—cont'd
  development of, 564-565
  significance of head and neck to, 565
Bone marrow
  cancer of; *see* Leukemia
  effects of radiation therapy on, 283
Bone pain, 386-387
Brain tumor(s)
  case study, 591-594
  diagnostic methods, 583-584
  incidence, 583
  multimodality treatment for, 240
  problems encountered by clients with
    appearance changes, 589-590
    isolation, 590-591
    mental status changes, 585-586
    motor and sensory function changes, 586
    side-effects and complications of treatment, 586-589
  signs and symptoms of, 582-583
  treatment of, 584-585
Breast cancer
  case study, 502-506
  drugs for treatment of, 318-319
  incidence, 488
  morbidity associated with
    from immunotherapy, 501
    from radiation therapy, 497-499
    secondary to chemotherapy, 499-501
    from surgery, 492-497
  multimodality treatment for, 237-238
  needs of client with, 491
  nursing interventions, 189-193
  risk factors, 141, 187-189, 488-491
Burkitt's lymphoma, 142, 346
Burnout
  antecedents of, 114-119
  definition of, 113-114
  intervention for, implementing individualized, 127-134
    recreate and relax, 131-132
    restore physical capacities, 132-133
    revamp communication styles, 129-131
    review cognitive basis for client care, 128-129
    revitalize work environment, 133-134
  manifestations of, 119-125
  strategies for prevention and interruption, 125-127
Busulfan, 298, 307

C

Cachexia, 513
Calusterone, 318
Cancer
  advanced
    care of child with, 431-440
    care of client with
      physiologic comfort, 376-380
      population characteristics, 374-375
      psychologic comfort, 375-376
      scientific basis for treating, 374

Cancer—cont'd
  advanced—cont'd
    care of client with—cont'd
      scope of problem, 373-374
  attitudes toward, changing, 4-5
  bladder, 204-206, 240, 598-600
  bone marrow; *see* Leukemia
  breast, 141, 187-193, 237-238, 488-507
  childhood, 240-241, 455-486
  as chronic illness, 551-552
  classifying, 25
  colorectal, 200-203, 239-240
  comparison with other diseases, 28
  complexities of, 114-115
  costs of, 31-34
  defining
    definition of, 20
    differentiating normal and malignant cells, 21-25
  detection and diagnosis, nursing opportunities in, 13-16
  diagnosis and staging of, improvements in, 241-244
  early detection of, 176-224
  endometrial, and exogenous estrogens, associations between, 158
  environmental chemicals and, 163-164
  etiology, 162-166
    cross-sectional studies, 159
    historic or reconstructed cohort study, 153-159
    prospective studies, 149-153
    protocols, 162
  gastric, 206-208, 240
  gastrointestinal, 508-523
  genitourinary, 595-612
  gynecologic, 211-221, 547-559
  head and neck, 240, 560-579
  iatrogenic, 166
  incidence, 25-28
    according to person, place, and time, 141-144
  kidney, 600-602
  larynx, 567-579
  life-style and, 164-166
  lung, 193-197
  multimodality treatment for, 237-250
  myths about, 365-366
  natural history of, 7
  nature and scope of, 20-34
  oral, 183-186
  organizations, institutional and national, 46-48
  ovarian, 239
  pain associated with, 384-403
  penile, 604
  prevention and carcinogenesis, nursing opportunities in, 12-13
  prostate, 197-200, 595-598
  quackery in treatment of, 357-369
  radioresponsiveness of, 263-265
  rates and ratios of, 144-146
  research and control, cost of, 32
  skin, 177-183
  societies, professional, 45-46

Cancer—cont'd
survival data, trends in, 29-31
survival following diagnosis, 28-31
terminal, and female sexuality, 555-556
testicular, 208-211, 238, 602-604
thyroid, 186-187
treatment
multimodal, 7
nursing opportunities in, 16-18
types of, 26
Cancer Care, Inc., 32
"Cancer personality," 54
Cancer Surveillance, Epidemiology, and End Results program (SEER), 28-29
Cancer surveillance programs, 171-172
CANSCREEN, 15
Carcin, CH-23, 359
Carcinoembryonic antigen, 202-203, 332
Carcinogenesis, 7, 337
Carcinoma(s), 25
bronchogenic, 194
of lip, 185-186
oat cell, 194, 195
small cell and epidermoid, of lung, 238-239
of spermatic epithelium, 208
squamous and basal cell, 179-180, 181
of tongue, 185-186
Cardiac toxicity, 313
Care and cure, conflicts between, 69
Carmustine, 298, 307, 584
Causal direction, 146-147
Causal relationships, special problems in assessing, 166-169
Causation and association, epidemiologic
causal, 148-149
criteria for causal, 146-147
noncausal, 147-148
Cell(s)
anaplastic, 21
cancer, differentiating normal and malignant, 21-25
cycle, 289-291
heterogeneity of, 22-23
kinetic processes of, in relation to cancer treatment, 291-294
replication of, 289
subpopulation, 23-25
Central gray stimulation, for control of pain, 394
Chemicals, environmental, and cancer, 163-164
Chemotherapy, 287-339, 457-458; *see also* Multimodality cancer treatment
agents for, in clinical use
alkylating, 295, 297-299, 306-308
antimetabolites, 299-301, 308-311
antitumor antibiotics, 303-304, 312-315
miscellaneous, 304-305, 315-317
plant alkaloids, 302, 311-312
biologic considerations, 289-295
for brain tumors, 584
for Burkitt's lymphoma, 330
combination, 328-332
Chemotherapy—cont'd
complications of, 333-336
drug development and clinical trials, 321-337
endocrine therapy, 317-321
for gynecologic cancer, and female sexuality, 554-555
immunosuppression, 336
long-term effects of, 336-337
morbidity associated with, 499-501
rationale for use, 294-295
research methodology, 337-339
for testicular cancer, 603
in treatment of acute leukemia, 527-528
Childhood cancer
care during, developmental approach to, 468-486
chemotherapy for, 457-458
modes of therapy for, 459-464
multimodality treatment for, 240-241
nursing care in, 431-440
philosophy of care, 466-468
radiation therapy for, 458-459
surgery for, 456-457
Chlorambucil, 298, 307
Chloroma, 221
Chlorotrianisene, 318
Choice of action, decision-making model to guide, 73-76
Choriocarcinoma, chemotherapy for, 331
Chromosomes, 262
Cigarette smoking, 13-15, 164-165
Cis-diamminedichloroplatinum II, 305, 316-317
Cisplatin, 458
Client(s)
with advanced cancer, control and comfort of, 373-380
with brain tumors, problems encountered by, 585-591
emotional support of, 367-368
establishing educational goals for, 84-86
and family
education, evaluating, 91-94
needs of, documentation of, 443-444
fears of, 364-365
identifying educational needs of, 83-84
needs
during surgery, 253, 254-256, 259
overview of, 445-453
physical care requirements, 115
providing information to, necessity of, 367
rationale for seeking cancer quackery methods, 361-366
reactions of, after cancer diagnosis, 406-409
role function of, 577-578
self-concept of, 576-577
spectrum of care for, 443-454
vulnerability of, 68-69
Client education, 368
justification for, 81-83
and male sexuality, 606
overview and background of, 79-80

Client education—cont'd
  principles of, 94-95
  rationale for, 80
  step-by-step development of, 83-94
  and stomal care, 607-612
Client-family advocate, 110-111
Client-family education, 17
Clinical practice, implications of research for, 107-111
Clinical trials, for drug development
  phase I, 323-324
  phase II, 325-326
  phase III, 326-328
Cobalt 60 machine, 266
Codeine, 398
Cohort, selection of, 150
Colitis, ulcerative, 200
Colorectal cancer
  multimodality treatment for, 239-240
  nursing interventions, 203
  recommended screening intervals and procedures for, 202
  risk factors, 200-203
Comfort, client's need for, 446-447
Committee for Freedom of Choice in Cancer Therapy, 362
Communication, 129-131, 366-367, 376, 405-418
Community, 7
Community diagnosis, 140
Conflicts
  between care and cure, 69
  value, in work context, 70-71
Confounding factors, 148
Conjugated equine estrogen, 318
Constipation, 334
Construction, cost of, 32
Consumer activism, 99
Consumer Product Safety Commission, 42
Consumers' rights movement, 79-80
Content knowledge, 83
Continuing education in cancer nursing, 620-621
Coordinating care, 17
Cordotomy, 393
Corticosteroids, 317, 321
  relative potencies of, 587
Corynebacterium parvum, 348-349
Costs of cancer
  direct, calculation of, 31-33
  indirect, calculation of, 34
  major categories, 31
Counseling, client-family, 109, 110
Counter-immunoelectrophoresis, and detection of prostate cancer, 198
Covariation, 146-147
Cryptorchidism, 208
Curriculum guidelines, 621
Cyclophosphamide, 297, 306-307, 458, 526
Cytoreductive surgery, 256
Cytosine arabinoside, 301, 311, 526

D

Dactinomycin, 303
Data analysis techniques, selection of, 105
Daunomycin hydrochloride, 304, 312-313, 526
Death
  fear of causing, nurse's, 422-423
  perception of, 426-427
Decision making, for burnout control, 128-129
Defense mechanisms, as sign of burnout, 121-122
Definitive therapy phase, 61-62
Deglutition, for larynx cancer patient, 574-575
Degree of sensitivity, 21
Delaney Clause, 40-41
Denial, 122
Dental regimen, for clients receiving radiation to head and neck, 277
Desquamation, 281
Developmental needs
  of adolescent, 480-481
  of infant, 469
  of preschooler, 473-474
  of school-age child, 476-477
  of toddler, 471-472
Dexamethasone, 319
Diagnosis
  of brain tumors, 583-584
  delay in, 57-58
  and staging
    clinical, 242-243
    surgical, 252-254
  survival following, 28-31
Diagnostic phase, providing client support during, 15
Diarrhea, 334
Diet
  and cancer, 165-166
  regulation, for clients receiving radiation therapy, 274-280
Diethylstilbestrol, 318
  and testicular cancer, 208
Differentiation, cell, degree of, 21
Dinitrochlorobenzene (DNCB), 350-351
Diphenhydramine hydrochloride, 354
Disease, 7
  differentiation of, 142-144
Displacement, 121
Division of Cancer Biology and Diagnosis, 39
Division of Cancer Control and Rehabilitation, 39
Division of Cancer Research Resources and Centers, 39
Division of Cancer Treatment, 39
DNA, 164, 261, 263, 289-291
DNCB skin test, 351
Dosage, calculation of, in chemotherapy, 324-325
Dose, radiation, as determinant of radioresponsiveness, 263-265
Dose-response relationship, 295
Double-blind trial, 160, 162
Down's syndrome, 223-224
Doxorubicin, 247, 303, 312-313, 457, 464, 526
Dromostanolone propionate, 318

Drugs, cytotoxic, 295-317
Drugs, nursing services, and home care, costs of, 33
Dying and death, confronting, as contribution to burnout, 117-118

E

Early detection of cancer, 176-224
Education
  cancer nursing, 620-621, 622-623
  client, 79-96
  client-family, 17, 108
Educational methods, selecting appropriate, 86-88
Educational program
  carrying out, 88-90
  minimum content of, 109
Elimination, 452
Emotions, change in, as sign of burnout, 123
Endorphins, 397
Enkephalins, 397
Environment, 7
  as antecedent of burnout, 115-116
Environmental Protection Agency, 41-42
Epidemiology
  causation and association, 146-149
  concepts of, 139-140
  screening, 169-171
  studies, policy implications from, 172-174
  and study of cancer
    cyclic nature of, 146
    descriptive approaches to, 141-146
Epipodophyllotoxins, 312
Erythroplakia, 186
Escherichia coli, 532
Estrogens, 318, 320
Ethical analysis, critical, proposed model for, 74-75
Ethical decision making, organizations conducive to, 76-77
Ethics, 67-77
Ethinyl estradiol, 318
Ewing's sarcoma, chemotherapy for, 331
Examination
  oral, maneuvers frequently omitted during, 186
  pelvic, 214-218
  physical, improvements in, 241
  self-breast, 189-191
  testicular self-, 210-211
Exercise, aerobic, 132-133
Expectations, in nurse-client relationship, 411
Experimentation, 147
Exposure, in epidemiologic study, 150-151, 155-156
Extracellular environment, as determinant of radioresponsiveness, 263
Extrapolation, animal-to-human, problems in, 167-169

F

Family, 7
  badgering, 414-416
  how home care affects, 435-437
  impact of cancer on, 100-105
Family—cont'd
  of infants with cancer, 470
  of toddler with cancer, 473
  as unit of care, 55
Fear, nurse's, 421-426
First-order kinetics, 295
Flexibility, decrease of, as sign of burnout, 123
5-Fluorouracil, 301, 310-311
Fluoxymesterone, 318
Folate antagonists, 308-310
Follow-up, in epidemiologic studies, 151
Food and Drug Administration, 40-41, 363
Furosemide, 349

G

Gardner's syndrome, 200
Gastrectomy, problems following, 516
Gastric cancer
  multimodality treatment for, 240
  nursing interventions, 207-208
  risk factors, 206-207
Gastrointestinal cancer
  care of clients with, phases of, 509-511
  case study, 520-522
  incidence, 508-509
  nutrition of clients with, 511-520
Gastrointestinal system, of client receiving radiation therapy, 274-275
Gap terminology of interphase, 289-290
Gate control theory of pain, 382-383
Genitourinary cancer, 595-612
Glover serum, 359
Glucocorticoids, 587-589
Graduate nursing education, 620
Granulocyte transfusions, 534-535
Grief, 62
  nurse's, 420-429
Growth and development, client, changes in, 449-450
Guaiac test, for determination of colorectal cancer, 201
Guilt, client, 61, 413-414
Gynecologic cancer; *see also* specific cancers
  drugs for treatment of, 319
  early symptoms, physical findings, and diagnostic procedures, 212-213
  and female sexuality, 547-559
  nursing interventions, 211-221
  risk factors, 211

H

Halstead radical mastectomy, 493, 494
Head and neck cancer
  characteristics of, 560-561
  estimated cases and deaths, 561
  multimodality treatment for, 240
  radiation therapy for, diet for clients receiving, 275-277
Heaf gun, for administration of BCG, 353-354
Health, 7

Health care
  cancer
    medical limitations of, 362-363
    organizational structure of
      cancer organizations, 43-48
      local cancer efforts, 48
      United States government agencies and branches, 35
  delivery, changes in, 80
Health care providers, 7, 9-10
  education of, 10-11
  training, cost of, 32
  increasing accountability of, 80
  prejudices of, in response to client pain, 391
Health-disease continuum, 6-8
  applied to health care system, 8-9
  general application of, 8
Helplessness, minimizing sense of, 82
Hematopoietic system, effect of radiation on, 263
Hematuria, 205
Hemorrhage, 528-529
Hepatic effects of chemotherapy, 336-337
Heterogeneity, cell, 22-23
Hexamethylmelamine, 305, 316
High-efficiency particulate air (HEPA) filters, 540
High-risk periods for client and family
  diagnostic period, 59-61
  end of life, 65
  period of treatment, 61-65
  prediagnostic period, 57-59
High-risk populations
  identifying, 14
  offering counsel to, 14-15
High-to-low dose extrapolation, 168-169
History taking, improvements in, 241
Hodgkin's disease, 261, 477
  chemotherapy for, 329, 330
  multimodality treatment, 247-250
Home care, for child with cancer, 432-439
Hope, fostering, 82-83
Hormonal receptors, 238
Hospice, 431-432
Hospital care, cost of, 31-32
Hospital discharge, initial, 62-63
Hoxsey chemotherapy, 358
Hydrocortisone, 319, 321, 354
Hydromorphone, 398
Hydroxyprogesterone caproate, 319
Hydroxyurea, 305, 316
Hygiene, for client with advanced cancer, 376-377
Hyperalimentation, intravenous, 519-520
Hyperpigmentation, 335
Hyperuricemia, 336
Hypnotism, 401
Hypophysectomy, 257
  client instructions following, 258

I

Illness, life-threatening, confrontation of, as contributor to burnout, 116
Immediate postconfirmation phase, characteristics of, 60-61
Immune ribonucleic acid, 350
Immunotherapy, tumor; *see also* Multimodality cancer treatment
  agents for
    bacillus Calmette-Guérin, 346-348
    Corynebacterium parvum, 348-349
    immune ribonucleic acid, 350
    levamisole, 349
    methanol-extracted residue (MER), 349-350
    thymosin, 350
    transfer factor, 350
  general limitations, 345
  morbidity associated with, 501
  nursing care during, 350-355
  scientific rationale for, 344-345
  types of
    active, 344-345
    passive, 345
Incidence of cancer, 25-28, 145
Infant, care needs of, 468-471
Infection control, 450-451
  in clients with acute leukemia, 524-546
Information
  client's need for, 447-448
  gathering, 62
  obtaining, assisting client and family in, 15-16
  providing, to client, 81-82
Informed consent, 80
Institutional and national organizations, 46-48
Institutional review board, 48
Intercalation, 313
International Association of Cancer Victims and Friends, 362
International Cancer Research Data Bank, 38
Interphase, 289-290
Interpretation, of results of cohort study, 153, 159
Interspecies extrapolation, 168
Intervention strategies, 58-59, 60-61
Interventions, effectiveness of, analytic approaches to studying, 159-162
Intradiagnostic phase, characteristics of, 59-60
Intrasil, 537
Iodine, as risk factor in thyroid cancer, 186
Ionizing radiation, 261-263
Isolation techniques, for prevention of infection in client with acute leukemia, 540
Isolation/withdrawal, 122

K

Karnofsky scale, 243
Kidney cancer
  nursing care for client with, 601-602
  staging of, 601
  treatment, 601
Kilovoltage machines, 265-266

Klebsiella, 532
Koch antitoxins, 359
Krebiozen (carcalon), 358
Kubler-Ross, theories of, 427-429

L

Laboratory studies, improvements in, 241-242
Laetrile (amygdalin), 358-359
Laminar airflow room (LAFR), 540-541
Laparotomy, diagnostic, 252-253
Larynx cancer, 567-579
  deglutition for client with, 574-575
  phonation for client with, 575-576
  respiration for client with, 575
Learning
  principles of, 94-95
  successful, impediments to, 109
Legislative branch of United States government, 41
Leukapheresis, 526
Leukemia
  acute
    in adults, multimodality treatment for, 239
    case study, 543-546
    clinical presentation, 525-526
    complications of, management of
      anemia, 527-528
      hemorrhage, 528-529
      infection, 529-535
    incidence, 524
    infection in clients with, 529-535, 541-546
    nursing interventions for, 535-538
    pathophysiology of, 524-525
    treatment of, 526-527
      specific measures, 538-541
  acute lymphocytic, 459-461
  chemotherapy for, 330
  nursing interventions, 221-224
  protocol for, 460
  risk factors, 221
  signs, symptoms, and physical findings, 222
Leukopenia, 335-336
Leukoplakia, 178, 185-186
Leucovorin, 309
Levamisole, 349
Levorphanol, 398
Life-style, cancer and, 164-166
Lomustine, 299, 307, 584
Lung cancer
  multimodality treatment for, 238-239
  nursing interventions, 194-197
  risk factors, 193-194
Lymph nodes, regional, importance of, in definitive surgery, 254-255
Lymphedema, 494
Lymphoma, 477
  diffuse histiocytic, chemotherapy for, 330
  non-Hodgkin's, multimodality treatment for, 239

M

Malignancy, 20
Malnutrition, deficiency, 514
Mammography, 188-189
Mastectomy, 492-497
Maximar, 266
Maxitron, 266
Mechlorethamine, 297, 306
Medical expertise, confusion between nonmedical questions and, 71-72
Meditation, 132
Medroxyprogesterone, 319
Megavoltage machines, 266-270
Megesterol acetate, 319
Melanoma, malignant, 180-183, 240
Mental status, changes in, in clients with brain tumors, 585-586
Meperidine, 398
6-Mercaptopurine, 300, 310, 526
Metastasis, removal of solitary, 256
Methadone, 398
Methanol-extracted residue (MER), 349-350
Methodological procedures, selection or development of, 105
Methotrexate, 299, 308-310, 526
Methyl CCNU, 299, 307, 308
Methylprednisolone, 319
Micrometastases, 245, 254
Mithramycin, 303, 312, 315
Mitomycin-C, 303, 312, 315
Mitosis, 289-291
Mitotic potential, as determinant of radioresponsiveness, 263
Mole, changes in, 182-183
MOPP drug combination, 249, 329
Moral art, nursing as, 67-70
Morbidity, 7, 34, 448
  minimizing treatment-related, 17-18
Morphine, 397, 399
Mortality, 25, 34, 145, 171, 288
Motor and sensory function changes, in clients with brain tumors, 586
Mucositis, 334-335
Multimodality cancer treatment, 332-333
  models of, 247-250
  reasons for improved client survival, 241-247
  recent advances in, 237-241
Mutation, radiation-induced, 262
Myelosuppression, 335

N

National Cancer Act, 36-37, 38
National Cancer Institute, 32, 36-40
National Disease and Therapeutic Index, 32
National Health Federation, 362
National Institute of Environmental Health Sciences, 42
National Institute of Occupational Safety and Health, 42
National Surgical Adjuvant Breast Project, 238

Nausea and vomiting, as side-effects of chemotherapy, 333-334
Negotiation, in nurse-client relationship, 411-412
Neoplasia, 289
Neoplasm, 20
Nephroblastoma, 27
Nerve blocks, for control of pain, 392-393
Neuroblastoma, 471-472
Neurologic involvement, pain associated with, 387
Neutropenia, 526
Nitrosureas, 307-308
Nonspuriousness, 146-147
Normality, concept of, 54-55
Nurse
  consultant roles, 619
  coordinator roles, 619-620
  home care provided by, 434
  personal stress factors of, as contributors to burnout, 118-119
  as provider, 10
  responsibility concerning cancer quackery, 366-369
  role as advocate, 368
  role in early detection of cancer, 176-224
  sexist stereotypes of, 71
  special role in client care, 67-69
Nurse practitioners, 176
Nursing
  cancer
    and body image alteration, 574-579
    and breast cancer clients, 496-497, 499, 500-501
    care of child, 431-440
    changing attitudes, 4-5
    for client with acute leukemia, 535-538
    for client with bladder cancer, 599-600
    for client with kidney cancer, 601-602
    for client with penile cancer, 604
    for client with prostate cancer, 597-598
    for client with testicular cancer, 603-604
    communication approaches in, 405-418
    conceptual framework for, 5-18, 72-76
    current progress and future trends, 617-624
    definition, 10-11
    ethical basis for, 618-619
    historical perspective, 3-4
    importance of, 444-445
    intervention, during surgery, 253-254, 256, 259
    management of pain, 381-403
    model, integrating adaptation and rehabilitation with, 11-12
    modification of techniques, 98-99
    multimodality treatment in, 237-250
    new roles in, 5
    and nutrition, assessment of, 379
    opportunities in, 13-18
    palliative cancer rehabilitation, 12
    preventive cancer rehabilitation, 11
    problem of grief in, 420-421
    psychosocial care, need for increased involvement in, 54
    psychosocial risks in, 55-56
Nursing—cont'd
  cancer—cont'd
    during radiation therapy, 273-285
    restorative cancer rehabilitation, 12
    significance of head and neck to body image, 565-567
    during tumor immunotherapy, 350-355
  ethical, conditions that inhibit, 70-72
  as moral art, 67-70
Nursing process, 7
Nursing research, 98-112, 621-622, 623
  in drug development and clinical trials, 321-339
  methodology for, 337-339
Nutrition, 450
  and cancer quackery, 360-361
  for client with advanced cancer, 379
  for clients with gastrointestinal cancer, 511-520
  routes of, 514-515

O

Obstruction
  pain caused by, 307
  surgical removal of, 256-257
Occupational Safety and Health Administration, 42
Office of Cancer Communication, 38
Office for Protection from Research Risks, 42
Oophorectomy, 317, 320
Opiate receptors, 397
Oral cancer
  nursing interventions, 184-186
  risk factors, 183-184
Orchiectomy, 603
Ortho para'-DDD, 305, 316
Osteogenic sarcoma, 238, 480-481
Outcome Standards For Cancer Nursing Practice, 80, 618, 622
Outpatients, leukemia, infections in, 541-543
Ovarian cancer
  chemotherapy for, 331
  multimodaliy treatment for, 239
Oxycodone, 399
Oxygen, function in tumor radioresponse, 263
Oxygenation, 452-453
  of client with advanced cancer, 379
Oxymorphone, 399

P

Paget's disease, 192
Pain
  administration of, as contributor to burnout, 116-117
  assessment of, in cancer, 388-391
  causes of, 386-388
  chronic versus acute, 383
  gate control theory of, 382-383
  incidence, in cancer, 384-386
  individual perceptions of, 383-384
  interventions for controlling
    biologically based techniques, 391-400
    psychosocially based techniques, 400-402

Pain—cont'd
neurosurgical management of, 257-259
overview and assessment of, 381-382
threshold and tolerance, 383
Palliative cancer rehabilitation nursing, 12
Pancreatomy, problems following, 516
Pap smear, 216, 218-220
Papanicolaou test, 15
Para-aminobenzoic acid (PABA), 178
Parenteral nutrition, 519-520
Passive immunotherapy, 345
Pathologist, role of, 243-244
Patient's Bill of Rights, 80
Penile cancer, 604
Pentazocine, 399
L-Phenylalanine mustard, 297, 307
Phonation, for client with larynx cancer, 575-576
Physical dysfunction, and breast cancer surgery, 494
Physical signs and symptoms of burnout, 123-125
Physician services, cost of, 32
Pigmentation effects of radiation therapy, 282-283
Plant alkaloids, 302, 311-312
Plasmapheresis, 346
Population
affected, characteristics of, 26-28
aging of, 79
captive, cancer clients as, 68-69
target, identification of, 105
Practitioners, educated for accountable nursing practice, 76
Prednisolone, 319, 321
Prednisone, 319, 321, 458, 526
Prepayment and administration, expenses of, 32-33
Preschooler, care needs of, 473-476
President's Cancer Panel, 38
Prevalence rates, 145
Prevention and early detection, 449
Preventive cancer rehabilitative nursing, 11
Problem analysis in clinical situations, 72-73
Problem solving, differentiated from research process, 100
Procarbazine, 305, 316, 584
Process knowledge, 83
Proctosigmoidoscopy, 201-202
Professional societies, 45-46
Progestins, 319, 320
Projection, 121-122
Propoxyphene, 399
Prostate cancer
drugs for treatment of, 318
nursing care for clients with, 597-598
nursing interventions, 198-200
risk factors, 197-198
staging of, 596
symptomatology, 595-596
treatment, 596-597
Protected environment, for client with acute leukemia, 540-541
Pseudomonas aeruginosa, 532, 533
Psychic and mystical methods of cancer quackery, 360
Psychologic dysfunction, and breast cancer surgery, 495-496
Psychosocial care, 53-66
dynamics of, 57
family as unit of, 55
high-risk periods for client and family, 56-65
normality, concept of, 54-55
nursing involvement, increased, need for, 54
risks to nurse, 55-56
Public policy and moral accountability, 77
Pulmonary effects of chemotherapy, 336-337
Purine antagonists, 310
Pyrimidine antagonists, 310-311

Q

Quackery, cancer
definitions of, 357-358
factors supporting, 361-366
forms of, 358-361
nurse's responsibility, 366-369

R

Radiation, 186
and skin cancer, 177, 178
Radiation therapy, 458-459; *see also* Multimodality cancer treatment
aims of, 261
for brain tumors, 584
complications of, in clients with brain tumors, 586-587
components of, and effect on tissue, 270-272
diet planning for clients receiving, 274-280
discovery of, 260-261
effects of, acute, intermediate, and late, 272-273
explanation of, and effects, 261-263
gynecologic, and female sexuality, 553-554
methods of delivering
external, 265-270
internal, 270
morbidity associated with, 497-499
myelosuppression for clients receiving, 283
for prostate cancer, 596
psychosocial issues in clients receiving, 283-285
responses of cancer to, 263-265
skin care for clients receiving, 280-283
in treatment of bone metastases, 245-246
Radioimmunoassay, and detection of prostate cancer, 198
Rashes, 335
Rationalization, 121
Recall antigen testing, 350-351
Recreation, 131
Rectal cancer; *see* Colorectal cancer
Refractiveness, 21
Rehabilitation, 7
after gynecologic cancer treatment, 556-559
Relaxation, 131-132
Renal effects of chemotherapy, 336-337

Reproduction, chemotherapeutic effect on, 336
Research, nursing, 98-112
  defined, 99-100
  findings, 105-107
  implications for clinical practice, 107-111
  process, 100
  proposal, development of, 100-105
  rationale for, 99
Residence, and incidence of cancer, 28
Resources, existing, promoting better utilization of, 14
Respiration, for larynx cancer client, 575
Rest and sleep, for client with advanced cancer, 377-378
Restorative cancer rehabilitation nursing, 12
Retinoblastoma, 468-469
Rhabdomyosarcoma, 474
Rubidazone, 526

S

Safety, client, 452
  with advanced cancer, 378-379
  and brain tumors, 582-594
Sarcomas, 25
  osteogenic, 238
  soft tissue, 239
Scarification method, for administration of BCG, 354
School-age child, care needs of, 476-480
Screening, epidemiologic, 169-171
Secondary association, 148
"Second-look" surgery, 253
SEER, 28-29, 172
Selection bias, 148
Self-assessment, to diagnose burnout, 125-127
Self-care agency, protection of, 72
Self-concept, of cancer clients, 576-577
Self-examination
  breast, 189-191
  oral/facial, 185
  testicular, 210-211
Self-image, decline of, as sign of burnout, 122-123
Sepsis and septic shock, in client with acute leukemia, 539-540
Serum acid phosphatase, and detection of prostate cancer, 198
Sex
  and incidence of cancer, 28
  and survival rate, 29-30
Sexist stereotypes of nurses, 71
Sexuality, 451
  assault to, cancer as, 549-556
  in clients with acute leukemia, 543
  concept of, 547-549
  female, and gynecologic cancer, 547-559
  following mastectomy, 495-496
  male, and genitourinary cancer, 595-612
Side-effects of chemotherapy, 587-589
  cutaneous and mucosal, 334-335
  gastrointestinal, 333-334
  hematologic, 335-336
Skin cancer
  chemotherapy for, 331
  incidence, clinical characteristics, and common sites of, 180
  nursing interventions, 178-183
  risk factors, 177-178
Smoking
  cessation of, available resources to aid in, 196
  cigarette, 13, 150, 164-165
Spectrum of care, 443-454
Staging, clinical, 242-243
Staphylococcus aureus, 532, 540
Statistics
  incidence, 25-26
  mortality, 25
Stomal care, 607-612
Stomatitis, 334-335, 377
Streptozoticin, 299, 308
Surgery, 456-457; *see also* Multimodality cancer treatment
  ablative, 257
  for brain tumors, 584
  current concepts in
    definitive, 254-256
    as diagnostic and staging procedure, 252-254
    neurosurgical management of pain, 257-259
    as palliation, 256-257
  cytoreductive, 256
  gynecologic, and female sexuality, 552-553
  history of, 251-252
  for kidney cancer, 601
  morbidity associated with, 492-497
  for prostate cancer, 596
Survival data, trends in, 29-31
Synergistic therapy, 328-329
System support, role in contributing to burnout, 118

T

Tamoxifen, 319
Teaching-learning process, 7
Technologic developments, 115
Test, Papanicoloau, 15
Testicular cancer
  chemotherapy for, 331
  multimodality treatment for, 238
  nursing care for client with, 603-604
  nursing intervention, 208-211
  risk factors, 208
  staging of, 602-603
  symptoms, 602
  treatment, 603
Testolactone, 318
Testosterone, 318
Therapy, adjuvant, 63-64
Thermography, 189
6-Thioguanine, 301, 310, 526
Thoracic involvement, diet for client receiving radiation therapy for, 277-280
Threshold limit values, 172-173
Thrombocytopenia, 335, 528-529

Thymosin, 350
Thyroid cancer
  nursing interventions, 187
  risk factors, 186-187
Thyroid hormones, 321
Tine technique, for administration of BCG, 353
Tissue tolerance, 270-272
TNM classification system, 242-243
Toddler, care needs of, 471-473
Transcutaneous nerve stimulator, 393-394
Transfer factor, 350
Transfusions, granulocyte, 534-535
Transillumination, in detection of testicular cancer, 210
Treatment
  multimodality, 237-250
  obtaining information about, 18
Triazenoimidazole carboxamide, 299, 308
Triethylenethiophosphoramide, 298, 307
Tube feeding, 518-519
Tumor
  growth, rate of, 21-22, 292-293
  site, and survival rate, 29
  Wilms', 27, 247, 331, 462-464

U

Urinary catheter, 597
Urinary diversion, 600

V

Values clarification, 128
Van de Graaff generator, 266
Variables, in research, selection and operationalization of, 104
Varian accelerator, 268
Vinblastine, 302, 311-312
Vincristine, 247, 302, 311-312, 458, 526, 584
VP-16, 302
Vulnerability, 68-69

W

Wilms' tumor, 27
  chemotherapy for, 331
  multimodality treatment of, 247
  protocol for, 462-464

X

Xeroderma pigmentosum, 177-178
Xerostomia, 277